Tourette Syndrome: Neurobiology and Genetics

Tourette Syndrome: Neurobiology and Genetics

Edited by Tommy Corbyn

STATES
ACADEMIC PRESS
www.statesacademicpress.com

States Academic Press,
109 South 5th Street,
Brooklyn, NY 11249, USA

Visit us on the World Wide Web at:
www.statesacademicpress.com

ISBN: 978-1-63989-527-4

Cataloging-in-Publication Data

Tourette syndrome : neurobiology and genetics / edited by Tommy Corbyn.
p. cm.
Includes bibliographical references and index.
ISBN 978-1-63989-527-4
1. Tourette syndrome. 2. Neurobiology. 3. Genetics. I. Corbyn, Tommy.
RC375 .T68 2022
616.83--dc23

Table of Contents

Preface

Tourette syndrome is a neurodevelopmental disorder that is characterized by multiple movement tics and at least one phonic tic. Tics are the repetitive and nonrhythmic motor movements or vocalizations involving different muscle groups. Common tics are coughing, blinking, sniffing, throat clearing and facial movements. The affected person feels an unwanted sensation in the affected muscles that sometimes can be suppressed temporarily and characteristically change in frequency, strength and location. Tourette syndrome is a more severe form of these tic disorders. There are no specific tests for the diagnosis of Tourette's syndrome. Most cases are mild and the severity of tics also decreases for most of children with age. This book brings forth some of the genetic and neurological aspects of Tourette syndrome. It presents researches and studies performed by experts across the globe. This book is meant for students who are looking for an elaborate reference text on Tourette syndrome.

Various studies have approached the subject by analyzing it with a single perspective, but the present book provides diverse methodologies and techniques to address this field. This book contains theories and applications needed for understanding the subject from different perspectives. The aim is to keep the readers informed about the progresses in the field; therefore, the contributions were carefully examined to compile novel researches by specialists from across the globe.

Indeed, the job of the editor is the most crucial and challenging in compiling all chapters into a single book. In the end, I would extend my sincere thanks to the chapter authors for their profound work. I am also thankful for the support provided by my family and colleagues during the compilation of this book.

Editor

1

Performance Monitoring in Medication-Naïve Children with Tourette Syndrome

Heike Eichele[1], Tom Eichele[1,2,3], Ingvar Bjelland[4,5], Marie F. Høvik[5], Lin Sørensen[1], Heidi van Wageningen[1], Marius Kalsås Worren[5], Kenneth Hugdahl[1,2,4] and Kerstin J. Plessen[2,6,7]*

[1] Department of Biological and Medical Psychology, University of Bergen, Bergen, Norway, [2] K.G. Jebsen Centre for Research on Neuropsychiatric Disorders, University of Bergen, Bergen, Norway, [3] Section for Neurophysiology, Department of Neurology, Haukeland University Hospital, Bergen, Norway, [4] Department of Psychiatry, Haukeland University Hospital, Bergen, Norway, [5] Department of Clinical Medicine, Faculty of Medicine and Dentistry, University of Bergen, Bergen, Norway, [6] Child and Adolescent Mental Health Center, Mental Health Services Capital Region, Copenhagen, Denmark, [7] Department of Clinical Medicine, Faculty of Health and Medical Sciences, University of Copenhagen, Copenhagen, Denmark

Edited by:
Peristera Paschou,
Democritus University of Thrace,
Greece

Reviewed by:
Georgina Jackson,
University of Nottingham, UK
Elizabeth Shephard,
King's College London, UK

***Correspondence:**
Heike Eichele
heike.eichele@uib.no

Background: Tourette syndrome (TS) is a childhood-onset neurodevelopmental disorder and its impact on cognitive development needs further study. Evidence from neuropsychological, neuroimaging and electrophysiological studies suggests that the decline in tic severity and the ability to suppress tics relate to the development of self-regulatory functions in late childhood and adolescence. Hence, tasks measuring performance monitoring might provide insight into the regulation of tics in children with TS.

Method: Twenty-five children with TS, including 14 with comorbid Attention-deficit/hyperactivity disorder (ADHD), 39 children with ADHD and 35 typically developing children aged 8–12 years were tested with a modified Eriksen-Flanker task during a 34-channel electroencephalography (EEG) recording. Task performance, as well as stimulus-locked and response-locked event-related potentials (ERP) were analyzed and compared across groups.

Results: Participants did not differ in their behavioral performance. Children with TS showed higher amplitudes of an early P3 component of the stimulus-locked ERPs in ensemble averages and in separate trial outcomes, suggesting heightened orienting and/or attention during stimulus evaluation. In response-locked averages, children with TS had a slightly higher positive complex before the motor response, likely also reflecting a late P3. Groups did not differ in post-response components, particularly in the error-related negativity (ERN) and error-related positivity (Pe).

Conclusions: These findings suggest that children with TS may employ additional attentional resources as a compensatory mechanism to maintain equal behavioral performance.

Keywords: Tourette syndrome, ADHD, children, P3, event-related potentials, performance monitoring

INTRODUCTION

Tourette Syndrome (TS) is a childhood onset neuropsychiatric disorder with multiple motor tics and at least one vocal tic for more than 1 year (American Psychiatric Association, 1994). Tics are often described as semi-voluntary, because children with TS can suppress their tics for a certain amount of time at the cost of increasing discomfort for the patient (Spessot et al., 2004). However, tic suppression is tiring and effortful, and may contribute to an increased feeling of "premonitory urge," which is an unpleasant bodily sensation preceding a tic and relieved by tic expression (Leckman, 2002). This reduction of unpleasant bodily sensation may contribute to a negative reinforcement of tic performance habit (Plessen, 2013).

Tic symptoms often attenuate in adolescence and about 40% of children are tic-free at the age of 18 (Leckman et al., 1998; Burd et al., 2001; Bloch and Leckman, 2009). This typical course of symptoms suggests that individuals with TS constantly, and often unconsciously, aim to suppress emerging tics to improve their psychosocial function (Eichele and Plessen, 2013). This process coincides with the development of self-regulatory control during childhood and adolescence (Davidson et al., 2006; Tau and Peterson, 2010) and maturation of the frontal cortex (Gogtay et al., 2004).

The ability to dynamically adapt the behavior to situational demands is a crucial part of adequate daily functioning (Ullsperger, 2006; Ullsperger et al., 2014). This requires a set of processing functions that localize to a broad network of brain areas encompassing frontal cortices, basal ganglia and thalamic nuclei, the cortico-striato-thalamo-cortical (CSTC) circuits. Activity in this network is elicited during performance monitoring and can be tested with the Eriksen-Flanker task (Eriksen and Eriksen, 1974).

Attention networks contribute to the perception of environmental cues that is essential for regulating behavior (Posner et al., 2014), and thus underlie the capacity of self-regulation (Rothbart et al., 2011). Different tasks of performance monitoring have been widely used to study this form of control (Fan et al., 2002). Recent work indicates that inhibitory control networks involving CSTC circuits are engaged during conflict trials to prevent attentional capture and interference (Tau and Peterson, 2010). Finally, imaging studies of individuals with TS implicate that inhibitory cognitive control processes might be altered (Worbe et al., 2015).

Due to the assumption that persons with TS show impairment of the CSTC circuits and the overlap of these networks with those involved in performance monitoring, the latter may also show impaired function. However, multiple studies report comparable, or even superior abilities of motor and cognitive control in children with TS compared with controls (Ozonoff and Jensen, 1999; Serrien et al., 2005; Mueller et al., 2006; Jackson et al., 2007, 2011; Eichele et al., 2010a). It is therefore of interest to investigate possible adaptive effects in this network. Many persons with TS are co-diagnosed with at least one further psychiatric disorder, with attention-deficit/hyperactivity disorder (ADHD) being the most common comorbid condition with 50–60% of all Tourette syndrome patients (Robertson, 2012; Hirschtritt et al., 2015). The reasons for the high co-occurrence have been widely discussed in the last decades but exact mechanisms still remain unclear. Evidence suggests that deficits in the basal portions of CSTC circuits represent shared neurobiological substrates for both disorders (Vloet et al., 2006; Sobel et al., 2010). Studies comparing children with TS with and without comorbid ADHD implied that children with comorbid ADHD showed impaired performance in tasks demanding cognitive control (Roessner et al., 2007; Greimel et al., 2008, 2011; Sukhodolsky et al., 2010). This is in line with findings suggesting altered behavioral and electrophysiological measures of performance monitoring tasks in persons with ADHD (Barry et al., 2003; Liotti et al., 2005; Johnstone and Galletta, 2013; Johnstone et al., 2013).

Different trial types modulate the sequence of stimulus- and response-locked event-related potentials (ERP) in the electroencephalogram (EEG) and outcomes indicate modulations of interference/conflict and control. The stimulus-locked N2 reflects early stages of conflict/mismatch detection (Folstein and Van Petten, 2008; Larson et al., 2014). This component is also reduced in children with ADHD (Albrecht et al., 2008). We decided to focus on the subsequent P3 that is thought to reflect a neural representation of a sensory process where the incoming stimulus is compared to the mental representation of the previous stimuli and the stimulus environment is updated. This is closely linked to concepts of orienting/surprise and predictive coding (Eichele et al., 2005). A later aspect of P3, the late positive complex (LPC) is thought to more closely represent working memory and response selection (Donchin, 1981; Donchin and Coles, 1998, 2010; Polich, 2007). Contingent upon this, the P3 is also sensitive to changes in conflict and control (Clayson and Larson, 2011a,b). Due to the ability of children with TS to react to the presence of internal cues (premonitory urges) we expected a superior function of this electrophysiological correlate for performance monitoring.

After errors, the error-related negativity (ERN) and error positivity (Pe) are detectable. The ERN arises immediately after error commission (Debener et al., 2005; Larson et al., 2014) and reflects automatic error detection in the mesial frontal cortex. Individuals with several neuropsychiatric disorders, including adolescents with ADHD (Albrecht et al., 2008) show a reduction of this early negativity. Finally, the ERN is followed by the Pe, a P3-like positive deflection, emerging approximately 300 ms after incorrect responses and is associated with evaluation and awareness, as well as the salience of errors. It is important to note here that the ERN is not fully established before adolescence and was therefore not focus in our study, whereas the Pe amplitude does not appear to change much with age (Davies et al., 2004; Ladouceur et al., 2007; Wiersema et al., 2007; Brydges et al., 2013; Tamnes et al., 2013; Dupuis et al., 2015).

To our knowledge, no prior ERP study has used this type of Flanker task in children with TS. However, one behavioral study reported that children with TS performed slightly less accurately on incompatible trials (Crawford et al., 2005). Only few ERP studies overall have included children with TS, mainly auditory oddball paradigms have been used with variable results (Van Woerkom et al., 1994; Oades et al., 1996; Zhu et al., 2006). A recent study using a Go/Nogo paradigm (Shephard et al., 2015) did not report significant differences in the ERP in children with TS compared with controls. However, here two distinct subcomponents of a P3 can be appreciated, which each show a differential amplitude modulation between the groups, where indeed the TS group grand average has highest amplitudes during an earlier subcomponent (Shephard et al., 2015) and thus add to motivate further study of this component in children with TS. Interestingly, this component seems reduced in children with ADHD (Albrecht et al., 2008). These independent observations motivate the focus on P3 in the current analysis.

A larger amount of data exists from children with ADHD, indicating either non-different or reduced N2, P3, ERN, and Pe amplitudes compared with controls (for an overview, see Barry et al., 2003; Johnstone et al., 2013). We aimed at investigating electrophysiological measures in the Flanker task related to attention, stimulus evaluation, conflict and control in medication-naïve children with TS, compared with medication-naïve children with ADHD and controls, primarily in the N2-P3 latency range and the post-response ERN-Pe. We hypothesized that participants with TS would show a typical or enhanced performance and ERP amplitudes similar to control participants, whereas participants with ADHD would show impaired performance (Willcutt et al., 2005; Mazaheri et al., 2014) and reduced ERP amplitudes. Due to the limited ERP-literature on children with TS we do not only present hypothesized effects but all components involved in the Flanker task for reference and discovery of knowledge in the field of child psychopathology (Loo et al., 2015). Comparisons between groups should not be limited to measurement of one component to ensure that significant differences between groups are not ceiling effects transporting smaller differences from one component to the next until adding up to a significant difference (Picton et al., 2000).

We focus on performance monitoring in children with TS, and, due to ADHD being a frequent comorbidity, we also included participants with TS and comorbid ADHD. This group is compared with children with ADHD, and a group of typically developing children. This allows to leverage the impact of comorbid ADHD in combination with TS, as well as to measure the specific contribution of TS on our main outcome variables. The recent attempt to collect data across the boundaries of diagnostic entities calls for the inclusion of contrastgroups to allow differentiating characteristics found in individuals with a specific disorder from more general markers present across conditions (Cuthbert, 2014).

MATERIALS AND METHODS

Participants

One hundred and two participants were recruited for a prospective longitudinal study of children with ADHD, Tourette syndrome, and control children aged 8–12 years. Participants with ADHD and TS were recruited from the Department of Child and Adolescent Psychiatry, Haukeland University Hospital, and from outpatient clinics in the greater Bergen area in the Hordaland County, Norway. Controls were recruited from local schools in the same geographic regions. The Regional Ethics Committee approved the study, and written consent in accordance with the Declaration of Helsinki was obtained from all parents. The diagnostic procedure consisted of a semi-structured interview, the K-SADS (Kiddie-Schedule for Affective Disorders and Schizophrenia for School-Aged Children; Kaufman et al., 1997); the Children Gobal Assessment Scale (CGAS; Shaffer et al., 1983), and the DuPaul ADHD-Rating Scale (ADHD-RS; Dupaul et al., 1998), along with a best estimate consensus procedure that considered all available study material (Leckman, 2002). TS and ADHD diagnoses, respectively, met the criteria set in Diagnostic and Statistical Manual of Mental Disorders, fourth edition (DSM-IV; American Psychiatric Association, 1994). Tic symptoms were measured with the Yale Global Tic Severity scale (YGTSS; Leckman et al., 1989). All children were native Norwegian speakers of Caucasian origin, were medication-naïve and had no prior treatment for ADHD. Exclusion criteria for the control group were a lifetime history of Tic disorder, Obsessive compulsive disorder (OCD), ADHD, or a current DSM-IV axis I disorder. Additional exclusion criteria for all groups were epilepsy, head trauma with loss of consciousness, autism spectrum disorder, prematurity (gestational age <36 weeks), or a full scale intelligence quotient (FSIQ) below 75, measured by the Wechsler Intelligence Scale for Children-IV (Wechsler, 2003). Children with ADHD had a diagnosis of ADHD, combined type ($n = 25$), inattentive type ($n = 11$) or hyperactive type ($n = 3$). Within the study groups, the following comorbid disorders were present: oppositional defiant disorder (ODD; ADHD $n = 17$, TS $n = 7$), and three children with ADHD also had conduct disorder (CD), chronic and transient tics (ADHD $n = 3$), OCD (TS $n = 2$), and elimination disorder (ADHD $n = 4$, TS $n = 3$, controls $n = 2$). Moreover, several children fulfilled criteria for phobia (ADHD $n = 7$, TS $n = 3$, control $n = 1$), separation anxiety (ADHD $n = 6$, TS $n = 1$) and general anxiety (ADHD $n = 3$, TS $n = 1$). Thirteen children with TS had an additional ADHD diagnosis (ADHD combined type $n = 7$, ADHD inattentive type $n = 6$), 1 of these had an additional OCD diagnosis.

Experimental Design

After instruction and training, participants performed a modified visual Eriksen-Flanker task implemented in E-prime 2 (Psychology Software Tools, Inc., Pittsburgh, PA, USA). Participants were instructed to fixate a dot presented in the center of a PC screen. Trials began with the presentation of 6 horizontal flanker arrows appearing below fixation. Participants should respond as fast as possible, and as accurate as possible with either a left or a right mouse button press following the direction of a central target arrow that appeared after 100 ms, pointing either into the same direction as the flanker arrows in compatible trials (<<< < <<<, >>> > >>>) or in the opposite direction in incompatible trials (<<< > <<<, >>> < >>>). The target- and flanker-arrows remained on screen until a response was registered. Trials were terminated by the motor response and followed by an 800-ms interval before onset of the next trial. Stimuli were presented in two blocks with 200 trials that were pseudorandomized separately for each participant. The overall probability of compatible and incompatible trials, as well as left and right responses were kept at 0.5. Performance feedback was given during the experiment when responses were erroneous or slower than an adaptive individual threshold value (mean response time plus 1.5 standard deviations (SD).

EEG Acquisition

EEG was recorded continuously in an electromagnetically shielded chamber. Data were sampled at 1000 Hz frequency with a time-constant of 10 s and a high cutoff at 250 Hz with Brain Amp amplifiers (BrainProducts, Munich, Germany). An elastic cap containing 34 Ag/AgCl electrodes placed at Fp1, Fp2, F7, F3, Fz, F4, F8, FT9, FC5, FC1, FC2, FC6, FT10, T7, C3, Cz, C4, T8, TP9, CP5, CP1, CP2, CP6, TP10, P7, P3, Pz, P4, P8, PO9, O1, O2, PO10, Iz was used. Channels were referenced to Fz. Vertical eye movements were recorded with a bipolar derivation between Fp1 and an additional electrode placed below the left eye, horizontal eye movement were recorded with a bipolar derivation between F7 and F8. Additionally, electrocardiogram was monitored. Impedances were kept below 10 kΩ.

EEG Processing

We preprocessed the EEG in Matlab (Mathworks, Natick, MA, USA) using the EEGLAB toolbox (Delorme and Makeig, 2004) and in-house scripts.

The continuous EEG data were resampled to 500 Hz. The data were then re-referenced to common average reference, and filtered from 0.5 to 45 Hz using a finite impulse response filter generated with the firfilt plugin (Widmann, 2006).

For artifact removal/reduction, the data were segmented into stimulus-locked (−0.5 to +1 s), and response-locked epochs (−1 to 0.5 s). The prestimulus period was used as baseline for both epochs. Epochs were excluded when exceeding a ±300 μV amplitude criterion. The remaining epochs were sorted using a summary score of root mean square amplitude across all channels and time points, spatial SD, power spectrum ratio between low and high frequencies, skewness and kurtosis, normalized to unit variance across epochs. Only epochs within ±1 SD were retained for further analysis. These epochs were concatenated and subjected to temporal independent component analysis (ICA) using the infomax algorithm (Bell and Sejnowski, 1995), and 32 components were estimated. We used spatial templates to identify horizontal and vertical eye movements and ECG artifacts, and removed these automatically (Viola et al., 2009). Following the rationale presented in COMPASS (Wessel and Ullsperger, 2011), we assumed that components of interest were broad, dipolar topographies with time-locked event-related responses, and we therefore generated scores based on the spatial smoothness of the component scalp maps and the root mean square of the event related average, and retained the top 15 components. These were then visually cross-checked, and components reminiscent of artifacts were marked. Between 10 and 15 components were kept and back-projected in this manner.

Averaging and Data Extraction

We sorted compatible, incompatible and erroneous trials and visually inspected the grand averaged data across all participants to generate ERP for further testing. Upon inspection of grand average ERP data and difference waves, we found that conditional effects on several components were consistently expressed around Cz/Vertex, which is in line with other work in this age group (Cycowicz, 2000; Stige et al., 2007). We therefore used regional averaging, for spatial data reduction, and controlling for inter-individual variability (Handy, 2005). This provides a better fit to the statistical models by collapsing together electrodes that commonly covary, in the same way that adding a spatial factor would do, however without complicating the analysis by additional terms of interaction. Moreover, it helps to control for variability (as seen in different age groups e.g., Cycowicz, 2000; Davies et al., 2004; Brydges et al., 2013) over locations by averaging across locations. This method addresses the objection to the large degrees of freedom that multiple electrode readings afford (Handy, 2005). We selected a central region of interest containing FC1, FC2, Cz, CP1, and CP2 with clear N1 (108 ms), P2 (196 ms), P3 (320 ms), and LPC (598 ms) waveforms in the stimulus-locked average, as well as LPC (−82 ms) in the response-locked average, and a clear modulation between outcomes (see **Figure 1**). ERN was identified as the first post-response negativity maximal on erroneous trials. The early positivity is defined as the first positive wave post-response—this common post-response component is labeled P2 or P90 elsewhere (Brunia and Van Boxtel, 2000). Error response generated an additional broad positivity Pe with peak latency at 268 ms post-response. Because latency jitter in ERP components between trials, especially in children, and peak amplitudes can be influenced by group differences in signal-noise-ratio, analyses of mean amplitudes were chosen (Luck, 2005). Amplitudes were extracted from 40 ms long windows centered on the grand average peak latency and were used for testing of group differences.

Statistics

Statistics were performed in Matlab and Statistica (Statsoft, Tulsa, OK, USA). Repeated measure analyses were conducted to test outcome effects in the behavioral and the ERP data

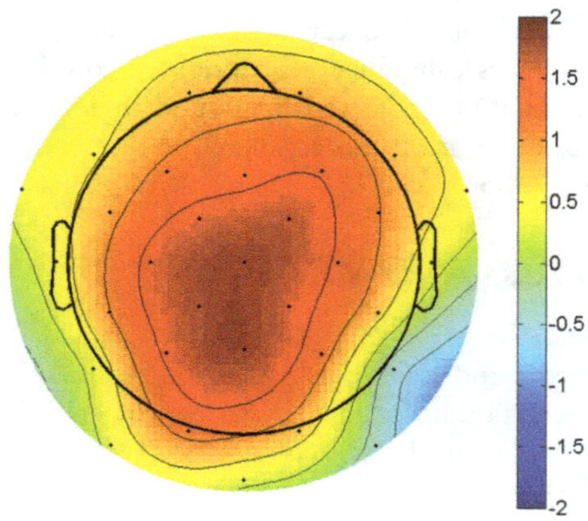

FIGURE 1 | P3 amplitude difference. Topographic plot of the amplitude difference between compatible and incompatible outcomes at 300 ms post stimulus. Scaling from -2 to 2 μV. Voltage maximum is at centro-parietal midline sites.

(congruent vs. incongruent vs. error trials) and "group." Additional univariate Analysis of Covariance (ANCOVA) were conducted for behavioral measures and ERP components as dependent variable, group as categorical factor and covariates as continuous predictors to test group differences. Significant or trend-significant effects were followed-up with additional *post-hoc* tests. All statistics were considered significant at $p < 0.05$. The effect size indicator partial eta squared (η_p^2) is reported for each significant/trend-significant statistical comparison as a measure of the strength of the effect, with of 0.01 representing a small effect, 0.06 a medium effect, and 0.14 a large effect (Cohen, 1988). To demonstrate the adequacy of pooling children with TS with and without comorbid ADHD, we also performed ANCOVAs with four groups, separating TS only and TS+ADHD, control group, ADHD, with the main behavioral and ERP result.

Response times (RT) and response accuracy (RACC) averages were generated for all possible outcomes. Premature responses faster than 200 ms and slow responses >2000 ms were not considered in the averages. RTs were analyzed with covariates:

Age: Because of substantial speeding of RT, and improvement of accuracy with age across the entire sample regardless of group, all analyses included age as a covariate.

FSIQ: We decided to analyze the behavioral data with FSIQ as covariate for the sake of consistency across behavioral- and ERP analyses. This appears to be the most sound practice in our case, however see relevant publications for a discussion on this issue (Willcutt et al., 2005; Dennis et al., 2009).

ERP components were analyzed with covariates:

Age: Groups did not differ in mean age. However, to control within group variation of electrophysiological measures we followed current guidelines (Picton et al., 2000). Age in particular influences many features in the EEG, resulting also in prominent maturational changes of ERP amplitudes and latencies (Davies et al., 2004; Wiersema et al., 2007; Brydges et al., 2013; Rojas-Benjumea et al., 2015).

FSIQ: Earlier research has also shown that IQ differences account for variability of ERP measures. We therefore decided to include IQ as a covariate in line with other studies in the field (Pelosi et al., 1992; Deary and Caryl, 1997; Jausovec and Jausovec, 2000; Ramchurn et al., 2014).

RT/ IIV: Response times and their variability substantially affect ERP features (Eichele et al., 2010b). This is partly due to task-induced amplitude modulation, and partly nuisance variability due to spatio-temporal overlap of stimulus and response-related components, see also (Ramchurn et al., 2014).

RACC: Average accuracy provides a gross measure of the effort that an individual invests in a task, therefore adjusting for ACC is useful to account for state and trait factors not specifically related to diagnosis/group.

ADHD symptom scores were included initially as a covariate in the statistical models for the behavioral and the ERP correlates, but proved non-significant and were subsequently removed from both models. Pairwise correlations were used to further investigate significant effects of the group factor and covariates. To test for post-error slowing (PES) and to compensate for confounders, we conducted a pairwise comparison of post-error and pre-error trials around each error (Dutilh et al., 2012) followed by an ANCOVA, including the covariates age and FSIQ.

Behavioral Characteristics

Data from two participants (with ADHD and with TS/ADHD, respectively) were discarded due to excessive EEG artifact, data from another participant (ADHD) were discarded due to performance on chance level, data from 99 participants thus were included, 39 children with a diagnosis of ADHD, 25 children with TS (11 TS "only" and 14 TS+ADHD), and 35 typically developing children. Children's age ranged from 8 to 12 years (M= 10.05; SD ± 1.21), 64 participants were boys and groups did not differ for age or sex. 15 participants were left-handed. Groups differed in FSIQ, similar to findings reported in other studies (Bornstein, 1991; Ozonoff et al., 1998; Baym et al., 2008; Debes et al., 2011), and FSIQ was employed as a covariate. Groups also differed in ADHD-RS total values. Current tic severity in the TS group was 11.3 ± 3.34 for motor and 8.00 ± 4.83 for vocal tics, and lifetime worst ever score 15.68 ± 3.44 for motor and 11.95 ± 5.0 for vocal tics (**Table 1**).

RESULTS

Behavioral Performance

We observed no significant differences between groups for premature responses, but a significant effect of FSIQ, with a weak correlation where lower FSIQ correlated with more premature responses ($r = -0.29$). Slow responses were more frequent in all groups compared with fast responses, also with a significant FSIQ effect, with correlations for lower FSIQ predicting more frequent slower responses ($r = -0.34$) and age ($r = -0.38$). (**Table 2**).

Reaction Times

A Repeated Measure Analysis revealed a typical RT pattern for the Flanker task with fast RT in compatible (CC) responses, slower incompatible (IC) responses and faster RT in erroneous trials in all three groups, and trend-significant group differences across all three outcomes [$F_{(2, 96)} = 2.85$, $p = 0.06$, $\eta_p^2 = 0.06$], without significant interactions of outcome-by-group. *Post-hoc* assessment revealed trend-significant differences for CC responses ($p = 0.07$) and erroneous responses ($p = 0.08$) between controls and ADHD and a significant difference in IC

TABLE 1 | Sample characteristics.

	Controls Mean ± *SD*	ADHD Mean ± *SD*	TS Mean ± *SD*	Statistics
FSIQ	105.82 ± 1.68	91.71 ± 1.59	97.96 ± 1.99	$F_{(2, 96)} = 18.51$, $p < 0.001$, $\eta_p^2 = 0.28$
Age (years)	10.04 ± 0.21	10.18 ± 0.19	9.87 ± 0.24	$F_{(2, 96)} = 0.49$, n.s.
Sex (% male)	57.14	69.23	68	$\chi 2 = 1.34$, n.s.
Handeness (% right handed)	91.43	84.62	76	$\chi 2 = 2.7$, n.s.
ADHD-RS total score	2.91 ± 1.33	30.73 ± 1.26	22.12 ± 1.57	$F_{(2, 96)} = 117.09$, $p < 0.001$, $\eta_p^2 = 0.62$

ADHD, attention-deficit/hyperactivity disorder; TS, Tourette syndrome; FSIQ, full scale intelligence quotient; ADHD-RS, attention-deficit/hyperactivity disorder rating scale; SD, standard deviation.

TABLE 2 | Behavioral performance.

	Controls	ADHD	TS	Repeated Measure ANOVA			ANCOVA	
	Mean ± *SD*	Mean ± *SD*	Mean ± *SD*	Outcome	Group	Outcome × group	Group	Covariates
RT CC (ms)	646.44 ± 19.69	677.37 ± 18.43	652.99 ± 21.26	$F_{(2,\ 192)} = 136.9$, $p < 0.001$, $\eta_p^2 = 0.59$	$F_{(2,\ 96)} = 2.85$, $p = 0.06$, $\eta_p^2 = 0.06$	$F_{(4,\ 192)} = 1.14$, n.s.	$F_{(2,\ 94)} = 0.65$, n.s.	FSIQ $F_{(1,\ 94)} = 11.77, p < 0.001$, $\eta_p^2 = 0.11$; Age $F_{(1,\ 94)} = 64.68$, $p < 0.001, \eta_p^2 = 0.41$
RT IC (ms)	773.11 ± 25.73	840.70 ± 24.01	789.58 ± 27.77				$F_{(2,\ 94)} = 1.77$, n.s.	FSIQ $F_{(1,\ 94)} = 10.19, p < 0.01$, $\eta_p^2 = 0.09$; Age $F_{(1,\ 94)} = 61.04$, $p < 0.001, \eta_p^2 = 0.39$
RT error (ms)	624.42 ± 29.70	644.70 ± 27.79	627.28 ± 32.06				$F_{(2,\ 94)} = 0.13$, n.s.	FSIQ $F_{(1,\ 94)} = 7.5, p < 0.01$, $\eta_p^2 = 0.07$; Age $F_{(1,\ 94)} = 34.06$, $p < 0.001, \eta_p^2 = 0.27$
IIV CC (ms)	209.48 ± 10.98	245.21 ± 10.27	231.66 ± 11.85	$F_{(2,\ 192)} = 25.46$, $p < 0.001$, $\eta_p^2 = 0.21$	$F_{(2,\ 96)} = 5.68$, $p < 0.01$, $\eta_p^2 = 0.11$	$F_{(4,\ 192)} = 0.71$, n.s.	$F_{(2,\ 94)} = 2.46$, n.s.	FSIQ $F_{(1,\ 94)} = 14.43, p < 0.001$, $\eta_p^2 = 0.13$; Age $F_{(1,\ 94)} = 32.72$, $p < 0.001, \eta_p^2 = 0.26$
IIV IC (ms)	245.13 ± 12.95	261.21 ± 12.12	266.46 ± 13.98				$F_{(2,\ 94)} = 0.66$, n.s.	FSIQ $F_{(1,\ 94)} = 12.66, p < 0.001$, $\eta_p^2 = 0.12$; Age $F_{(1,\ 94)} = 22.48$, $p < 0.001, \eta_p^2 = 0.19$
IIV error (ms)	271.01 ± 20.41	309.89 ± 19.09	290.70 ± 22.03				$F_{(2,\ 94)} = 0.83$, n.s.	FSIQ $F_{(1,\ 94)} = 7.75, p < 0.01$, $\eta_p^2 = 0.08$; Age $F_{(1,\ 94)} = 26.73$, $p < 0.001, \eta_p^2 = 0.22$
Compatible errors(%)	6.57 ± 1.07	7.85 ± 1.01	9.32 ± 1.26	$F_{(1,\ 96)} = 142.14$, $p < 0.001$, $\eta_p^2 = 0.6$	$F_{(2,\ 96)} = 2.46$, $p = 0.09$, $\eta_p^2 = 0.05$	$F_{(2,\ 96)} = 3.01$, $p = 0.06$, $\eta_p^2 = 0.06$	$F_{(2,\ 92)} = 1.47$, n.s.	FSIQ $F_{(1,\ 94)} = 7.12, p < 0.01$, $\eta_p^2 = 0.07$
Incompatible errors (%)	18.96 ± 2.37	20.65 ± 2.21	21.78 ± 2.56				$F_{(2,\ 92)} = 0.32$, n.s.	FSIQ $F_{(1,\ 92)} = 9.53, p < 0.01$, $\eta_p^2 = 0.003$
Responses <200 ms (n)	6.79 ± 2.64	4.77 ± 2.47	9.01 ± 2.85				$F_{(2,\ 94)} = 0.63$, n.s.	FSIQ $F_{(1,\ 94)} = 8.35, p < 0.01$, $\eta_p^2 = 0.08$
Responses >2000 ms (n)	12.49 ± 3.59	21.65 ± 3.36	11.73 ± 3.87				$F_{(2,\ 94)} = 2.29$, n.s.	FSIQ $F_{(1,\ 94)} = 7.22, p < 0.01$, $\eta_p^2 = 0.07$; Age $F_{(1,\ 94)} = 23.22$, $p < 0.001, \eta_p^2 = 0.19$
PES (ms)	79.47 ± 20.71	87.11 ± 19.38	36.73 ± 22.36				$F_{(2,\ 94)} = 1.67$, n.s.	
Overall RT (ms)	695.49 ± 22.16	735.80 ± 20.73	690.72 ± 23.92				$F_{(2,\ 94)} = 1.21$, n.s.	FSIQ $F_{(1,\ 94)} = 8.01, p < 0.01$, $\eta_p^2 = 0.08$; Age $F_{(1,\ 94)} = 56.71$, $p < 0.001, \eta_p^2 = 0.38$
Overall IIV (ms)	255.11 ± 11.26	286.59 ± 10.53	270.25 ± 12.15				$F_{(2,\ 94)} = 1.8$, n.s.	FSIQ $F_{(1,94)} = 17.21, p < 0.001$, $\eta_p^2 = 0.15$; Age $F_{(1,\ 94)} = 38.29$, $p < 0.001, \eta_p^2 = 0.29$
Overall RACC (%)	86.68 ± 1.63	86.54 ± 1.52	84.64 ± 1.75				$F_{(2,\ 92)} = 0.25$, n.s.	FSIQ $F_{(1,\ 92)} = 10.05, p < 0.01$, $\eta_p^2 = 0.10$

CC, compatible correct; IC, incompatible correct; PES, post-error slowing; RT, reaction time; IIV, intraindividual variability; RACC, response accuracy; ANCOVA, analysis of covariance; ANOVA, analysis of variance, ADHD, attention-deficit/hyperactivity disorder; TS, Tourette syndrome; SD, standard deviation; n.s., not significant; Responses >2000 ms are considered equivalent to omissions, Responses <200 ms are considered false alarms.

trials ($p < 0.01$) between controls and ADHD. No differences between children with TS and controls.

When controlling for covariates in a follow-up ANCOVA, the CC, IC or erroneous RTs did not differ between groups (**Table 2**).

Response Accuracy

Errors were defined as incorrect key presses to compatible and incompatible trials. As expected, significantly more errors occurred to incompatible than compatible trials [$F_{(1, 96)} = 142.14$, $p < 0.001$, $\eta_p^2 = 0.6$]. A repeated measure analysis revealed a trend-significant group difference [$F_{(2, 96)} = 2.46$, $p = 0.09$, $\eta_p^2 = 0.05$] and a trend-significant outcome-by-group difference [$F_{(2, 96)} = 3.01$, $p = 0.06$, $\eta_p^2 = 0.06$] which was due to higher incompatible error rates in children with ADHD ($p < 0.01$) and TS ($p < 0.05$) than controls.

After controlling for covariates (ANCOVA), groups did not differ in in error rates for either CC or IC responses, or for overall RACC with a significant effect of FSIQ (**Table 2**).

Post Error Slowing

ANCOVA for PES yielded no significant group differences (**Table 2**).

Intraindividual Variability

A repeated measure analysis of IIV showed smaller IIV for compatible trials, larger IIV in incompatible trials and largest IIV in erroneous trials, and significant group differences across all three outcomes [$F_{(2, 96)} = 5.68$, $p < 0.01$, $\eta_p^2 = 0.11$]. No significant interaction for outcome-by-group was found.

When controlling for covariates in the follow-up ANCOVA groups did not differ with respect to IIV, but the relevant covariates FSIQ and age reached significance in the overall IIV, as well as in the separate CC, IC and error trials (**Table 2**).

Electrophysiological Results

After inspection of the grand averages of the stimulus-locked (**Figure 2**) and response-locked (**Figure 3**) ERP data, we conducted repeated measure analyses for the components separately to test the presence of the typical compatibility/conflict effects considering the factors "outcome," "group" and the "outcome x group" interaction. We observed significant "outcome" effects for the stimulus-locked P3 and LPC and the response-locked LPC, ERN and Pe. Trend-significant effects of "outcome" were seen in the P2, no significant effects of outcomes were seen for N1 and response-locked early positivity. We also did observe "group" and "outcome x group" effects, which were followed-up by appropriate ANCOVA designs controlling for confounds (**Tables 3, 4**).

Stimulus-Locked ERPs (Table 3)

N1 (108 ms)

ANCOVA showed no group differences in compatible, incompatible, and error outcomes. A significant effect of RT and IIV was present in incompatible correct outcomes.

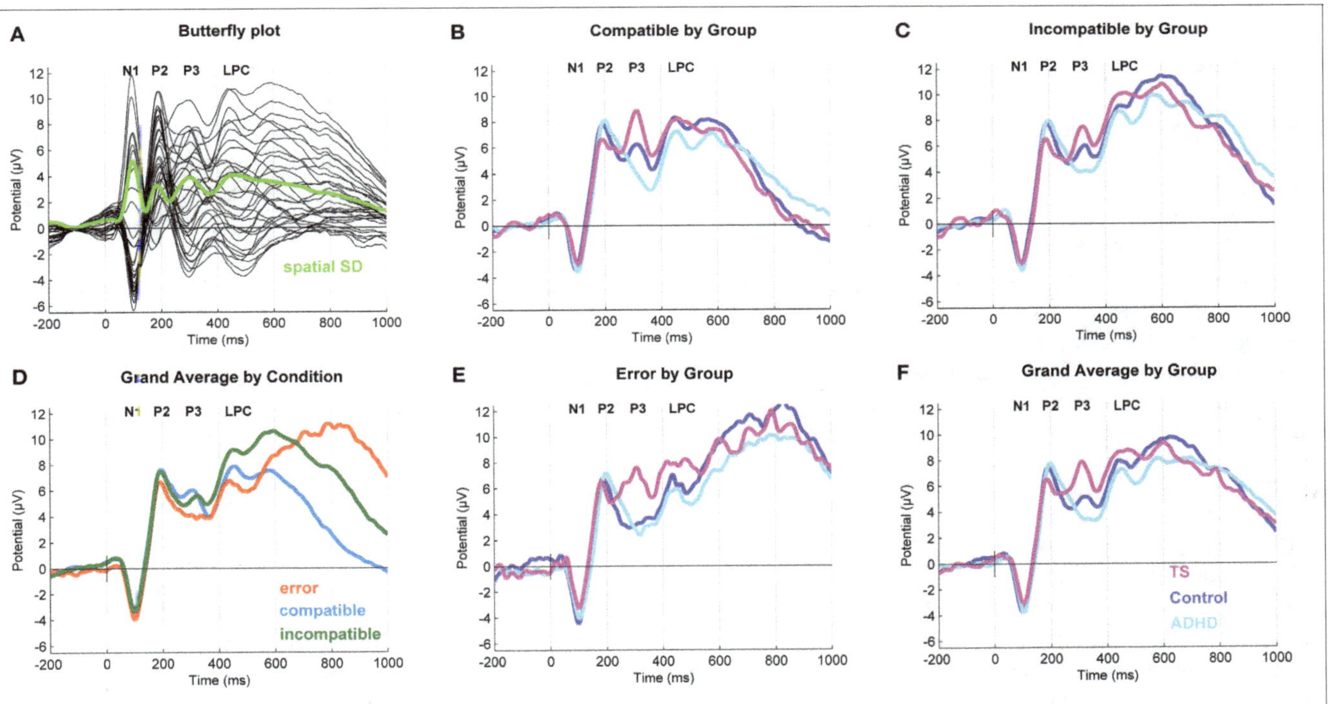

FIGURE 2 | Stimulus-locked event-related potentials (ERP). (A) Butterfly plot. Topographical distribution of the P3 component across outcomes. **(D)** Grand average ERP by Outcome at a central region of interest for compatible (blue), incompatible (green) and erroneous (red) trials. **(B,C,E)** Grand average ERPs at a central region of interest with a N1 (108 ms), P2 (196 ms), P3 (320 ms), and a Late Positive Component (598 ms) for compatible, incompatible and erroneous trials. **(F)** Grand average ERP by Group. Group differences for Tourette syndrome (TS) (pink), attention-deficit/hyperactivity disorder (ADHD) (turquoise) and control children (blue) at a central region of interest.

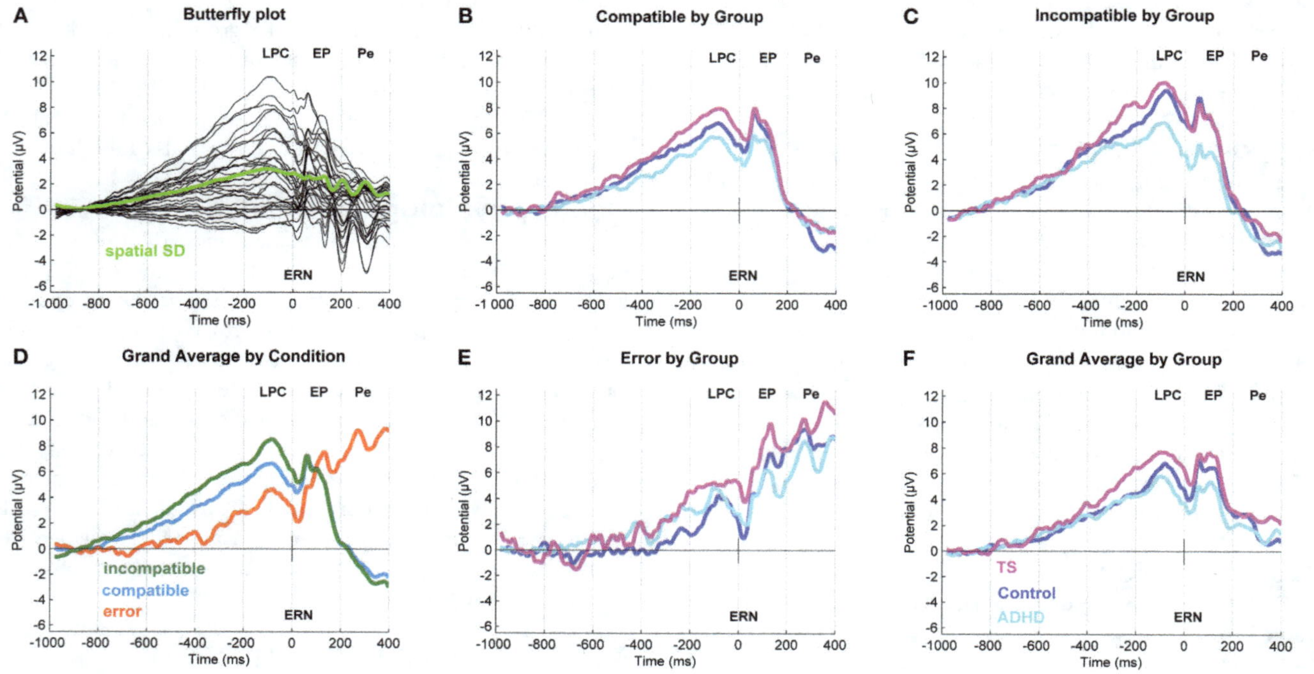

FIGURE 3 | Response-locked event-related potentials (ERP). (A) Butterfly plot. Topographical distribution of the Late Positive Component across outcomes. **(D)** Grand average ERP by Outcome at a central region of interest for compatible (blue), incompatible (green) and erroneous (red) trials. **(B,C,E)** Linked mastoid referenced grand average ERPs at a central region of interest with a Late Positive Component (−80 ms) and early positivity (60 ms). In erroneous trials (bottom middle) also seen an ERN (20 ms) and a Pe (268 ms). **(F)** Grand average ERP by Group. Group differences for Tourette syndrome (TS) (pink), attention-deficit/hyperactivity disorder (ADHD) (turquoise) and control children (blue) at a central region of interest.

P2 (196 ms)

No group effects were found in ANCOVA for compatible, incompatible, and erroneous P2 amplitudes.

P3 (320 ms)

ANCOVA yielded a significant group effect for compatible correct [$F_{(2,\ 91)} = 4.62, p = 0.01, \eta_p^2 = 0.09$] and erroneous responses [$F_{(2,\ 91)} = 5.17, p < 0.01, \eta_p^2 = 0.10$]. Incompatible correct outcomes also approached significance [$F_{(2,\ 91)} = 2.82$, $p = 0.06, \eta_p^2 = 0.06$], and a significant effect of RACC and IIV was observed. A *post-hoc* assessment revealed that, P3 amplitudes across outcomes were higher in children with TS compared to both controls ($p < 0.05$), and those with ADHD ($p < 0.05$). No significant differences were found between participants with ADHD and controls.

LPC (600 ms)

ANCOVA showed no significant group difference in compatible correct outcomes, there was a significant effect of RACC. Similarly, no differences were present in incompatible correct outcomes, while a significant covariate-effect of IIV was present. No differences were found in erroneous LPC amplitudes.

Response-Locked ERPs (Table 4)

LPC (−80 ms)

ANCOVA showed no significant group differences in compatible and erroneous amplitudes. Incompatible amplitudes showed a trend-significant group effect [$F_{(2,\ 91)} = 2.5, p = 0.08, \eta_p^2 = 0.05$], with a significant effect of RACC and RT. *Post-hoc* tests showed higher amplitudes in TS vs. controls ($p = 0.04$), and a similar trend between TS and ADHD ($p = 0.09$), but no difference between controls and ADHD.

ERN (20 ms)

In this sample, we did not observe a distinct negative ERN in this age group, consistent with Davies (Davies et al., 2004). However, the most negative amplitudes during the post-response period were seen for erroneous trials, and a trend-significant outcome-by-group effect [$F_{(4,\ 192)} = 2.09, p = 0.08, \eta_p^2 = 0.04$]. However, this was due to higher incompatible amplitudes for controls than ADHD ($p = 0.03$) and similarly for TS compared to ADHD ($p = 0.06$), whereas no differences were seen between TS and controls. Note though that there is a substantial carry-over of the amplitude modulation from the preceding LPC into this time-window, especially for correct responses.

When controlling for covariates, ANCOVA showed no group differences in any trial outcome, whereas clear effects of age and RT were present for incompatible correct.

Early positivity (60 ms)

ANCOVA showed no significant group differences across outcomes. Significant effect of RT and age were present only for incompatible outcomes.

TABLE 3 | Stimulus-locked ERP amplitudes.

	Controls	ADHD	TS	Repeated Measure ANOVA			ANCOVA	
Stimulus-locked	**Mean ± *SD* (μV)**	**Mean ± *SD* (μV)**	**Mean ± *SD* (μV)**	**Outcome**	**Group**	**Outcome x Group**	**Group**	**Covariates**
N1 (108 ms)								
Compatible	−2.72 ± 0.70	−3.04 ± 0.65	−2.42 ± 0.75	$F_{(2,\ 192)} = 1.89$, n.s.	$F_{(2,\ 96)} = 0.22$, n.s.	$F_{(4,\ 192)} = 0.43$, n.s.	$F_{(2,\ 91)} = 0.19$, n.s.	RT $F_{(1,\ 91)} = 5.95, p = 0.02, \eta_p^2 = 0.06$;IIV $F_{(1,\ 91)} = 7.06, p < 0.01, \eta_p^2 = 0.07$
Incompatible	−2.49 ± 0.68	−3.47 ± 0.63	−2.36 ± 0.73				$F_{(2,\ 91)} = 0.74$, n.s.	
Error	−3.07 ± 0.90	−4.03 ± 0.84	−2.79 ± 0.97				$F_{(2,\ 91)} = 0.5$, n.s.	
Mean	−2.80 ± 0.69	−3.44 ± 0.65	−2.57 ± 0.75					
P2 (196 ms)								
Compatible	7.19 ± 0.91	7.05 ± 0.84	6.36 ± 0.96	$F_{(2,\ 192)} = 2.69$, $p = 0.06, \eta_p^2 = 0.03$	$F_{(2,\ 96)} = 0.21$, n.s.	$F_{(4,\ 192)} = 0.35$, n.s.	$F_{(2,\ 91)} = 0.23$, n.s.	
Incompatible	7.23 ± 0.98	6.73 ± 0.92	6.33 ± 1.05				$F_{(2,\ 91)} = 0.19$, n.s.	
Error	6.53 ± 1.06	5.82 ± 0.99	5.99 ± 1.13				$F_{(2,\ 91)} = 0.11$, n.s.	
Mean	6.89 ± 0.91	6.64 ± 0.85	6.19 ± 0.97					
P3 (320 ms)								
Compatible	5.26 ± 1.04	4.70 ± 0.93	8.69 ± 1.07	$F_{(2,\ 192)} = 11.71$, $p < 0.001, \eta_p^2 = 0.11$	$F_{(2,\ 96)} = 3.61$, $p = 0.03, \eta_p^2 = 0.07$	$F_{(4,\ 192)} = 2.21$, $p = 0.06, \eta_p^2 = 0.04$	$F_{(2,\ 91)} = 4.62$, $p = 0.01, \eta_p^2 = 0.09$	RACC $F_{(1,\ 91)} = 4.43, p = 0.04, \eta_p^2 = 0.05$; IIV $F_{(1,\ 91)} = 5.21, p = 0.03, \eta_p^2 = 0.05$
Incompatible	4.60 ± 1.03	4.46 ± 0.97	7.61 ± 1.12				$F_{(2,91)} = 2.82$, $p = 0.06, \eta_p^2 = 0.06$	
Error	2.84 ± 1.15	2.89 ± 1.07	7.47 ± 1.23				$F_{(2,\ 91)} = 5.17$, $p < 0.01, \eta_p^2 = 0.10$	
Mean	4.09 ± 0.99	4.22 ± 0.93	7.81 ± 1.06					
LPC (598 ms)								
Compatible	7.12 ± 0.96	7.78 ± 0.89	8.46 ± 1.02	$F_{(2,\ 192)} = 14.35$, $p < 0.001, \eta_p^2 = 0.13$	$F_{(2,\ 192)} = 0.61$, n.s.	$F_{(4,\ 192)} = 0.48$, n.s.	$F_{(2,\ 91)} = 0.45$, n.s.	RACC $F_{(1,\ 91)} = 3.96, p = 0.05, \eta_p^2 = 0.04$
Incompatible	8.11 ± 1.03	8.89 ± 0.96	10.86 ± 1.11				$F_{(2,\ 91)} = 1.79$, n.s.	IIV $F_{(1,\ 91)} = 9.01, p < 0.01, \eta_p^2 = 0.09$
Error	5.95 ± 1.39	5.73 ± 1.31	8.13 ± 1.50				$F_{(2,91)} = 0.88$, n.s.	
Mean	6.83 ± 1.00	7.72 ± 0.94	9.07 ± 1.08					

ERP, event-related potentials; SD, standard deviation; ANOVA, analysis of variance; ADHD, attention-deficit/hyperactivity disorder; TS, Tourette syndrome; LPC, Late positive component; n.s., not significant.

TABLE 4 | Response-locked ERP amplitudes.

	Controls	ADHD	TS	Repeated measure ANOVA			ANCOVA	
Response-locked	**Mean ± *SD* (μV)**	**Mean ± *SD* (μV)**	**Mean ± *SD* (μV)**	**Outcome**	**Group**	**Outcome × Group**	**Group**	**Covariates**
LPC (−82 ms)								
Compatible	6.37 ± 0.88	5.88 ± 0.82	8.14 ± 0.93	$F_{(2, 192)} = 26.92$, $p < 0.001$, $\eta_p^2 = 0.22$	$F_{(2, 96)} = 1.21$, n.s.	$F_{(4, 192)} = 2.01$, $p = 0.09$, $\eta_p^2 = 0.04$	$F_{(2, 91)} = 1.84$, n.s.	RACC $F_{(1, 91)} = 8.21$, $p < 0.01$, $\eta_p^2 = 0.08$; RT $F_{(1, 91)} = 16.46$, $p < 0.001$, $\eta_p^2 = 0.15$
Incompatible	7.46 ± 0.87	8.24 ± 0.82	10.23 ± 0.94				$F_{(2, 91)} = 2.5$, $p = 0.08$, $\eta_p^2 = 0.05$	
Error	4.41 ± 1.25	4.34 ± 1.17	5.29 ± 1.34				$F_{(2, 91)} = 0.17$, n.s.	
Mean	6.09 ± 0.86	6.19 ± 0.81	7.79 ± 0.92					
ERN (20 ms)								
Compatible	4.55 ± 0.89	4.25 ± 0.84	5.71 ± 0.96	$F_{(2, 192)} = 13.04$, $p < 0.001$, $\eta_p^2 = 0.12$	$F_{(2, 96)} = 1.46$, n.s.	$F_{(4, 192)} = 2.09$, $p = 0.08$, $\eta_p^2 = 0.04$	$F_{(2, 91)} = 0.74$, n.s.	RT $F_{(1, 91)} = 16.45$, $p < 0.001$, $\eta_p^2 = 0.15$; Age $F_{(1, 91)} = 6.57$, $p = 0.01$, $\eta_p^2 = 0.07$
Incompatible	4.85 ± 0.90	5.28 ± 0.85	6.52 ± 0.98				$F_{(2, 91)} = 0.87$, n.s.	
Error	1.93 ± 1.50	1.73 ± 1.40	4.24 ± 1.61				$F_{(2, 91)} = 0.84$, n.s.	
Mean	3.77 ± 0.96	3.80 ± 0.80	5.42 ± 1.03					
EARLY POSITIVITY (62 ms)								
Compatible	6.47 ± 0.96	6.02 ± 0.89	7.23 ± 1.02	$F_{(2, 192)} = 1.72$, n.s.	$F_{(2, 96)} = 1.53$, n.s.	$F_{(4, 192)} = 1.69$, n.s.	$F_{(2, 91)} = 0.41$, n.s.	RT $F_{(1, 91)} = 14.17$, $p < 0.001$, $\eta_p^2 = 0.13$; Age $F_{(1, 91)} = 4.35$, $p = 0.04$, $\eta_p^2 = 0.05$
Incompatible	5.80 ± 0.98	6.12 ± 0.93	7.49 ± 1.06				$F_{(2, 91)} = 0.78$, n.s.	
Error	5.12 ± 1.51	4.59 ± 1.41	7.15 ± 1.62				$F_{(2, 91)} = 0.78$, n.s.	
Mean	5.81 ± 1.02	5.61 ± 0.96	7.20 ± 1.09					
Pe (268 ms)								
Compatible	−0.07 ± 0.99	−1.45 ± 0.92	−0.88 ± 1.05	$F_{(2, 192)} = 115.16$, $p < 0.001$, $\eta_p^2 = 0.55$	$F_{(2, 96)} = 0.31$, n.s.	$F_{(4, 192)} = 0.12$, n.s.	$F_{(2, 91)} = 0.44$, n.s.	RT $F_{(1, 91)} = 8.58$, $p < 0.01$, $\eta_p^2 = 0.08$; Age $F_{(1, 91)} = 4.27$, $p = 0.04$, $\eta_p^2 = 0.04$
Incompatible	−1.13 ± 0.94	−1.31 ± 0.88	−0.99 ± 1.01				$F_{(2, 91)} = 0.03$, n.s.	FSIQ $F_{(1, 91)} = 5.39$, $p = 0.02$, $\eta_p^2 = 0.06$; RACC $F_{(1, 91)} = 8.84$, $p < 0.01$, $\eta_p^2 = 0.09$
Error	9.31 ± 1.68	8.08 ± 1.56	10.42 ± 1.79				$F_{(2, 91)} = 0.48$, n.s.	
Mean	2.58 ± 1.01	1.93 ±.94	2.78 ± 1.08					

ERP, event-related potentials; SD, standard deviation; ANOVA, analysis of variance; ADHD, attention-deficit/hyperactivity disorder; TS, Tourette syndrome; LPC, Late positive component; ERN, error-related negativity; Pe, error positivity; n.s., not significant.

Pe (268 ms)

ANCOVA showed no group differences throughout. Incompatible ERPs showed a significant effect of RT and age, during erroneous trials with we saw a significant effect of FSIQ and RACC.

Correlation with Symptoms

We found no robust correlations between behavioral or ERP measurements and YGTSS scores.

Grouping of Children with TS Only and with TS and Comorbid ADHD

To demonstrate the adequacy of pooling children with TS with and without ADHD, we performed ANCOVAs with four groups, separating TS only and TS+ADHD, control group, ADHD, with the main behavioral and ERP result.

For RT, this analysis showed no group difference [$F_{(3, 93)} = 1.21$, $p = 0.31$, $\eta_p^2 = 0.03$]. Comorbid ADHD in the TS group resulted in marginally different RTs compared to TS only ($p = 0.99$) and controls ($p = 0.78$). Children with ADHD showed high RTs, but no significant differences to other groups ($p > 0.2$).

Also for the IIV, no group differences were found [$F_{(3, 93)} = 1.21$, $p = 0.31$, $\eta_p^2 = 0.03$] and a *post-hoc* comparison revealed no significant differences between the groups (all $p \geq 0.1$).

For the P3 this analysis repeats a significant group difference [$F_{(3, 90)} = 2.99$, $p = 0.04$, $\eta_p^2 = 0.09$], and showed that comorbid ADHD resulted in marginally lower amplitude values in ERPs compared to participants with TS only without significant differences ($p = 0.63$). Children with TS+ADHD showed trends toward higher amplitudes than controls ($p = 0.06$) and children with ADHD ($p = 0.06$), whereas TS only had significantly larger amplitudes than ADHD ($p = 0.03$), and controls ($p = 0.02$).

Based on these additional analyses, the fact that the sample sizes in analyses of these subsamples are small, and the pattern of results redundant and the high clinical relevance of a comorbid group, we merged all participants with TS into one group.

DISCUSSION

This study investigated electrophysiological differences in a Flanker task in children with TS compared with children with ADHD and with typically developing children. We expected that children with TS would perform comparable or better than controls, whereas children with ADHD would show impairments of behavior and ERP measures.

Our results confirmed that children with TS performed behaviorally on the same level as control children. This finding is consistent with previous studies of behavioral performance (Serrien et al., 2005; Roessner et al., 2008; Eichele et al., 2010a; Greimel et al., 2011). In contrast to our expectations, the present study did not find group behavioral differences between children with ADHD and control children when controlling for relevant covariates, which stands in contrast to some previous findings (Albrecht et al., 2008), but not others (Johnstone and Galletta, 2013).

Children with TS, however, showed higher amplitudes in the stimulus-locked ERPs in the early P3 amplitude compared with children with ADHD and control children across task outcomes, which was sustained through the later positive complex. We speculate therefore, that this increased amplitude might reflect a process that may help children with TS to maintain their behavioral performance. The increase in P3 amplitude might reflect greater sustained effort in the TS group in processing the stimuli (Isreal et al., 1980; Luck, 2005) yielding in turn increased attentional resource allocation during stimulus processing. This is supported by the fact that the P3 in children with TS consistently higher across outcomes. Moreover, the increase in P3 in the TS group might indicate that children with TS displayed enhanced processes to update working memory. Together with the increase in the response-locked LPC amplitude, this might reflect an altered sustained attention/orienting pattern of whether the first decision of stimulus classification has led to appropriate steps of processing (Verleger et al., 2005) in children with TS.

Here, TS children show the largest peak of all groups in the earlier P3 subcomponent around 300–350 ms after flanker onset. A recent study using a Go/Nogo-paradigm (Shephard et al., 2015) in a similar cohort with a broader age range did not report differences in ERP correlates between children with TS and control children. The authors analyzed the P3 complex in a longer time-window from 300 to 650 ms. Interestingly, two distinct subcomponents of the P3 can be appreciated during this period, which each show a differential amplitude pattern between the groups, where indeed the TS group grand average has highest amplitudes during the earlier subcomponent (see Figure 3 in Shephard et al., 2015). Similarly, another experiment from the same group, the authors assessed goal directed learning and showed distinct P3 peaks, where the earlier peak consistently had higher amplitudes in TS (Shephard, 2013, pp. 102–103). With respect to children with ADHD who showed the smallest amplitude across outcomes here, it is interesting to note that the data presented by a prior study had the same pattern for this component at the central site around 300ms after flanker onset, as well as across flanker conditions (see figure 2 and 4 at Cz in Albrecht et al., 2008). Interestingly, in this dataset, the P3 component seemed reduced in children with ADHD (Albrecht et al., 2008, personal communication).

While there are some notable exceptions (Albrecht et al., 2008), many studies using simple choice response tasks in children do not find specific differences in N2 between ADHD and controls (e.g., Banaschewski et al., 2004; Broyd et al., 2005; Wiersema et al., 2006; Spronk et al., 2008). In our data, we saw a small frontal N2 component (not shown), but we did not find any clear negative modulation for incompatible and erroneous trials, or any group differences in the location and latency range of N2 that is typically present in flanker tasks in healthy young adults (e.g., Eichele et al., 2010b). Similarly, in this data we did not see a distinct ERN, or specific group differences therein, which may be explained by the clear developmental effect in this component, in the sense that our sample on average has an immature response (Davies et al., 2004). Due to the close interrelation between the ERN and the midfrontal N2, we can also speculate that frontal lobe maturation might affect N2 in the same way (Brydges et al., 2012; Tamnes et al., 2013).

We did separate analyses of the P3 subcomponents here to disentangle processing related to an early P3 component, representing more likely the orienting of attention to stimuli (Polich, 2007), and the later P3b/LPC reflecting response selection and other response-related processing (Falkenstein et al., 1994). The separation of stimulus- and response-locked LPC allows to study response selection/ orienting and response preparation separately (Verleger et al., 2005), which gives further insight into motor control in children with TS. It is possible that the greater increase in P3/LPC amplitude in the TS group reflects a stronger consolidation of the Flanker task in children with TS than in children with ADHD and control children (Johnson, 1984) and may suggest that children with TS employ greater resources in this process to maintain performance.

Individuals with TS frequently need to suppress emerging tics to achieve adequate psychosocial function. Other research has shown that children with TS have a generalized increase in cognitive control over motor activity (Mueller et al., 2006; Jackson et al., 2007) and enhanced control over their manual responses on a task-switching paradigm (Jackson et al., 2011), probably as a consequence of tic suppression. Here, we show that these adaptive effects already may happen earlier during stimulus evaluation, where an adaptation of the attentional system may result in higher attentional levels toward salient stimuli and an increased ability to suppress distracting information. This would in turn improve response selection.

The earlier discordant findings in the few previous studies of P3 in TS children may relate to different methods of recruiting the subjects (comorbidities, medication), and to differences in task selection (passive, active, visual, auditory, response mode; Luck, 2005), as well as different EEG/ERP post-processing and analysis. Here, use of ICA for artifact correction, and region of interest averaging allows for a clearer representation of a small, but robust ERP difference that is appreciable already in earlier work (Albrecht et al., 2008; Shephard et al., 2015).

We found smallest P3/LPC component amplitudes in the ADHD group, albeit not reaching significant difference levels compared with controls. This appears generally consistent with existing literature from several choice response tasks in this age group, including the Flanker task (Johnstone et al., 2010; Kratz et al., 2011). A reduced P3 in ADHD is considered reflective of diminished evaluative and processing capabilities (Brandeis et al., 2002; Lawrence et al., 2005; Johnstone et al., 2010; Kratz et al., 2011). Results from this group are heterogeneous however, for example a recent study using a Flanker task did not find differences on ERP or behavioral measures in children with ADHD compared to a control group (Johnstone and Galletta, 2013). Some inconsistencies may be related to study design, i.e., use of different compositions of clinical samples regarding age-range, sample size, medication status/type, gender distribution or comorbid disorders (Johnstone et al., 2013). However, amplitudes of children with ADHD become more like those of controls when motivated to perform well (Groom et al., 2010) and might have resulted in typical amplitude findings in our study.

We did not find that children with TS used a different strategy in prioritizing either speed or accuracy in compatible or incompatible trials and with respect to symptoms measured with the YGTSS, nor could we find significant correlations for speed or accuracy.

Strengths and Limitations of the Study

All children were medication-naïve. Age and FSIQ differences did not readily explain group differences because groups were matched for age, as well as age and FSIQ were also used as covariates. The inclusion of children with ADHD is a strength of the study, because it allowed to illustrate the specificity of a higher P3 in children with TS, with and without comorbidity.

A limitation here is the relatively small sample size given the incidence, which led us to group TS+ADHD and TS only together. Ideally, the impact of comorbid conditions should be assessed separately, and in more detail, requiring larger sample sizes in future studies, probably best achievable through collaborative multi-site consortia. However, the fact that we did not find any significant differences between these subsamples in the dependent measures reported here justified the inclusion of children with TS only and those with additional ADHD in the same group. The relative lack of negative impact of comorbid ADHD on TS in our sample seems at variance with previous work reporting impaired ERPs (Shephard et al., 2015) and behavior (Roessner et al., 2007; Sukhodolsky et al., 2010; Greimel et al., 2011; Shephard et al., 2015) in participants with TS and ADHD. However, differences in mean age and gender distribution of the samples, as well as use of medication are different. Differences in task design and time on task may also play a role.

Many executive tasks are influenced by global changes in response caution, and motivation and error rates might fluctuate. The skills implemented to solve cognitive challenges may differ considerably in typically developing children from children with ADHD or TS. However, we tried to minimize these influences by keeping the time-on-trial to a minimum, and providing individual feedback after slow and after erroneous trials, respectively. During the experiment and upon debriefing there was no reason to suspect differences in motivation, attention or fatigue across groups and order of tasks was counterbalanced. Also, we used a robust estimate of PES (Dutilh et al., 2012), that discounts slow drifts.

CONCLUSION

These findings provide further evidence that TS is not associated with widespread executive impairments, but presents robust evidence that adaptive changes, such as a heightened attentional capacity, are a core component of the TS disorder. In particular, we report a differential modulation of a P3-subcomponent that has not received much attention so far.

AUTHOR CONTRIBUTIONS

Conception and design: HE, TE, IB, LS, KH, KP. Acquisition of data: HE, TE, MH, LS, HW, MW, KP. Analysis and interpretation: HE, TE, KP. Writing of article: HE, TE, KP. Critical review of article: HE, TE, IB, MH, LS, HW, MW, KH, KP. Final approval for publication: HE, TE, IB, MH, LS, HW, MW, KH, KP. Agreement to be accountable for all aspects of the work: HE, TE, IB, MH, LS, HW, MW, KH, KP.

ACKNOWLEDGMENTS

This work was supported by the Research Council of Norway (190544/H110), the Western Norway Health Authority (MoodNet and the Network for Anxiety Disorders; 911435, 911607, 911827), and the National Norwegian ADHD network grants to KP, the K.G. Jebsen Foundation to TE, and the University of Bergen to HE.

REFERENCES

Albrecht, B., Brandeis, D., Uebel, H., Heinrich, H., Mueller, U. C., Hasselhorn, M., et al. (2008). Action monitoring in boys with attention-deficit/hyperactivity disorder, their nonaffected siblings, and normal control subjects: evidence for an endophenotype. *Biol. Psychiatry* 64, 615–625. doi: 10.1016/j.biopsych.2007.12.016

American Psychiatric Association (1994). *Diagnostic and Statistical Manual of Mental Disorders*. Washington, DC: American Psychiatric Press.

Banaschewski, T., Brandeis, D., Heinrich, H., Albrecht, B., Brunner, E., and Rothenberger, A. (2004). Questioning inhibitory control as the specific deficit of ADHD–evidence from brain electrical activity. *J. Neural Transm. (Vienna)* 111, 841–864. doi: 10.1007/s00702-003-0040-8

Barry, R. J., Johnstone, S. J., and Clarke, A. R. (2003). A review of electrophysiology in attention-deficit/hyperactivity disorder: II. Event-related potentials. *Clin. Neurophysiol.* 114, 184–198. doi: 10.1016/S1388-2457(02)00363-2

Baym, C. L., Corbett, B. A., Wright, S. B., and Bunge, S. A. (2008). Neural correlates of tic severity and cognitive control in children with Tourette syndrome. *Brain* 131, 165–179. doi: 10.1093/brain/awm278

Bell, A. J., and Sejnowski, T. J. (1995). An information-maximization approach to blind separation and blind deconvolution. *Neural Comput.* 7, 1129–1159. doi: 10.1162/neco.1995.7.6.1129

Bloch, M. H., and Leckman, J. F. (2009). Clinical course of Tourette syndrome. *J. Psychosom. Res.* 67, 497–501. doi: 10.1016/j.jpsychores.2009.09.002

Bornstein, R. A. (1991). Neuropsychological correlates of obsessive characteristics in Tourette syndrome. *J. Neuropsychiatry Clin. Neurosci.* 3, 157–162. doi: 10.1176/jnp.3.2.157

Brandeis, D., Banaschewski, T., Baving, L., Georgiewa, P., Blanz, B., Warnke, A., et al. (2002). Multicenter P300 brain mapping of impaired attention to cues in hyperkinetic children. *J. Am. Acad. Child Adolesc. Psychiatry* 41, 990–998. doi: 10.1097/00004583-200208000-00018

Broyd, S. J., Johnstone, S. J., Barry, R. J., Clarke, A. R., McCarthy, R., Selikowitz, M., et al. (2005). The effect of methylphenidate on response inhibition and the event-related potential of children with attention deficit/hyperactivity disorder. *Int. J. Psychophysiol.* 58, 47–58. doi: 10.1016/j.ijpsycho.2005.03.008

Brunia, C. H. M., and Van Boxtel, G. J. M. (2000). "Motor preparation," in *Handbook of Psychophysiology*, eds J. T. Cacioppo, L. G. Tassinary, and G. G. Bernston (Cambridge: Cambridge University Press), 507–532.

Brydges, C. R., Anderson, M., Reid, C. L., and Fox, A. M. (2013). Maturation of cognitive control: delineating response inhibition and interference suppression. *PLoS ONE* 8:e69826. doi: 10.1371/journal.pone.0069826

Brydges, C. R., Clunies-Ross, K., Clohessy, M., Lo, Z. L., Nguyen, A., Rousset, C., et al. (2012). Dissociable components of cognitive control: an event-related potential (ERP) study of response inhibition and interference suppression. *PLoS ONE* 7:e34482. doi: 10.1371/journal.pone.0034482

Burd, L., Kerbeshian, P. J., Barth, A., Klug, M. G., Avery, P. K., and Benz, B. (2001). Long-term follow-up of an epidemiologically defined cohort of patients with Tourette syndrome. *J. Child Neurol.* 16, 431–437. doi: 10.1177/088307380101600609

Clayson, P. E., and Larson, M. J. (2011a). Conflict adaptation and sequential trial effects: support for the conflict monitoring theory. *Neuropsychologia* 49, 1953–1961. doi: 10.1016/j.neuropsychologia.2011.03.023

Clayson, P. E., and Larson, M. J. (2011b). Effects of repetition priming on electrophysiological and behavioral indices of conflict adaptation and cognitive control. *Psychophysiology* 48, 1621–1630. doi: 10.1111/j.1469-8986.2011.01265.x

Cohen, J. (1988). *Statistical Power Analysis for the Behavioral Sciences*. Hillsdale: Lawrence Erlbaum Associates.

Crawford, S., Channon, S., and Robertson, M. M. (2005). Tourette's syndrome: performance on tests of behavioural inhibition, working memory and gambling. *J. Child Psychol. Psychiatry* 46, 1327–1336. doi: 10.1111/j.1469-7610.2005.01419.x

Cuthbert, B. N. (2014). The RDoC framework: facilitating transition from ICD/DSM to dimensional approaches that integrate neuroscience and psychopathology. *World Psychiatry* 13, 28–35. doi: 10.1002/wps.20087

Cycowicz, Y. M. (2000). Memory development and event-related brain potentials in children. *Biol. Psychol.* 54, 145–174. doi: 10.1016/S0301-0511(00)00055-7

Davidson, M. C., Amso, D., Anderson, L. C., and Diamond, A. (2006). Development of cognitive control and executive functions from 4 to 13 years: evidence from manipulations of memory, inhibition, and task switching. *Neuropsychologia* 44, 2037–2078. doi: 10.1016/j.neuropsychologia.2006.02.006

Davies, P. L., Segalowitz, S. J., and Gavin, W. J. (2004). Development of response-monitoring ERPs in 7- to 25-year-olds. *Dev. Neuropsychol.* 25, 355–376. doi: 10.1207/s15326942dn2503_6

Deary, I. J., and Caryl, P. G. (1997). Neuroscience and human intelligence differences. *Trends Neurosci.* 20, 365–371. doi: 10.1016/S0166-2236(97)01070-9

Debener, S., Ullsperger, M., Siegel, M., Fiehler, K., Von Cramon, D. Y., and Engel, A. K. (2005). Trial-by-trial coupling of concurrent electroencephalogram and functional magnetic resonance imaging identifies the dynamics of performance monitoring. *J. Neurosci.* 25, 11730–11737. doi: 10.1523/JNEUROSCI.3286-05.2005

Debes, N. M., Lange, T., Jessen, T. L., Hjalgrim, H., and Skov, L. (2011). Performance on Wechsler intelligence scales in children with Tourette syndrome. *Eur. J. Paediatr. Neurol.* 15, 146–154. doi: 10.1016/j.ejpn.2010.07.007

Delorme, A., and Makeig, S. (2004). EEGLAB: an open source toolbox for analysis of single-trial EEG dynamics including independent component analysis. *J. Neurosci. Methods* 134, 9–21. doi: 10.1016/j.jneumeth.2003.10.009

Dennis, M., Francis, D. J., Cirino, P. T., Schachar, R., Barnes, M. A., and Fletcher, J. M. (2009). Why IQ is not a covariate in cognitive studies of neurodevelopmental disorders. *J. Int. Neuropsychol. Soc.* 15, 331–343. doi: 10.1017/S1355617709090481

Donchin, E. (1981). Surprise!...Surprise? *Psychophysiology* 18, 493–513. doi: 10.1111/j.1469-8986.1981.tb01815.x

Donchin, E., and Coles, M. G. H. (1998). Context updating and the P300. *Behav. Brain Sci.* 21, 152. doi: 10.1017/S0140525X98230950

Donchin, E., and Coles, M. G. H. (2010). Is the P300 component a manifestation of context updating? *Behav. Brain Sci.* 11, 357. doi: 10.1017/S0140525X00058027

Dupaul, G. J., Power, T. J., and Anastopoulos, A. D. (1998). *ADHD Rating Scale-IV: Checklist, Norms, and Clinical Interpretation*. New York, NY: Guilford Press.

Dupuis, D., Ram, N., Willner, C. J., Karalunas, S., Segalowitz, S. J., and Gatzke-Kopp, L. M. (2015). Implications of ongoing neural development for the measurement of the error-related negativity in childhood. *Dev. Sci.* 18, 452–468. doi: 10.1111/desc.12229

Dutilh, G., Van Ravenzwaaij, D., Nieuwenhuis, S., Van Der Maas, H. L., Forstmann, B. U., and Wagenmakers, E. J. (2012). How to measure post-error slowing: a confound and a simple solution. *J. Math. Psychol.* 56, 208–216. doi: 10.1016/j.jmp.2012.04.001

Eichele, H., Eichele, T., Hammar, A., Freyberger, H. J., Hugdahl, K., and Plessen, K. J. (2010a). Go/NoGo performance in boys with Tourette syndrome. *Child Neuropsychol.* 16, 162–168. doi: 10.1080/09297040903150182

Eichele, H., Juvodden, H. T., Ullsperger, M., and Eichele, T. (2010b). Maladaptation of event-related EEG responses preceding performance errors. *Front. Hum. Neurosci.* 4:65. doi: 10.3389/fnhum.2010.00065

Eichele, H., and Plessen, K. J. (2013). Neural plasticity in functional and anatomical MRI studies of children with Tourette syndrome. *Behav. Neurol.* 27, 33–45. doi: 10.1155/2013/376590

Eichele, T., Specht, K., Moosmann, M., Jongsma, M. L., Quiroga, R. Q., Nordby, H., et al. (2005). Assessing the spatiotemporal evolution of neuronal activation with single-trial event-related potentials and functional MRI. *Proc. Natl. Acad. Sci. U.S.A.* 102, 17798–17803. doi: 10.1073/pnas.0505508102

Eriksen, B. A., and Eriksen, C. W. (1974). Effects of noise letters upon identification of a target letter in a nonsearch task. *Percept. Psychophys.* 16, 143–149. doi: 10.3758/BF03203267

Falkenstein, M., Hohnsbein, J., and Hoormann, J. (1994). Effects of choice complexity on different subcomponents of the late positive complex of the event-related potential. *Electroencephalogr. Clin. Neurophysiol.* 92, 148–160. doi: 10.1016/0168-5597(94)90055-8

Fan, J., McCandliss, B. D., Sommer, T., Raz, A., and Posner, M. I. (2002). Testing the efficiency and independence of attentional networks. *J. Cogn. Neurosci.* 14, 340–347. doi: 10.1162/089892902317361886

Folstein, J. R., and Van Petten, C. (2008). Influence of cognitive control and mismatch on the N2 component of the ERP: a review. *Psychophysiology* 45, 152–170. doi: 10.1111/j.1469-8986.2007.00602.x

Gogtay, N., Giedd, J. N., Lusk, L., Hayashi, K. M., Greenstein, D., Vaituzis, A. C., et al. (2004). Dynamic mapping of human cortical development during childhood through early adulthood. *Proc. Natl. Acad. Sci. U.S.A.* 101, 8174–8179. doi: 10.1073/pnas.0402680101

Greimel, E., Herpertz-Dahlmann, B., Gunther, T., Vitt, C., and Konrad, K. (2008). Attentional functions in children and adolescents with attention-deficit/hyperactivity disorder with and without comorbid tic disorder. *J. Neural Transm. (Vienna)* 115, 191–200. doi: 10.1007/s00702-007-0815-4

Greimel, E., Wanderer, S., Rothenberger, A., Herpertz-Dahlmann, B., Konrad, K., and Roessner, V. (2011). Attentional performance in children and adolescents with tic disorder and co-occurring attention-deficit/hyperactivity disorder: new insights from a 2 x 2 factorial design study. *J. Abnorm. Child Psychol.* 39, 819–828. doi: 10.1007/s10802-011-9493-7

Groom, M. J., Scerif, G., Liddle, P. F., Batty, M. J., Liddle, E. B., Roberts, K. L., et al. (2010). Effects of motivation and medication on electrophysiological markers of response inhibition in children with attention-deficit/hyperactivity disorder. *Biol. Psychiatry* 67, 624–631. doi: 10.1016/j.biopsych.2009.09.029

Handy, T. C. (2005). *Event-Related Potentials: A Methods Handbook.* Cambridge: MIT Press.

Hirschtritt, M. E., Lee, P. C., Pauls, D. L., Dion, Y., Grados, M. A., Illmann, C., et al. (2015). Lifetime prevalence, age of risk, and genetic relationships of comorbid psychiatric disorders in Tourette syndrome. *JAMA Psychiatry* 72, 325–333. doi: 10.1001/jamapsychiatry.2014.2650

Isreal, J. B., Chesney, G. L., Wickens, C. D., and Donchin, E. (1980). P300 and tracking difficulty: evidence for multiple resources in dual-task performance. *Psychophysiology* 17, 259–273. doi: 10.1111/j.1469-8986.1980.tb00146.x

Jackson, G. M., Mueller, S. C., Hambleton, K., and Hollis, C. P. (2007). Enhanced cognitive control in Tourette Syndrome during task uncertainty. *Exp. Brain Res.* 182, 357–364. doi: 10.1007/s00221-007-0999-8

Jackson, S. R., Parkinson, A., Jung, J., Ryan, S. E., Morgan, P. S., Hollis, C., et al. (2011). Compensatory neural reorganization in Tourette syndrome. *Curr. Biol.* 21, 580–585. doi: 10.1016/j.cub.2011.02.047

Jausovec, N., and Jausovec, K. (2000). Correlations between ERP parameters and intelligence: a reconsideration. *Biol. Psychol.* 55, 137–154. doi: 10.1016/S0301-0511(00)00076-4

Johnson, R. Jr. (1984). P300: a model of the variables controlling its amplitude. *Ann. N.Y. Acad. Sci.* 425, 223–229. doi: 10.1111/j.1749-6632.1984.tb23538.x

Johnstone, S. J., Barry, R. J., and Clarke, A. R. (2013). Ten years on: a follow-up review of ERP research in attention-deficit/hyperactivity disorder. *Clin. Neurophysiol.* 124, 644–657. doi: 10.1016/j.clinph.2012.09.006

Johnstone, S. J., and Galletta, D. (2013). Event-rate effects in the flanker task: ERPs and task performance in children with and without AD/HD. *Int. J. Psychophysiol.* 87, 340–348. doi: 10.1016/j.ijpsycho.2012.07.170

Johnstone, S. J., Watt, A. J., and Dimoska, A. (2010). Varying required effort during interference control in children with AD/HD: task performance and ERPs. *Int. J. Psychophysiol.* 76, 174–185. doi: 10.1016/j.ijpsycho.2010.03.010

Kaufman, J., Birmaher, B., Brent, D., Rao, U., Flynn, C., Moreci, P., et al. (1997). Schedule for affective disorders and schizophrenia for school-age children-present and lifetime version (K-SADS-PL): initial reliability and validity data. *J. Am. Acad. Child Adolesc. Psychiatry* 36, 980–988. doi: 10.1097/00004583-199707000-00021

Kratz, O., Studer, P., Malcherek, S., Erbe, K., Moll, G. H., and Heinrich, H. (2011). Attentional processes in children with ADHD: an event-related potential study using the attention network test. *Int. J. Psychophysiol.* 81, 82–90. doi: 10.1016/j.ijpsycho.2011.05.008

Ladouceur, C. D., Dahl, R. E., and Carter, C. S. (2007). Development of action monitoring through adolescence into adulthood: ERP and source localization. *Dev. Sci.* 10, 874–891. doi: 10.1111/j.1467-7687.2007.00639.x

Larson, M. J., Clayson, P. E., and Clawson, A. (2014). Making sense of all the conflict: a theoretical review and critique of conflict-related ERPs. *Int. J. Psychophysiol.* 93, 283–297. doi: 10.1016/j.ijpsycho.2014.06.007

Lawrence, C. A., Barry, R. J., Clarke, A. R., Johnstone, S. J., McCarthy, R., Selikowitz, M., et al. (2005). Methylphenidate effects in attention deficit/hyperactivity disorder: electrodermal and ERP measures during a continuous performance task. *Psychopharmacology* 183, 81–91. doi: 10.1007/s00213-005-0144-y

Leckman, J. F. (2002). Tourette's syndrome. *Lancet* 360, 1577–1586. doi: 10.1016/S0140-6736(02)11526-1

Leckman, J. F., Riddle, M. A., Hardin, M. T., Ort, S. I., Swartz, K. L., Stevenson, J., et al. (1989). The yale global tic severity scale: initial testing of a clinician-rated scale of tic severity. *J. Am. Acad. Child Adolesc. Psychiatry* 28, 566–573. doi: 10.1097/00004583-198907000-00015

Leckman, J. F., Zhang, H., Vitale, A., Lahnin, F., Lynch, K., Bondi, C., et al. (1998). Course of tic severity in Tourette syndrome: the first two decades. *Pediatrics* 102, 14–19. doi: 10.1542/peds.102.1.14

Liotti, M., Pliszka, S. R., Perez, R., Kothmann, D., and Woldorff, M. G. (2005). Abnormal brain activity related to performance monitoring and error detection in children with ADHD. *Cortex* 41, 377–388. doi: 10.1016/S0010-9452(08)70274-0

Loo, S. K., Lenartowicz, A., and Makeig, S. (2015). Research review: use of EEG biomarkers in child psychiatry research - current state and future directions. *J. Child Psychol. Psychiatry* 57, 4–17. doi: 10.1111/jcpp.12435

Luck, S. J. (2005). *An Introduction to the Event-Related Potential Technique.* MIT Press.

Mazaheri, A., Fassbender, C., Coffey-Corina, S., Hartanto, T. A., Schweitzer, J. B., and Mangun, G. R. (2014). Differential oscillatory electroencephalogram between attention-deficit/hyperactivity disorder subtypes and typically developing adolescents. *Biol. Psychiatry* 76, 422–429. doi: 10.1016/j.biopsych.2013.08.023

Mueller, S. C., Jackson, G. M., Dhalla, R., Datsopoulos, S., and Hollis, C. P. (2006). Enhanced cognitive control in young people with Tourette's syndrome. *Curr. Biol.* 16, 570–573. doi: 10.1016/j.cub.2006.01.064

Oades, R. D., Dittmann-Balcar, A., Schepker, R., Eggers, C., and Zerbin, D. (1996). Auditory event-related potentials (ERPs) and mismatch negativity (MMN) in healthy children and those with attention-deficit or tourette/tic symptoms. *Biol. Psychol.* 43, 163–185. doi: 10.1016/0301-0511(96)05189-7

Ozonoff, S., and Jensen, J. (1999). Brief report: specific executive function profiles in three neurodevelopmental disorders. *J. Autism Dev. Disord.* 29, 171–177. doi: 10.1023/A:1023052913110

Ozonoff, S., Strayer, D. L., McMahon, W. M., and Filloux, F. (1998). Inhibitory deficits in Tourette syndrome: a function of comorbidity and symptom severity. *J. Child Psychol. Psychiatry* 39, 1109–1118. doi: 10.1111/1469-7610.00415

Pelosi, L., Holly, M., Slade, T., Hayward, M., Barrett, G., and Blumhardt, L. D. (1992). Event-related potential (ERP) correlates of performance of intelligence tests. *Electroencephalogr. Clin. Neurophysiol.* 84, 515–520. doi: 10.1016/0168-5597(92)90040-I

Picton, T. W., Bentin, S., Berg, P., Donchin, E., Hillyard, S. A., Johnson, R. Jr., et al. (2000). Guidelines for using human event-related potentials to study cognition: recording standards and publication criteria. *Psychophysiology* 37, 127–152. doi: 10.1111/1469-8986.3720127

Plessen, K. J. (2013). Tic disorders and Tourette's syndrome. *Eur. Child Adolesc. Psychiatry* 22(Suppl. 1), S55–S60. doi: 10.1007/s00787-012-0362-x

Polich, J. (2007). Updating P300: an integrative theory of P3a and P3b. *Clin. Neurophysiol.* 118, 2128–2148. doi: 10.1016/j.clinph.2007.04.019

Posner, M. I., Rothbart, M. K., Sheese, B. E., and Voelker, P. (2014). Developing attention: behavioral and brain mechanisms. *Adv. Neurosci. (Hindawi)* 2014, 405094. doi: 10.1155/2014/405094

Ramchurn, A., De Fockert, J. W., Mason, L., Darling, S., and Bunce, D. (2014). Intraindividual reaction time variability affects P300 amplitude rather than latency. *Front. Hum. Neurosci.* 8:557. doi: 10.3389/fnhum.2014.00557

Robertson, M. M. (2012). The Gilles de la Tourette syndrome: the current status. *Arch. Dis. Child. Educ. Pract. Ed.* 97, 166–175. doi: 10.1136/archdischild-2011-300585

Roessner, V., Albrecht, B., Dechent, P., Baudewig, J., and Rothenberger, A. (2008). Normal response inhibition in boys with Tourette syndrome. *Behav. Brain Funct.* 4, 29. doi: 10.1186/1744-9081-4-29

Roessner, V., Becker, A., Banaschewski, T., and Rothenberger, A. (2007). Executive functions in children with chronic tic disorders with/without ADHD: new insights. *Eur. Child Adolesc. Psychiatry* 16(Suppl. 1), 36–44. doi: 10.1007/s00787-007-1005-5

Rojas-Benjumea, M. A., Sauque-Poggio, A. M., Barriga-Paulino, C. I., Rodriguez-Martinez, E. I., and Gomez, C. M. (2015). Development of behavioral parameters and ERPs in a novel-target visual detection paradigm in children, adolescents and young adults. *Behav. Brain Funct.* 11, 22. doi: 10.1186/s12993-015-0067-7

Rothbart, M. K., Sheese, B. E., Rueda, M. R., and Posner, M. I. (2011). Developing mechanisms of self-regulation in early life. *Emot. Rev.* 3, 207–213. doi: 10.1177/1754073910387943

Serrien, D. J., Orth, M., Evans, A. H., Lees, A. J., and Brown, P. (2005). Motor inhibition in patients with Gilles de la Tourette syndrome: functional activation patterns as revealed by EEG coherence. *Brain* 128, 116–125. doi: 10.1093/brain/awh318

Shaffer, D., Gould, M. S., Brasic, J., Ambrosini, P., Fisher, P., Bird, H., et al. (1983). A children's global assessment scale (CGAS). *Arch. Gen. Psychiatry* 40, 1228–1231. doi: 10.1001/archpsyc.1983.01790100074010

Shephard, E. (2013). *Electrophysiological Correlates of Learning and Cognitive Control in Children with Tics with and without ADHD Symptoms.* Doctor of Philosophy, University of Nottingham.

Shephard, E., Jackson, G. M., and Groom, M. J. (2015). The effects of co-occurring ADHD symptoms on electrophysiological correlates of cognitive control in young people with Tourette syndrome. *J. Neuropsychol.* doi: 10.1111/jnp.12071. [Epub ahead of print].

Sobel, L. J., Bansal, R., Maia, T. V., Sanchez, J., Mazzone, L., Durkin, K., et al. (2010). Basal ganglia surface morphology and the effects of stimulant medications in youth with attention deficit hyperactivity disorder. *Am. J. Psychiatry* 167, 977–986. doi: 10.1176/appi.ajp.2010.09091259

Spessot, A. L., Plessen, K. J., and Peterson, B. S. (2004). Neuroimaging of developmental psychopathologies: the importance of self-regulatory and neuroplastic processes in adolescence. *Ann. N.Y. Acad. Sci.* 1021, 86–104. doi: 10.1196/annals.1308.010

Spronk, M., Jonkman, L. M., and Kemner, C. (2008). Response inhibition and attention processing in 5- to 7-year-old children with and without symptoms of ADHD: An ERP study. *Clin. Neurophysiol.* 119, 2738–2752. doi: 10.1016/j.clinph.2008.09.010

Stige, S., Fjell, A. M., Smith, L., Lindgren, M., and Walhovd, K. B. (2007). The development of visual P3a and P3b. *Dev. Neuropsychol.* 32, 563–584. doi: 10.1080/87565640701361096

Sukhodolsky, D. G., Landeros-Weisenberger, A., Scahill, L., Leckman, J. F., and Schultz, R. T. (2010). Neuropsychological functioning in children with Tourette syndrome with and without attention-deficit/hyperactivity disorder. *J. Am. Acad. Child Adolesc. Psychiatry* 49, 1155–1164. doi: 10.1016/j.jaac.2010.08.008

Tamnes, C. K., Walhovd, K. B., Torstveit, M., Sells, V. T., and Fjell, A. M. (2013). Performance monitoring in children and adolescents: a review of developmental changes in the error-related negativity and brain maturation. *Dev. Cogn. Neurosci.* 6, 1–13. doi: 10.1016/j.dcn.2013.05.001

Tau, G. Z., and Peterson, B. S. (2010). Normal development of brain circuits. *Neuropsychopharmacology* 35, 147–168. doi: 10.1038/npp.2009.115

Ullsperger, M. (2006). Performance monitoring in neurological and psychiatric patients. *Int. J. Psychophysiol.* 59, 59–69. doi: 10.1016/j.ijpsycho.2005.06.010

Ullsperger, M., Danielmeier, C., and Jocham, G. (2014). Neurophysiology of performance monitoring and adaptive behavior. *Physiol. Rev.* 94, 35–79. doi: 10.1152/physrev.00041.2012

Van Woerkom, T. C., Roos, R. A., and Van Dijk, J. G. (1994). Altered attentional processing of background stimuli in Gilles de la Tourette syndrome: a study in auditory event-related potentials evoked in an oddball paradigm. *Acta Neurol. Scand.* 90, 116–123. doi: 10.1111/j.1600-0404.1994.tb02690.x

Verleger, R., Jaœkowski, P., and Wascher, E. (2005). Evidence for an integrative role of P3b in linking reaction to perception. *J. Psychophysiol.* 19, 165–181. doi: 10.1027/0269-8803.19.3.165

Viola, F. C., Thorne, J., Edmonds, B., Schneider, T., Eichele, T., and Debener, S. (2009). Semi-automatic identification of independent components representing EEG artifact. *Clin. Neurophysiol.* 120, 868–877. doi: 10.1016/j.clinph.2009.01.015

Vloet, T. D., Neufang, S., Herpertz-Dahlmann, B., and Konrad, K. (2006). [Neuroimaging data of ADHD, tic-disorder and obsessive-compulsive-disorder in children and adolescents]. *Z. Kinder Jugendpsychiatr. Psychother.* 34, 343–355. doi: 10.1024/1422-4917.34.5.343

Wechsler, D. (2003). *Wechlser Intelligence Scale for Children-Fourth Edition (WISC-IV).* Stockholm: Pearson Assessment.

Wessel, J. R., and Ullsperger, M. (2011). Selection of independent components representing event-related brain potentials: a data-driven approach for greater objectivity. *Neuroimage* 54, 2105–2115. doi: 10.1016/j.neuroimage.2010.10.033

Widmann, A. (2006). *Firfilt EEGLAB Plugin, 1.5.1. Edn.* Leipzig: University of Leipzig.

Wiersema, J. R., Van Der Meere, J. J., and Roeyers, H. (2007). Developmental changes in error monitoring: an event-related potential study. *Neuropsychologia* 45, 1649–1657. doi: 10.1016/j.neuropsychologia.2007.01.004

Wiersema, R., Van Der Meere, J., Roeyers, H., Van Coster, R., and Baeyens, D. (2006). Event rate and event-related potentials in ADHD. *J. Child Psychol. Psychiatry* 47, 560–567. doi: 10.1111/j.1469-7610.2005.01592.x

Willcutt, E. G., Doyle, A. E., Nigg, J. T., Faraone, S. V., and Pennington, B. F. (2005). Validity of the executive function theory of attention-deficit/hyperactivity disorder: a meta-analytic review. *Biol. Psychiatry* 57, 1336–1346. doi: 10.1016/j.biopsych.2005.02.006

Worbe, Y., Marrakchi-Kacem, L., Lecomte, S., Valabregue, R., Poupon, F., Guevara, P., et al. (2015). Altered structural connectivity of cortico-striato-pallido-thalamic networks in Gilles de la Tourette syndrome. *Brain* 138, 472–482. doi: 10.1093/brain/awu311

Zhu, Y., Liu, P. Z., Leung, K. M., Su, L. Y., Wu, D. X., and Zhou, M. (2006). P300 differences exist between Tourette's syndrome with and without attention deficiency and hyperactivity disorder in children. *World J. Biol. Psychiatry* 7, 91–98. doi: 10.1080/15622970500492723

2

New Insights into Clinical Characteristics of Gilles de la Tourette Syndrome: Findings in 1032 Patients from a Single German Center

Tanvi Sambrani[1,2]*, *Ewgeni Jakubovski*[2] *and Kirsten R. Müller-Vahl*[2]

[1] *Department of Education, Monash University, Melbourne, VIC, Australia,* [2] *Clinic of Psychiatry, Social Psychiatry, and Psychotherapy, Hannover Medical School, Hannover, Germany*

Edited by:
Ashok Mysore,
St. John's Medical College Hospital,
India

Reviewed by:
Rajshekhar Bipeta,
Gandhi Medical College and Hospital,
India
Kerstin Jessica Plessen,
University of Copenhagen, Denmark
Janardhan Y. C. Reddy,
National Institute of Mental Health and
Neurosciences, India

***Correspondence:**
Tanvi Sambrani
tsam14@student.monash.edu

Background: Gilles de la Tourette syndrome (TS) is a complex neuropsychiatric disorder defined by the presence of motor and phonic tics, but often associated with psychiatric comorbidities. The main objective of this study was to explore the clinical presentation and comorbidities of TS.

Method: We analyzed clinical data obtained from a large sample (n = 1032; 529 children and 503 adults) of patients with tic disorders from one single German TS center assessed by one investigator. Data was collected with the help of an expert-reviewed semi-structured interview, designed to assess tic severity and certain comorbidities. Group comparisons were carried out via independent sample t-tests and chi-square tests.

Results: The main findings of the study are: (1) tic severity is associated with the presence of premonitory urges (PU), copro-, echo-, and paliphenomena and the number of comorbidities, but not age at tic onset; it is higher in patients with comorbid obsessive-compulsive disorder (OCD) than in patients with comorbid attention deficit/hyperactivity disorder (ADHD). (2) PU were found to be highly associated with "not just right experiences" and to emerge much earlier than previously thought alongside with the ability to suppress tics (PU in >60% and suppressibility in >75% at age 8–10 years). (3) Self-injurious behavior (SIB) is highly associated with complex motor tics and coprophenomena, but not with OCD/obsessive-compulsive behavior (OCB). While comorbid ADHD is associated with a lower ability to suppress tics, comorbid depression is associated with sleeping problems.

Discussion: Our results demonstrate that tic severity is not influenced by age at onset. From our data, it is suggested that PU represent a specific type of "not just right experience" that is not a prerequisite for tic suppression. Comorbid ADHD reduces patients' ability of successful tic suppression. Our data suggest that SIB belongs to the coprophenomena spectrum and hence should be conceptualized as a complex tic rather than a compulsion. Finally, this study strongly supports the hypothesis that TS+OCD is a more severe form of TS and that comorbid OCD/OCB, depression, and anxiety belong to the TS spectrum, while ADHD should be better conceptualized as a separate problem.

Keywords: Tourette syndrome, tics, comorbidities, ADHD, OCD, premonitory urges, self-injurious behavior, depression

INTRODUCTION

A part of the broad spectrum of tic disorders—including provisional tic disorder and persistent (chronic) tic disorder—Gilles de la Tourette syndrome (TS) is a neuropsychiatric disorder with an onset in childhood. This developmental disorder is characterized by the presence of multiple motor tics and at least one phonic tic for a minimum period of 1 year, beginning before 18 years of age and occurring in bouts (American Psychiatric Association, 2013). Typically, tics begin to appear between 5–7 years of age, follow a waxing and waning course, reach their peak severity between 10 and 12 years of age, and decline drastically or even vanish completely by the end of adolescence (Leckman et al., 1998). Not only is TS found among people in all countries, cultures, and ethnic groups, but its main characteristics are also mostly similar across such different populations (Tanner and Goldman, 1997), with the estimated prevalence ranging between 1% (Robertson et al., 2009) and 5.26% (Cubo et al., 2011), the latter relatively high percentage conveying that TS in the general community is milder and more ubiquitous than its prevalence estimates based on its occurrence in clinical settings (Robertson, 2000). Relevant literature also points toward a clear sex difference in prevalence of TS, with it being approximately four times more common in males than in females (Robertson, 1994; Tanner and Goldman, 1997; Freeman et al., 2000).

The vast majority of individuals with TS report a certain discomfort or feeling of pressure before a tic occurs—either focal and specific to a particular anatomical location or more generalized—called "premonitory urge" (PU), that tends to intensify before the tic occurs and is usually mitigated temporarily once the individual performs the tic (Leckman et al., 1993).

Particularly in more severely affected patients, simple motor and phonic tics are often accompanied by different forms of complex tics including coprophenomena—such as making socially inappropriate gestures (copropraxia) or verbal expressions (coprolalia)—in which symptoms tend to manifest during the preadolescent period when tics are at their most severe (Freeman et al., 2009), echophenomena such as imitating gestures (echopraxia) and words or phrases (echolalia), and paliphenomena such as phonic blocking and repetition (palilalia). Additionally, TS is considerably comorbid with attention deficit/hyperactivity disorder (ADHD), obsessive-compulsive disorder (OCD) or (subclinical) obsessive-compulsive behavior (OCB), anxiety disorders, depression, self-injurious behavior (SIB), rage attacks, and to a lesser extent with learning disorders, personality disorders, and other behavioral disorders (Robertson, 2000). Freeman et al. (2000) found that at all ages, a mere 12% of the clinical population with TS have no reported comorbidity.

Robertson and Baron-Cohen (1998) have provided a relatively clear clinical division of TS: (i) "pure TS," including almost only motor and phonic tics; (ii) "full blown TS," consisting of related echo-, copro-, and paliphenomena; and (iii) "TS plus" (first coined by Packer, 1997), which includes cases of those who also have SIB, ADHD, severe OCB, or OCD, as well as other severe psychopathologies such as depression, anxiety, and antisocial behaviors. Another classification was proposed by Robertson and Cavanna (2007), in which "cluster 1" consisted of only simple tics, "cluster 2" involved tics, ADHD, and aggression, whilst "cluster 3" included tics, and affective disorders such as OCD/OCB, depression, and anxiety. The second classification is in line with research indicating that depression, anxiety, OCD, and OCB are all a part of the TS spectrum, whereas ADHD is somewhat separate (Lebowitz et al., 2012; Hirschtritt et al., 2015; Trillini and Müller-Vahl, 2015).

In their multisite study, Freeman et al. (2000) analyzed data obtained from 3500 individuals diagnosed with TS obtained from 64 different centers across 22 countries, and established several findings. They reported that the mean age at onset of tics was 6.4 years. The most common reported comorbidity was ADHD at 60% followed by history of sleeping problems (37%) and OCB (32%). In terms of gender differences, they confirmed not only the well-known male:female ratio (4.3:1), but also found that males are more likely to have comorbid disorders such as conduct disorder (CD)/oppositional defiant disorder (ODD), ADHD, pervasive developmental disorders, anger control problems, specific learning disability, stuttering, social skills problems, and pre-/perinatal-problems than females, whereas females showed significantly higher rates for SIB and trichotillomania. Males were also found to have a significantly higher comorbidity score (2.06) than females (1.83). Symptoms such as sleeping problems, coprolalia, SIB, and anger control problems were found to be positively associated with the comorbidity score. With respect to associated psychopathology, their results also showed that sleeping problems were twice as likely to occur in the comorbid group as opposed to the "TS only" group (without comorbidities).

Through this study, we aim to extend our knowledge of possible differences in the clinical presentation and nature of TS-related phenomena/various tic symptoms based on gender, age groups, and single comorbidity subgroups of TS, and thereby achieve a better understanding of the factors producing variations in order to engage in better subtyping of TS. Therefore, we used a large database—consisting purely of data gathered during the first evaluation of every patient at the TS center—as a suitable starting point for studying a large sample ($n = 1032$) from a single research site, thereby controlling for inter-site variance. We also posit a more specific hypothesis that whilst comorbidities such as OCD, anxiety, depression, and SIB are more related to the TS spectrum, comorbidities like ADHD and rage attacks tend to be slightly independent of it, as has been suggested earlier (Lebowitz et al., 2012; Hirschtritt et al., 2015; Trillini and Müller-Vahl, 2015).

METHODS

This study bases on a large data set obtained from only one single large German TS center at the Clinic of Psychiatry, Socialpsychiatry, and Psychotherapy at the Hannover Medical School (MHH). It is the largest TS center in all of Germany with an outpatient clinic which treats both adults and children. The waiting time for an appointment ranges between 2 and 3 months. The administration of this institution allows patients to visit the outpatient clinic without the need for a referral by another medical professional. The medical costs incurred by the patients' families are covered by health insurance. Thus, patients from all over Germany—and in some cases even from abroad—present at this TS center. All patients included in this study had not only been personally seen by one of the authors (KMV), but their medical history was also personally looked into by her in each case. KMV is both a neurologist and an adult psychiatrist and a well-experienced specialist for tic disorders.

Clinical data was elicited over a period of nearly 20 years (1995–2013) from 1032 patients consisting of 529 children and 503 adults (median age = 17; *SD* = 12.91) with various tic disorders. The diagnoses of different form of tic disorders were made according to DSM criteria valid at that time (DSM-III-R–DSM-IV-TR). All subjects were prospectively interviewed using a clinician-reviewed semi-structured interview assessing several different aspects including tics and comorbidities. This schedule closely resembles the National Hospital Interview Schedule, developed by Robertson and Eapen (1996), and its credibility was established based on the expertise of one of the authors (KMV). Lifetime data for 9 motor and phonic tic symptoms were obtained: simple motor (MT) and phonic tics (PT), complex MT and PT (including all different forms of complex tics), and specifically coprolalia, copropraxia, echolalia, echopraxia, and palilalia (each symptom was scored as either present or absent). In addition, we asked for age at tic onset (separately for MT and PT), suppressibility of tics (yes/no), and presence of PU (yes/no), including the nature/localization of the PU (local, diffused, or uncertain).

Current tic severity was assessed on the day of diagnosis at MHH using the Shapiro Tourette-Syndrome Severity Scale (STSS), which contains five variables with matching rating scales as follows: (1) tics noticeable to others (0–3), (2) tics elicit comments or curiosity (0–1), (3) patient considered odd or bizarre (0–2), (4) tics interfere with functioning (0–2), (5) incapacitated, homebound or hospitalized (0–1). The total score ranges from 0 to 9 with the following interpretation: 0 = none, $0 - <1$ = very mild, $1 - <2$ = mild, $2 - <4$ = moderate, $4 - <6$ = marked, $6 - 8$ = severe, and $>8 - 9$ = very severe (Shapiro et al., 1988). The corresponding Global Severity Ratings (GSR) range from 0 (indicating "none") to 6 (indicating "very severe").

Lifetime prevalence for the following comorbidities was evaluated based on the semi-structured clinical interview: hyperactivity, inattention, rage attacks, anxiety (including different forms of anxiety disorders including phobias, panic disorders, and general anxiety disorder), depression, OCD, SIB, and sleeping problems. ADHD was diagnosed for each participant based on the presence of either hyperactivity or inattention, and hence these two are considered one comorbidity. OCB, being a mild form of OCD, was assessed, but not considered as a comorbidity. Specific obsessive-compulsive (OC) symptoms such as obsessions and compulsions—particularly those of counting, checking, ordering, washing, and "not just right experiences"—were also assessed. For the assessment of comorbidities, no validated rating scales were used. Diagnoses of psychiatric comorbidities were based either on patients' history or—in case of current symptomatology—on DSM criteria. A comorbidity score was calculated by adding up the total number of comorbidities for each patient as suggested earlier (Freeman et al., 2000), ranging from 0 to 6 (including OCD, ADHD, rage attacks, anxiety, depression, and SIB).

Several group comparisons were undertaken. Patients diagnosed with TS according to DSM ("TS group") were categorized as "TS only"—consisting of those individuals with no comorbidities (as defined above)—and "TS + comorbidities" (equivalent of the "TS plus" sub-group coined by Packer, 1997)—comprised those TS patients with ≥1 comorbidity (including OCD, ADHD, rage attacks, anxiety, depression, and SIB). In addition, we conducted two further subgroup comparisons: (i) TS+OCD (excluding ADHD but including other comorbidities) vs. TS+ADHD (excluding OCD/OCB but including other comorbidities) in order to further investigate the hypothesis that OCD, but not ADHD, is part of the TS spectrum; and (ii) TS+OCD/OCB/anxiety/depression/SIB vs. TS+ADHD+rage attacks in order to verify the validity of the classification of TS suggested by Robertson and Cavanna (2007).

All data analyses were carried out using the Statistical Package for Social Sciences (V.21.0 for Mac, SPSS Inc.) and Microsoft Excel Mac 2011. *Z*-score tests of proportion were carried out to measure gender differences for various clinical features of TS and associated disorders. Pearson's Chi-square tests were conducted to test for associations between categorical variables measuring the presence of several comorbidities. ANOVA and *t*-tests were conducted to test for gender differences and differences in tic severity in continuous variables. Alpha value was set at 0.05 (two-tailed). Due to a few issues related to data collection, some of the fields in the database were left blank, thereby resulting in an incomplete database and consequently certain missing values, the absolute numbers and percentages of which have been mentioned at the appropriate parts of the results section.

RESULTS

Of the entire sample of 1032 patients, 529 (51.3%) were children (<18 years of age) whilst 503 (48.7%) were adults (≥18 years of age). Nine hundred and seventy-eight patients had TS, 40 patients were diagnosed with chronic motor tics (CMT), and the remaining 14 had other tic disorders, such as transient (provisional) or chronic (persistent) vocal or other tic disorders. Unless otherwise specified, all the results pertain to the entire sample. Further, details for the CMT group will be provided elsewhere (Müller-Vahl et al., in preparation). Depending on the presence of comorbidities we found: "TS only" (n = 75; 7.2%), "TS + comorbidities" (n = 898; 87.0%), TS+OCD (n = 45; 4.4%), TS+ADHD (n = 102; 9.9%), TS+OCD/OCB/anxiety/depression/SIB (n = 209; 20.3%), and TS+ADHD+rage attacks (n = 56; 5.4%).

Tics: Age at Onset and Tic Severity

The mean age at time of assessment was 20.9 years (range 4–72; *SD*: 12.91). The mean age at onset of tics was 6.97 years (range, 0–21; *SD*: 3.17). Only one of the 978 participants claimed that his tics started at the age of 21 years, although all other respective DSM criteria were met. The mean age at onset for MT was 7.51 years (range, 0–53; *SD*: 3.95) whereas that for PT was 9.76 years (range, 0–48; *SD*: 5.58). The mean age at diagnosis was 18.9 years (range, 4–72; *SD*: 12.72). Mean tic severity ratings (GSR) according to STSS were 2.79 when considering the entire sample (range, 1–6; *SD*: 1.17) and 2.83 within the TS group (range, 1–6; *SD*: 1.17). **Table 1** shows tic severity across the entire sample demonstrating that even in a tertiary referral center like ours, tic severity is very mild to moderate in almost three-quarter of patients. No significant relationship was found between age at onset of tics and tic severity as measured by the STSS [$F_{(5)} = 0.817$; n.s.]. **Table 2** shows percentages of the total sample developing tics at various age ranges.

TABLE 1 | Tic severity according to STSS-GSR (range, 1–6) across the sample (n = 1032).

STSS-GSR	Number (%)
1 = very mild	120 (12.0)
2 = mild	343 (34.3)
3 = medium	265 (26.5)
4 = marked	176 (17.6)
5 = severe	90 (9.0)
6 = very severe	5 (0.5)

STSS-GSR, Global Severity Rating of the Shapiro Tourette-Syndrome Severity Scale.

TABLE 2 | Age range at tic onset.

Age range [years]	Tic onset *N* (%)
<6	352 (34.1)
6–10	543 (52.6)
11–15	119 (11.6)
16–18	17 (1.6)
>18	1 (0.1)

N = number of cases.

Considering the three age groups (based on current age of the patient) according to age dependency of tic severity provided by Bloch et al. (2006), we found a significant positive association between mean tic severity and age groups [$F_{(2)} = 31.658$; $p < 0.001$]: age <10 years (n = 184): mean STSS-GSR = 2.33, age 10–12 years (n = 198): mean STSS-GSR = 2.52, and age >12 years (n = 650): mean STSS-GSR = 3.00. For the purpose of finding the age group where tics reach their worst severity, in addition, for the following age groups mean STSS-GSR were calculated and again demonstrated a significant positive relationship between STSS-GTS and age groups [$F_{(5)} = 12.688$; $p < 0.001$]: <6 years (n = 13): mean STSS-GSR = 2.31, 6–10 years (n = 251): mean STSS-GSR = 2.38, 11–15 years (n = 205): mean STSS-GSR = 2.66, 16–20 years (n = 141): mean STSS-GSR = 2.99, 21–25 years (n = 100): mean STSS-GSR = 3.02, >25 years (n = 322): mean STSS-GSR = 3.06.

In addition, mean tic severity (STSS-GSR) was found to be highly associated with the comorbidity score [$F_{(6)} = 19.945$; $p < 0.001$; **Table 3**]. Mean STSS-GTS was significantly lower in the "TS only" group (2.20) compared to the "TS + comorbidity" group [2.88, [$t_{(945)} = -4.937$; $p < 0.001$]]. Further, details regarding tic severity depending on the presence of one or more comorbidities are given in **Table 4**.

Coprophenomena, Echophenomena, Palilalia

With regards to specific complex tics ("full blown TS"), 290 patients (28.1%) reported coprophenomena, of which 247 (24%) reported coprolalia and 160 (15.5%) copropraxia, 290 patients (28.1%) claimed to have echolalia and 238 (23.1%) echopraxia, and 339 patients (33%) reported palilalia. Results showing associations between presence of various complex tics and tic severity are shown in **Table 5**.

In addition, we found a significant association between coprophenomena and comorbidity score (X^2 = 126.823;

TABLE 3 | Association between number of comorbidities (=comorbidity score) and mean tic severity*.

Number of comorbidities	*N*	Mean tic severity	*SD*	Std. Error	95% Confidence Interval for Mean	
					Lower bound	Upper bound
0	82	2.11	0.817	0.09	1.93	2.29
1	179	2.38	1.006	0.075	2.23	2.53
2	206	2.71	1.083	0.075	2.56	2.86
3	217	2.82	1.147	0.078	2.67	2.97
4	170	3.02	1.186	0.091	2.84	3.20
5	107	3.38	1.264	0.122	3.14	3.63
6	36	3.69	1.091	0.182	3.33	4.06

**comorbidity score including OCD, anxiety, depression, SIB, rage attacks, and ADHD, mean tic severity (according to SPSS-GSR; missing data: n = 35).*
OCD, obsessive-compulsive disorder; OCB, obsessive-compulsive behavior; ADHD, attention-deficit hyperactivity disorder; SIB, self-injurious behavior; STSS-GSR, Global Severity Rating of the Shapiro Tourette-Syndrome Severity Scale; N, number of cases; SD, standard deviation; Std., Standard.

TABLE 4 | Tic severity depending on the presence (±) of different comorbidities*.

Comorbidity		N	Mean tic severity	SD	Std. Error Mean	t-value	Significance
OCD†	+	97	3.15	1.143	0.038	3.266	$p < 0.001$
	−	901	2.74	1.307	0.133		
Anxiety	+	314	3.05	1.106	0.042	4.88	$p < 0.001$
	−	684	2.67	1.250	0.071		
Depression	+	228	3.15	1.130	0.041	5.453	$p < 0.001$
	−	771	2.68	1.218	0.081		
SIB	+	392	3.19	1.039	0.042	9.201	$p < 0.001$
	−	604	2.52	1.235	0.062		
Rage attacks	+	577	2.96	1.081	0.053	5.642	$p < 0.001$
	−	420	2.54	1.198	0.050		
ADHD†	+	449	2.92	1.174	0.050	3.256	$p < 0.001$
	−	550	2.68	1.146	0.054		
TS only		75	2.20	0.870	0.100	−4.937	$p < 0.001$
TS + comorbidities		872	2.88	1.172	0.04		
TS+OCD		45	3.07	1.388	0.209	2.434	$p < 0.05$
TS+ADHD		102	2.57	0.956	0.099		
TS+OCD/OCB/Anxiety/Depression/SIB		205	2.66	0.908	0.125	1.424	n.s.
TS+ADHD+rage attacks		53	2.42	1.155	0.081		

*comorbidities including OCD, anxiety, depression, SIB, rage attacks, and ADHD, mean tic severity according to SPSS-GSR (missing data: $n = 35$).

†groups include patients having other miscellaneous comorbidities and are therefore larger in number than the "TS+OCD" and "TS+ADHD" groups, which indicate a purer form of the stated comobidity.

OCD, obsessive-compulsive disorder; OCB, obsessive-compulsive behavior; ADHD, attention-deficit hyperactivity disorder; SIB, self-injurious behavior; STSS-GSR, Global Severity Rating of the Shapiro Tourette-Syndrome Severity Scale; N, number of cases; SD, standard deviation; Std., Standard.

TABLE 5 | Tic severity* depending on presence (±) of certain complex tics.

Complex tic		N	Mean STSS-GSR	SD	Std. error	t-value	Significance
Coprophenomena	+	278	3.36	1.255	0.075	−10.093	$p < 0.001$
	−	721	2.57	1.052	0.039		
Coprolalia	+	239	3.46	1.262	0.082	−10.742	$p < 0.001$
	−	757	2.58	1.050	0.038		
Copropraxia	+	154	3.49	1.280	0.103	−8.473	$p < 0.001$
	−	843	2.66	1.096	0.038		
Echolalia	+	280	3.21	1.220	0.073	−7.438	$p < 0.001$
	−	717	2.62	1.100	0.041		
Echopraxia	+	227	3.19	1.292	0.086	−6.101	$p < 0.001$
	−	770	2.67	1.098	0.040		
Palilalia	+	325	3.22	1.175	0.065	−8.406	$p < 0.001$
	−	670	2.58	1.104	0.043		

*according to STSS-GSR.

STSS-GSR, Global Severity Rating of the Shapiro Tourette-Syndrome Severity Scale; N, number of cases; SD, standard deviation; Std., Standard.

$p < 0.001$), echophenomena and comorbidity score ($X^2 = 76.14$; $p < 0.001$), and paliphenomena and comorbidity score ($X^2 = 87.38$; $p < 0.001$). Prevalence rates of coprophenomena demonstrated a significant association with age ($X^2 = 23.227$; $p < 0.001$): <10 years = 36 (19.6%), 10–12 years = 46 (23.2%), and >12 years = 208 (32%). There were also significant associations between age group and other complex tics such as echolalia ($X^2 = 7.736$; $p < 0.05$), echopraxia ($X^2 = 24.737$; $p < 0.001$), and palilalia ($X^2 = 7.111$; $p < 0.05$). In terms of individual comorbidities, coprophenomena were most highly associated with SIB ($X^2 = 60.302$; $p < 0.001$; with both coprolalia and copropraxia having similarly significant associations), followed by depression ($X^2 = 34.484$; $p < 0.001$), rage attacks ($X^2 = 33.800$; $p < 0.001$); ADHD ($X^2 = 30,856$; $p < 0.001$); anxiety ($X^2 = 27.122$; $p < 0.001$), OCD ($X^2 = 17.341$; $p < 0.001$), and lastly OCB ($X^2 = 13.551$; $p < 0.001$).

Premonitory Urges (PU) and Tic Suppressibility

Of the total sample of 1032 participants, 291 (29.4%) individuals did not report a PU [missing data, $n = 41$ (3.97%)]. Amongst the 700 (67.82%) patients who did report the experience of a PU, 446 (46%) participants experienced a localized PU, 113 (11.6%) a diffused PU, and for the remaining 141 (13.7%), although the PU was present, its precise nature was uncertain. With regards to tic suppression, 853 (85.4%) participants mentioned that they were able to suppress their tics whereas 146 (14.6%) claimed that they were unable to do so (missing data, $n = 33$).

In order to investigate age dependencies for both PU and suppressibility, we used different age ranges: on the one hand we used ranges based on the natural course of tics with the worst period between ages 10 and 12 (Bloch et al., 2006)—<10 years, 10–12 years, >12 years (**Table 6**)—and on the other hand age groups as suggested by Banaschewski et al. (2003): 8–10, 11–14,

15–19 years. In addition to the latter age ranges, we looked at PU and suppressibility in very young children (age <8 years) and adults (age >19 years) to further investigate age dependency and possible habituation (**Table 7**). Both classifications demonstrated clear age dependencies for PU as well as tic suppression. Patients who reported a PU suffered from significantly more severe tics compared to those without PU [mean STSS-GSR = 2.87 vs. 2.62, ($t = -3.164$; $p < 0.005$)]. In contrast, tic severity was not different in patients who were able to suppress their tics compared to those who were unable to do so [mean STSS-GSR = 2.83 vs. 2.63, ($t = -1.830$; n.s.)]. A significant positive association was found between PU and the ability to suppress tics ($X^2 = 96.691$; $p < 0.001$).

While no significant association was found between PU and OCD ($X^2 = 3.085$; n.s.), we found a highly significant ($X^2 = 15.379$; $p < 0.001$) positive association between PU and OCB. In particular, there was a strong direct association between PU and "not just right experiences" ($X^2 = 20.871$; $p < 0.001$). Certain other such significant positive associations were also found between PU and obsessions ($X^2 = 11.218$; $p < 0.01$), compulsions in general ($X^2 = 26.769$; $p < 0.01$), and various specific OC symptoms including counting ($X^2 = 15.571$; $p < 0.01$), checking ($X^2 = 18.897$; $p < 0.01$), ordering ($X^2 = 13.979$; $p < 0.01$), but not washing ($X^2 = 0.854$; n.s.). Tic suppression was found to have a significant and direct association with inattention ($X^2 = 6.056$; $p < 0.05$), rage attacks ($X^2 = 5.062$; $p < 0.05$), and hyperactivity ($X^2 = 4.838$; $p < 0.05$).

TABLE 6 | PU, tic suppression, comorbidity score, and tic severity* based on age ranges suggested by Bloch et al. (2006).

Age group (years; N)	PU reported (%)	Ability to suppress tics (%)	Mean comorbidity score (entire age group)	Mean tic severity (entire age group)
<10 (181)	46.7	65.5	2.35	2.33
10–12 (195)	61.3	78.8	2.21	2.52
>12 (623)	79.7	92.6	2.91	3

*according to STSS-GSR
PU, premonitory urge, STSS-GSR, Global Severity Rating of the Shapiro Tourette-Syndrome Severity Scale; N, numbers.

Comorbidities

Comorbidity Score

Across the entire sample, following were the percentages of different comorbidity scores: 84 patients (8.2%) had no comorbidity ("TS only"), 186 (18.1%) had one, 211 (20.5%) had two, 226 (22%) had three, 175 (17%) had four, 109 (10.6%) had five, and 36 (3.5%) had all six comorbidities as defined above (OCD, anxiety, depression, SIB, rage attacks, and ADHD; missing data: $n = 5$; see also **Table 3**). The mean comorbidity score was 2.67 (range, 0–6; $SD = 1.57$). A significant positive relationship was found between age groups and comorbidity score [$F_{(2)} = 20.579$; $p < 0.001$; **Tables 6, 7**]. Only 75 (7.67%) of the individuals from the "TS group" presented with "TS only." **Table 4** shows that in all those with a comorbidity score ≥1 (indicating the presence of any of the six comorbidities), the mean tic severity tended to be significantly higher than in those with no comorbidity. We also ran a test to compare the presence of comorbidities in patients based on the following age groups: <25, ≥25 and <50, and ≥50 years at the time of assessment. This was done to check for recall issues in describing comorbidities before and after a certain age. However, no significant differences were found between the various age groups.

OCD/OCB

Whilst only 103 (10%) patients of the sample had been clinically diagnosed with OCD according to DSM, 637 (61.8%) suffered from mild to moderate OCB without fulfilling diagnostic criteria for OCD. **Table 8** shows prevalence rates for different forms of OC symptoms amongst those with OCD and OCB. The most often reported OC symptom was a "not just right experience" [in 575 (55.9%) patients across the entire sample].

ADHD, Rage Attacks

Hyperactivity was reported by 291 (28.4%) participants, inattention by 405 (39.4%), and the diagnosis of ADHD according to DSM was made in 463 (44.9%) individuals. As expected, ADHD was significantly associated with hyperactivity ($X^2 = 499.818$; $p < 0.001$), inattention ($X^2 = 816.434$; $p < 0.001$), and rage attacks ($X^2 = 67.331$; $p < 0.01$). However, the association with rage attacks was comparatively much weaker than that with the other two variables. Of the 594 patients (57.8%) who were diagnosed with rage attacks, 261 (43.94%) did

TABLE 7 | PU, tic suppression, comorbidity score, and tic severity* compared to results provided by Banaschewski et al. (2003).

Age group years (N)	Presence of premonitory feeling		Ability to suppress tics		Mean comorbidity score (entire age group)	Mean tic severity (entire age group)
	Banaschewski et al. (%)	Current study (%)	Banaschewski et al. (%)	Current study (%)		
<8 (80)	–	34.8	–	56.5	2.23	2.34
8–10 (180)	34	61.8	48	75.1	2.36	2.39
11–14 (174)	56	61.8	66	82.8	2.35	2.66
15–19 (136)	68	76.6	79	90.6	2.62	2.92
>19 (429)	–	81.3	–	93.4	3.03	3.05

*according to STSS-GSR, comorbidity score including OCD, anxiety, depression, SIB, rage attacks, and ADHD.
PU, premonitory urge; STSS-GSR, Global Severity Rating of the Shapiro Tourette-Syndrome Severity Scale.

TABLE 8 | Prevalence rates of different forms of OC symptoms in TS patients with comorbid OCD compared to those with comorbid OCB.

OC Symptom	OCD (*N*; %)	OCB (*N*; %)	*Z*-score	Significance
Compulsions	101 (98.1)	603 (94.9)	1.41	n.s.
-Not just right experiences	87 (85.3)	467 (73.3)	2.38	n.s.
-Checking	77 (76.2)	279 (43.9)	5.02	$p < 0.001$
-Ordering	57 (55.9)	181 (28.4)	3.80	$p < 0.001$
-Washing	35 (34.7)	50 (7.8)	3.12	$p < 0.01$
-Counting	28 (27.7)	96 (15.1)	1.53	n.s.
Obsessions	92 (91.1)	262 (41.3)	8.25	$p < 0.001$

OC, obsessive-compulsive; OCD, obsessive-compulsive disorder; OCB, obsessive-compulsive behavior; TS, Tourette Syndrome; N, numbers; n.s., not significant.

not suffer from either hyperactivity or inattention, thus giving rise to the new and significant observation of the prevalence of rage attacks in Tourette patients, often even in the absence of ADHD.

Sleeping Problems

Sleeping problems (lifetime prevalence) were reported by 273 (26.7%) patients in the sample. Sleeping problems were found to have strong direct associations with depression ($X^2 = 24.548$; $p < 0.001$), followed by ADHD ($X^2 = 14.785$; $p < 0.001$), anxiety ($X^2 = 12.088$; $p < 0.005$), and OCD ($X^2 = 7.214$; $p < 0.001$). Its associations with tic severity ($X^2 = 5.097$; $p < 0.05$) and OCB were very weak ($X^2 = 4.879$; $p < 0.05$). Accordingly, sleeping problems were significantly more common in the "TS + comorbidity" group [$n = 256$ (28.7%)] compared to patients with TS only [$n = 4$ (5.3%); $Z = 4.3905$; $p < 0.01$]. There was also a significant positive association between the presence of sleeping problems and the comorbidity score ($X^2 = 53.569$; $p < 0.001$).

Anxiety

The clinical lifetime diagnosis of any kind of an anxiety disorder was made in 323 patients (31.4%). Prevalence rates for anxiety were significantly higher amongst those with TS+OCD (55.6%, $n = 45$) compared to those with TS+ADHD (16.8%, $n = 102$; $Z = 4.794$; $p < 0.01$; refer to **Table 4**).

Depression

The lifetime diagnosis of depression was made in 236 patients (22.9%). However, depression was found in 55.6% of the patients with TS+OCD, but only in 9.9% of the TS+ADHD group, resulting in a significant difference ($Z = 5.988$; $p < 0.01$; refer to **Table 4**). A significant positive association was also found between the prevalence of depression and anxiety ($X^2 = 69.083$; $p < 0.001$).

SIB

Lifetime prevalence of SIB was reported by 405 (39.4%) patients. SIB was found to have a significant positive associations with the presence of complex motor tics ($X^2 = 57.551$; $p < 0.01$), OCB ($X^2 = 32.026$; $p < 0.01$), and anxiety ($X^2 = 31.634$; $p < 0.01$), in a descending order of the strength of the association (refer to **Table 4**). For association with coprophenomena, see above.

Sub-Classification of TS

For the purpose of further exploring Robertson and Cavanna's (2007) sub-classification of TS and common comorbidities, the three clusters provided by them were examined for expected differences in certain variables: (i) cluster 1, which consists of only tics ("TS only"; $n = 75$), (ii) cluster 2, which consists of TS and comorbid ADHD and rage attacks ($n = 56$), and (iii) cluster 3, which consists of TS and comorbid OCD, OCB, anxiety, depression, and SIB ($n = 209$). Since we included only those patients in clusters 2 and 3 who had all of the aforementioned comorbidities (e.g., cluster 2 consisted of TS patients with both comorbid ADHD and rage attacks, and not just one of the two), only one-third of the total number of patients could be classified using Robertson and Cavanna's (2007) sub-classification criteria. The rate of copropraxia in cluster 2 was 16.1 vs. 4.8% in cluster 3 and 2.7% in cluster 1, the difference between cluster 2 and cluster 3 being significant in the direction of the hypothesis ($X^2 = 25.887$; $p < 0.001$). The ability for tic suppression in the "TS only" group was 91.7%, and was significantly higher than that in cluster 2 (78.2%) ($Z = 2.1983$; $p < 0.05$), but not significantly different from that in cluster 3 (89.7%) ($Z = 0.5004$; n.s.). The percentage of patients reporting PU based on the different clusters was the following: cluster 1 ("TS only"): 57.7%, cluster 2: 62.3%, and cluster 3: 75.1%. PU reported in cluster 3 was significantly higher than that reported in cluster 1 ($Z = 2.835$; $p < 0.001$) but was not significantly higher than PU reported in cluster 2 ($Z = 1.9029$; n.s.).

Gender Differences

The male-to-female ratio in the current TS group is 3.4:1. **Table 9** shows results of gender-based comparisons of TS-related phenomena from data obtained from all patients in the sample demonstrating that males suffer more often from coprolalia, copropraxia, palilalia, OCB, hyperactivity, and inattention. They are also more likely to experience PU. Females, on the other hand, are more likely than males to suffer from sleeping problems. No significant gender differences were found with regards to age at onset of both tic types in general, [$t_{(963)} = 0.022$; n.s.], MT [$t_{(542)} = -1.216$; n.s.], and PT [$t_{(951)} = 1.489$; n.s.]. No significant relationship was found between comorbidity score and gender [$t_{(1025)} = 1.398$; n.s.].

DISCUSSION

In this study, we report clinical information collected from a large sample of 1032 patients with different forms of primary tic disorder. As two of the primary objectives of this study were the exploration of the TS spectrum and the verification of the accuracy of the sub-group classifications propounded by other researchers, we concentrated on TS in association to its various comorbidities.

Age at Onset and Tic Severity

The mean age at onset of tics in general, and MT and PT in particular, were all found to be consistent with findings of other studies (Freeman et al., 2000), but somewhat above the data in TS literature. This could be because there was a high number of adult participants in our study and since such data are always

TABLE 9 | Gender differences in various TS-related aspects.

	Males *n* (%)	Mean STSS-GSR	Females *n* (%)	Mean STSS-GSR	*Z*-Score	*p*-value	Significance	Dominant Gender
Coprophenomena	242 (30.4)	3.4	48 (20.3)	3.35	3.0205	0.002	$p < 0.01$	m > f
-Coprolalia	205 (25.9)	3.48	42 (17.8)	3.36	2.5161	0.01	$p < 0.05$	m > f
-Copropraxia	141 (17.8)	3.45	19 (8.1)	3.83	3.6019	0.0003	$p < 0.01$	m > f
Palilalia	278 (35.1)	3.19	68 (25.8)	3.35	1.7465	0.08	$p < 0.01$	m > f
Echolalia	231 (29.1)	3.22	59 (25)	3.18	1.2067	0.22	n.s.	–
Echopraxia	183 (23.1)	3.19	55 (23.3)	3.22	−0.1009	0.92	n.s.	–
OCD	72 (9.1)	3.04	31 (13.1)	3.41	−1.8411	0.06	n.s.	–
OCB	509 (64)	2.91	128 (54.2)	2.94	2.6946	0.007	$p < 0.01$	m > f
Compulsions	552 (69.7)	2.83	153 (65.1)	2.97	1.3097	0.19	n.s.	–
-Non Just Right Experiences	446 (56.2)	2.94	129 (54.7)	2.06	0.3719	0.71	n.s.	–
-Ordering	185 (23.3)	3.18	53 (22.5)	3.17	0.251	0.80	n.s.	–
-Checking	281 (35.5)	3.08	81 (34.3)	3.14	0.2769	0.77	n.s.	–
-Counting	97 (12.3)	3.03	28 (11.9)	3.41	0.133	0.89	n.s.	–
-Washing	66 (8.3)	2.72	20 (8.5)	3.05	−0.0894	0.92	n.s.	–
Obsessions	273 (34.6)	3.02	84 (35.7)	2.93	−0.3115	0.75	n.s.	–
Hyperactivity	294 (31.4)	2.97	42 (17.9)	2.97	5.51	<0.0000	$p < 0.01$	m > f
Inattention	337 (42.4)	2.9	68 (29.1)	3.03	3.5378	0.0004	$p < 0.01$	m > f
ADHD	387 (48.6)	2.92	76 (32.2)	2.92	4.4449	<0.0000	$p < 0.01$	m > f
Sleeping problems	198 (25.1)	2.97	75 (32.1)	3.11	−2.1122	0.03	$p < 0.05$	f > m
Anxiety	246 (31)	3.06	7 (32.8)	3.03	−0.5012	0.60	n.s.	–
Depression	177 (22.3)	3.1	59 (25)	3.32	−0.8879	0.37	n.s.	–
Rage attacks	460 (58)	2.93	134 (57)	3.07	0.2755	0.77	n.s.	–
SIB	310 (38.9)	3.2	97 (41.1)	3.15	−0.5955	0.54	n.s.	–
Severity of Tics* (severe)	67 (8.7)	–	28 (12.2)	–	−1.6104	0.10	n.s.	–
Premonitory urges	551 (72.3)	2.85	149 (65.1)	2.99	2.133	0.03	$p < 0.05$	m > f
Tic suppression	655 (85.2)	2.82	198 (86.1)	2.85	−0.3439	0.72	n.s.	–

**according to STSS-GSR, severe, 5; very severe, 6 (range, 0–6).*
OCD, obsessive-compulsive disorder; OCB, obsessive-compulsive behavior; ADHD, attention-deficit hyperactivity disorder; SIB, self-injurious behavior; TS, Tourette Syndrome; STSS-GSR, Global Severity Rating of the Shapiro Tourette-Syndrome Severity Scale; n.s., not significant.

based on patient reports and memory, it is possible that there was a recollection bias toward slightly greater age at onset, because tic onset goes back many years, and thus could not be dated precisely.

We found no association between tic severity and age at onset, which is contradictory to previous research (Khalifa and von Knorring, 2005). To the best of our knowledge, there is almost no data available investigating specifically the association between age at tic onset and tic severity, although this is an important clinical question that is often asked by parents of affected children. From our results, it is strongly—and for the first time—suggested that there is no such association, although one could easily expect this. This finding is in line with results of the large clinical database by Freeman et al. (2000): although not specifically mentioned, it can be concluded that in this dataset there was also no association between age at tic onset and tic severity, since they found no difference with respect to age at tic onset depending on the presence of comorbidities (but more severe tics in patients with comorbidities compared to those without). When looking at the data by Khalifa and von Knorring (2005) in more detail, the suggested correlation between tic severity and age at onset appears questionable, since this was found only in the very small group of patients with TS ($n = 25$), but not in the larger group diagnosed with chronic motor/vocal tics ($n = 58$).

We also found that for a majority of the participants in our study, tic onset was much earlier than the age of 18 (refer to **Table 2**). This is consistent with Freeman et al.'s (2000) finding, where in 92.7% of the sample, tic onset was before 10 years of age, and in 99% of the sample, it was before 16 years. Thus, data from these two large datasets clearly confirm that the "18-year maximum age of onset criterion" used in DSM-5 is well-founded and should be maintained. In our sample, the median for tic severity was found to be mild to moderate (median STSS-GSR = 3; 25th percentile = 2, 75th percentile = 4), which demonstrates how rare extremely severe TS is, since even in a highly specialized outpatient unit such as our center, 904 (87.6%) patients had mild to moderate tics and only 95 (9.2%) had severe or very severe tics. Our data do not demonstrate the well-known age dependency of tic severity, but a continuous tic increase with increasing age. However, this should be interpreted as a bias stemming from the fact that this was a cross-sectional and not a longitudinal study, tic assessment was done only once during the first medical examination, and patients tend to come to the clinic when their tics get worse and usually not when their tics reduce. At our center several patients present for the first only at adult age (with or without having received the correct diagnosis of TS before). It can be assumed that the majority of these patients belong to the small group of those patients who suffer not only from persistent tics, but also from more severe tics. This selection bias may be the reason why we failed to demonstrate the well-known age dependency of tics.

Completely in line with available data (Freeman et al., 2000), tic severity was positively related to the comorbidity score in that greater the number of comorbidities, higher the tic severity, and also that those with one or more comorbidities had significantly more severe tics than those without comorbid disorders. Comorbid SIB was found to have the highest impact on tic severity, followed by rage attacks, depression, anxiety, OCD, and lastly, ADHD. In line with our hypothesis and TS literature (Lebowitz et al., 2012), we also found that tic severity was significantly greater in those with comorbid OCD but no ADHD than in those with comorbid ADHD but no OCB/OCD. These findings further corroborate the hypothesis that TS plus OCD is a more severe form of TS, that OCB/OCD is part of the TS spectrum, and that ADHD should be better conceptualized as a separate problem (Trillini and Müller-Vahl, 2015).

Coprophenomena, Echophenomena, and Paliphenomena

The prevalence rates of both coprolalia and copropraxia were higher as compared to the percentages reported in Freeman et al.'s study on coprophenomena, where the rate of coprolalia ever was 18.5% and that of copropraxia was 5.7% (Freeman et al., 2009), but were lower than those reported by Cavanna et al. (2011), in which coprolalia and copropraxia were reported by 30.4 and 21.1% of the sample, respectively. The relatively high prevalence rates reported in our study are possible due to the fact that ours is a highly specialized clinic, where mostly patients with several complex tics are referred. In addition, almost half of our sample comprised adult patients. This might be another reason for the higher prevalence rates of coprophenomena in our sample, since the prevalence of coprophenomena increases with age. Finally, all patients were specifically asked for the presence of copro-, echo-, and paliphenomena.

The presence of all, coprophenomena, echophenomena, and paliphenomena were associated with both tic severity and the number of comorbidities, corroborating the hypothesis that "full blown TS" is a more severe form of TS as suggested by Robertson and Baron-Cohen (1998).

We also found that for both copro- and echophenomena, the prevalence of the respective PT form (i.e. copro- and echolalia) was higher than their corresponding MT form (copro- and echopraxia). This is well-known (Freeman et al., 2000, 2009) and suggests that copro- and echophenomena are, in a way, different from simple tics, in which the frequency is vice-versa (MT > PT). Assuming that tics present "fragments of innate behavioral routines" as suggested recently (Leckman et al., 2013), it can be speculated that copro-/echolalia are more common than copro-/echopraxia, because swearing and repeating noises (such as coughing) is nearer to "normal behavior" than performing obscene gestures and the repetition of movements. However, and in contrast, excessive brief movements such as eye blinking and grimacing are "nearer to normal" than excessive fast and meaningless noises.

In agreement with results from Freeman et al.'s database (2009), we found that both coprolalia and copropraxia were most highly associated with SIB, while associations with other comorbidities were much weaker. The strong association of coprophenomena with SIB, along with the equally high association between SIB and complex motor tics suggests that SIB in TS belongs to the coprophenomena spectrum and is a complex tic rather than an OC symptom, as has previously been suggested (Mathews et al., 2004). However, Mathews et al. (2004) found a correlation between OC symptoms and "mild SIB," while "severe SIB" correlated with tic severity and, therefore, they suggested the presence of two distinct forms of SIB. In this study, no distinction was made with respect to severity in a mild form (including hand banging, compulsive skin picking, self-hitting, and lip biting) and a severe form with serious injuries. In line with Mathews et al.'s results (2004), we found no strong association between SIB and rage attacks. Our finding that SIB had a higher impact on tic severity than all other comorbidities (rage attacks, depression, anxiety, OCD, and ADHD), in addition with the well-known correlation between coprophenomena and tic severity (Freeman et al., 2009), further suggests that SIB is a specific form of a complex tic rather than an OC symptom. Our findings may have important implications for the clinical management of SIB and suggest the use of both behavioral therapy and antipsychotics instead of serotonin reuptake inhibitors.

Prevalence rates of echolalia and echopraxia were found to be lower than the rates reported by Eapen et al. in their 2004 paper (echolalia: 37.4%, $n = 34$; echopraxia: 29.9%, $n = 27$) as well as those reported by Cavanna et al. (2011) [echolalia: 40.3%; echopraxia: 36.9%; (numbers not provided)], but higher compared to other samples: echolalia: 16% ($n = 32$; Cardoso et al., 1996) and echolalia: 21% and echopraxia: 18% ($n = 71$; Neal and Cavanna, 2013). In our sample, the prevalence rate for palilalia was found to be similar to that in Eapen et al.'s (2004) sample (29.7%) as well as to Cavanna et al.'s (2011) sample (31.7%). These differences may be due to the fact that the prevalence rate for echophenomena and palilalia in any study depends on whether the examiner asks the patient for relevant symptoms, or only records what (s)he observes in the patient. Furthermore, the way in which these questions are framed by the examiner may also affect the prevalence rate. In the case of echophenomena, the examiner in the present study specifically asked all patients "when you see movements and hear noises from other people—independent of whether these are tics or normal movements, or noises like coughing, or even noises from animals or machines—have you ever felt that you had to imitate this?" Only when the patient responded in the affirmative and said that (s)he had acted accordingly was (s)he recorded as positive for the echophenomenon. In any case, our data confirm the assumption that echophenomena are a core symptom of TS (Ganos et al., 2012).

Premonitory Urges and Tic Suppression

Banaschewski et al. (2003) conducted a study to determine if there is any age dependency of the presence of PU as well as of tic suppression (refer to **Table 7**). In our study, we aimed to replicate these findings. Our results were mixed in terms of support for Banaschewski et al.'s findings. In general, PU and tic suppression showed a clear age dependency. Secondly, although PU and the ability to suppress tics were strongly associated, in each age group, the percentage of patients who were capable of tic suppression was greater than the percentage of those who experienced a PU, indicating that tic suppression is possible without necessarily being aware of a PU. However, there were also some relevant differences between our results and those of Banaschewski et al. Firstly, our results did not show "jumps" for the development of either PUs or the ability to suppress tics, unlike Banaschewski et al.'s findings, which suggested that children develop the ability for tic suppression at around the age of 10 years, and for PU around age 14. Secondly and most important, the percentages of those patients who experience a PU as well as those who could suppress their tics were much higher at each age group compared to Banaschewski et al.'s study. We found that both PU and tic suppressing ability is already present in a high number of TS patients before the age of 8 (refer to **Table 7**)—much earlier than previously thought. This indicates that PU and suppression exist right from the beginning, and do not develop during the course of TS. From our data, therefore, it is suggested that the only reason that PU and tic suppression cannot be seen in (very) young children is because they are unable to either introspect or express them well-enough. This has important implications with respect to the treatment with habit reversal training and is in line with efficacy of this treatment even in younger children as was demonstrated by Piacentini et al. (2010).

On considering the age dependency based on the natural history as described by Bloch et al. (2006), we found high percentages of those who experienced PU and had the ability to suppress tics at every age category. Here too, we observed a clear age dependency, with a consistent increase of around 12–20% at every successive age category.

Finally, our results also show that the higher the tic severity, the more likely it is that the patient experiences a PU. However, no such association was observed between tic severity and tic suppression ability. With respect to Robertson and Cavanna's (2007) classification, we found that patients in cluster 3 (comorbid OCD/anxiety/depression/SIB) were almost equally able to suppress their tics compared to those in cluster 1 ("TS only"). However, a significant difference exists in tic suppression between patients with TS only and patients in cluster 2 (comorbid ADHD/rage attacks). This suggests that tic suppression is independent from comorbid OCD/anxiety/depression/SIB, but patients who suffer from ADHD are less able to suppress their tics. Results also showed that PU was higher in the "TS + comorbidity" group than in the "TS only" group, which is supported by past findings (Eddy and Cavanna, 2013). Particularly, it was highest in cluster 3 (including patients with OCD/OCB/SIB/anxiety/depression), followed by cluster 2 (including patients with ADHD/rage attacks) and finally by the group of patients having no comorbidities (cluster 1, "TS only"). This too is in line with Eddy and Cavanna's (2013) finding that comorbidities such as anxiety, OCD, and ADHD are strongly correlated with PU. Finally, our results also showed a strong positive association between PU and "not just right experiences" (and to a relatively lesser degree with OCB, but not OCD), which indicates that PU may be a form of this specific and very common form of OCB in TS. This further corroborates the hypothesis that "not just right experiences" are intrinsic to the phenomenology of TS (Neal and Cavanna, 2013).

Influence of Comorbidities

The fact that only a small percentage of the TS sub-group had not reported or were diagnosed with any comorbidity is consistent with relevant literature (Freeman et al., 2000; Khalifa and von Knorring, 2006; Cavanna et al., 2011; Robertson et al., 2015). However, relative to the total TS population, this could be a bias arising out of the method of data collection; the sample is a clinical one and mostly, only patients with more severe tics and more comorbidities come for a referral. This could be because the quality of one's life is impaired by common comorbidities of TS far more than the tics themselves, as has been consistently demonstrated in past literature (Pringsheim et al., 2009; Müller-Vahl et al., 2010; Jalenques et al., 2012). Research has shown that quality of life (Eddy et al., 2012) and psychosocial health (Pringsheim et al., 2009) was most adversely affected on all domains in those TS patients suffering from both comorbid OCD and comorbid ADHD, whereas having only one of the two comorbidities causes domain-specific impairment. Rizzo et al. (2014) found a significantly lower quality of life among those patients having TS+OCD/TS+ADHD/TS+OCD+ADHD as compared to patients with pure TS. Studies have also found comorbid depression to be one of the most significant independent factors impairing the quality of life of TS patients (Müller-Vahl et al., 2010; Jalenques et al., 2012).

In our sample, rage attacks were found to be the most common comorbidity followed by ADHD. In contrast to this, Freeman et al. (2000) found ADHD (60%) to be the most highly occurring comorbidity. With respect to anxiety, depression, and SIB, the sample in the current study showed much higher prevalence rates compared to Freeman et al.'s sample, where 18, 12.1, and 14% had anxiety, depression, and SIB respectively. All these differences in prevalence rates of different comorbidities can probably be best explained by age differences between our sample and Freeman et al.'s sample (mean age = 18.9 vs. 13.2 years), as the older the patients, the more likely it is that they have comorbidities such as depression and sleeping problems and the younger they are, the more likely it is that they have ADHD. The prevalence rate of depression was also much higher than the 6.0% found by Khalifa and von Knorring (2006), but this could be because their sample consisted only of school children in the 7–15 years age range. Our results, however, were very similar to the 27.8% reported by Robertson et al. (2006). Cavanna et al. (2009), in their review of the literature on the phenotype of TS stated that among the 5295 patients with TS who presented at specialist clinics, the prevalence rate of depressive symptomatology was found to range from 13 to 76%.

With respect to OC symptoms, we found a lower prevalence rate for OCD compared to the Freeman et al.'s (2000) sample in their 2000 paper (27%). This might be explained by the fact that the evaluator (KMV) was extremely particular whilst diagnosing OCD and often made the diagnosis of OCB, unless all symptoms matched the prerequisites. However, the by far most often reported OC symptom in both groups OCD and OCB was a "non-just right experience" (refer to **Table 8**), which corroborates recent findings suggesting that "not just right experiences" are intrinsic to the clinical phenomenology of TS (Neal and Cavanna, 2013). As described above, in this context again it is worth mentioning that from our findings it is suggested that premonitory urges (PU) prior to the occurrence of tics may also be a form of a "non-just right experience." In addition, we found that among those who had either OCD or OCB in our sample, compulsions such as checking and ordering were much higher, whereas those of counting and washing tended to be lower. This is in line with past research in TS related OCD/OCB (Worbe et al., 2010). According to Stewart et al. (2008), there are four factors for OCD: factor 1 (aggressive/sexual/religious/somatic/checking); factor 2 (symmetry/ordering/counting/repeating); factor 3 (contamination/cleaning), and factor 4 (hoarding). Of these, only factor 2 was found to be common in TS, which further supports the hypothesis that OCD/OCB in TS is different form pure OCD.

We found that almost half the total number of patients diagnosed with rage attacks did not have either hyperactivity or inattention, which is consistent with the finding that rage attacks, as compared to hyperactivity and inattention, is highly common and represents one symptom of the typical spectrum of disinhibited behaviors in TS that occurs in a substantial number of patients independently from the presence of ADHD (Frank et al., 2011). The assumption that rage attacks in TS are slightly separate from and independent of the ADHD spectrum is further supported by our finding that in our sample both inattention and hyperactivity, but not rage attacks were more common in males than in females.

Sleeping problems among the patients in our sample were very common, and were found to be about five times as common in the "TS + comorbidity" group as compared to the "TS only" group. Such problems were most highly associated with depression, indicating the well-stated finding that in TS depression has a strong adverse effect on the patients' quality of life (Müller-Vahl et al., 2010; Eddy et al., 2011; Jalenques et al., 2012). Other comorbidities (such as ADHD, anxiety, and OCD, in a descending order of the strength of the association) as well as tics (with lesser strength of association) may also have an impact, but these associations were found to be much weaker in comparison to depression. The strong association between sleeping problems and depression has important clinical implication: TS patients suffering from sleeping problems should be screened for depression and, if necessary, treated for this disorder. We found sleeping problems in the comorbid group as twice as common in the comorbid group studied by Freeman et al. (2000). This can be explained by the age difference between both samples with more children in the Freeman et al.'s group and the strong association with depression. Significantly higher prevalence rates of both anxiety and depression in the TS+OCD group as compared to the TS+ADHD group are in line with previous research findings (Lebowitz et al., 2012; Trillini and Müller-Vahl, 2015) and also provide support to our hypothesis that TS is more closely related with OCD, anxiety, and depression as compared to ADHD.

Influence of Gender

The male-to-female ratio in our sample was 3.4:1 and therefore comparable to several other studies (Erenberg et al., 1986; Freeman et al., 2000). In addition, results showed significant predominance of males over females with respect to coprophenomena (coprolalia, copropraxia, and overall), OCB, hyperactivity, inattention, ADHD, and PU. A significantly greater percentage of females in the sample had sleeping problems. In contrast to our findings, past research in non-TS samples has consistently shown twofold higher prevalence of anxiety and depression in females over males (Bijl et al., 2002). In agreement with recent studies in larger samples in both children (Robertson et al., 2006) and mixed groups (Freeman et al., 2000), we did not find gender differences with respect to anxiety and depression. In contrast, in a recent internet-based survey (n = 460 adults) women reported more often about both depressive symptoms and non-OCD anxiety disorders (35.6 and 33.7%, respectively) compared to men (23.2 and 15.5%, respectively; Lewin et al., 2012). However, these results should be interpreted with caution not only due to the well-known limitations related to such a study design, but also other findings (e.g., insignificantly higher prevalence rate for self-reported ADHD in female compared to male). Thus, our results as well as past research (Freeman et al., 2000; Robertson et al., 2006) suggest that the nature of both depression and anxiety disorders in patients with TS differs from that found in the general population. These disorders are a part of the TS spectrum and are not only secondary due to tics and an impaired quality of life. This, in addition, also supports the assumption that the TS subgroup with comorbid OCD, anxiety, and depression represents a more severe form of the disease.

We found no gender differences in the prevalence of rage attacks. Since there is a general predominance of males over females with respect to the prevalence of ADHD in ADHD-only samples (Kessler et al., 2006), TS+ADHD samples (Freeman et al., 2000), as well as in the current study sample, our finding of similar prevalence rates of rage attacks for both genders is in line with relevant literature (Frank et al., 2011) which shows that in TS, rage attacks are independent and separate from ADHD.

Limitations

Our study has some noticeable limitations. Primarily, there was an absence of a standardized assessment procedure and diagnoses were made based on judgments of a single expert clinician, thereby increasing the likelihood of errors caused by various biases in evaluation. However, KMV is a highly trained expert in both neurology and psychiatry and thus had a rich experience in diagnosing movement disorders from the very start of her career. Since most studies are carried out by clinicians with less expertise in diagnosing TS, we do not see this is being any major disadvantage of our study. Another limitation is a lack of temporal stability, since data was collected over almost two decades and the diagnoses were made based on the version of the DSM valid at that time. It should be noted though, that the core criteria of tic disorders did not change over time, therefore this should not be too much of a concern. The cross-sectional nature of our data also makes it difficult to learn about the temporal progression of tic severity. Lastly, the possible effects of various medications on tic suppression were not controlled for. It can be assumed that using medication would improve one's ability to suppress tics, and therefore we cannot dismiss the idea that its use by some of the patients influenced our results. However, to the best of our knowledge, there is no study that looks particularly into such an influence.

CONCLUSION

We believe that this study is the first single-site study on TS and TS-related phenomena involving such a large sample. For the first time, our results suggest that an early age of tic onset is not necessarily associated with higher tic severity at subsequent ages.

Secondly, it has revealed that PU and tic suppression are factors that are present from earlier than previously assumed in past literature (Banaschewski et al., 2003). Both phenomena seem to emerge in parallel to the tics rather than later in the course of the disorder. Therefore, our data corroborate more recent findings suggesting that PU is not a prerequisite for tic suppression.

Thirdly, our data suggests that PU could represent of specific type of OCB and in particular a "not just right experience."

Fourthly, our data suggest that SIB belongs to the coprophenomena spectrum and hence should be conceptualized as a complex tic rather than a compulsion. This has important implications for the treatment of severe SIB.

Fifthly, our results suggest that both depression and anxiety disorders in patients with TS differ from their presentation in non-TS samples. Sleeping problems are common in (adult) patients with TS and are most often caused by comorbid depression. Therefore, patients with TS reporting about sleeping problems should be screened for comorbid depression.

Sixthly, rage attacks represent a typical symptom of disinhibited behaviors in patients with TS. For clinicians it is important to classify rage attacks as a manifestation of the disease that often occur even in the absence of comorbid ADHD.

Seventhly, patients with TS and comorbid ADHD are less able to suppress their tics when compared with those without attention deficits.

Finally, our data demonstrate that TS+OCD is a more severe form of the disease. Furthermore, our clinical data adds to other clinical observations that subjects with ADHD may not be able to suppress tics as well as those without ADHD. Synthesizing all our data, we find support for the hypothesis that comorbid OCD/OCB, depression, and anxiety belong to the TS spectrum, while ADHD needs to be considered an independent diagnosis.

AUTHOR CONTRIBUTIONS

TS engaged mainly data analysis, data interpretation, writing of the manuscript. EJ provided advice on statistical analysis, and participated in manuscript preparation. KM managed data collection, formulated the study design, supervised data analysis and manuscript preparation.

ACKNOWLEDGMENTS

We wish to thank Lars Makowski, Sarah Bottor, and Anna-Sophie Ellinghausen for helping us build up the extensive database used in our study. Special thanks also to all the participants for their effort.

REFERENCES

American Psychiatric Association (2013). *Diagnostic and statistical manual of mental disorders 5th Edn.* Washington, DC.

Banaschewski, T., Woerner, W., and Rothenberger, A. (2003). Premonitory sensory phenomena and suppressibility of tics in Tourette syndrome: developmental aspects in children and adolescents. *Dev. Med. Child Neurol.* 45, 700–703. doi: 10.1017/s0012162203001294

Bijl, R. V., De Graaf, R., Ravelli, A., Smit, F., and Vollebergh, W. A. (2002). Gender and age-specific first incidence of DSM-III-R psychiatric disorders in the general population. *Soc. psychiatry psychiatr. Epidemiol.* 37, 372–379. doi: 10.1007/s00127-002-0566-3

Bloch, M. H., Peterson, B. S., Scahill, L., Otka, J., Katsovich, L., Zhang, H., et al. (2006). Adulthood outcome of tic and obsessive-compulsive symptom severity in children with Tourette syndrome. *Arch.Pediatr. Adolesc. Med.* 160, 65–69. doi: 10.1001/archpedi.160.1.65

Cardoso, F., Veado, C. C., and de Oliveira, J. T. (1996). A Brazilian cohort of patients with Tourette's syndrome. *J. Neurol. Neurosurg. Psychiatry* 60, 209–212. doi: 10.1136/jnnp.60.2.209

Cavanna, A. E., Critchley, H. D., Orth, M., Stern, J. S., Young, M. B., and Robertson, M. M. (2011). Dissecting the Gilles de la Tourette spectrum: a factor analytic study on 639 patients. *J. Neurol. Neurosurg. Psychiatry* 82, 1320–1323. doi: 10.1136/jnnp.2010.225029

Cavanna, A. E., Servo, S., Monaco, F., and Robertson, M. M. (2009). The behavioral spectrum of Gilles de la Tourette syndrome. *J. Neuropsychiatry Clin. Neurosci.* 21, 13–23. doi: 10.1176/jnp.2009.21.1.13

Cubo, E., Gabriely Galán, J. M., Villaverde, V. A., Velasco, S. S., Benito, V. D., Macarrón, J. V., et al. (2011). Prevalence of tics in schoolchildren in central Spain: a population-based study. *Pediatr. Neurol.* 45, 100–108. doi: 10.1016/j.pediatrneurol.2011.03.003

Eapen, V., Fox-Hiley, P., Banerjee, S., and Robertson, M. (2004). Clinical features and associated psychopathology in a Tourette syndrome cohort. *Acta Neurol. Scand.* 109, 255–260. doi: 10.1046/j.1600-0404.2003.00228.x

Eddy, C. M., and Cavanna, A. E. (2013). Premonitory urges in adults with complicated and uncomplicated Tourette syndrome. *Behav. Modif.* 8, 264–275. doi: 10.1177/0145445513504432

Eddy, C. M., Cavanna, A. E., Gulisano, M., Agodi, A., Barchitta, M., Calì, P., et al. (2011). Clinical correlates of quality of life in Tourette syndrome. *Mov. Disord.* 26, 735–738. doi: 10.1002/mds.23434

Eddy, C. M., Cavanna, A. E., Gulisano, M., Calì, P., Robertson, M. M., and Rizzo, R. (2012). The effects of comorbid obsessive-compulsive disorder and attention-deficit hyperactivity disorder on quality of life in tourette syndrome. *J. Neuropsychiatry Clin. Neurosci.* 24, 458–462. doi: 10.1176/appi.neuropsych.11080181

Erenberg, G., Cruse, R. P., and Rothner, A. D. (1986). Tourette syndrome: an analysis of 200 pediatric and adolescent cases. *Cleve Clin. Q.* 53, 127–131. doi: 10.3949/ccjm.53.2.127

Frank, M. C., Piedad, J., Rickards, H., and Cavanna, A. E. (2011). The role of impulse control disorders in Tourette syndrome: an exploratory study. *J. Neurol. Sci.* 310, 276–278. doi: 10.1016/j.jns.2011.06.032

Freeman, R. D., Fast, D. K., Burd, L., Kerbeshian, J., Robertson, M. M., and Sandor, P. (2000). An international perspective on Tourette syndrome: selected findings from 3500 individuals in 22 countries. *Develop. Med. Child Neurol.* 42, 436–447. doi: 10.1017/S0012162200000839

Freeman, R. D., Zinner, S. H., Müller-Vahl, K. R., Fast, D. K., Burd, L. J., Kano, Y., et al. (2009). Coprophenomena in Tourette syndrome. *Develop. Med. Child Neurol.* 51, 218–227. doi: 10.1111/j.1469-8749.2008.03135.x

Ganos, C., Ogrzal, T., Schnitzler, A., and Münchau, A. (2012). The pathophysiology of echopraxia/echolalia: relevance to Gilles de la Tourette syndrome. *Mov. Disord.* 27, 1222–1229. doi: 10.1002/mds.25103

Hirschtritt, M. E., Lee, P. C., Pauls, D. L., Dion, Y., Grados, M. A., Illmann, C., et al. (2015). Lifetime prevalence, age of risk, and genetic relationships of comorbid psychiatric disorders in Tourette syndrome. *JAMA Psychiatry* 72, 325–333. doi: 10.1001/jamapsychiatry.2014.2650

Jalenques, I., Galland, F., Malet, L., Morand, D., Legrand, G., Auclair, C., et al. (2012). Quality of life in adults with Gilles de la Tourette Syndrome. *BMC psychiatry* 12:109. doi: 10.1186/1471-244X-12-109

Kessler, R. C., Adler, L., Barkley, R., Biederman, J., Conners, C. K., Demler, O., et al. (2006). The prevalence and correlates of adult ADHD in the United States: results from the National Comorbidity Survey Replication. *Am. J. Psychiatry* 163, 716–723. doi: 10.1176/ajp.2006.163.4.716

Khalifa, N., and von Knorring, A. L. (2005). Tourette syndrome and other tic disorders in a total population of children: clinical assessment and background. *Acta Paediatr.* 94, 1608–1614. doi: 10.1111/j.1651-2227.2005.tb01837.x

Khalifa, N., and von Knorring, A. L. (2006). Psychopathology in a Swedish population of school children with tic disorders. *J. Am. Acad. Child Adolesc. Psychiatry* 45, 1346–1353. doi: 10.1097/01.chi.0000251210.98749.83

Lebowitz, E. R., Motlagh, M. G., Katsovich, L., King, R. A., Lombroso, P. J., Grantz, H., et al. (2012). Tourette syndrome in youth with and without obsessive compulsive disorder and attention deficit hyperactivity disorder. *Eur. Child Adolesc. Psychiatry* 21, 451–457. doi: 10.1007/s00787-012-0278-5

Leckman, J. F., Bloch, M. H., Sukhodolsky, D. G., Scahill, L., and King, R. A. (2013). "Phenomenology of tics and sensory urges: the self under siege," in *Tourette Syndrome*, ed D. Martino (New York, NY: Oxford University Press), 3–25.

Leckman, J. F., Walker, D. E., and Cohen, D. J. (1993). Premonitory urges in Tourette's syndrome. *Am. J. Psychiatry* 150, 98–102. doi: 10.1176/ajp.150.1.98

Leckman, J. F., Zhang, H., Vitale, A., Lahnin, F., and Lynch, K., Bondi, C., et al. (1998). Course of tic severity in Tourette syndrome: the first two decades. *Pediatrics* 102, 14–19. doi: 10.1542/peds.102.1.14

Lewin, A. B., Murphy, T. K., Storch, E. A., Conelea, C. A., Woods, D. W., Scahill, L. D., et al. (2012). A phenomenological investigation of women with Tourette or other chronic tic disorders. *Compr. Psychiatry* 53, 525–534. doi: 10.1016/j.comppsych.2011.07.004

Mathews, C. A., Waller, J., Glidden, D., Lowe, T. L., Herrera, L., Budman, C., et al. (2004). Self injurious behaviour in Tourette syndrome: correlates with impulsivity and impulse control. *J. Neurol. Neurosurg. Psychiatry* 75, 1149–1155. doi: 10.1136/jnnp.2003.020693

Müller-Vahl, K., Dodel, I., Müller, N., Münchau, A., Reese, J. P., Balzer-Geldsetzer, M., et al. (2010). Health-related quality of life in patients with Gilles de la Tourette's syndrome. *Mov. Disord.* 25, 309–314. doi: 10.1002/mds.22900

Neal, M., and Cavanna, A. E. (2013). "Not just right experiences" in patients with Tourette syndrome: complex motor tics or compulsions?. *Psychiatry Res.* 210, 559–563. doi: 10.1016/j.psychres.2013.06.033

Packer, L. E. (1997). Social and educational resources for patients with Tourette syndrome. *Neurol. Clin.* 15, 457–473. doi: 10.1016/S0733-8619(05)70326-1

Piacentini, J., Woods, D. W., Scahill, L., Wilhelm, S., Peterson, A. L., Chang, S., et al. (2010). Behavior therapy for children with Tourette disorder: a randomized controlled trial. *JAMA* 303, 1929–1937. doi: 10.1001/jama.2010.607

Pringsheim, T., Lang, A., Kurlan, R., Pearce, M., and Sandor, P. (2009). Understanding disability in Tourette syndrome. *Develop. Med. Child Neurol. 51*, 468–472. doi: 10.1111/j.1469-8749.2008.03168.x

Rizzo, R., Gulisano, M., Pellico, A., Calì, P. V., and Curatolo, P. (2014). Tourette syndrome and comorbid conditions a spectrum of different severities and complexities. *J. Child Neurol.* 29, 1383–1389. doi: 10.1177/0883073814534317

Robertson, M. M. (1994). Annotation: Gilles De La Tourette Syndrome—an update. *J. Child Psychol. Psychiatry* 35, 597–611. doi: 10.1111/j.1469-7610.1994.tb01209.x

Robertson, M. M. (2000). Tourette syndrome, associated conditions and the complexities of treatment. *Brain* 123, 425–462. doi: 10.1093/brain/123.3.425

Robertson, M. M., and Baron-Cohen, V. (1998). *Tourette Syndrome: The Facts, 1st Edn*. London: Oxford Press.

Robertson, M. M., and Cavanna, A. E. (2007). The Gilles de la Tourette syndrome: a principal component factor analytic study of a large pedigree.*Psychiatr. Genet.* 17, 143–152. doi: 10.1097/YPG.0b013e328015b937

Robertson, M. M., Cavanna, A. E., and Eapen, V. (2015). Gilles de la Tourette syndrome and disruptive behavior disorders: prevalence, associations, and explanation of the relationships. *J. Neuropsychiatry Clin. Neurosci.* 27, 33–41. doi: 10.1176/appi.neuropsych.13050112

Robertson, M. M., and Eapen, V. (1996). The National Hospital Interview Schedule for the assessment of Gilles de la Tourette syndrome. *Int. J. Methods Psychiatr. Res.* 6, 203–226.

Robertson, M. M., Eapen, V., and Cavanna, A. E. (2009). The international prevalence, epidemiology, and clinical phenomenology of Tourette syndrome: a cross-cultural perspective. *J. Psychosom. Res.* 67, 475–483. doi: 10.1016/j.jpsychores.2009.07.010

Robertson, M. M., Williamson, F., and Eapen, V. (2006). Depressive symptomatology in young people with Gilles de la Tourette Syndrome—A comparison of self-report scales. *J. Affect. Disord.* 91, 265–268. doi: 10.1016/j.jad.2005.12.046

Shapiro, A. K., Shapiro, E. S., Young, J. G., and Feinberg, T. E. (1988). *Gilles De La Tourette Syndrome, 2nd Edn.* New York, NY: Raven Press.

Stewart, S. E., Rosario, M. C., Baer, L., Carter, A. S., Brown, T. A., Scharf, J. M., et al. (2008). Four-factor structure of obsessive-compulsive disorder symptoms in children, adolescents, and adults. *J. Am. Acad. Child Adolesc. Psychiatry* 47, 763–772. doi: 10.1097/CHI.0b013e318172ef1e

Tanner, C. M., and Goldman, S. M. (1997). Epidemiology of Tourette syndrome. *Neurol. Clin.* 15, 395–402. doi: 10.1016/S0733-8619(05)70320-0

Trillini, M. O., and Müller-Vahl, K. R. (2015). Patients with Gilles de la Tourette syndrome have widespread personality differences. *Psychiatry Res.* 228, 765–773. doi: 10.1016/j.psychres.2015.04.043

Worbe, Y., Mallet, L., Golmard, J. L., Béhar, C., Durif, F., Jalenques, I., et al. (2010). Repetitive behaviours in patients with Gilles de la Tourette syndrome: tics, compulsions, or both. *PLoS ONE* 5:e12959. doi: 10.1371/journal.pone.0012959

3

Comorbidities, Social Impact, and Quality of Life in Tourette Syndrome

Valsamma Eapen[1,2], Andrea E. Cavanna[3,4,5] and Mary M. Robertson[6,7,8]*

[1] School of Psychiatry, University of New South Wales, Sydney, NSW, Australia, [2] Academic Unit of Child Psychiatry, Ingham Institute, Sydney South Western Local Health District, Sydney, NSW, Australia, [3] Department of Neuropsychiatry, Birmingham and Solihull Mental Health NHS Foundation Trust, Birmingham, UK, [4] Aston Brain Centre, School of Life and Health Sciences, Aston University, Birmingham, UK, [5] Sobell Department of Motor Neuroscience and Movement Disorders, Institute of Neurology, University College London (UCL), London, UK, [6] Neuropsychiatry, University College London (UCL), London, UK, [7] St Georges Hospital and Medical School, London, UK, [8] Department of Psychiatry, University of Cape Town, Cape Town, South Africa

Edited by:
Peristera Paschou,
Democritus University of Thrace, Greece

Reviewed by:
Roger Dante Freeman,
University of British Columbia, Canada
Carol A. Mathews,
University of Florida, USA

****Correspondence:***
Valsamma Eapen
v.eapen@unsw.edu.au

Tourette syndrome (TS) is more than having motor and vocal tics, and this review will examine the varied comorbidities as well as the social impact and quality of life (QoL) in individuals with TS. The relationship between any individual and his/her environment is complex, and this is further exaggerated in the case of a person with TS. For example, tics may play a significant role in shaping the person's experiences, perceptions, and interactions with the environment. Furthermore, associated clinical features, comorbidities, and coexisting psychopathologies may compound or alter this relationship. In this regard, the common comorbidities include attention-deficit hyperactivity disorder and disruptive behaviors, obsessive compulsive disorder, and autism spectrum disorder, and coexistent problems include anxiety, depression, and low self-esteem, which can all lead to poorer psychosocial functioning and QoL. Thus, the symptoms of TS and the associated comorbid conditions may interact to result in a vicious cycle or a downward spiraling of negative experiences and poor QoL. The stigma and social maladjustment in TS and the social exclusion, bullying, and discrimination are considered to be caused in large part by misperceptions of the disorder by teachers, peers, and the wider community. Improved community and professional awareness about TS and related comorbidities and other psychopathologies as well as the provision of multidisciplinary services to meet the complex needs of this clinical population are critical. Future research to inform the risk and resilience factors for successful long-term outcomes is also warranted.

Keywords: Tourette syndrome, attention-deficit hyperactivity disorder, obsessive compulsive disorder, autism spectrum disorder, comorbidity, psychopathology, psychosocial, quality of life

INTRODUCTION

There are significant social and emotional sequelae to living with Tourette syndrome (TS), which can adversely affect the quality of life (QoL). Although majority of TS patients with mild forms of the disorder adapt to their symptoms and lead fulfilling lives, those with severe and persistent symptoms may experience significant negative impact on overall health and well-being. For example, an individual with TS may suffer from physical consequences such as the pain and discomfort of the repetitive movements and the stigma of the severe, violent, or socially inappropriate movements, vocalizations, or actions. Furthermore, they may become anxious particularly thinking about having the tics in front of others or become depressed from difficulties at school or lack of educational/

vocational or employment opportunities. Lack of response to treatment or medication side effects as well as comorbidities may also add unique challenges.

THE IMPACT OF COMORBIDITIES AND COEXISTENT PSYCHOPATHOLOGIES

The common comorbidities in TS include attention-deficit hyperactivity disorder (ADHD), obsessive compulsive disorder or behaviors (OCD/B), and autism spectrum disorder (ASD), whereas some of the common coexistent problems include anxiety, depression, substance abuse, childhood conduct disorder, and adult personality disorder (1). All of these can lower self-esteem directly or have consequences that may lead to poorer psychosocial functioning and QoL. For example, tics and comorbid ADHD may interact to create a vicious cycle of distractibility and inability to focus, due to both the efforts in trying to control the tics and due to inattention of ADHD; similarly, tics and comorbid severe obsessive compulsive disorder (OCD) may render an individual to check repeatedly, striving for perfection, and thus unable to finish school or office work (2). This may limit academic progress, while at the same time, negatively affecting the social outcomes and opportunities due to lack of education and under or unemployment. This may in turn create a downward spiraling of events compounded by poor frustration tolerance, impulsivity, and rage with consequent social exclusion, poor interpersonal, and family relationships. All of these can also precipitate or maintain comorbid mental health problems, drug and alcohol abuse, and even forensic encounters. Furthermore, the individual's and their families' QoL may be affected due to blame from delayed diagnosis or guilt from genetic etiology or wrong attributions about "parenting" or their own "TS" related behaviors including ADHD and obsessive compulsive features (clinical or subclinical) impacting on their ability to "parent" or "care" for the individual with TS.

One way of understanding the personal and social experiences of individuals with TS comes from the stories of people who have lived with TS for many years such as Joseph Bliss (3), and the writings of professionals with TS such as the neuroscientist Peter Hollenbeck (4), and physicians Lance Turtle (5), and Sam Zinner (6). Despite having marked symptoms, Bliss (3) received his diagnosis only at the age of 67 years. While identification and diagnosis of TS have improved in the last four decades since Bliss's experience, clinicians working in the field continue to hear such stories about delay in diagnosis or misdiagnosis compounded by the lack of information, knowledge, and awareness about TS in the community, including among health professionals. Although tics remain the core feature of TS in the diagnostic classificatory systems (7), the presence of tics in the absence of other associated features and comorbidities occurs in only around 13% of cases ("pure-TS") while the remaining (i.e., around 87%) have a number of associated features and comorbid disorders ("TS-plus") (8). Comorbidities in TS can adversely affect the overall outcome and QoL in TS, and hence early recognition and appropriate management of the associated comorbidities and coexistent psychopathologies are critical.

THE SOCIAL IMPACT OF TS ON AN INDIVIDUAL'S AND FAMILY'S LIFE

About one-third of TS patients have been reported to have social problems particularly due to potentially socially disabling features of TS, such as coprophenomena and also non-obscene socially inappropriate behaviors (NOSI), which is usually directed at a family member or familiar person at home or in a familiar setting (9). Other patients have self-injurious behaviors (10, 11) which can be difficult to treat and may compound social difficulties. These difficulties, plus shame, and embarrassment can also lead to difficulties outside the home or familiar settings and can have a negative impact on friendships and interpersonal relationships. For example, young people with TS have been found to have poorer peer relationships compared with their classmates and those with diabetes mellitus (12). Furthermore, in a clinical cohort of 16- to 54-year-old TS patients, problems with family relationships were reported in 29%, difficulties in making friends in 27%, social life in 20%, and being self-conscious in 15% (13). It has been found that parents of those with TS and comorbid behavioral disorder experience a greater impact on the family than those with uncomplicated TS (14). In this regard, increased Care Giver Burden and psychopathology have been reported in parents of young people with TS as compared with those with asthma (15). In addition, parents of young children with TS have been found to be significantly more likely to fall into the "parenting aggravation index" (e.g., feeling that their child is more difficult to care for than other children their age, feeling bothered by their child, and feeling angry with their child) category compared with those without TS (16). Moreover, another study observed that aggression and delinquency in the context of TS added unique contributions to impairment in social and family functioning, controlling for age, gender, and diagnostic status (17).

School problems have been noted in a number of clinic and community studies (18–20), and these have stressed the importance of teacher understanding and flexibility, as well as parent/school communication. It has also been found that the parents of children with TS considered tics to be the main cause of social maladaptation (21); finally, school-based intervention to improve knowledge and attitudes about TS has been found to enable prosocial behaviors in classmates while helping children with TS to embrace their condition (22).

A recent study comparing parental reports of TS youngsters with that of peers without TS found significantly higher rates of insecure peer attachment, problems in peer relationships, difficulty making friends, stigmatization, and lower levels of social functioning in the TS group, in particular, higher rates of the personality dimension "Neuroticism" acted as a significant barrier to friendship for individuals with TS (23). It has also been observed that parental perception of both tic frequency and intensity predicted tic-related functional impairment in several areas including family and peer relationships, school interference, and social endeavors with tic intensity predicting more variance across more domains than tic frequency (24). Another study (25) found that over half of the parents of TS patients reported one significant problem area due to the presence of tics, whereas over one-third reported two or more problem areas. The rate of non-tic-related impairment was very high, with 70% of parents reporting at least one problem area in the domains of school, home, or social activities (e.g., concentrating on school work, being prepared for class, taking tests or exams, or writing in class, doing household chores, sleeping at night, making new friends, and being with a group of strangers). In a UK study (26), significantly worse QoL was reported in a TS cohort compared with that of children in a normative sample with four main themes; "TS can be distressing and disabling," "struggling to fit into society's expectations of normal behavior," "needing to control tics," and "TS is one part of who I am." Furthermore, high peer victimization and bullying have been reported in TS patients (27) as well as discrimination due to tics (28). Yet, another study (29) identified several main themes of social impact: these included more adverse experiences with TS than positive ones, pervasive misconceptions about TS symptoms, a desire for more understanding of TS by the public and understanding and supportive families, experiencing increased stress, academic challenges requiring accommodations, the active suppression of tics in school and in pubic, and finally, more complex social interactions with peers. It has also been observed that while young people felt the presence of their TS constantly, they often learnt to cope with their symptoms and other people's reactions to them (30). Although they encountered problems when interacting with the wider peer network and expressed concerns around meeting new people and future employment, most of them had developed supportive friendships. The adolescents also described specific ways in which TS affects QoL and social interactions, and the effort it can take to cope successfully. Furthermore, low self-esteem has been linked with decreased QoL in all areas except for academic functionality (31). Considerable difficulties in socialization in TS patients have been reported, and it has been pointed out that the therapeutic elements must be identified by a change not only in environment but only in a child's adaptation ability (32). In the light of these observations, it appears that treating both tic and non-tic-related impairments concurrently may improve functioning more so than treating the tic symptoms in isolation. In this regard, it has been noted (33) that treatment success should not only be assessed with the classic "tic-scales" but also with the global assessment of functioning (GAF) and TS-specific QoL scales. It is also important to control clinical symptoms and improve family environment to achieve better outcomes (34).

Moreover, Tourette syndrome patients have been found to exhibit insecure attachment with significantly higher scores in relationship anxiety and relationship avoidance and significantly higher aggression scores (35). A recent study of parents of young people with TS found that youth with TS are at increased risk for insecure peer attachment, which, in turn, might adversely affect the QoL outcomes (36). This study also observed that accurate identification of comorbidities is critical along with multidisciplinary support, as half of the parents of young people with TS had experienced stigmatization due to poor understanding about TS in the community including among those in the educational and health services (23, 37–39).

QUALITY OF LIFE IN TOURETTE SYNDROME

The wide-ranging impact of TS on health-related QoL of patients of all ages has been investigated in a number of dedicated studies since the turn of the millennium (13, 40) with the first study by Elstner et al. suggesting lower QoL in TS patients than in the general population (9). There is no consensus on the exact definition of QoL as it is affected by health; in addition, the relationship between clinical symptoms and QoL is neither simple nor direct (41). From an operational perspective, it has been proposed that subjective QoL can be conceptualized as the discrepancy between patients' expectations about life and their actual experiences (42). Such a construct provides a useful framework for implementation in routine clinical practice; it is therefore not surprising that QoL is increasingly being used as a primary outcome measure for both health monitoring and active interventions for a range of medical conditions (43). Research has mainly focused on the burden of tic disorders and comorbid behavioral problems; the few controlled studies conducted to date have consistently shown that patients with TS have a poorer QoL than general population samples (13, 44, 45). Understandably, both the direct consequences of tic expression and the constant efforts related to their active suppression can be intrusive experiences affecting the individual's well-being and their social interactions. Moreover, the high prevalence of comorbid behavioral problems in patients with TS is known to be associated with significant disease burden resulting in the subjective perception of poorer QoL (13).

The many clinical studies conducted in both children/adolescents (17, 24, 26, 28, 36, 39, 44–59) and admittedly fewer in adults (13, 60–66) with TS have, in general, shown similar results with lower QoL in TS. However, when examined in detail it becomes apparent that the different studies have yielded heterogeneous findings, especially with regard to the reciprocal contributions of tics and behavioral problems to specific domains of QoL. It is to be noted that the changes in arbitrary diagnostic criteria (e.g., DSM 111 > DSM-IV → DSM-IV-TR → DSM-5) over the long time period in which cited research has taken place may have contributed to the discrepancy in the findings, but taken together, the results of these studies suggest impairment across six general QoL themes as follows: physical, psychological, occupational, social, obsessional, and cognitive domains.

Severe tics have been reported to result in physical pain and in actual injuries. For example, findings from the Tourette Syndrome Impact Survey study, which involved both children and adults with TS, showed that the majority of respondents reported at least one tic that caused pain and indeed physical damage (64 and 60%, respectively), with significant correlations to reported tic severity (28, 65). Difficulties in carrying out activities of daily living, including self care, have also been documented among the consequences of problems in functional mobility and ability to perform exercises, especially as children mature to adolescence and adulthood (67). The presence of comorbid ADHD and OCD has been found to further affect the physical aspects of QoL, especially in children (44, 47), with few exceptions (48). Taken together, these findings suggest that the physical components of QoL should not be overlooked throughout the lifespan.

Psychological distress, feelings of frustration, and low mood in general are commonly experienced by patients with TS. The psychological domain of QoL has consistently been found to be significantly affected in the TS population compared with healthy controls. For example, 57% of adult patients with TS from a clinical sample reported problems with coexistent anxiety and depressive symptoms, with an odds ratio of 13 compared with age-matched controls (61). A study conducted in a clinical sample of children with TS showed that anxiety and depression were significantly more prevalent than in both healthy individuals (controls) and epilepsy control groups (44). It is thought that the increased prevalence of affective symptoms in TS, although not genetically linked, is probably multifactorial (68) rather than purely reactive to the psychosocial impairment and frustration caused by the chronic presence of tic symptoms (63). Psychological symptoms have been shown to be among the most important determinants of overall QoL (69), especially in adulthood (54, 60).

The negative impact of TS on QoL in children at school and in adults at work environment has also been investigated. The presence of comorbid conditions, particularly ADHD, has consistently been shown to affect school life (46, 47, 53). In addition, the spontaneous improvement or at least reduction of some of this comorbidity with age may contribute to explain the less pronounced impairment of QoL reported in adult working life (70, 71). For example, findings from the Tourette Syndrome Impact Survey study have shown that adults report milder interference with work productivity compared with the level of academic interference noted by the child population (28, 65). The development of coping strategies through adolescence has been found to improve satisfaction in the workplace (30), although dissatisfaction with school experiences can have far-reaching implications, possibly influencing future career or occupational choices or even employment status (72).

Relationships with family and friends are also important in life and indeed are also components of the social domain of QoL. Specifically, healthy family functioning has been recognized as integral to long-term social and emotional stability in children with TS (73). Multiple studies have shown that younger patients can often feel responsible for family arguments as a result of their TS symptoms and can therefore be more likely to avoid communication with their parents (44, 48, 57), possibly resulting in increased insecurity and exacerbated problems over time (57). In turn, one study conducted in adult patients with TS showed that 29% of participants had felt unsupported by their family about their condition (13). Of importance is that patients of all ages have reported a higher interference from TS within peer friendships than in family relationships (28, 65). The former way will result in potential difficulties in the formation of intimate or meaningful relationships which are an important part of adult life (63). However, the full extent of the social impact of the comorbidities of TS remains difficult to determine and quantify, especially in the case of adults with comorbid OCD (40, 74).

Nevertheless, the development of disease-specific QoL measures, such as the GTS-QoL in adults and the GTS-QoL-C&A in children, has enabled researchers to more sensitively assess the impact of repetitive behaviors and comorbid OCD on the overall perception of QoL in patients with TS (54, 60). Results from studies using disease-specific measures seem to indicate a decrease in the perceived impact of OCD on QoL as patients develop to adulthood, in the absence of decreased symptom severity, possibly suggesting the development of more effective coping strategies over time (51, 64).

Reduced concentration, forgetfulness, and inability to complete important tasks are important cognitive aspects of QoL. Although age-dependent improvement of comorbid ADHD seems likely to have a significant impact on cognitive functioning (71), results from the Tourette Syndrome Impact Survey study highlighted a significant correlation between tic severity and cognitive domain scores (65). Studies conducted using the GTS-QoL further suggested that QoL perception in adulthood is more deeply affected by cognitive factors than in children (54, 60). These findings suggest that complex interaction between tics and cognitive function in determining QoL across the lifespan deserves further investigation in future studies.

CONCLUSION

The social impact of TS is varied, and there are a number of TS patients who are known to us and are reported in the literature who cope and adapt well, with many using creativity or humor to their advantage, or by focusing on something that they are good at or enjoy doing such as leisure activities, sports, or academic or artistic pursuits. However, in those with severe forms of the disorder and with severe comorbidities, TS may interfere with the individual's everyday life and activities of school, home, or work, such as being educated to their full potential, obtaining a job/career, gaining independence, and having meaningful relationships with family and friends. There are a number of factors that contribute to outcomes in terms of social adjustment and QoL, although treatment for tics or better coping strategies may be positively correlated with functional improvement, particular attention to the complex interaction with comorbidities is critical to successful outcomes. For example, fidgetiness may be part of tics or due to ADHD or both; coprolalia and disruptive behaviors may well attract negative consequences such as disciplinary action in children or stigma and social embarrassment in adults (2). In this regard, supportive environments, anticipatory guidance, as well as appropriate emotional, behavioral, and learning supports are indicated to overcome the challenges confronting those with TS. Education of health and other professionals as well as implementation of community awareness programs are needed along with research to gain better understanding of the factors that contribute to better long-term outcomes. Thus, we suggest that future research should examine the possible influence of successful treatment on outcomes such as pharmacological intervention for symptom control or indeed improving a sense of personal mastery through skill building in comprehensive behavioral intervention for tics (CBIT); this must be conducted in tandem with research on the quality, duration, and effect of early supportive services on later QoL.

AUTHOR CONTRIBUTIONS

VE, AC, and MR jointly wrote the manuscript, each taking charge of a subsection.

ACKNOWLEDGMENTS

The authors acknowledge our own patients for their continuing and insightful feedback on the central topics of this article. This article was motivated by the first World Congress on Tourette Syndrome and Tic Disorders (June 24-26, 2015) and was supported by the Tourette Association of America.

REFERENCES

1. Robertson M. A personal 35 year perspective on Gilles de la Tourette syndrome: assessment, investigations, and management. *Lancet Psychiatry* (2015) 2(1):88–104. doi:10.1016/S2215-0366(14)00132-1
2. Eapen V, Črnčec R, McPherson S, Snedden C. Tic disorders and learning disability: clinical characteristics, cognitive performance and comorbidity. *Australas J Spec Educ* (2013) 37(02):162–72. doi:10.1017/jse.2013.2
3. Bliss J. Sensory experiences of Gilles de la Tourette syndrome. *Arch Gen Psychiatry* (1980) 37(12):1343–7. doi:10.1001/archpsyc.1980.01780250029002
4. Hollenbeck P. How life imitates Tourette syndrome: reflections of an afflicted neuroscientist. *CNS Spectr* (1999) 4(02):22–3.
5. Turtle L, Robertson M. Tics, twitches, tales: the experiences of Gilles de la Tourette's syndrome. *Am J Orthopsychiatry* (2008) 78(4):449. doi:10.1037/a0014329
6. Zinner S. Tourette disorder. *Pediatr Rev/American Acad of Pediatr* (2000) 21(11):372.
7. Robertson M, Eapen V. Tourette's: syndrome, disorder or spectrum? Classificatory challenges and an appraisal of the DSM criteria. *Asian J Psychiatr* (2014) 11:106–13. doi:10.1016/j.ajp.2014.05.010
8. Eapen V, Robertson M. Are there distinct subtypes in Tourette syndrome? Pure-Tourette syndrome versus Tourette syndrome-plus, and simple versus complex tics. *Neuropsychiatr Dis Treat* (2015) 11:1431. doi:10.2147/NDT.S72284
9. Kurlan R, Daragjati C, Como P, McDermott M, Trinidad K, Roddy S, et al. Non-obscene complex socially inappropriate behavior in Tourette's syndrome. *J Neuropsychiatry Clin Neurosci* (1996) 8(3):311–7. doi:10.1176/jnp.8.3.311
10. Robertson M, Trimble M, Lees A. Self-injurious behaviour and the Gilles de la Tourette syndrome: a clinical study and review of the literature. *Psychol Med* (1989) 19(03):611–25. doi:10.1017/S0033291700024211
11. Mathews CA, Waller J, Glidden D, Lowe TL, Herrera LD, Budman CL, et al. Self injurious behaviour in Tourette syndrome: correlates with impulsivity and impulse control. *J Neurol Neurosurg Psychiatry* (2004) 75(8):1149–55. doi:10.1136/jnnp 2003.020693
12. Bawden H, Stokes A, Camfield C, Camfield P, Salisbury S. Peer relationship problems in children with Tourette's disorder or diabetes mellitus. *J Child Psychol Psychiatry* (1998) 39(5):663–8. doi:10.1111/1469-7610.00366
13. Elstner K, Selai CE, Trimble MR, Robertson MM. Quality of life (QoL) of patients with Gilles de la Tourette's syndrome. *Acta Psychiatr Scand* (2001) 103(1):52–9. doi:10.1034/j.1600-0447.2001.00147.x
14. Wilkinson B, Newman M, Shytle R, Silver A, Sanberg P, Sheehan D. Family impact of Tourette's syndrome. *J Child Fam Stud* (2001) 10:477–83. doi:10.1023/A:1016713508665
15. Cooper C, Robertson M, Livingston G. Psychological morbidity and caregiver burden in parents of children with Tourette's disorder and psychiatric comorbidity. *J Am Acad Child Adolesc Psychiatry* (2003) 42(11):1370–5. doi:10.1097/01.CHI.0000085751.71002.48
16. Robinson L, Bitsko R, Schieve L, Visser S. Tourette syndrome, parenting aggravation, and the contribution of co-occurring conditions among a nationally representative sample. *Disabil Health J* (2013) 6(1):26–35. doi:10.1016/j.dhjo.2012.10.002
17. Sukhodolsky D, Scahill L, Zhang H, Peterson B, King R, Lombroso P, et al. Disruptive behavior in children with Tourette's syndrome: association with ADHD comorbidity, tic severity, and functional impairment. *J Am Acad Child Adolesc Psychiatry* (2003) 42:98–105. doi:10.1097/00004583-200301000-00016
18. Khalifa N, von Knorring A. Prevalence of tic disorders and Tourette syndrome in a Swedish school population. *Dev Med Child Neurol* (2003) 45:315–9. doi:10.1111/j.1469-8749.2003.tb00402.x
19. Hornsey H, Banerjee S, Zeitlin H, Robertson M. The prevalence of Tourette syndrome in 13-14-year-olds in mainstream schools. *J Child Psychol Psychiatry* (2001) 42(8):1035–9. doi:10.1111/1469-7610.00802
20. Grace R, Russell C. Tourette's syndrome and the school experience: a qualitative study of children's and parents' perspectives. *Australas J Spec Educ* (2005) 29(1):40–59. doi:10.1080/1030011050290104
21. Rivera-Navarro J, Cubo E, Almazán J. The impact of Tourette's syndrome in the school and the family: perspectives from three stakeholder groups. *Int J Adv Couns* (2014) 36(1):96–113. doi:10.1007/s10447-013-9193-9
22. Nussey C, Pistrang N, Murphy T. Does it help to talk about tics? An evaluation of a classroom presentation about Tourette syndrome. *Child Adolesc Ment Health* (2014) 19(1):31–8. doi:10.1111/camh.12000
23. O'Hare D, Eapen V, Helmes E, McBain K, Reece J, Grove R. Factors impacting the quality of peer relationships of youth with Tourette's syndrome. *BMC Psychol* (2015) 3(1):34. doi:10.1186/s40359-015-0090-3
24. Espil F, Capriotti M, Conelea C, Woods D. The role of parental perceptions of tic frequency and intensity in predicting tic-related functional impairment in youth with chronic tic disorders. *Child Psychiatry Hum Dev* (2014) 45(6):657–65. doi:10.1007/s10578-013-0434-2
25. Storch E, Lack C, Simons L, Goodman W, Murphy T, Geffken G. A measure of functional impairment in youth with Tourette's syndrome. *J Pediatr Psychol* (2007) 32(8):950–9. doi:10.1093/jpepsy/jsm034
26. Cutler D, Murphy T, Gilmour J, Heyman I. The quality of life of young people with Tourette syndrome. *Child Care Health Dev* (2009) 35:496–504. doi:10.1111/j.1365-2214.2009.00983.x
27. Zinner SH, Conelea C, Glew G, Woods D, Budman C. Peer victimization in youth with Tourette syndrome and other chronic tic disorders. *Child Psychiatry Hum Dev* (2012) 43(1):124–36. doi:10.1007/s10578-011-0249-y
28. Conelea C, Woods D, Zinner S, Budman C, Murphy T, Scahill L, et al. Exploring the impact of chronic tic disorders on youth: results from the Tourette syndrome impact survey. *Child Psychiatry Hum Dev* (2011) 42(2):219–42. doi:10.1007/s10578-010-0211-4
29. Happich R. *Tourette Syndrome in Adolescence: How it Impacts an Adolescent's Experience of Their Family, Peers, School, Self-Concept and View of the Future*. New Brunswick: Rutgers University-Graduate School of Applied and Professional Psychology (2012).
30. Wadman R, Tischler V, Jackson G. 'Everybody just thinks I'm weird': a qualitative exploration of the psychosocial experiences of adolescents with Tourette syndrome. *Child Care Health Dev* (2013) 39(6):880–6. doi:10.1111/cch.12033
31. Hesapçıoğlu S, Tural M, Kandil S. Quality of life and self-esteem in children with chronic tic disorder. *Turk Pediatri Ars* (2014) 49(4):323–32. doi:10.5152/tpa.2014.1947
32. Meucci P, Leonardi M, Zibordi F, Nardocci N. Measuring participation in children with Gilles de la Tourette syndrome: a pilot study with ICF-CY. *Disabil Rehabil* (2009) 31(S1):S116–20. doi:10.3109/09638280903317773
33. Dehning S, Leitner B, Schennach R, Müller N, Bötzel K, Obermeier M, et al. Functional outcome and quality of life in Tourette's syndrome after deep brain stimulation of the posteroventrolateral globus pallidus internus: long-term follow-up. *World J Biol Psychiatry* (2014) 15(1):66–75. doi:10.3109/15622975.2013.849004
34. Yi M, Sun Z, Ran N. Subjective quality of life in children with Tourette syndrome. *Zhongguo Dang Dai Er Ke Za Zhi* (2011) 13(9):732–5.
35. Dehning S, Burger M, Krause D, Jobst A, Yundina E, Müller N, et al. Tourette syndrome is associated with insecure attachment and higher aggression. *Int J Neurosci* (2014) 125(7):521–5. doi:10.3109/00207454.2014.951040
36. O'Hare D, Helmes E, Eapen V, Grove R, McBain K, Reece J. The impact of tic severity, comorbidity and peer attachment on quality of life outcomes and

functioning in Tourette's syndrome: parental perspectives. *Child Psychiatry Hum Dev* (2015) 6:1–11. doi:10.1007/s10578-015-0590-7

37. O'Hare D, Eapen V, Grove R, Helmes E, McBain K, Reece J. Youth with Tourette syndrome: parental perceptions and experiences in the Australian context. *Aust J Psychol* (2016). doi:10.1111/ajpy.12111
38. O'Hare D, Eapen V, Helmes E, McBain K, Reece J, Grove R. Recognising and treating Tourette's in young Australians: a need for informed multidisciplinary support. *Aust Psychol* (2016) 51:238–45. doi:10.1111/ap.12170
39. O'Hare D, Helmes E, Reece J, Eapen V, McBain K. The differential impact of Tourette syndrome and comorbid diagnosis on the quality of life and functioning of diagnosed children and adolescents. *J Child Adolesc Psychiatr Nurs* (2016) 29(1):30–6. doi:10.1111/jcap.12132
40. Cavanna A, David K, Bandera V, Termine C, Balottin U, Schrag A, et al. Health-related quality of life in Gilles de la Tourette syndrome: a decade of research. *Behav Neurol* (2013) 27(1):83–93. doi:10.3233/BEN-120296
41. Carr A, Gibson B, Robinson P. Is quality of life determined by expectations or experience? *Br Med J* (2001) 322(7296):1240–3. doi:10.1136/bmj.322.7296.1240
42. Calman K. Quality of life in cancer patients – an hypothesis. *J Med Ethics* (1984) 10(3):124–7. doi:10.1136/jme.10.3.124
43. Higginson I, Carr A. Using quality of life measures in the clinical setting. *Br Med J* (2001) 322(7297):1297–300. doi:10.1136/bmj.322.7297.1297
44. Eddy C, Rizzo R, Gulisano M, Agodi A, Barchitta M, Calì P, et al. Quality of life in young people with Tourette syndrome: a controlled study. *J Neurol* (2011) 258(2):291–301. doi:10.1007/s00415-010-5754-6
45. Gutierrez-Colina A, Eaton C, Lee J, LaMotte J, Blount R. Health-related quality of life and psychosocial functioning in children with Tourette syndrome parent-child agreement and comparison to healthy norms. *J Child Neurol* (2014) 30(3):326–32. doi:10.1177/0883073814538507
46. Storch E, Merlo L, Lack C, Milsom V, Geffken G, Goodman W, et al. Quality of life in youth with Tourette's syndrome and chronic tic disorder. *J Clin Child Adolesc Psychol* (2007) 36(2):217–27. doi:10.1080/15374410701279545
47. Bernard B, Stebbins G, Siegel S, Schultz T, Hays C, Morrissey M, et al. Determinants of quality of life in children with Gilles de la Tourette syndrome. *Mov Disord* (2009) 24:1070–3. doi:10.1002/mds.22487
48. Pringsheim T, Lang A, Kurlan R, Pearce M, Sandor P. Understanding disability in Tourette syndrome. *Dev Med Child Neurol* (2009) 51:468–72. doi:10.1111/j.1469-8749.2008.03168.x
49. Hao Y, Tian Q, Lu Y, Chai Y, Rao S. Psychometric properties of the Chinese version of the pediatric quality of life inventory 4.0 generic core scales. *Qual Life Res* (2010) 19(8):1229–33. doi:10.1007/s11136-010-9672-y
50. Eddy C, Cavanna A, Gulisano M, Calì P, Robertson M, Rizzo R. The effects of comorbid obsessive-compulsive disorder and attention-deficit hyperactivity disorder on quality of life in Tourette syndrome. *J Neuropsychiatry Clin Neurosci* (2012) 24(4):458–62. doi:10.1176/appi.neuropsych.11080181
51. Rizzo R, Gulisano M, Calì P, Curatolo P. Long term clinical course of Tourette syndrome. *Brain Dev* (2012) 34(8):667–73. doi:10.1016/j.braindev.2011.11.006
52. Cavanna A, Luoni C, Selvini C, Blangiardo R, Eddy C, Silvestri P, et al. Disease-specific quality of life in young patients with Tourette syndrome. *Pediatr Neurol* (2013) 48(2):111–4. doi:10.1016/j.pediatrneurol.2012.10.006
53. Cavanna AE, Luoni C, Selvini C, Blangiardo R, Eddy CM, Silvestri PR, et al. Parent and self-report health-related quality of life measures in young patients with Tourette syndrome. *J Child Neurol* (2013) 28(10):1305–8. doi:10.1177/0883073812457462
54. Cavanna A, Luoni C, Selvini C, Blangiardo R, Eddy C, Silvestri P, et al. The Gilles de la Tourette syndrome-quality of life scale for children and adolescents (C&A-GTS-QoL): development and validation of the Italian version. *Behav Neurol* (2013) 27(1):95–103. doi:10.1155/2013/140210
55. McGuire J, Hanks C, Lewin A, Storch E, Murphy T. Social deficits in children with chronic tic disorders: phenomenology, clinical correlates and quality of life. *Compr Psychiatry* (2013) 54(7):1023–31. doi:10.1016/j.comppsych.2013.04.009
56. Rizzo R, Gulisano M, Pellico A, Calì P, Curatolo P. Tourette syndrome and comorbid conditions a spectrum of different severities and complexities. *J Child Neurol* (2014) 29(10):1383–9. doi:10.1177/0883073814534317
57. Liu S, Zheng L, Zheng X, Zhang X, Yi M, Ma X. The subjective quality of life in young people with Tourette syndrome in China. *J Atten Disord* (2014) 1–7. doi:10.1177/1087054713518822
58. McGuire J, Park J, Wu M, Lewin A, Murphy T, Storch E. The impact of tic severity dimensions on impairment and quality of life among youth with chronic tic disorders. *Child Health Care* (2015) 44(3):277–92. doi:10.1080/02739615.2014.912944
59. Eapen V, Snedden C, Črnčec R, Pick A, Sachdev P. Tourette syndrome, co-morbidities and quality of life. *Aust N Z J Psychiatry* (2015) 50(1):82–93. doi:10.1177/0004867415594429
60. Cavanna A, Schrag A, Morley D, Orth M, Robertson M, Joyce E, et al. The Gilles de la Tourette syndrome-quality of life scale (GTS-QoL) development and validation. *Neurology* (2008) 71(18):1410–6. doi:10.1212/01.wnl.0000327890.02893.61
61. Müller-Vahl K, Dodel I, Müller N, Münchau A, Reese J, Balzer-Geldsetzer M, et al. Health-related quality of life in patients with Gilles de la Tourette's syndrome. *Mov Disord* (2010) 25:309–14. doi:10.1002/mds.22900
62. Eddy C, Cavanna A, Gulisano M, Agodi A, Barchitta M, Calì P, et al. Clinical correlates of quality of life in Tourette syndrome. *Mov Disord* (2011) 26(4):735–8. doi:10.1002/mds.23434
63. Jalenques I, Galland F, Malet L, Morand D, Legrand G, Auclair C, et al. Quality of life in adults with Gilles de la Tourette syndrome. *BMC Psychiatry* (2012) 12(1):109. doi:10.1186/1471-244X-12-109
64. Cavanna A, David K, Orth M, Robertson M. Predictors during childhood of future health-related quality of life in adults with Gilles de la Tourette syndrome. *Eur J Paediatr Neurol* (2012) 16(6):605–12. doi:10.1016/j.ejpn.2012.02.004
65. Conelea C, Woods D, Zinner S, Budman C, Murphy T, Scahill L, et al. The impact of Tourette syndrome in adults: results from the Tourette syndrome impact survey. *Community Ment Health J* (2013) 49(1):110–20. doi:10.1007/s10597-011-9465-y
66. Crossley E, Cavanna A. Sensory phenomena: clinical correlates and impact on quality of life in adult patients with Tourette syndrome. *Psychiatry Res* (2013) 209(3):705–10. doi:10.1016/j.psychres.2013.04.019
67. Parisi J. Engagement in adulthood: perceptions and participation in daily activities. *Act Adapt Aging* (2010) 34(1):1–16. doi:10.1080/01924780903552246
68. Robertson M. Mood disorders and Gilles de la Tourette's syndrome: an update on prevalence, etiology, comorbidity, clinical associations, and implications. *J Psychosom Res* (2006) 61(3):349–58. doi:10.1016/j.jpsychores.2006.07.019
69. Lewin A, Storch E, Conelea C, Woods D, Zinner S, Budman C, et al. The roles of anxiety and depression in connecting tic severity and functional impairment. *J Anxiety Disord* (2011) 25(2):164–8. doi:10.1016/j.janxdis.2010.08.016
70. Robertson M. Attention deficit hyperactivity disorder, tics and Tourette's syndrome: the relationship and treatment implications. A commentary. *Eur Child Adolesc Psychiatry* (2006) 15(1):1–11. doi:10.1007/s00787-006-0505-z
71. Haddad A, Umoh G, Bhatia V, Robertson M. Adults with Tourette's syndrome with and without attention deficit hyperactivity disorder. *Acta Psychiatr Scand* (2009) 120(4):299–307. doi:10.1111/j.1600-0447.2009.01398.x
72. Shady G, Broder R, Staley D, Furer P, Brezden Papadopolos R. Tourette syndrome and employment: descriptors, predictors, and problems. *Psychiatr Rehabil J* (1995) 19(1):35. doi:10.1037/h0095462
73. Carter A, O'Donnell D, Schultz R, Scahill L, Leckman J, Pauls D. Social and emotional adjustment in children affected with Gilles de la Tourette's syndrome: associations with ADHD and family functioning. *J Child Psychol Psychiatry* (2000) 41:215–23. doi:10.1111/1469-7610.00602
74. Eddy C, Cavanna A. Tourette syndrome and obsessive compulsive disorder: compulsivity along the continuum. *J Obsessive Compuls Relat Disord* (2014) 3(4):363–71. doi:10.1016/j.jocrd.2014.04.003

4

Animal Models of Tourette Syndrome—From Proliferation to Standardization

*Dorin Yael†, Michal Israelashvili† and Izhar Bar-Gad**

The Leslie and Susan Goldschmied (Gonda) Multidisciplinary Brain Research Center, Bar-Ilan University, Ramat-Gan, Israel

Edited by:
Peristera Paschou, Democritus University of Thrace, Greece

Reviewed by:
Csaba Barta, Semmelweis University, Hungary
Bastian Hengerer, Boehringer Ingelheim Pharma GmbH & Co.KG, Germany

Ester Nespoli contributed to the review of Bastian Hengerer

***Correspondence:**
Izhar Bar-Gad
izhar.bar-gad@biu.ac.il

†These authors have contributed equally to this work.

Tourette syndrome (TS) is a childhood onset disorder characterized by motor and vocal tics and associated with multiple comorbid symptoms. Over the last decade, the accumulation of findings from TS patients and the emergence of new technologies have led to the development of novel animal models with high construct validity. In addition, animal models which were previously associated with other disorders were recently attributed to TS. The proliferation of TS animal models has accelerated TS research and provided a better understanding of the mechanism underlying the disorder. This newfound success generates novel challenges, since the conclusions that can be drawn from TS animal model studies are constrained by the considerable variation across models. Typically, each animal model examines a specific subset of deficits and centers on one field of research (physiology/genetics/pharmacology/etc.). Moreover, different studies do not use a standard lexicon to characterize different properties of the model. These factors hinder the evaluation of individual model validity as well as the comparison across models, leading to a formation of a fuzzy, segregated landscape of TS pathophysiology. Here, we call for a standardization process in the study of TS animal models as the next logical step. We believe that a generation of standard examination criteria will improve the utility of these models and enable their consolidation into a general framework. This should lead to a better understanding of these models and their relationship to TS, thereby improving the research of the mechanism underlying this disorder and aiding the development of new treatments.

Keywords: Tourette syndrome, animal model, standardization, validation, striatum

TOURETTE SYNDROME AND THE BASAL GANGLIA

Tourette syndrome (TS) is a neurodevelopmental disorder characterized by vocal and motor tics in the form of rapid, repetitive, non-rhythmic vocalizations or movements (American Psychiatric Association, 2013). The standard pharmacological treatment consists of the administration of antipsychotic drugs which act mainly as D2 dopamine receptor antagonists. However, this treatment has significant side effects and is typically not sufficient for complete tic suppression (Eddy et al., 2011). Unlike other motor disorders, tics are not completely involuntary. More than 90% of all TS patients report experiencing premonitory urges preceding the tic. These patients describe tics as voluntary actions which alleviate these uncomfortable urges (Leckman et al., 1993). While tics are the defining symptom of TS, most patients (>90%) suffer from additional symptoms classically associated with other disorders, such as attention deficit hyperactivity disorder (ADHD) and obsessive-compulsive behavior and disorder (OCD), each affecting roughly half of the patients (Freeman et al., 2000). Genetic factors were found to play a role in TS etiology (Price et al., 1985; Bertelsen et al., 2016). Nevertheless, most of the identified genes are rare, and to date no gene is known to have a major effect on TS etiology (Godar et al., 2014). The underlying pathophysiology of TS is currently unknown. Many different systems, brain regions and neuronal circuits are considered likely candidates, with most current studies linking the disorder to abnormalities in the cortico-basal ganglia (CBG) pathway.

The basal ganglia are a group of interconnected nuclei forming partially closed loops leading from most cortical areas back to frontal cortical areas. The loops are functionally divided into domains based on the cortical regions which send their input to the BG. The domains include the motor, associative (executive), and limbic areas. The role of the CBG pathway in TS has been hypothesized to be related with abnormal inhibition of undesired actions (Albin and Mink, 2006). This lack of inhibition has been attributed to local deficits within the striatum, which serves as the primary input nucleus of the BG. Most neurons in the striatum are the medium spiny projection neurons (MSNs) whose activity is modulated by interneurons such as GABAergic fast spiking interneurons (FSIs) and cholinergic tonically active neurons (TANs) (Kita et al., 1990; Bennett and Bolam, 1994; English et al., 2011) as well as by neuromodulatory afferents including dopaminergic, histaminergic, and adrenergic inputs (Holmberg et al., 1999; Surmeier et al., 2007; Ellender et al., 2011).

Converging evidence point to the involvement of the CBG loop, and specifically the striatum, in the pathology of TS: A small decrease in overall volume (Peterson et al., 2003) and a substantial reduction in the cell count of FSIs and TANs (Kalanithi et al., 2005; Kataoka et al., 2010) have been observed in the striatum of TS patients. Tic severity in early adulthood was found to be correlated with the extent of volume reduction of the caudate nucleus in childhood (Bloch et al., 2005). Further, correlations have been found between the severity of tics and the structural connectivity between the motor cortex and the striatum (Worbe et al., 2015), and between the supplementary motor area and the BG (Cheng et al., 2014). Abnormalities in neuronal transmission including decreased $GABA_A$ receptor binding in the striatum (Lerner et al., 2012) and increased putamen dopamine release (Singer et al., 2002) have been reported in TS patients.

ANIMAL MODELS OF TOURETTE SYNDROME

TS is a multifaceted disorder associated with a wide spectrum of clinical symptoms involving multiple underlying neuronal systems (Yael et al., 2015). In this perspective we focus on TS animal models related to the striatum since most findings from TS patients and most modern animal models are associated directly or indirectly with deficits within this brain region.

Motor and vocal tics, the primary symptom of TS, may be evoked by a disruption of GABAergic transmission within the striatum. Local microinjections of different $GABA_A$ antagonists (such as bicuculline and picrotoxin) into the motor domain of the striatum have been shown to induce tics in both rodents (Marsden et al., 1975; Tarsy et al., 1978; Bronfeld et al., 2013b) and primates (Crossman et al., 1988; McCairn et al., 2009). The location of the disinhibition within the striatum determines the properties of the tics; injections in the motor striatum induce motor tics expressed in the body region associated with the somatotopic location of the striatal injection (Bronfeld et al., 2013b), whereas injections in the limbic striatum induce vocal tics (McCairn et al., 2016). Disinhibition in non-motor functional domains of the striatum induces behaviors similar to hyperactivity and compulsive symptoms (Worbe et al., 2009), thus exposing an intriguing link between tics and their comorbid symptoms. Additional support to the role of the striatum in TS and its comorbid disorders arise from a transgenic mouse model affecting the limbic cortico-striatal connectivity. This model demonstrates multiple symptoms such as OCD-like behaviors and sensorimotor gating deficits (Campbell et al., 1999; Nordstrom and Burton, 2002; Godar et al., 2015).

The identification of specific striatal neuronal subpopulations whose number is altered in TS (Kalanithi et al., 2005; Kataoka et al., 2010) inspired the development of animal models that target these subpopulations exclusively. Models have mimicked the selective suppression of the population of FSIs (using IEM-1460) thereby inducing abnormal movements (Gittis et al., 2011). The decline in the population of TANs has been modeled using viral-targeted cell ablation that leads to a highly specific reduction in this neuronal subpopulation in the dorsolateral striatum in mice (Xu et al., 2015). The ablation led to an increase in the expression of stereotypic behavior following stress and amphetamine treatment. However, although the animals displayed motor and behavioral abnormalities, no tics were observed in either model.

Other TS animal models are based on the dopaminergic model. This widely used model was originally related to other disorders such as schizophrenia, ADHD and OCD. Based on the "dopamine hypothesis," which argues that the pathophysiology leading to TS involves hyper activation of the dopaminergic system (Singer et al., 1982), this model was associated with TS. Systemic (Randrup and Munkvad, 1967; Taylor et al., 2010) and intrastriatal (Kelley et al., 1988) administration of dopamine agonists (such as amphetamine and apomorphine) was shown to induce behavioral stereotypies and sensorimotor gating disruption (Mansbach et al., 1988; Swerdlow et al., 2003) but not motor or vocal tics. Dopamine induced behavioral stereotypies may be enhanced when other neuromodulator systems are disrupted, as has been recently illustrated in the histidine decarboxylase (HDC) knockout TS mouse model (Castellan Baldan et al., 2014).

VALIDATION OF TOURETTE SYNDROME ANIMAL MODELS

The validation of animal models for human disorders is based upon three factors: face, predictive and construct validity. (1)

Face validity is defined as the phenomenological similarity between the human clinical condition symptoms and symptoms expressed in the animal model. (2) Predictive validity refers to the ability of the model to predict some aspects of the disorder. Specifically, this validation is usually based on the extent to which the animals' response to medication can predict the human response. (3) Construct validity refers to the theoretical rationale of the model, based on the known pathophysiology of the disorder (Jinnah and Hess, 2005; Bronfeld et al., 2013a).

In TS animal models, assessment of face validity is complicated by the wide spectrum of features associated with the disorder due in part to the fact that TS lies in a gray area between movement disorders (based on the existence of motor tics) and psychiatric disorders (based on the premonitory urges and comorbid symptoms). The primary feature associated with the movement disorder aspect of TS is the ability to induce tic-like movements. Currently, the striatal disinhibition model is the only one expressing motor tic-like movements (Marsden et al., 1975; Crossman et al., 1988; McCairn et al., 2009; Bronfeld et al., 2013b) and/or vocal tic-like sounds (McCairn et al., 2016). Other animal models typically elicit other forms of abnormal movements such as dyskinesia and dystonia (Gittis et al., 2011). Assessing TS as a psychiatric disorder complicates the evaluation of face validity. It is impossible to directly assess the existence of premonitory urges in animals; however, it was suggested these can reflect deficits in sensory motor gating (Swerdlow et al., 1999). Thus, indirectly these urges can be assessed by the pre-pulse inhibition (PPI) paradigm. Using PPI, deficits in the sensory motor gating have been reported in several dopamine related animal models (Mansbach et al., 1988; Castellan Baldan et al., 2014) but have not been tested in other models. Another aspect of TS is the high rates of comorbid conditions. Dopaminergic, cholinergic (TANs) and HDC models (subsequent to stress and/or amphetamine injection) were found to show an increase in stereotypic behaviors (Randrup et al., 1963; Kelley et al., 1988; Castellan Baldan et al., 2014; Xu et al., 2015) whereas the striatal disinhibition model demonstrated both hyperactivity and stereotypy following manipulation of non-motor (limbic and associative) areas in the striatum (Worbe et al., 2009).

The predictive validation of TS animal models is restricted by the non-specific medication for TS which is mostly based on responses to antipsychotic drugs (Shapiro and Shapiro, 1968). Due to the common definition, the dopaminergic animal models have a high predictive validity, as this model is based on the effectiveness of these drugs. Other models have not been explicitly tested for response to antipsychotics as well as to other drug treatments.

Evaluating the construct validity of TS animal models is currently speculative because the underlying pathophysiology of TS is still unclear. Typically the construct validity of TS animal models is based on their relationship to the small subset of currently known differences identified in TS patients compared to controls. Striatal animal models have been linked to current evidence from human studies, including dopamine dysfunction (Singer et al., 1991, 2002; Cheon et al., 2004; Minzer et al., 2004; Steeves et al., 2010), genetic abnormalities in a small subpopulation of TS patients (HDC model; Ercan-Sencicek et al., 2010), and a reduction in the cell count of striatal FSIs and TANs (Kalanithi et al., 2005; Kataoka et al., 2010). Another approach to assessing the construct validity of TS animal models is their relationship to theoretical functional models of information processing in the BG in both normal and pathological states. The "box and arrow" model of the BG describes their function based on their main anatomical connectivity (Albin et al., 1989; DeLong, 1990). According to this model, dopaminergic innervation to the striatum modulates striatal activity and consequently increases the overall cortical activation, leading to hyperkinetic symptoms. Consistent with this model, the dopaminergic model yields increased movement in the form of stereotypic behavior (Randrup and Munkvad, 1967; Kelley et al., 1988). This behavior was also observed in HDC knockout (Castellan Baldan et al., 2014) and TAN ablated (Xu et al., 2015) mouse models of TS which demonstrated enhanced stereotypic behavior in response to dopamine agonists. The "action selection" model contemplates that the BG chooses a single action while inhibiting competing actions (Mink, 1996). A loss of inhibition in a specific area within the striatum would thus prevent the selection process (Mink, 2001). This coincides with the animal model of focal disinhibition of the striatum using local blocking of GABA which prevents input from all inhibitory sources, including FSIs and neighboring MSNs (McCairn et al., 2009; Worbe et al., 2013). This functional model may also explain the behavioral and neuronal effects observed in the animal model based on selective suppression of FSIs (Gittis et al., 2011).

STANDARDIZATION OF TOURETTE SYNDROME ANIMAL MODELS

Over the last decade, rapid progress has been made in TS animal models studies, leading to a proliferation of novel models. Accumulating results from imaging, genetic, and anatomic studies performed on TS patients, provided solid foundation for the development of novel models with high construct validity, such as the TANs, FSIs, and HDC models. In addition, animal models which were previously attributed to other disorders have been recently considered valid models of TS. These include the striatal disinhibition model previously attributed to myoclonus (Marsden et al., 1975) and the dopaminergic models previously attributed to OCD and/or schizophrenia (Swerdlow and Geyer, 1998; Korff and Harvey, 2006). The use of different species of animals has made it possible to investigate multiple properties of the disorder by utilizing the relative advantages of each species. Mouse studies have enabled the investigation of genetic manipulation, rat studies explore the relationship between pharmacology, physiology, and behavior, and primate studies serve the study of complex behaviors linking the motor and psychiatric aspects of the disorder. Studies utilizing animal models significantly improved our understanding of the underlying mechanisms of specific properties of TS. For example, key questions such as "when" and "where" tics are expressed were recently addressed in animal model studies (Bronfeld et al., 2013b; Israelashvili and Bar-Gad, 2015). Similarly, data pointing to a common pathophysiology of TS and its comorbid conditions were experimentally supported when the same manipulation yielded a variety of behavioral symptoms (Worbe et al., 2009). This progress has led to a situation where finally basic and clinical science can co-contribute to the study of this disorder.

This major progress generates new challenges faced by TS animal models studies. The complexity of TS research which results from the myriad of symptoms and the fact that the pathophysiology leading to the disorder is still largely unknown have resulted in high variability in the study of mechanisms and behavioral symptoms in animal models of TS. Naturally, each of the current animal models focuses on a small subset of symptoms associated with the disorder which are examined using specific, non-standard and non-overlapping tests. Typically, these early-stage models were developed and studied by teams with specific expertise such as pharmacology, electrophysiology and genetics, thus creating a situation in which different models are studied with a high degree of focus into one field with significantly less effort in others. As a result, under the broad title of a "TS animal model study," a variety of models exist, that vary widely as regards to the scientific basis, methods used and the features examined. This issue is evident even when different models examine the same feature. The description of motor deficits does not adhere to an accepted classification, which leads to unclear (and in some cases ill-defined) definitions such as tic-like movement, tic-like stereotypy, and tic-like dyskinesia, without a robust kinematic evaluation. While this variability may contribute to a better understanding and characterization of different aspects of the disorder, it hinders the comparison across results of different models and the evaluation of the relevance, uniqueness, and contribution of each model. Furthermore, the use of this wide nomenclature is not necessarily supported by a large variety of underlying behavioral symptoms. A standardization of the examination criteria of TS animal models could help overcome these challenges.

Standardization is a widely used procedure in multiple fields to ensure consistency and comparability between processes or products. Evaluation criteria defined in standard protocols assist in the assessment of relevant information and allow uniformity within and between different users. In the clinic the necessity of standard protocols for diagnosis and treatment was raised for TS and other disorders, leading to the development of multiple standardized guidelines. The consistency and comparability enabled by these guidelines are highly beneficial in terms of the ability to properly diagnose and treat individual patients. More broadly it provides a uniform database enabling future study and the existence of a worldwide discourse. The reasons that led to the establishment of guidelines in the clinic apply to the development of standardized assessment of TS animal models that are still lacking in the field.

A standardization process defining the gold standard for the evaluation of TS animal model will improve the utility of these models and their use in both basic science as well as drug and treatment discovery. Standardized parameters will explicitly define the major components of a TS animal model evaluation, by providing an organized list detailing the range of characteristics of a valid TS animal model. In addition, a standardization process will allow an evaluation of the studied model's coverage, pointing to features that were studied using a specific model and those that were not. The standard definitions arrived at through this process will provide a clear differentiation between behavioral, pharmacological or physiological characteristics which are qualitatively different. These definitions will provide well-defined guidelines for classification of parameters while avoiding a use of fuzzy definitions. Thus, it will enable categorizing behaviors into either different categories if these behaviors resemble distinct symptoms or into a merged category if they resemble similar symptoms. This common terminology will allow both the evaluation of each model by standardized categories, and more importantly, a comparison between different models using the same vocabulary. The process of standardization in TS animal model research will help combine information from different studies into a general framework describing the mechanisms and their behavioral outcomes. It will enable a transition in TS research from small, local attempts typically confined to a single lab into a global effort. The development and implementation of such standards by a single lab or a small group of cooperating labs is prone to generate a partial picture biased by the inherent properties of this group. Thus, the standard criteria for TS animal model evaluation should be developed by a diverse committee including experts from various fields, reflecting a broad and comprehensive perspective, including both basic scientists developing and studying animal models, scientists conducting studies with TS patients and the clinicians working with these patients. This committee should be responsible for both writing the guidelines and maintaining a worldwide database summarizing results from different studies. We believe that such an effort should be managed by research-supporting international associations such as the Tourette Association of America (TAA) and/or the European Society for the Study of Tourette Syndrome (ESSTS), which hold the ability to direct international efforts. This standardization process, previously shown to be highly beneficial in other fields, has the potential to translate the rapidly accumulating results into a comprehensive framework for experimental studies of TS.

AUTHOR CONTRIBUTIONS

All authors listed, have made substantial, direct and intellectual contribution to the work, and approved it for publication.

ACKNOWLEDGMENTS

This article was motivated by the 1st World Congress on Tourette Syndrome and Tic Disorders (London, June 24-26, 2015) and was supported by the Tourette Association of America.

REFERENCES

Albin, R. L., and Mink, J. W. (2006). Recent advances in Tourette syndrome research. *Trends Neurosci.* 29, 175–182. doi: 10.1016/j.tins.2006.01.001

Albin, R. L., Young, A. B., and Penney, J. B. (1989). The functional anatomy of basal ganglia disorders. *Trends Neurosci.* 12, 366–375. doi: 10.1016/0166-2236(89)90074-X

American Psychiatric Association (2013). *DSM-5*. Arlington, TX: American Psychiatric Association Publishing.

Bennett, B. D., and Bolam, J. P. (1994). Synaptic input and output of parvalbumin-immunoreactive neurons in the neostriatum of the rat. *Neuroscience* 62, 707–719. doi: 10.1016/0306-4522(94)90471-5

Bertelsen, B., Stefánsson, H., Riff Jensen, L., Melchior, L., Mol Debes, N., Groth, C., et al. (2016). Association of AADAC deletion and gilles de la tourette syndrome in a large European cohort. *Biol. Psychiatry* 79, 383–391. doi: 10.1016/j.biopsych.2015.08.027

Bloch, M. H., Leckman, J. F., Zhu, H., and Peterson, B. S. (2005). Caudate volumes in childhood predict symptom severity in adults with Tourette syndrome. *Neurology* 65, 1253–1258. doi: 10.1212/01.wnl.0000180957.98702.69

Bronfeld, M., Israelashvili, M., and Bar-Gad, I. (2013a). Pharmacological animal models of Tourette syndrome. *Neurosci. Biobehav. Rev.* 37, 1101–1119. doi: 10.1016/j.neubiorev.2012.09.010

Bronfeld, M., Yael, D., Belelovsky, K., and Bar-Gad, I. (2013b). Motor tics evoked by striatal disinhibition in the rat. *Front. Syst. Neurosci.* 7:50. doi: 10.3389/fnsys.2013.00050

Campbell, K. M., de Lecea, L., Severynse, D. M., Caron, M. G., McGrath, M. J., Sparber, S. B., et al (1999). OCD-Like behaviors caused by a neuropotentiating transgene targeted to cortical and limbic D1+ neurons. *J. Neurosci.* 19, 5044–5053.

Castellan Baldan, L., Williams, K. A., Gallezot, J. D., Pogorelov, V., Rapanelli, M., Crowley, M., et al. (2014). Histidine decarboxylase deficiency causes tourette syndrome: parallel findings in humans and mice. *Neuron* 81, 77–90. doi: 10.1016/j.neuron.2013.10.052

Cheng, B., Braass, H., Ganos, C., Treszl, A., Biermann-Ruben, K., Hummel, F. C., et al. (2014). Altered intrahemispheric structural connectivity in Gilles de la Tourette syndrome. *NeuroImage Clin.* 4, 174–181. doi: 10.1016/j.nicl.2013.11.011

Cheon, K.-A., Ryu, Y.-H., Namkoong, K., Kim, C.-H., Kim, J.-J., and Lee, J. D. (2004). Dopamine transporter density of the basal ganglia assessed with [123I]IPT SPECT in drug-naive children with Tourette's disorder. *Psychiatry Res.* 130, 85–95. doi: 10.1016/j.pscychresns.2003.06.001

Crossman, A. R., Mitchell, I. J., Sambrook, M. A., and Jackson, A. (1988). Chorea and myoclonus in the monkey induced by gamma-aminobutyric acid antagonism in the lentiform complex. *Brain* 111, 1211–1233. doi: 10.1093/brain/111.5.1211

DeLong, M. R. (1990). Primate models of movement disorders of basal ganglia origin. *Trends Neurosci.* 13, 281–285. doi: 10.1016/0166-2236(90)90110-V

Eddy, C. M., Rickards, H. E., and Cavanna, A. E. (2011). Treatment strategies for tics in Tourette syndrome. *Ther. Adv. Neurol. Disord.* 4, 25–45. doi: 10.1177/1756285610390261

Ellender, T. J., Huerta-Ocampo, I., Deisseroth, K., Capogna, M., and Bolam, J. P. (2011). Differential modulation of excitatory and inhibitory striatal synaptic transmission by histamine. *J. Neurosci.* 31, 15340–15351. doi: 10.1523/JNEUROSCI.3144-11.2011

English, D. F., Ibanez-Sandoval, O., Stark, E., Tecuapetla, F., Buzsáki, G., Deisseroth, K., et al. (2011). GABAergic circuits mediate the reinforcement-related signals of striatal cholinergic interneurons. *Nat. Neurosci.* 15, 123–130. doi: 10.1038/nn.2984

Ercan-Sencicek, A. G., Stillman, A. A., Ghosh, A. K., Bilguvar, K., O'Roak, B. J., Mason, C. E., et al. (2010). L-histidine decarboxylase and Tourette's syndrome. *N. Engl. J. Med.* 362, 1901–1908. doi: 10.1056/NEJMoa0907006

Freeman, R. D., Fast, D. K., Burd, L., Kerbeshian, J., Robertson, M. M., and Sandor, P. (2000). An international perspective on Tourette syndrome: selected findings from 3,500 individuals in 22 countries. *Dev. Med. Child Neurol.* 42, 436–447. doi: 10.1017/S0012162200000839

Gittis, A. H., Leventhal, D. K., Fensterheim, B. A., Pettibone, J. R., Berke, J. D., and Kreitzer, A. C. (2011). Selective inhibition of striatal fast-spiking interneurons causes dyskinesias. *J. Neurosci.* 31, 15727–15731. doi: 10.1523/JNEUROSCI.3875-11.2011

Godar, S. C., Mosher, L. J., Di Giovanni, G., and Bortolato, M. (2014). Animal models of tic disorders: a translational perspective. *J. Neurosci. Methods* 238, 54–69. doi: 10.1016/j.jneumeth.2014.09.008

Godar, S. C., Mosher, L. J., Strathman, H. J., Gochi, A. M., Jones, C. M., Fowler, S. C., et al. (2015). *The D1CT-7* mouse model of Tourette syndrome displays sensorimotor gating deficits in response to spatial confinement. *Br. J. Pharmacol.* doi: 10.1111/bph.13243. [Epub ahead of print].

Holmberg, M., Scheinin, M., Kurose, H., and Miettinen, R. (1999). Adrenergic alpha2C-receptors reside in rat striatal GABAergic projection neurons: comparison of radioligand binding and immunohistochemistry. *Neuroscience* 93, 1323–1333. doi: 10.1016/S0306-4522(99)00260-2

Israelashvili, M., and Bar-Gad, I. (2015). Corticostriatal divergent function in determining the temporal and spatial properties of motor tics. *J. Neurosci.* 35, 16340–16351. doi: 10.1523/JNEUROSCI.2770-15.2015

Jinnah, H. A., and Hess, E. J. (2005). "Assessment of movement disorders in rodents," in *Animal Models of Movement Disorders*, ed M. LeDoux (Amsterdam: Elsevier Academic Press), 55–72.

Kalanithi, P. S. A., Zheng, W., Kataoka, Y., DiFiglia, M., Grantz, H., Saper, C. B., et al. (2005). Altered parvalbumin-positive neuron distribution in basal ganglia of individuals with Tourette syndrome. *Proc. Natl. Acad. Sci. U.S.A.* 102, 13307–13312. doi: 10.1073/pnas.0502624102

Kataoka, Y., Kalanithi, P. S. A., Grantz, H., Schwartz, M. L., Saper, C., Leckman, J. F., et al. (2010). Decreased number of parvalbumin and cholinergic interneurons in the striatum of individuals with Tourette syndrome. *J. Comp. Neurol.* 518, 277–291. doi: 10.1002/cne.22206

Kelley, A. E., Lang, C. G., and Gauthier, A. M. (1988). Induction of oral stereotypy following amphetamine microinjection into a discrete subregion of the striatum. *Psychopharmacology (Berl).* 95, 556–559. doi: 10.1007/BF00172976

Kita, H., Kosaka, T., and Heizmann, C. W. (1990). Parvalbumin-immunoreactive neurons in the rat neostriatum: a light and electron microscopic study. *Brain Res.* 536, 1–15. doi: 10.1016/0006-8993(90)90002-S

Korff, S., and Harvey, B. H. (2006). Animal models of obsessive-compulsive disorder: rationale to understanding psychobiology and pharmacology. *Psychiatr. Clin. North Am.* 29, 371–390. doi: 10.1016/j.psc.2006.02.007

Leckman, J. F., Walker, D. E., and Cohen, D. J. (1993). Premonitory urges in Tourette's syndrome. *Am. J. Psychiatry* 150, 98–102. doi: 10.1176/ajp.150.1.98

Lerner, A., Bagic, A., Simmons, J. M., Mari, Z., Bonne, O., Xu, B., et al. (2012). Widespread abnormality of the γ-aminobutyric acid-ergic system in Tourette syndrome. *Brain* 135, 926–1936. doi: 10.1093/brain/aws104

Mansbach, R. S., Geyer, M. A., and Braff, D. L. (1988). Dopaminergic stimulation disrupts sensorimotor gating in the rat. *Psychopharmacology (Berl).* 94, 507–514. doi: 10.1007/BF00212846

Marsden, C. D., Meldrum, B. S., Pycock, C., and Tarsy, D. (1975). Focal myoclonus produced by injection of picrotoxin into the caudate nucleus of the rat. *J. Physiol. (Lond).* 246, 96P.

McCairn, K. W., Bronfeld, M., Belelovsky, K., and Bar-Gad, I. (2009). The neurophysiological correlates of motor tics following focal striatal disinhibition. *Brain* 132, 2125–2138. doi: 10.1093/brain/awp142

McCairn, K. W., Nagai, Y., Hori, Y., Ninomiya, T., Kikuchi, E., Lee, J.-Y., et al. (2016). A primary role for nucleus accumbens and related limbic network in vocal tics. *Neuron* 89, 300–307. doi: 10.1016/j.neuron.2015.12.025

Mink, J. W. (1996). The basal ganglia: focused selection and inhibition of competing motor programs. *Prog. Neurobiol.* 50, 381–425. doi: 10.1016/S0301-0082(96)00042-1

Mink, J. W. (2001). Basal ganglia dysfunction in Tourette's syndrome: a new hypothesis. *Pediatr. Neurol.* 25, 190–198. doi: 10.1016/S0887-8994(01)00262-4

Minzer, K., Lee, O., Hong, J. J., and Singer, H. S. (2004). Increased prefrontal D2 protein in Tourette syndrome: a postmortem analysis of frontal cortex and striatum. *J. Neurol. Sci.* 219, 55–61. doi: 10.1016/j.jns.2003.12.006

Nordstrom, E. J., and Burton, F. H. (2002). A transgenic model of comorbid Tourette's syndrome and obsessive-compulsive disorder circuitry. *Mol. Psychiatry* 7, 617–625. doi: 10.1038/sj.mp.4001144

Peterson, B. S., Thomas, P., Kane, M. J., Scahill, L., Zhang, H., Bronen, R., et al. (2003). Basal Ganglia volumes in patients with Gilles de la Tourette syndrome. *Arch. Gen. Psychiatry* 60, 415–424. doi: 10.1001/archpsyc.60.4.415

Price, R. A., Kidd, K. K., Cohen, D. J., Pauls, D. L., and Leckman, J. F. (1985). A twin study of Tourette syndrome. *Arch. Gen. Psychiatry* 42, 815–820. doi: 10.1001/archpsyc.1985.01790310077011

Randrup, A., and Munkvad, I. (1967). Stereotyped activities produced by amphetamine in several animal species and man. *Psychopharmacologia* 11, 300–310. doi: 10.1007/BF00404607

Randrup, A., Munkvad, I., and Udsen, P. (1963). Adrenergic mechanisms and amphetamine induced abnormal behaviour. *Acta Pharmacol. Toxicol. (Copenh).* 20, 145–157. doi: 10.1111/j.1600-0773.1963.tb01731.x

Shapiro, A. K., and Shapiro, E. (1968). Treatment of Gilles de la Tourette's Syndrome with haloperidol. *Br. J. Psychiatry* 114, 345–350. doi: 10.1192/bjp.114.508.345

Singer, H. S., Butler, I. J., Tune, L. E., Seifert, W. E. Jr., and Coyle, J. T. (1982). Dopaminergic dsyfunction in Tourette syndrome. *Ann. Neurol.* 12, 361–366. doi: 10.1002/ana.410120408

Singer, H. S., Hahn, I. H., and Moran, T. H. (1991). Abnormal dopamine uptake sites in postmortem striatum from patients with Tourette's syndrome. *Ann. Neurol.* 30, 558–562. doi: 10.1002/ana.410300408

Singer, H. S., Szymanski, S., Giuliano, J., Yokoi, F., Dogan, A. S., Brasic, J. R., et al. (2002). Elevated intrasynaptic dopamine release in Tourette's syndrome measured by PET. *Am. J. Psychiatry* 159, 1329–1336. doi: 10.1176/appi.ajp.159.8.1329

Steeves, T. D. L., Ko, J. H., Kideckel, D. M., Rusjan, P., Houle, S., Sandor, P., et al. (2010). Extrastriatal dopaminergic dysfunction in tourette syndrome. *Ann. Neurol.* 67, 170–181. doi: 10.1002/ana.21809

Surmeier, D. J., Ding, J., Day, M., Wang, Z., and Shen, W. (2007). D1 and D2 dopamine-receptor modulation of striatal glutamatergic signaling in striatal medium spiny neurons. *Trends Neurosci.* 30, 228–235. doi: 10.1016/j.tins.2007.03.008

Swerdlow, N. R., Braff, D. L., and Geyer, M. A. (1999). Cross-species studies of sensorimotor gating of the startle reflex. *Ann. N. Y. Acad. Sci.* 877, 202–216. doi: 10.1111/j.1749-6632.1999.tb09269.x

Swerdlow, N. R., and Geyer, M. A. (1998). Using an animal model of deficient sensorimotor gating to study the pathophysiology and new treatments of schizophrenia. *Schizophr. Bull.* 24, 285–301. doi: 10.1093/oxfordjournals.schbul.a033326

Swerdlow, N. R., Shoemaker, J. M., Platten, A., Pitcher, L., Goins, J., and Crain, S. (2003). Heritable differences in the effects of amphetamine but not DOI on startle gating in albino and hooded outbred rat strains. *Pharmacol. Biochem. Behav.* 75, 191–197. doi: 10.1016/S0091-3057(03)00078-9

Tarsy, D., Pycock, C. J., Meldrum, B. S., and Marsden, C. D. (1978). Focal contralateral myoclonus produced by inhibition of GABA action in the caudate nucleus of rats. *Brain* 101, 143–162. doi: 10.1093/brain/101.1.143

Taylor, J. L., Rajbhandari, A. K., Berridge, K. C., and Aldridge, J. W. (2010). Dopamine receptor modulation of repetitive grooming actions in the rat: potential relevance for Tourette syndrome. *Brain Res.* 1322, 92–101. doi: 10.1016/j.brainres.2010.01.052

Worbe, Y., Baup, N., Grabli, D., Chaigneau, M., Mounayar, S., McCairn, K., et al. (2009). Behavioral and movement disorders induced by local inhibitory dysfunction in primate striatum. *Cereb. Cortex* 19, 1844–1856. doi: 10.1093/cercor/bhn214

Worbe, Y., Marrakchi-Kacem, L., Lecomte, S., Valabregue, R., Poupon, F., Guevara, P., et al. (2015). Altered structural connectivity of cortico-striato-pallido-thalamic networks in Gilles de la Tourette syndrome. *Brain* 138, 472–482. doi: 10.1093/brain/awu311

Worbe, Y., Sgambato-Faure, V., Epinat, J., Chaigneau, M., Tandé, D., François, C., et al. (2013). Towards a primate model of Gilles de la Tourette syndrome: anatomo-behavioural correlation of disorders induced by striatal dysfunction. *Cortex* 49, 1126–1140. doi: 10.1016/j.cortex.2012.08.020

Xu, M., Kobets, A., Du, J.-C., Lennington, J., Li, L., Banasr, M., et al. (2015). Targeted ablation of cholinergic interneurons in the dorsolateral striatum produces behavioral manifestations of Tourette syndrome. *Proc. Natl. Acad. Sci. U.S.A.* 112, 893–898. doi: 10.1073/pnas.1419533112

Yael, D., Vinner, E., and Bar-Gad, I. (2015). Pathophysiology of tic disorders. *Mov. Disord.* 30, 1171–1178. doi: 10.1002/mds.26304

5

Mild White Matter Changes in Un-medicated Obsessive-Compulsive Disorder Patients and their Unaffected Siblings

Siyan Fan[1,2,3], Odile A. van den Heuvel[1,2,4,5], Danielle C. Cath[3,6], Ysbrand D. van der Werf[1,4,7], Stella J. de Wit[1,2,4,5], Froukje E. de Vries[1,2,4], Dick J. Veltman[2,4] and Petra J. W. Pouwels[4,8]*

[1] Department of Anatomy and Neurosciences, VU University Medical Center, Amsterdam, Netherlands, [2] Department of Psychiatry, VU University Medical Center, Amsterdam, Netherlands, [3] Department of Social and Behavioural Science, Utrecht University, Utrecht, Netherlands, [4] Neuroscience Campus Amsterdam, VU/VU University Medical Center, Amsterdam, Netherlands, [5] The OCD Team, Haukeland University Hospital, Bergen, Norway, [6] Academic Anxiety Center Altrecht, Utrecht, Netherlands, [7] Netherlands Institute for Neuroscience, Amsterdam, Netherlands, [8] Department of Physics and Medical Technology, VU University Medical Center, Amsterdam, Netherlands

Edited by:
Kirsten R. Müller-Vahl, Medical Doctor, Germany

Reviewed by:
Kerstin Jessica Plessen, University of Copenhagen, Denmark
Tino Prell, University Hospital Jena, Germany

***Correspondence:**
Odile A. van den Heuvel
oa.vandenheuvel@vumc.nl

Objective: Obsessive-compulsive disorder (OCD) is a common neuropsychiatric disorder with moderate genetic influences and white matter abnormalities in frontal-striatal and limbic regions. Inconsistencies in reported white matter results from diffusion tensor imaging (DTI) studies can be explained, at least partly, by medication use and between-group differences in disease profile and stage. We used a family design aiming to establish whether white matter abnormalities, if present in un-medicated OCD patients, also exist in their unaffected siblings.

Method: Forty-four OCD patients, un-medicated for at least the past 4 weeks, 15 of their unaffected siblings, and 37 healthy controls (HC) underwent DTI using a 3-Tesla MRI-scanner. Data analysis was done using tract-based spatial statistics (TBSS). Fractional anisotropy (FA), axial diffusivity (AD), radial diffusivity (RD), and mean diffusivity (MD) values were compared within seven skeletonised regions of interest (ROIs), i.e., corpus callosum, bilateral cingulum bundle, bilateral inferior longitudinal fasciculus/frontal-occipital fasciculus (ILF/FOF) and bilateral superior longitudinal fasciculus (SLF).

Results: Un-medicated OCD patients, compared with HC, had significantly lower FA in the left cingulum bundle. FA was trend-significantly lower in all other ROIs, except for the corpus callosum. Significant three-group differences in FA (and in RD at trend-significant level) were observed in the left cingulum bundle, with the unaffected siblings representing an intermediate group between OCD patients and HC.

Conclusions: OCD patients showed lower FA in the left cingulum bundle, partly driven by trend-significantly higher values in RD. Since the unaffected siblings were found to be an intermediate group between OCD patients and HC, this white matter alteration may be considered an endophenotype for OCD.

Keywords: diffusion tensor imaging, fractional anisotropy, obsessive-compulsive disorder, endophenotype

INTRODUCTION

Obsessive-compulsive disorder (OCD) is a debilitating neuropsychiatric disorder characterized by obsessions (intrusive recurrent thoughts) and/or compulsions (repetitive behaviors). OCD is moderately heritable (Hudziak et al., 2004; Van Grootheest et al., 2007), with heritability rates between 40 and 45% (Hudziak et al., 2004) and first degree relatives of the patients having a 4–10 times higher risk of developing OCD (Nestadt et al., 2000), depending on age of the proband. At the same time, the genetic basis of OCD is complex, multi-factorial, and under strong environmental influence (Grisham et al., 2008). Both structural and functional neural correlates of OCD have been found in the unaffected first-degree relatives of OCD patients (Chamberlain et al., 2008; Menzies et al., 2008b; de Wit et al., 2012; de Vries et al., 2014), suggesting that at least in part, the alterations are state-independent and might be regarded as correlates of genetic vulnerability, also called endophenotypes (Gottesman and Gould, 2003).

In contrast to the large literature on gray matter alterations in OCD (Radua and Mataix-Cols, 2009; Rotge et al., 2009; de Wit et al., 2014), white matter abnormalities in OCD have caught relatively less attention. A recent OCD Brain Imaging Consortium mega-analysis (de Wit et al., 2014), involving 412 OCD patients and 368 healthy controls (HC), reported decreased white matter volumes in frontal regions in the patient group, suggesting abnormalities of white matter connections between the prefrontal and subcortical regions within the frontal-striatal circuits. These results were consistent with some previous studies on white matter volume (van den Heuvel et al., 2009; Togao et al., 2010). White matter volume alterations have also been reported for the parietal and occipital lobes (Riffkin et al., 2005; Lázaro et al., 2009, 2011).

Although potentially related to white matter volume, the microstructure of the white matter tracts may provide additional insights into the pathophysiology of OCD. Diffusion tensor imaging (DTI) is a widely used neuroimaging technique to study brain tissue microstructure by quantification of the diffusion characteristics of water molecules (Le Bihan et al., 2001). Anisotropy, generally expressed as fractional anisotropy (FA), is a directionally dependent property of water diffusivity. FA in white matter reflects the underlying characteristics of microstructure, such as fiber density, axonal diameter, thickness of the myelin sheaths, and directionality of the fibers (Koch et al., 2014). FA is derived from the three eigenvalues of the diffusion tensor: $\lambda 1$, $\lambda 2$, and $\lambda 3$. The largest eigenvalue ($\lambda 1$), or axial diffusivity (AD), has been found to be a possible marker for axonal injury. The average of the two smaller eigenvalues $\lambda 2$ and $\lambda 3$, or radial diffusivity (RD) has been suggested as an indicator of myelin damage (Song et al., 2003; Fan et al., 2012). Mean diffusivity (MD) is the average of all three eigenvalues.

A recent DTI meta-analysis by Radua et al., comparing 204 OCD patients with 231 matched HC, showed reduced FA in the corpus callosum, the cingulum bundle, the inferior longitudinal fasciculi (ILF)/the frontal-occipital fasciculi (FOF), and the superior longitudinal fasciculi (SLF). Whether these alterations reflect state or trait effects (i.e., are the result of adaptive changes as a consequence of disease) or underlie disease vulnerability (and thus can be considered an endophenotype of OCD), cannot be deduced from the classical case-control studies. Therefore, extension to a family-based approach is warranted.

Menzies et al. (2008b) were the first to show that both OCD patients and their first-degree relatives had reduced FA in the right inferior parietal white matter and increased FA in the right medial frontal region. However, their results may have been partly confounded by suboptimal matching between the groups and medication use. Also, they did not explore differences in diffusivity parameters underlying the FA alterations. A combined DTI/voxel-based morphometry study using a monozygotic (MZ) twin design reported white matter characteristics of MZ twins who were concordant and discordant on obsessive-compulsive traits (den Braber et al., 2011). This study reported effects for environmental as opposed to genetic influences on regional white matter volume: the predominant FA decrease found in inferior frontal regions in the MZ concordant-high vs. concordant-low twins was suggested to reflect genetic (trait) effects, whereas the within MZ discordant twin comparison revealed increased dorsolateral prefrontal white matter changes in the high scoring twins, thought to reflect changes due to environmental effects. More recently, Shaw et al. investigated adult and adolescent OCD patients and their unaffected siblings and found similar morphological abnormalities in cortical and subcortical regions of caudate nucleus, thalamus and the right orbitofrontal cortex. Besides, both OCD patients and unaffected siblings, as compared with healthy controls, showed increased thickness of the right precuneus (Shaw et al., 2015).

In summary, available evidence for white matter abnormalities in OCD is largely inconsistent. We suggest several possible reasons for the reported discrepancies: (1) in OCD, white matter alterations might be subtle thus difficult to detect; (2) medication effects seem to confound the findings (Yoo et al., 2007; Fan et al., 2012; Benedetti et al., 2013; Radua et al., 2014); (3) results are highly variable across pediatric, adolescent and adult patients due to changes in white matter architecture throughout brain development (Peters et al., 2012); (4) debate has risen recently on whether FA alone is sufficient and sufficiently representative to indicate changes in white matter microstructure (Hasan, 2006; Fan et al., 2012; Szczepankiewicz et al., 2014); and (5) small samples and inconsistent methodologies have been used (Radua et al., 2014).

In this study, we aimed to replicate and extend previous findings, by exploring white matter microstructure in a group of un-medicated adult OCD patients, their unaffected siblings and gender and age-matched HC. By using tract-based spatial statistics (TBSS), we first aimed to investigate whether there were any abnormalities of FA in OCD patients compared with HC, and to investigate whether these between-group differences could be explained by any of the diffusivity measures (i.e., AD and RD). Finally, we aimed to explore whether alterations in diffusion parameters also existed in the unaffected siblings, to disentangle whether white matter changes are cause or consequence of the disease.

We used a region-of-interest (ROI) approach by selecting 7 ROIs, based on the results from the meta-analysis of Radua et al. (2014), corpus callosum, the bilateral cingulum bundle, the bilateral ILF/FOF and the bilateral SLF. We hypothesized that OCD patients compared with HC would show lower FA with changes in diffusivity values in the ROIs. Moreover, based on the familiality of OCD we expected that these abnormalities would be shared (as a trait), at least partly, in the unaffected siblings of the patients.

METHODS AND MATERIALS

Participants

Forty-four OCD patients who were un-medicated for at least 4 weeks when participating in the study (mean age 38.5 year, SD = 9.9), 15 of their unaffected siblings (mean age 38.1 year, SD = 14.1), and 37 HC (mean age 39.5 year, SD = 11.5) were included. The groups were matched on age, gender, handedness, and education level. OCD patients were recruited from the outpatient clinics within the Netherlands OCD Association cohort (Schuurmans et al., 2012), the Academic Anxiety Center Altrecht (Utrecht, the Netherlands), and by online advertisements. HC were recruited by local and online community advertisements.

All participants were screened on axis I psychiatric disorders using the Structured Clinical Interview for DSM-IV-TR Axis I Disorders (First et al., 2002). OCD symptom characteristics and severity were assessed with the Yale-Brown Obsessive Compulsive Scale (Y-BOCS, symptom list and severity scale) (Goodman et al., 1989) and the/Inventory-Revised (OCI-R) (Foa et al., 2002). Depressive symptoms were assessed with the Montgomery-Åsberg Depression Rating Scale (MADRS) (Montgomery and Asberg, 1979) and handedness with the Edinburgh Handedness Inventory (Oldfield, 1971).

Current psychoactive medication use, current or past psychosis, major physical illness, a history of a major neurological illness, and MRI contra-indications served as exclusion criteria. All the OCD patients were un-medicated for at least 4 weeks. No patients were excluded due to their psychiatric comorbidity (including tic disorder) and they could participate if they had a primary diagnosis of OCD without predominant hoarding. Siblings were included provided that they did not meet lifetime criteria for OCD and had no current DSM-IV-TR axis I diagnosis. Healthy control subjects had no current DSM-IV-TR axis I diagnosis and no family history of OCD. The local ethical review board of VU university medical center approved all procedures and all subjects provided written informed consent.

MRI Acquisition

MRI was performed using a whole-body 3-Tesla MR system (Signa HDxt, GE Healthcare, Milwaukee, USA) equipped with an eight-channel phased-array head coil. Diffusion weighted echo-planar imaging was collected in 30 diffusion weighted ($b = 1000$ s/mm^2) and five reference ($b = 0$ s/mm^2) volumes with 49 contiguous axial slices of 2.4 mm slice thickness for covering the whole brain (repetition time TR 14 s, echo time TE 85 ms). The acquired in-plane resolution was 2.0 × 2.0 mm, which was reconstructed to 1.0 × 1.0 mm. Parallel imaging was applied with an acceleration factor of 2.

Data Processing

The diffusion MRI data were preprocessed for motion and eddy-current correction by using the FMRIB Software Library (FSL5; http://fsl.fmrib.ox.ac.uk/fsl). By fitting a tensor model to the raw diffusion data voxel-wise values of FA, AD, RD, and MD were obtained. All subjects' FA data were aligned to MNI standard space by using the non-linear image registration tool (FNIRT). Next, the mean FA image was created and thinned to create a mean FA skeleton, which represents the centers of all tracts common to the group. Each subject's aligned FA data was then projected onto this skeleton and the resulting data were fed into voxel-wise cross-subject statistics. The same non-linear registration was applied to the diffusivity parameters AD, RD and MD.

Statistical Analysis

We compared the skeletonized diffusion parameters between OCD patients, the unaffected siblings and healthy controls using a ROI approach, including the 7 ROI's (i.e., the corpus callosum, the bilateral cingulum bundle, the bilateral ILF/FOF, and the bilateral SLF) based on the results from the meta-analysis of Radua et al. (2014). The Johns Hopkins University (JHU) ICBM-DTI-81 white-matter labels atlas provided by FSL was chosen to define the ROIs. Permutation-based testing (5000 permutations) was carried out with Randomise, using Threshold-Free Cluster Enhancement (Smith and Nichols, 2009), and p-values were corrected for family wise error rate (FWE) taking into account multiple spatial comparisons. In addition to the ROI approach, for exploratory reasons, we performed whole-brain skeletonized voxel-wise statistics in order to check for group differences in the brain areas outside the ROIs. Corrected $p < 0.05$ was considered significant, and uncorrected $p < 0.05$ was considered a trend. Age and gender were added as covariates.

Randomise was used to compare FA values between OCD and HC. For each skeletonised ROI that had significantly different FA values between the two groups, we performed a three-group comparison, now including the unaffected siblings, using Randomise. Of voxels that showed difference in the three-group comparison, the mean diffusion parameters (for FA, AD, RD, and MD) were extracted for each subject (at uncorrected $p < 0.05$). Subsequently, One-way ANOVA analysis was performed to investigate the overall group effect (three groups) of AD, RD, and MD ($p < 0.05$). *Post-hoc* 2-sample-T tests were conducted to explore differences within groups. Within-group (OCD patients only) multiple regression analyses were carried out to investigate the relationship between FA and patients' disease severity (i.e., YBOCS severity scores).

RESULTS

Demographic and Clinical Characteristics

Age, sex, education level and handedness did not differ significantly between OCD patients, unaffected siblings, and HC (see **Table 1**). A main effect of group was found for Y-BOCS (symptom list and severity scale), the OCI-R and MADRS. OCD patients scored higher compared with HC and the unaffected siblings ($p < 0.01$); the sibling group did not significantly differ from the HC group on these measures. Twenty-five OCD patients (57%) also met criteria for one or more comorbid current axis I diagnosis. No significant difference was found between OCD patients with ($n = 25$) or without ($n = 19$) comorbid diagnoses on demographic or other clinical measures ($p > 0.16$) (see **Table 1**).

TBSS Analysis: FA Differences between OCD and HC

OCD patients, compared with HC, had significantly lower FA in the left cingulum bundle (peak MNI coordinates $x = -24$, $y = -13$, $z = -32$; ROI-corrected $p < 0.05$) as shown in **Figure 1** and **Table 2**. At trend-significance level (uncorrected $p < 0.05$) OCD patients showed a lower FA in a larger area of the left and in parts of the right cingulum bundle, bilateral ILF, and bilateral SLF (see **Figures 2A,B** and **Table 2**). No difference in FA was found in corpus callosum (uncorrected $p > 0.14$). There were no areas in which OCD patients had higher FA than HC. TBSS analysis of the whole brain skeleton revealed no significant differences in FA between OCD and HC at the corrected level.

YBOCS and OCI-R scores were found neither positively nor negatively correlated with FA within the OCD patients group.

Three Group Comparisons—Endophenotype Analysis

FA of the left cingulum bundle showed a significant effect of group (peak MNI coordinates $x = -28$, $y = -13$, $z = -31$; ROI-corrected $p < 0.05$) as shown in **Figure 1**. Mean diffusion parameters values from the left cingulum bundle were extracted

TABLE 1 | Demographic and clinical characteristics of obsessive compulsive disorder patients, unaffected siblings, and healthy controls.

	OCD Patients (N = 44)		Siblings (N = 15)		HC (N = 37)		Analysis	
	N	%	*N*	%	*N*	%	X^2 (df = 2) *p*	
DEMOGRAPHIC MEASURES								
Gender (men)	22	50	11	73	18	49		0.231
Handedness (right)	37	84	12	80	32	86		0.841
	Mean	**SD**	**Mean**	**SD**	**Mean**	**SD**	**F (df = 2, 93) *p***	
Age (years)	38.5	9.9	38.1	14.1	39.5	11.5	0.1	0.893
Education level[a]	5.9	1.9	6.0	1.5	5.8	1.9	0.1[b]	0.953
CLINICAL MEASURES								
Y-BOCS severity (range 0–40)	21.48	6.16	0.33	0.03	0	0	84.96[b]	<0.001
OCI-R								
Total score	23.75	12.27	3.27	3.35	3.22	4.80	59.23[b]	<0.001
Washing score	2.77	3.84	0.20	0.41	0.30	0.62	14.17[b]	<0.001
Checking score	6.25	3.85	0.47	0.74	0.49	0.93	52.66[b]	<0.001
Order score	4.75	3.85	0.87	1.41	0.81	1.53	31.07[b]	<0.001
Obsession score	5.36	3.83	0.53	0.92	0.32	1.36	50.20[b]	<0.001
MADRS	11.66	8.54	1.93	3.77	0.89	1.51	52.60[b]	<0.001

[a]Education level was recorded in nine levels ranging from 1 (no finished education) to 9 (university training). [b]Kruskal-Wallis test, H (df = 2, 93). Y-BOCS, Yale-Brown Obsessive Compulsive Scale; OCI-R, Obsessive-Compulsive Inventory-Revised; MADRS, Montgomery-Åsberg Depression Rating Scale; HC, Healthy Controls.

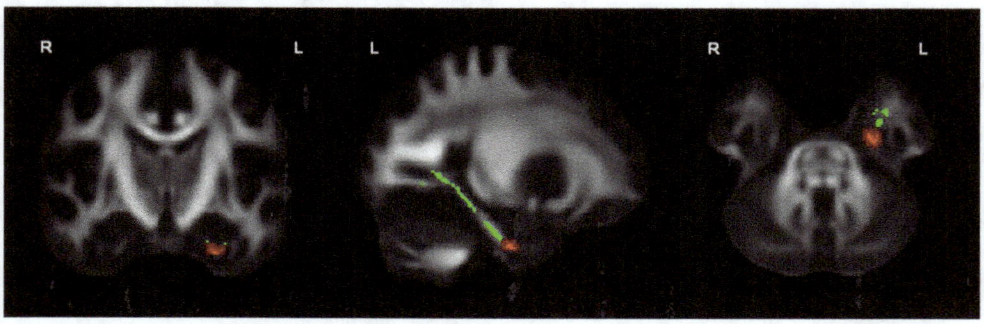

FIGURE 1 | OCD patients ($n = 44$) showed significantly lower FA than healthy controls ($n = 37$) in the left cingulum bundle, significant at $p < 0.05$ (in red; corrected for multiple comparisons); for illustration purposes, the displayed skeletonized results were thickened. In green the parts of the skeleton within the pre-defined ROI.

TABLE 2 | Locations of decreased FA in OCD patients compared to healthy controls.

ROIs	Peak coordinates			Cluster/Area	OCD < HC *p*-value (uncorrected)
	x	*Y*	*z*		
Left * cingulum bundle	−24	−13	−32	38	0.001*
Right cingulum bundle	25	−5	−33	28	0.003
Left ILF/FOF	−37	−61	2	61	0.011
Right ILF/FOF	43	−50	−17	110	0.003
Left SLF	−51	−20	30	131	0.05
Right SLF	56	−12	−22	105	0.03

*Peak MNI coordinates, cluster sizes and p-values (uncorrected). *indicates significance at $p < 0.05$ corrected for multiple comparisons for ROI. FA, fractional anisotropy; IFO/FOF, inferior longitudinal fasciculus/frontal occipital fasciculus; SLF, superior longitudinal fasciculus; HC, healthy controls.*

for all subjects based on voxels identified at uncorrected $p < 0.05$ in the [FA (three-group comparison)] F-contrast. We selected values within this larger area of the left cingulum bundle (167 voxels), since the significant area at corrected $p < 0.05$ is a relatively small cluster of 38 voxels located close to the inferior border of the cingulum bundle (see **Figure 1**). **Figure 3** and **Table 3** show that, after correction for multiple comparisons, mean FA was significantly lower in OCD patients compared with HC [$F_{(2, 93)} = 6.40, p < 0.001$]; mean FA values of unaffected siblings were intermediate between those of the OCD patients and of the HC, although *post-hoc* 2-sample-T comparisons did not show a significant difference between siblings and either the OCD patients or the HC ($p = 0.223$ and $p = 1.000$ respectively).

Mean values of AD and MD in the left cingulum bundle (see **Table 3**) did not significantly differ across groups. RD values in this region showed a reverse pattern compared to FA values, with the OCD patients showing trend-significantly higher RD compared with HC and the unaffected siblings representing an intermediate group (see **Table 3** and **Figure 3**). Although no effect of group was found for these diffusivity values after correction for multiple comparisons, a trend-significant effect of group was observed for the RD values [$F_{(2, 93)} = 3.34, p = 0.04$ uncorrected]. To test laterality of these results, we performed the same procedure for the diffusivity values in the right cingulum bundle, showing a similar pattern, although it does not surpass the trend-significant level.

DISCUSSION

The main finding of the present study is lower FA in the left cingulum bundle in un-medicated OCD patients compared with HC, which partially replicates the findings from the meta-analysis conducted by Radua et al. (2014). We also found, in line with Radua et al., although at uncorrected significance level, lower FA in the other ROIs (except for the corpus callosum), i.e., the right cingulum bundle, the bilateral ILF/FOF, and the bilateral SLF. Lower FA appeared to be associated with higher RD. The three-group comparison showed that the unaffected siblings seemed to represent an intermediate group between the OCD patients and HC with respect to FA in the left cingulum bundle.

Lower FA in the cingulum bundle has been reported by most studies that investigated adult OCD patients (Koch et al., 2014; Radua et al., 2014). Increasing evidence from structural and functional neuroimaging research in recent years has emphasized the impact of deficits in temporo-parietal-occipital regions in the pathophysiology of OCD besides the frontal-striatal and fronto-limbic neurocircuitries (Menzies et al., 2008a; Piras et al., 2013). The cingulum bundle contains many short and long association fibers linking the frontal lobe with the temporal lobe (Schmahmann and Pandya, 2006), supporting communication between the prefrontal, parietal, and temporal regions (Jones et al., 2012). The finding of lower FA in the left cingulum bundle in OCD supports the suggested involvement of temporal and parietal regions in the pathophysiology of the disorder.

Although FA values in the right cingulum bundle, ILF/IFOF and SLF were only trend-wise lower in OCD patients compared with HC, these findings may still be relevant since these differences were observed in all a-priori hypothesized regions bilaterally.

In general, the changes in diffusion parameters observed in these un-medicated OCD patients were subtle. Although Radua et al. (2014) in their meta-analyses reported widespread white matter abnormalities in OCD, no clear evidence so far has suggested OCD as a typical white matter disease (Koch et al., 2014). Furthermore, the lack of consistent DTI findings in the OCD literature may be explained, at least partly, by the impact of medication in OCD. Radua et al. (2014) reported that the lower FA was most prominent in samples with more medicated OCD patients. Benedetti et al. (2013) found that medicated OCD patients had higher RD in the corpus callosum and adjacent cingulate gyrus when compared to drug-naïve OCD patients and HC. Other studies in OCD also showed pharmacological treatment effects on white matter alterations (Yoo et al., 2007; Fan et al., 2012). Therefore, the subtle white matter abnormalities found in our un-medicated patient sample suggests that medication might be a potential confounder in most previous studies.

The here reported (trend-) significantly lower FA values all concern white matter regions that are spatially connected to temporal-parietal-occipital regions. Structural abnormalities found in both gray matter and white matter regions in posterior parts of the brain of OCD patients mainly concern the parietal lobe extending to the temporal and occipital lobes (Piras et al., 2013). These posterior regions are associated with cognitive functions including visuo-spatial functions, which have been consistently found to be impaired in OCD patients (Cohen et al., 1996; Savage et al., 1999). Our findings thus indirectly suggest abnormalities in these white matter microstructures might also be contributors to the cognitive impairments in visuo-spatial abilities.

The three-group comparison on FA in the left cingulum bundle showed a significant effect of group, with the unaffected siblings showing intermediate FA values. Mean AD and MD

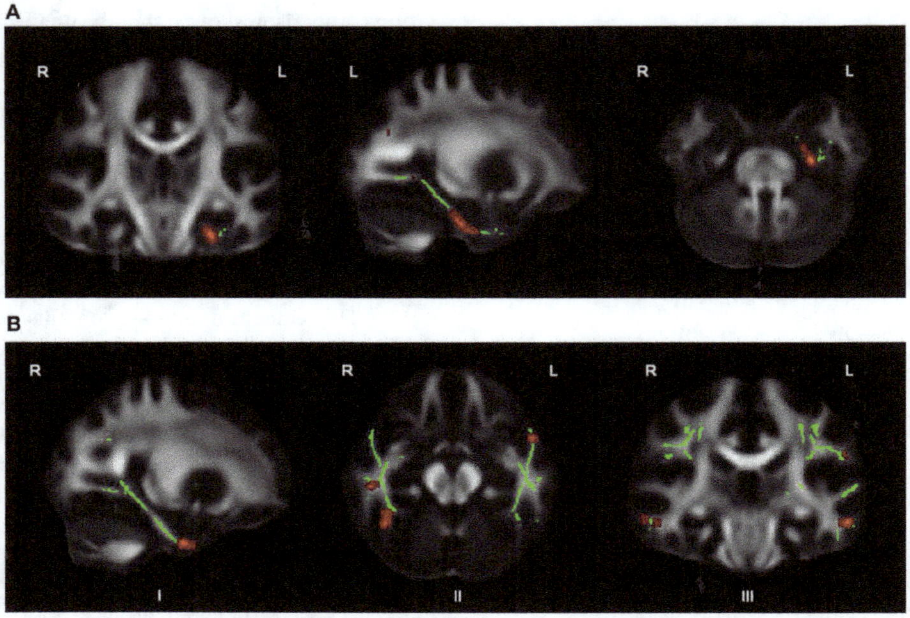

FIGURE 2 | OCD patients ($n = 44$) compared with healthy controls ($n = 37$) showed trend-significantly decreased FA in a larger part of the left cingulum bundle (A), in parts of the right cingulum bundle (I), bilateral ILF (II), and bilateral SLF (III) (in red; at $p \leq 0.05$ uncorrected) (B); for illustration purposes, the displayed skeletonized results were thickened. In green the parts of the skeleton within the pre-defined ROIs.

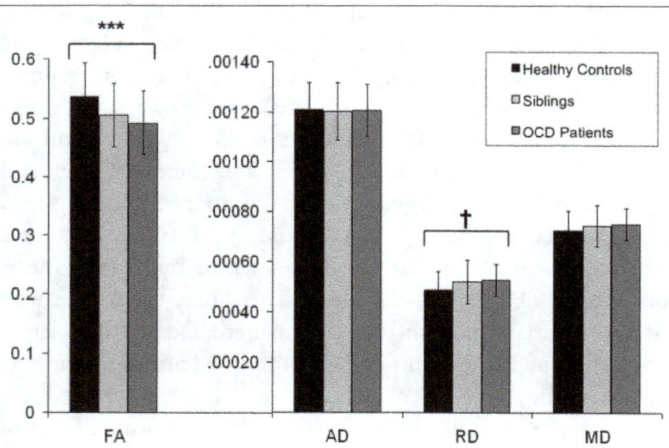

FIGURE 3 | Mean FA, AD, RD, and MD values from the extracted voxels in the left cingulum bundle across groups. Y-axis indicates the mean FA, AD, RD, and MD values; along the X-axis are the three subject groups (healthy controls, unaffected siblings, and OCD patients). Solid dark bard represent healthy controls. Striped bars represent unaffected siblings. Light bars represent OCD patients. *** indicates $p < 0.001$. † indicates $p < 0.05$ (trend significant). Error Bars: ± 1 SD. FA, fractional anisotropy; AD, axial diffusivity; RD, radial diffusivity; MD, mean diffusivity; OCD, obsessive-compulsive disorder.

TABLE 3 | Means and standard deviations of FA, AD, RD, and MD values for subject groups of healthy controls, unaffected siblings and OCD patients in the left cingulum bundle.

Left cingulum bundle	HC	Siblings	OCD patients
	$N = 37$	$N = 15$	$N = 44$
	Mean ± SD	Mean ± SD	Mean ± SD
FA	0.54 ± 0.06	0.51 ± 0.05	0.49 ± 0.05***
AD	120.9 ± 10.9	120.2 ± 11.4	120.8 ± 10.3
RD	48.5 ± 7.3	51.8 ± 8.6	52.5 ± 6.4
MD	72.6 ± 7.7	74.6 ± 8.3	75.2 ± 6.3

*Diffusivities AD, MD, and RD are given in units of 10^{-5} mm^2/s. ***indicates $p<.001$ compared with healthy controls. AD, axial diffusivity; RD, radial diffusivity; MD, mean diffusivity; OCD, obsessive-compulsive disorder; HC, healthy controls.*

values did not differ across groups. Mean RD revealed a reverse pattern to that seen for FA: RD was trend-significantly higher in OCD patients compared to HC, with intermediate values in unaffected siblings. Such changes in diffusion parameters are in line with findings from previous DTI studies in OCD (Bora et al., 2011; Fan et al., 2012). Although Song et al. (2003) suggested a higher RD to be associated with demyelination, others have shown that the interpretation of changes in RD and AD needs careful consideration, due to the inherent disbalance between fiber thickness and imaging resolution (Wheeler-Kingshott and Cercignani, 2009). Although a few genetic studies suggested myelination in the OCD pathophysiology (Zai et al., 2004; Stewart et al., 2007), we can only speculate about possible disruption of myelin integrity contributing to the white matter abnormalities in the left cingulum bundle. A similar pattern of lower FA in combination with higher RD (and normal AD values) has also been reported for autism, schizophrenia, and depression (Alexander et al., 2007;

Ashtari et al., 2007; Lee et al., 2007; Michael et al., 2008; Seal et al., 2008; Whitford et al., 2010; Korgaonkar et al., 2011).

With regard to both FA and RD, the unaffected siblings seem to represent an intermediate group between patients and HC, suggesting that white matter alterations can be considered, at least partly, an endophenotype of OCD. The identification of disease endophenotypes can help to identify possible genetic risk factors of diseases and environmental effects. Menzies et al. (2008b) also found abnormal FA values in OCD patients as well as their first-degree relatives, although in that study abnormalities were mainly reported in the parietal and medial frontal regions.

To our knowledge, this is the first study investigating the white matter endophenotype of un-medicated OCD by exploring FA in combination with AD and RD. The sample sizes of the OCD and control groups were fairly large compared to previous studies and the ROIs were selected based on the most recent meta-analysis (Radua et al., 2014). An important limitation of the present study is that the reported findings were not corrected for multiple comparisons as we identified 7 ROIs *a priori*. In addition, we can't exclude the long-term effects of past medication use, although a 4-week washout period is thought as a sufficient time period for wearing off direct medication effects. Finally, only 15 unaffected siblings were included in the study. Due to the limited sample size, we can't rule out the possibility that the observation that the unaffected siblings were neither significantly different from OCD patients nor the HC might be due to the limited statistical power.

In conclusion, this DTI study shows white matter alterations in OCD patients, un-medicated for at least 4 weeks, compared with HC, mainly in the left cingulum bundle. A lower FA seems to be related to trend-wise higher RD, suggesting potential disruption of myelin integrity in this region. The fact that the unaffected siblings represent an intermediate group between OCD patients and HC is suggestive for a white matter endophenotype of OCD, reflecting genetic vulnerability.

AUTHOR CONTRIBUTIONS

SF contributed to data analysis and paper writing. OH contributed to daily supervision on the research analyses and paper writing. DC, YV, and DV contributed to supervision on the research. SD and FD contributed to data collection. PP contributed to technical supports and daily supervision on the research analyses and paper writing.

ACKNOWLEDGMENTS

This study was supported by FP7-People-2012-ITN grant (316978, project: TS-Eurotrain), the Dutch Organization for Scientific Research (NWO) with a ZonMW VENI grant (916-86-038 to OV) and ZonMW AGIKO grant (920-03-542 to FD), a NARSAD young investigators award of the Brain & Behavior Research Foundation (to OV), the Amsterdam Brain Imaging Platform, the Netherlands Brain Foundation (2010(1)-50 to OV), the Stichting tot Steun VCVGZ (STO957 to DC).

REFERENCES

Alexander, A. L., Lee, J. E., Lazar, M., Boudos, R., DuBray, M. B., Oakes, T. R., et al. (2007). Diffusion tensor imaging of the corpus callosum in Autism. *Neuroimage* 34, 61–73. doi: 10.1016/j.neuroimage.2006.08.032

Ashtari, M., Cottone, J., Ardekani, B. A., Cervellione, K., Szeszko, P. R., Wu, J., et al. (2007). Disruption of white matter integrity in the inferior longitudinal fasciculus in adolescents with schizophrenia as revealed by fiber tractography. *Arch. Gen. Psychiatry* 64, 1270–1280. doi: 10.1001/archpsyc.64.11.1270

Benedetti, F., Giacosa, C., Radaelli, D., Poletti, S., Pozzi, E., Dallaspezia, S., et al. (2013). Widespread changes of white matter microstructure in obsessive-compulsive disorder: effect of drug status. *Eur. Neuropsychopharmacol.* 23, 581–593. doi: 10.1016/j.euroneuro.2012.07.002

Bora, E., Harrison, B. J., Fornito, A., Cocchi, L., Pujol, J., Fontenelle, L. F., et al. (2011). White matter microstructure in patients with obsessive-compulsive disorder. *J. Psychiatry Neurosci.* 36, 42–46. doi: 10.1503/jpn.100082

Chamberlain, S. R., Menzies, L., Hampshire, A., Suckling, J., Fineberg, N. A., del Campo, N., et al. (2008). Orbitofrontal dysfunction in patients with obsessive-compulsive disorder and their unaffected relatives. *Science* 321, 421–422. doi: 10.1126/science.1154433

Cohen, L. J., Hollander, E., DeCaria, C. M., Stein, D. J., Simeon, D., Liebowitz, M. R., et al. (1996). Specificity of neuropsychological impairment in obsessive-compulsive disorder: a comparison with social phobic and normal control subjects. *J. Neuropsychiatry Clin. Neurosci.* 8, 82–85. doi: 10.1176/jnp.8.1.82

de Vries, F. E., de Wit, S. J., Cath, D. C., van der Werf, Y. D., van der Borden, V., van Rossum, T. B., et al. (2014). Compensatory frontoparietal activity during working memory: an endophenotype of obsessive-compulsive disorder. *Biol. Psychiatry* 76, 878–887. doi: 10.1016/j.biopsych.2013.11.021

de Wit, S. J., Alonso, P., Schweren, L., Mataix-Cols, D., Lochner, C., Menchón, J. M., et al. (2014). Multicenter voxel-based morphometry mega-analysis of structural brain scans in obsessive-compulsive disorder. *Am. J. Psychiatry* 171, 340–349. doi: 10.1176/appi.ajp.2013.13040574

de Wit, S. J., de Vries, F. E., van der Werf, Y. D., Cath, D. C., Heslenfeld, D. J., Veltman, E. M., et al. (2012). Presupplementary motor area hyperactivity during response inhibition: a candidate endophenotype of obsessive-compulsive disorder. *Am. J. Psychiatry* 169, 1100–1108. doi: 10.1176/appi.ajp.2012.12010073

den Braber, A., van't Ent, D., Boomsma, D. I., Cath, D. C., Veltman, D. J., Thompson, P. M., et al. (2011). White matter differences in monozygotic twins discordant or concordant for obsessive-compulsive symptoms: a combined diffusion tensor imaging/voxel-based morphometry study. *Biol. Psychiatry* 70, 969–977. doi: 10.1016/j.biopsych.2011.03.029

Fan, Q., Yan, X., Wang, J., Chen, Y., Wang, X., Li, C., et al. (2012). Abnormalities of white matter microstructure in unmedicated obsessive-compulsive disorder and changes after medication. *PLoS ONE* 7:e35889. doi: 10.1371/journal.pone.0035889

First, M. B. S. R., Gibbon, M., and Williams, J. B. W. (2002). *Structured Clinical Interview for DSM-IV-TR Axis I Disorder, Research Version* . Patient Edition (SCID-I/P) ed. (New York, NY: Biometrics Research; New York State Psychiatric Institute).

Foa, E. B., Huppert, J. D., Leiberg, S., Langner, R., Kichic, R., Hajcak, G., et al. (2002). The Obsessive-Compulsive Inventory: development and validation of a short version. *Psychol. Assess.* 14, 485–496. doi: 10.1037/1040-3590.14.4.485

Goodman, W. K., Price, L. H., Rasmussen, S. A., Mazure, C., Delgado, P., Heninger, G. R., et al. (1989). The yale-brown obsessive compulsive scale. II. Validity. *Arch Gen Psychiatry* 46, 1012–1016. doi: 10.1001/archpsyc.1989.01810110054008

Gottesman, I. I., and Gould, T. D. (2003). The endophenotype concept in psychiatry: etymology and strategic intentions. *Am. J. Psychiatry* 160, 636–645. doi: 10.1176/appi.ajp.160.4.636

Grisham, J. R., Anderson, T. M., and Sachdev, P. S. (2008). Genetic and environmental influences on obsessive-compulsive disorder. *Eur. Arch. Psychiatry Clin. Neurosci.* 258, 107–116. doi: 10.1007/s00406-00 7-0789-0

Hasan, K. M. (2006). Diffusion tensor eigenvalues or both mean diffusivity and fractional anisotropy are required in quantitative clinical diffusion tensor MR reports: fractional anisotropy alone is not sufficient. *Radiology* 239, 611–612; author reply 612–613. doi: 10.1148/radiol.2392051172

Hudziak, J. J., Van Beijsterveldt, C. E., Althoff, R. R., Stanger, C., Rettew, D. C., Nelson, E. C., et al. (2004). Genetic and environmental contributions to the Child Behavior Checklist Obsessive-Compulsive Scale: a cross-cultural twin study. *Arch. Gen. Psychiatry* 61, 608–616. doi: 10.1001/archpsyc.6 1.6.608

Jones, D. K., Christiansen, K. F., Chapman, R. J., and Aggleton, J. P. (2012). Distinct subdivisions of the cingulum bundle revealed by diffusion MRI fibre tracking: implications for neuropsychological investigations. *Neuropsychologia* 51, 67–78. doi: 10.1016/j.neuropsychologia.2012.11.018

Koch, K., Reess, T. J., Rus, O. G., Zimmer, C., and Zaudig, M. (2014). Diffusion tensor imaging (DTI) studies in patients with obsessive-compulsive disorder (OCD): a review. *J. Psychiatr. Res.* 54, 26–35. doi: 10.1016/j.jpsychires.2014.03.006

Korgaonkar, M. S., Grieve, S. M., Koslow, S. H., Gabrieli, J. D., Gordon, E., and Williams, L. M. (2011). Loss of white matter integrity in major depressive disorder: evidence using tract-based spatial statistical analysis of diffusion tensor imaging. *Hum. Brain Mapp.* 32, 2161–2171. doi: 10.1002/hbm. 21178

Lázaro, L., Bargalló, N., Castro-Fornieles, J., Falcón, C., Andrés, S., Calvo, R., et al. (2009). Brain changes in children and adolescents with obsessive-compulsive disorder before and after treatment: a voxel-based morphometric MRI study. *Psychiatry Res.* 172, 140–146. doi: 10.1016/j.pscychresns.2008.12.007

Lázaro, L., Castro-Fornieles, J., Cullell, C., Andrés, S., Falcón, C., Calvo, R., et al. (2011). A voxel-based morphometric MRI study of stabilized obsessive-compulsive adolescent patients. *Prog. Neuropsychopharmacol. Biol. Psychiatry* 35, 1863–1869. doi: 10.1016/j.pnpbp.2011.07.016

Le Bihan, D., Mangin, J. F., Poupon, C., Clark, C. A., Pappata, S., Molko, N., et al. (2001). Diffusion tensor imaging: concepts and applications. *J. Magn. Reson. Imaging* 13, 534–546. doi: 10.1002/jmri.1076

Lee, J. E., Bigler, E. D., Alexander, A. L., Lazar, M., DuBray, M. B., Chung, M. K., et al. (2007). Diffusion tensor imaging of white matter in the superior temporal gyrus and temporal stem in autism. *Neurosci. Lett.* 424, 127–132. doi: 10.1016/j.neulet.2007.07.042

Menzies, L., Chamberlain, S. R., Laird, A. R., Thelen, S. M., Sahakian, B. J., and Bullmore, E. T. (2008a). Integrating evidence from neuroimaging and neuropsychological studies of obsessive-compulsive disorder: the orbitofronto-striatal model revisited. *Neurosci. Biobehav. Rev.* 32, 525–549. doi: 10.1016/j.neubiorev.2007.09.005

Menzies, L., Williams, G. B., Chamberlain, S. R., Ooi, C., Fineberg, N., Suckling, J., et al. (2008b). White matter abnormalities in patients with obsessive-compulsive disorder and their first-degree relatives. *Am. J. Psychiatry* 165, 1308–1315. doi: 10.1176/appi.ajp.2008.07101677

Michael, A. M., Calhoun, V. D., Pearlson, G. D., Baum, S. A., and Caprihan, A. (2008). Correlations of diffusion tensor imaging values and symptom scores in patients with schizophrenia. *Conf. Proc. IEEE Eng. Med. Biol. Soc.* 2008, 5494–5497. doi: 10.1109/iembs.2008.4650458

Montgomery, S. A., and Asberg, M. (1979). A new depression scale designed to be sensitive to change. *Br. J. Psychiatry* 134, 382–389. doi: 10.1192/bjp.13 4.4.382

Nestadt, G., Grados, M., and Samuels, J. F. (2000). Genetics of obsessive-compulsive disorder. *Psychiatr. Clin. North Am.* 33, 141–158. doi: 10.1016/j.psc.2009.11.001

Oldfield, R. C. (1971). The assessment and analysis of handedness: the Edinburgh inventory. *Neuropsychologia* 9, 97–113. doi: 10.1016/0028-3932(71)90067-4

Peters, B. D., Szeszko, P. R., Radua, J., Ikuta, T., Gruner, P., DeRosse, P., et al. (2012). White matter development in adolescence: diffusion tensor imaging and meta-analytic results. *Schizophr. Bull.* 38, 1308–1317. doi: 10.1093/schbul/sbs054

Piras, F., Piras, F., Chiapponi, C., Girardi, P., Caltagirone, C., and Spalletta, G. (2013). Widespread structural brain changes in OCD: a systematic review of voxel-based morphometry studies. *Cortex* 62, 89–108. doi: 10.1016/j.cortex.2013.01.016

Radua, J., Grau, M., van den Heuvel, O. A., Thiebaut de Schotten, M., Stein, D. J., Canales-Rodríguez, E. J., et al. (2014). Multimodal voxel-based meta-analysis of white matter abnormalities in obsessive-compulsive disorder. *Neuropsychopharmacology* 39, 1547–1557. doi: 10.1038/npp.2014.5

Radua, J., and Mataix-Cols, D. (2009). Voxel-wise meta-analysis of grey matter changes in obsessive-compulsive disorder. *Br. J. Psychiatry* 195, 393–402. doi: 10.1192/bjp.bp.108.055046

Riffkin, J., Yücel, M., Maruff, P., Wood, S. J., Soulsby, B., Olver, J., et al. (2005). A manual and automated MRI study of anterior cingulate and orbito-frontal cortices, and caudate nucleus in obsessive-compulsive disorder: comparison with healthy controls and patients with schizophrenia. *Psychiatry Res.* 138, 99–113. doi: 10.1016/j.pscychresns.2004.11.007

Rotge, J. Y., Guehl, D., Dilharreguy, B., Tignol, J., Bioulac, B., Allard, M., et al. (2009). Meta-analysis of brain volume changes in obsessive-compulsive disorder. *Biol. Psychiatry* 65, 75–83. doi: 10.1016/j.biopsych.2008.06.019

Savage, C. R., Baer, L., Keuthen, N. J., Brown, H. D., Rauch, S. L., and Jenike, M. A. (1999). Organizational strategies mediate nonverbal memory impairment in obsessive-compulsive disorder. *Biol. Psychiatry* 45, 905–916. doi: 10.1016/S0006-3223(98)00278-9

Schmahmann, J., and Pandya, D. (2006). *Fiber Pathways of the Brain.* New York, NY: Oxford University Press.

Schuurmans, J., van Balkom, A. J., van Megen, H. J., Smit, J. H., Eikelenboom, M., Cath, D. C., et al. (2012). The Netherlands Obsessive Compulsive Disorder Association (NOCDA) study: design and rationale of a longitudinal naturalistic study of the course of OCD and clinical characteristics of the sample at baseline. *Int. J. Methods Psychiatr. Res.* 21, 273–285. doi: 10.1002/mpr.1372

Seal, M. L., Yücel, M., Fornito, A., Wood, S. J., Harrison, B. J., Walterfang, M., et al. (2008). Abnormal white matter microstructure in schizophrenia: a voxelwise analysis of axial and radial diffusivity. *Schizophr. Res.* 101, 106–110. doi: 10.1016/j.schres.2007.12.489

Shaw, P., Sharp, W., Sudre, G., Wharton, A., Greenstein, D., Raznahan, A., et al. (2015). Subcortical and cortical morphological anomalies as an endophenotype in obsessive-compulsive disorder. *Mol. Psychiatry* 20, 224–231. doi: 10.1038/mp.2014.3

Smith, S. M., and Nichols, T. E. (2009). Threshold-free cluster enhancement: addressing problems of smoothing, threshold dependence and localisation in cluster inference. *Neuroimage* 44, 83–98. doi: 10.1016/j.neuroimage.2008.03.061

Song, S. K., Sun, S. W., Ju, W. K., Lin, S. J., Cross, A. H., and Neufeld, A. H. (2003). Diffusion tensor imaging detects and differentiates axon and myelin degeneration in mouse optic nerve after retinal ischemia. *Neuroimage* 20, 1714–1722. doi: 10.1016/j.neuroimage.2003.07.005

Stewart, S. E., Platko, J., Fagerness, J., Birns, J., Jenike, E., Smoller, J. W., et al. (2007). A genetic family-based association study of OLIG2 in obsessive-compulsive disorder. *Arch. Gen. Psychiatry* 64, 209–214. doi: 10.1001/archpsyc.64.2.209

Szczepankiewicz, F., Lasic, S., van Westen, D., Sundgren, P. C., Englund, E., Westin, C. F., et al. (2014). Quantification of microscopic diffusion anisotropy disentangles effects of orientation dispersion from microstructure: applications in healthy volunteers and in brain tumors. *Neuroimage* 104, 241–252. doi: 10.1016/j.neuroimage.2014.09.057

Togao, O., Yoshiura, T., Nakao, T., Nabeyama, M., Sanematsu, H., Nakagawa, A., et al. (2010). Regional gray and white matter volume abnormalities in obsessive-compulsive disorder: a voxel-based morphometry study. *Psychiatry Res.* 184, 29–37. doi: 10.1016/j.pscychresns.2010.06.011

van den Heuvel, O. A., Remijnse, P. L., Mataix-Cols, D., Vrenken, H., Groenewegen, H. J., Uylings, H. B., et al. (2009). The major symptom dimensions of obsessive-compulsive disorder are mediated by partially distinct neural systems. *Brain* 132, 853–868. doi: 10.1093/brain/ awn267

Van Grootheest, D. S., Cath, D. C., Beekman, A. T., and Boomsma, D. I. (2007). Genetic and environmental influences on obsessive-compulsive symptoms in adults: a population-based twin-family study. *Psychol. Med.* 37, 1635–1644. doi: 10.1017/s0033291707000980

Wheeler-Kingshott, C. A., and Cercignani, M. (2009). About "axial" and "radial" diffusivities. *Magn. Reson. Med.* 61, 1255–1260. doi: 10.1002/mrm.21965

Whitford, T. J., Kubicki, M., Schneiderman, J. S., O'Donnell, L. J., King, R., Alvarado, J. L., et al. (2010). Corpus callosum abnormalities and their association with psychotic symptoms in patients with schizophrenia. *Biol. Psychiatry* 68, 70–77. doi: 10.1016/j.biopsych.2010.03.025

Yoo, S. Y., Jang, J. H., Shin, Y. W., Kim, D. J., Park, H. J., Moon, W. J., et al. (2007). White matter abnormalities in drug-naive patients with obsessive-compulsive disorder: a diffusion tensor study before and after citalopram treatment. *Acta Psychiatr. Scand.* 116, 211–219. doi: 10.1111/j.1600-0447.2007.01046.x

Zai, G., Bezchlibnyk, Y. B., Richter, M. A., Arnold, P., Burroughs, E., Barr, C. L., et al. (2004). Myelin oligodendrocyte glycoprotein (MOG) gene is associated with obsessive-compulsive disorder. *Am. J. Med. Genet. B Neuropsychiatr. Genet.* 129B, 64–68. doi: 10.1002/ajmg.b.30077

6

The Genetic Etiology of Tourette Syndrome: Large-Scale Collaborative Efforts on the Precipice of Discovery

Marianthi Georgitsi[1,2], A. Jeremy Willsey[3], Carol A. Mathews[4], Matthew State[3], Jeremiah M. Scharf[5]* and Peristera Paschou[1]**

[1] Department of Molecular Biology and Genetics, Democritus University of Thrace, Alexandroupoli, Greece, [2] Department of Medicine, Aristotle University of Thessaloniki, Thessaloniki, Greece, [3] Department of Psychiatry, University of California, San Francisco, San Francisco, CA, USA, [4] Department of Psychiatry, University of Florida School of Medicine, Gainesville, FL, USA, [5] Departments of Neurology and Psychiatry, Massachusetts General Hospital, Harvard Medical School, Boston, MA, USA

Edited by:
John Vijay Sagar Kommu, National Institute of Mental Health and Neurosciences, India

Reviewed by:
Katerina Maniadaki, Technological Educational Institute of Athens, Greece
Preeti Kandasamy, Jawaharlal Institute of Postgraduate Medical Education and Research, Puducherry (JIPMER), India

***Correspondence:**
Matthew State
matthew.state@ucsf.edu
Jeremiah M. Scharf
jscharf@partners.org
Peristera Paschou
ppaschou@mbg.duth.gr

Gilles de la Tourette Syndrome (TS) is a childhood-onset neurodevelopmental disorder that is characterized by multiple motor and phonic tics. It has a complex etiology with multiple genes likely interacting with environmental factors to lead to the onset of symptoms. The genetic basis of the disorder remains elusive. However, multiple resources and large-scale projects are coming together, launching a new era in the field and bringing us on the verge of discovery. The large-scale efforts outlined in this report are complementary and represent a range of different approaches to the study of disorders with complex inheritance. The Tourette Syndrome Association International Consortium for Genetics (TSAICG) has focused on large families, parent-proband trios and cases for large case-control designs such as genomewide association studies (GWAS), copy number variation (CNV) scans, and exome/genome sequencing. TIC Genetics targets rare, large effect size mutations in simplex trios, and multigenerational families. The European Multicentre Tics in Children Study (EMTICS) seeks to elucidate gene-environment interactions including the involvement of infection and immune mechanisms in TS etiology. Finally, TS-EUROTRAIN, a Marie Curie Initial Training Network, aims to act as a platform to unify large-scale projects in the field and to educate the next generation of experts. Importantly, these complementary large-scale efforts are joining forces to uncover the full range of genetic variation and environmental risk factors for TS, holding great promise for identifying definitive TS susceptibility genes and shedding light into the complex pathophysiology of this disorder.

Keywords: Gilles de la Tourette syndrome, genetics of complex disorders, neurodevelopmental disorders, GWAS (genomewide association study), gene-environment interactions, next generation sequencing, collaborative studies

INTRODUCTION

Gilles de la Tourette Syndrome (TS; OMIM #137580) is a childhood-onset neurodevelopmental disorder, characterized by motor and vocal tics. Previous prevalence estimates ranged from 0.4 to 3.8% (Robertson, 2008); however, a recent meta-analysis refined the prevalence estimate to 0.3–0.9% (Scharf et al., 2015). TS often presents with co-morbidities such as attention deficit hyperactivity disorder (ADHD) and obsessive-compulsive disorder (OCD) (Swain et al., 2007), but autism spectrum disorders (ASD), depressive, and anxiety disorders may be also present (Hirschtritt et al., 2015). This overlap across disorders supports the hypothesis of a shared neurological background and genetic susceptibility (Mathews and Grados, 2011; Yu et al., 2015). Twin and family studies have long established that TS bears a strong genetic component (Pauls et al., 2014). However, TS is a complex disorder and has been associated with several environmental factors as well, with Group-A Streptococcal (GAS) infection and psychosocial stress being the most prominent among them (Hoekstra et al., 2013; Mathews et al., 2014). Despite the extensive research to unravel the genetic basis of TS, the field is still in its nascence. A simple PubMed search for "tic disorders" (26/3/2016) yields 5200 articles, far behind in comparison to those found for other childhood-onset neurodevelopmental disorders, such as ADHD (27,706 articles) and autism (33,167 articles), or related disorders such as OCD (16,445 articles). However, as presented at the First World Congress on Tourette Syndrome and Tic Disorders (London, June 24–26, 2015), and as described further here, the field of TS genetics stands at the precipice of discovery, thanks to the concerted efforts of multiple researchers from around the world and the coordination of multiple large-scale collaborative projects funded by the European Commission and the US National Institutes of Health.

The large-scale efforts outlined in this report, are complementary and represent a range of different approaches for the study of multifactorial disorders. The Tourette Syndrome Association International Consortium for Genetics (TSAICG) focuses on large families, sibpairs, trios, and cases for large case-control designs such as genomewide association studies (GWAS), copy number variation (CNV) scans, and exome/genome sequencing. TIC Genetics studies simplex trios as well as multigenerational families targeting rare, large effect size mutations. The European Multicentre Tics in Children Study (EMTICS) seeks to elucidate gene-environment interactions including the involvement of infection and immune mechanisms in TS etiology. Finally, TS-EUROTRAIN is a training network, aiming to act as a platform to unify large-scale projects in the field and educate the next generation of experts. To set the stage for the description of the aims of these consortia we briefly report the most notable findings that have shaped our current knowledge for TS genetic susceptibility (excellent exhaustive reviews are available in the literature) (State, 2011; Deng et al., 2012; Paschou, 2013; Sun et al., 2016).

Candidate Gene Association Studies

Based on findings from pathophysiological studies, hypotheses about the neuroanatomical regions affected in TS, and therapeutic response to neuroleptics, the first TS candidate genes were members of the dopaminergic, serotonergic, and glutamatergic pathways (Peterson et al., 2003; Kalanithi et al., 2005; Hartmann and Worbe, 2013; **Table 1**). Despite years of effort, results have been inconsistent, possibly owing to the small sample size of each individual study, the restricted number of variants explored in each study, and the inherent difficulties of candidate gene studies in genetically heterogenous disorders.

Chromosomal Aberration Studies

SLITRK1 has become the focus of debate in the TS literature following the discovery of a *de novo* inversion in a TS patient (Abelson et al., 2005). Although follow-up studies could not find novel *SLITRK1* mutations in a large number of patients (Deng et al., 2006; Chou et al., 2007; Scharf et al., 2008; Zimprich et al., 2008; Miranda et al., 2009), tagging-SNP-based association studies supported the implication of unidentified *SLITRK1* regulatory variants (Miranda et al., 2009; Karagiannidis et al., 2012). Tracing chromosomal aberrations in TS patients, *IMMP2L* has also been implicated in TS (Boghosian-Sell et al., 1996; Kroisel et al., 2001; Petek et al., 2001; Patel et al., 2011; Katuwawela, 2012) and other neurodevelopmental disorders, such as ASD, ADHD and dyslexia (Elia et al., 2010; Maestrini et al., 2010; Pagnamenta et al., 2010; Girirajan et al., 2011); yet *IMMP2L* coding mutations have not been identified (Petek et al., 2007). Other cytogenetic abnormalities associated with TS have implicated signal transduction and cell-adhesion proteins, such as CNTNAP2 (Verkerk et al., 2003; Poot et al., 2010) and NLGN4 (Lawson-Yuen et al., 2008; **Table 1**).

CNV Studies

Scans of structural variations in relation to TS have revealed *de novo* or recurrent rare CNVs in multiple genes (**Table 1**). Of particular interest is the significant overlap of rare CNVs observed in TS individuals with patients of other neuropsychiatric and neurodevelopmental disorders, including OCD, autism, ASD, and schizophrenia, suggesting shared etiology (Sundaram et al., 2010; Fernandez et al., 2012; McGrath et al., 2014).

Linkage Analysis Studies

Early linkage studies on large multigenerational pedigrees failed to identify a major TS susceptibility gene (Deng et al., 2012; Paschou, 2013), and the single-gene hypothesis was soon abandoned. Recently, Ercan-Sencicek et al. identified an extremely rare non-sense mutation in *HDC*, in a unique family with several affected siblings, spurring again the interest for monogenic TS and introducing the involvement of the, until recently, ignored histaminergic pathway and its role in striatal dopamine regulation (Ercan-Sencicek et al., 2010; Castellan Baldan et al., 2014; Rapanelli et al., 2014). Although *HDC* mutations have been extremely rare in the literature (Lei et al., 2012), there is still evidence for association of the histaminergic pathway genes and TS (Fernandez et al., 2012; Karagiannidis et al., 2013).

GWAS Studies

The first TS GWAS was published in 2013, including 1285 cases and 4964 ancestry-matched controls. While no marker achieved a genomewide significance threshold, the strongest signal was observed for an intronic single nucleotide polymorphism (SNP) in *COL27A1* (Scharf et al., 2013). Moreover, a replication study of 42 top-signal SNPs from the first TS GWAS in 609 independent cases and 610 ancestry-matched controls, revealed the most significant association to date with a

TABLE 1 | List of genes that have so far been implicated in TS etiology.

Experimental approach by which the gene was initially identified	Gene	Protein function	Study sample size	References
CANDIDATE GENE				
Dopamine receptor D2	*DRD2*	Dopamine receptor	147 TS cases/314 controls 225 TS cases/67 controls 151 TS cases/183 controls 69 trios	Comings et al., 1991 Comings et al., 1996 Lee et al., 2005 Herzberg et al., 2010
Dopamine receptor D4	*DRD4*	Dopamine receptor	12 trios/3 large families 61 OCD cases with and without tics 110 trios	Grice et al., 1996 Cruz et al., 1997 Díaz-Anzaldúa et al., 2004
Dopamine transporter [Solute carrier family 6 (neurotransmitter transporter), member 3]	*DAT1 (SLC6A3)*	Dopamine transporter	225 TS cases/67 controls 103 trios 266 TS cases/236 controls 110 trios	Comings et al., 1996 Tarnok et al., 2007 Yoon et al., 2007 Díaz-Anzaldúa et al., 2004
Dopamine beta hydroxylase	*DBH*	Dopamine metabolism (transformation of dopamine to norepinephrine)	352 TS cases/148 controls	Comings et al., 1996
Monoamine oxidase-A	*MAOA*	Dopamine and serotonin metabolism (inactivation)	229 TS cases/90 relatives of TS/57 controls 110 trios	Gade et al., 1998 Díaz-Anzaldúa et al., 2004
Serotonin receptor 1A	*HTR1A*	Serotonin receptor	56 TS cases/20 controls	Lam et al., 1996
Serotonin receptor 2C	*HTR2C*	Serotonin receptor	87 TS cases/311 controls	Dehning et al., 2010
Serotonin transporter [Solute carrier family 6 (neurotransmitter transporter), member 4]	*SERT (SLC6A4)*	Serotonin transporter	151 TS cases/858 controls	Moya et al., 2013
	5-HTTLPR locus	–	151 TS cases/858 controls	Moya et al., 2013
Tryptophan hydroxylase	*TPH2*	Serotonin metabolism (synthesis)	98 TS cases/178 controls	Mössner et al., 2007
Glutamate transporter [Solute carrier family 1 (glial high affinity glutamate transporter), member 3]	*EAAT1 (SLC1A3)*	Glutamate transporter	256 TS cases/224 controls	Adamczyk et al., 2011
CHROMOSOMAL ABERRATIONS				
Slit and Trk-like, Family Member 1	*SLITRK1*	Neurite outgrowth	175 TS cases/2148 controls 222 trios	Abelson et al., 2005 Karagiannidis et al., 2012
Inner mitochondrial membrane protein 2L	*IMMP2L*	Targets proteins to the inner mitochondrial membrane (exact role unknown)	*De novo* duplication in one TS patient *De novo* duplication in one TS patient *De novo* translocation in one TS patient	Petek et al., 2001 Kroisel et al., 2001 Patel et al., 2011
Contactin associated protein-like 2	*CNTNAP2*	Cell-cell interaction (myelinated axon-glia junction) and membrane potential (interaction with voltage-activated potassium channel)	One family 460 TS cases/1131 controls	Verkerk et al., 2003 Fernandez et al., 2012

(Continued)

TABLE 1 | Continued

Experimental approach by which the gene was initially identified	Gene	Protein function	Study sample size	References
Neuroligin 4	*NLGN4*	Post-synaptic cell adhesion (synaptogenesis and synapse remodeling)	One family	Lawson-Yuen et al., 2008
COPY NUMBER VARIANTS				
Neurexin 1	*NRXN1*	Pre-synaptic cell adhesion (synapse formation)	111 TS cases/73 controls 460 TS cases/1131 controls 210 TS cases/285 controls	Sundaram et al., 2010 Fernandez et al., 2012 Nag et al., 2013
Arylacetamide deacetylase	*AADAC*	Detoxification (drug metabolism)—Unknown function in the brain	111 TS cases/73 controls 243 TS cases/1571 controls (initial study) 1181 TS cases/118730 controls (meta-analysis)	Sundaram et al., 2010; Bertelsen et al., 2015
Catenin alpha 3	*CTNNA3*	Cytoskeleton modeling (actin fillament assembly)	111 TS cases/73 controls 460 TS cases/1131 controls	Sundaram et al., 2010 Fernandez et al., 2012
Fibrous sheath CABYR binding protein	*FSCB*	Ca^{2+}-binding protein involved in fibrous sheath biogenesis	111 TS cases/73 controls	Sundaram et al., 2010
Voltage-gated potassium channel (*KCNE1*, *KCNE2*) and regulator of calcineurin 1 (*RCAN1*)	*KCNE1-KCNE2-RCAN1* locus	Neuronal cell membrane repolarization (*KCNE1*, *KCNE2*) and intracellular calcineurin-mediated signaling (*RCAN1*)	111 TS cases/73 controls	Sundaram et al., 2010
Collagen, type VIII, alpha 1	*COL8A1*	Connective tissue and basement membrane component (extracellular matrix collagen)	210 TS cases/285 controls	Nag et al., 2013
LINKAGE STUDIES				
Histidine decarboxylase	*HDC*	Histidine metabolism (synthesis)	One large family 520 trios	Ercan-Sencicek et al., 2010 Karagiannidis et al., 2013
GENOMEWIDE ASSOCIATION STUDIES				
Collagen, type XXVII, alpha 1	*COL27A1**	Connective tissue component (extracellular matrix collagen)	1285 TS cases/4964 controls (initial GWAS) 1496 TS cases/5249 controls (meta-analysis)	Scharf et al., 2013
Netrin 4	rs2060546 (proximal to *NTN4*)	Extracellular protein that directs axon outgrowth and guidance	609 TS cases/610 controls (initial analysis) 1894 TS cases/5574 controls (meta-analysis)	Paschou et al., 2014

As described in detail in the text, associations still remain inconclusive with difficulties in replicating original positive findings. To date, the heterogeneity of the disorder and small sample sizes have been hampering the identification of TS susceptibility genes and, large scale studies like the ones described in this perspective, hold the promise to unravel the genetic basis of TS.

**Only the top hit is shown here. No SNP reached genomewide significance levels.*

SNP lying closest to *NTN4*, an axon guidance molecule expressed in the developing striatum (Paschou et al., 2014). The first ever epigenome-wide association study of tic disorders revealed association signals nearby genes previously associated with neurological disorders that warrant further investigation (Zilhão et al., 2015).

THE TOURETTE SYNDROME ASSOCIATION INTERNATIONAL CONSORTIUM FOR GENETICS (TSAICG)—GENOMEWIDE ASSOCIATION STUDIES FOR TS

The TSAICG was founded in 1986 by TS genetic researchers in the United States and The Netherlands and brought together by the TSA-USA to exchange ideas and share preliminary data with the goal of identifying TS susceptibility genes. Early studies focused on parametric linkage analyses in large, multi-generational TS families (Pakstis et al., 1991; Barr et al., 1999) under the assumption that TS was a monogenic disorder. However, as evidence mounted to indicate the presence of non-Mendelian inheritance (Kurlan et al., 1994; Hasstedt et al., 1995), the TSAICG expanded to 11 clinical sites in USA, Canada, Germany, the UK, and the Netherlands to collect TS affected sibling pairs for non-parametric analyses using a standardized phenotypic assessment for TS, OCD, and ADHD, still used today by the three international TS consortia discussed here. The TSAICG was awarded NIH funding in 2000 to collect additional small nuclear families and completed a high-density linkage study of all existing affected sibpairs and multi-generational families (TSAICG, 2007). These analyses of over 2000 individuals identified a genomewide significant non-parametric linkage signal on chromosome 2p (TSAICG, 2007), though subsequent analyses have demonstrated significant heterogeneity across this locus, consistent with the presence of multiple distinct signals within the linkage region (O'Rourke et al., 2009). With the advent of the GWAS era, the TSAICG changed its collection goals to focus on association studies using both parent-proband trios and individual TS cases. These collections served as the basis for the first TS GWAS and parallel CNV analysis as described above (Scharf et al., 2013; McGrath et al., 2014). As it became clear that sample size is the major hindrance to gene discovery for complex neuropsychiatric traits, the TSAICG added additional recruitment sites and novel recruitment and assessment methods, such as web-based assessments of previously diagnosed TS cases and remote DNA collection using commercial laboratories across the US (Egan et al., 2012; Darrow et al., 2015). These online protocols facilitated collection of 1600 independent TS cases over the course of 2 years, a sample that served as the basis for the second TS GWAS and CNV studies whose preliminary results were presented at the First World Congress on Tourette Syndrome and Tic Disorders (to be published by fall 2016).

Each of these large-scale TS genetic studies have relied heavily on extended collaborations and data sharing, both within the TSAICG as well as across additional US and European research groups. The Gilles de la Tourette Syndrome GWAS Replication Initiative (GGRI) consists of multiple TS research groups across USA, Canada, France, Germany, Austria, Hungary, Italy, Greece and Poland, and formed out of an NIH TS Genetics Workshop following completion of the first TS GWAS. The GGRI collaborative resulted in both the targeted replication study described above (Paschou et al., 2014) and acted as another major contributing source for the second international TS GWAS and CNV studies. Similarly, TIC Genetics has contributed data from over 400 TS parent-proband trios to the latest TS GWAS. TSAICG and TIC Genetics are also currently collaborating in a joint analysis of exome sequencing data aimed at identifying recurrent, *de novo* mutations in TS parent-proband trio families (see below). Most recently, all of the above collaborative groups have also contributed their GWAS data to the Psychiatric Genomics Consortium (PGC) and formed the TS component of the TS and OCD Working Group of the PGC.

THE TOURETTE INTERNATIONAL COLLABORATIVE GENETICS (TIC GENETICS) STUDY—WHOLE EXOME SEQUENCING IN FAMILIES WITH TS

The TIC Genetics Study is a large, multi-center effort established in 2011 (http://tic-genetics.org) with several goals, including (1) to create a large, central repository for sharing clinical data and biomaterials from genotypically and phenotypically well-characterized affected individuals and their relatives; (2) to increase our understanding of the genetic architecture of tic disorders through identification of risk genes and loci, and enumeration of the number of these genes and loci that contribute risk; and (3) to leverage these findings alongside systems biological approaches to provide insights into the neurobiology underlying these disorders (Dietrich et al., 2014).

Patients are recruited at more than 20 sites from USA, Europe, and South Korea, including academic research and mental health care centers (Dietrich et al., 2014). Recruiting focusses on both multiplex families and apparently-simplex trios. Following extensive phenotyping, blood is drawn and processed at the NIMH Center for Collaborative Genomics Research on Mental Disorders at RUCDR (http://www.rucdr.org) for DNA and RNA extraction, lymphocytes cryopreservation, and lymphoblastoid cell lines establishment. Anonymized clinical data and biomaterials are stored in a sharing repository located within the National Institute for Mental Health Center for Collaborative Genomics Research on Mental Disorders (www.nimhgenetics.org). Importantly, this study has been designed to optimize compatibility with other TS genetic consortia and researchers, as this will be critical to advancing our understanding of this disorder (Dietrich et al., 2014).

The TIC Genetics study leverages multiple genomewide approaches for identifying rare, large effect size variants, focusing both on identifying highly penetrant genetic variants segregating in multiply affected pedigrees and on *de novo* mutations identified in simplex families. Genomewide methods include genotyping microarrays for linkage analysis (Ercan-Sencicek et al., 2010) and CNV detection (Fernandez et al., 2012), and whole-exome sequencing (WES) for SNP and insertion-deletion variant (indel) detection. Efforts of TIC Genetics investigators led to the implication of histaminergic pathway genes in TS etiology (Ercan-Sencicek et al., 2010; Fernandez et al., 2012).

TIC Genetics is currently finishing analysis of WES data from 325 simplex TS trios. The main focus is the detection of *de novo* SNPs and indels, largely due to the success of this gene discovery approach in ASD (Sanders et al., 2015). Because of the rarity of *de novo* mutations and their large effect size, recurrent mutations can be leveraged to identify risk genes with high confidence. Excitingly, the identification of risk genes, in a hypothesis-free manner, facilitates systems biological analyses aimed at answering critical questions about the underlying neurobiology of TS. Systems approaches alongside gene-expression data from the developing human brain may have already been quite fruitful in this regard (Willsey et al., 2013).

EMTICS: EUROPEAN MULTICENTRE TICS IN CHILDREN STUDY; EXPLORING GENE-ENVIRONMENT INTERACTIONS THAT UNDERLIE TS ETIOLOGY

EMTICS is a multi-national study funded by the European Commission under the Seventh Framework Programme, including 17 clinical sites from across Europe (http://emtics.eu). It is prospectively designed to offer, for the first time, the opportunity to evaluate environmental risk factors that may lead to tic exacerbation but also, new tic onset, while correlating to genomic background. Two unique patient cohorts form the core of EMTICS: The ONSET study involves follow-up of 375 high-risk children aged 3–10 years who have a first degree relative with a diagnosis of TS and at study entry have no tics. The COURSE study includes and follows for up to 3 years, 700 children, and adolescents aged 3–16 years with a known chronic tic disorder or TS.

Individual genetic background alone cannot predict the risk for TS and a role of exposure to psychosocial stress, pre- and perinatal difficulties, and GAS infections (Hoekstra et al., 2013; Mathews et al., 2014) in TS etiology has been shown. The human pathogen GAS is a major cause of common pharyngitis, but also of significant post-streptococcal autoimmune multi-organ sequelae associated with the existence of host autoantibodies against GAS antigens, including rheumatic fever and Sydenham's chorea (Church et al., 2002). In the 1990s, Swedo et al. (1998) described a clinical phenotype, named Paediatric Autoimmune Neuropsychiatric Disorders Associated with Streptococcal Infections (PANDAS). Although it is still controversial whether PANDAS criteria can be used to designate a unique clinical entity, further research into the potential role of the innate and adaptive immune systems in the pathogenesis of tics and OCD is warranted (Martino et al., 2009; Murphy et al., 2010). The etiological link between GAS infections and TS/OCD may be related to an autoimmune process, following the model of molecular mimicry, according to which structural similarity between streptococcal and cerebral antigens might elicit a pathogenic cross-reactivity of antibodies originally targeting GAS antigens to host antigens.

Within EMTICS, the main hypothesis is that the onset of TS is dependent on identifiable genetic factors interacting with identifiable environmental factors. The study aims to test the likelihood that the development of new tics or tic exacerbation in individuals with a specific genetic background, is increased by recent exposure to pharyngeal GAS carriage or infection. The study investigates the genomic background of studied individuals through genomewide genotyping, in relation to new tic onset and tic exacerbation, correlating to the presence of GAS in throat swabs, comorbidities, pre- and perinatal difficulties, psychosocial stress (also measured via cortisol levels in hair follicles), and immunological measures. Transcriptome-wide gene-expression profiles of patients at points of tic exacerbation and tic remission as well as before and after tic onset in newly-diagnosed patients will also reveal, for the first time, pathways that are activated during the course or onset of TS. The first patient was enrolled in March 2013 and the study will conclude in 2017. The potential observation of a pathogenic link between an environmental immune-activating factor and risk for the development of a tic disorder and/or OCD may pave the way to the application of immune-modulating prophylactic and treatment approaches in these conditions.

TS-EUROTRAIN—COORDINATING LARGE-SCALE STUDIES AND TRAINING THE NEXT GENERATION OF EXPERTS FOR TS

In an effort to address the need for large-scale collaboration in order to tackle the multi-faceted etiology of TS but also train the next generation of young experts in the field, the Marie Curie Initial Training Network TS-EUROTRAIN was established, supported by the European Commission (http://ts-eurotrain.eu). Collaborative efforts of 14 academic institutes along with 12 PhD students form a highly multidisciplinary and inter-sectorial team, with the European experts in the study of TS collaborating with leading scientists in the USA. Building bridges between academia and industry is key to the network with two industrial partners providing pioneering expertise to the network: deCODE Genetics, a large genetic services and research provider and Boehringer Ingelheim PHARMA, one of the 20 largest pharmaceutical companies in the world. Twelve individual, yet complementary, projects interact to form a comprehensive study of TS and comorbidities from genetics and epigenetics through to physiology, brain anatomy, and function. These projects can roughly be divided into three groups by their main approach; genetic (and epigenetic), animal models, and human neuroimaging, respectively.

TS-EUROTRAIN aspires to act as an interface bringing together multiple large-scale efforts in the field. The main scientific goals are to assemble and interrogate a large genetic database for the evaluation of the genetic architecture of TS, to explore the role of gene-environment interactions in TS etiology including, for the first time, the effects of epigenetic phenomena, and to gain new insights into the neurobiological mechanisms of TS via cross-sectional and longitudinal neuroimaging studies and animal studies. Among the main expected outcomes of TS-EUROTRAIN will be the largest meta-analysis of European patient cohorts, resulting in a total of about 3000 patients with TS analysed for about 700,000 genetic markers across the genome as well as genomewide CNV studies in European patient cohorts. Furthermore, already, TS-EUROTRAIN has produced the first ever epigenome-wide association study for tics, analysing data from the Netherlands Twin Register (Zilhão et al., 2015). This study interrogated 411,469 autosomal methylation sites in 1678 individuals. Although no site reached genomewide significance, the top hits include several genes and regions previously associated with neurological disorders and warrant further investigation (Zilhão et al., 2015). Systems biology approaches and integration of data from multiple sources are main aspects of TS-EUROTRAIN methodology. Thus, large-scale data analysis and novel algorithm development for integration of data from "omics" platforms but also clinical and neuroimaging data are important parts of the study.

The academic and industrial partners form a unified training infrastructure to provide interdisciplinary training for TS. Specialized training covers cutting-edge scientific areas ranging from basic neuroscience and genomics to bioinformatics and computer science. Direct interaction of the network with European patient groups (Tourette-Gesellschaft Deutschland e.V., Germany and Netherlands Foundation of patients with TS, Netherlands) provides a unique opportunity to learn from patients and disseminate scientific knowledge of TS to large non-scientific audiences. Undertaking a comprehensive scientific and outreach programme, TS-EUROTRAIN aims to build Pan-European infrastructure and render TS into an example disorder for the study of other neurodevelopmental disorders and the development of European policies for the promotion of childhood mental health.

CONCLUSIONS

Collaborative efforts of dedicated researchers from around the world have brought us on the verge of a new era, promising exciting, and rapid discoveries in the field of TS genetics. Multiple resources are coming together for TS genetic research; large well-characterized patient cohorts, specialized epidemiological databases, novel genomics technologies, and sophisticated methodology for the analysis of large-scale datasets. Systems biology approaches and integration of data from multiple sources and "omics" platforms can be expected to reveal novel facets of TS etiology, while cross-disorder meta-analysis for the identification of overlapping risk factors is shifting our view toward a whole spectrum of neurodevelopmental phenotypes. Importantly, the individual large-scale efforts described here, are ultimately joining their powers with the goal to boost power and identify definitive susceptibility genes for TS. These scientific alliances in concert with parallel large scale efforts in psychiatric genetics such as the PGC hold the promise to get us over the "precipice" and enter a new phase in TS gene discovery that may lead us to new pathophysiologic mechanisms underlying the disorder.

AUTHOR CONTRIBUTIONS

All authors listed, have made substantial, direct and intellectual contribution to the work, and approved it for publication.

ACKNOWLEDGMENTS

We would like to thank all the patients and families who participated in these studies in the hope of increasing knowledge about the causes of TS and identifying new treatments. This article was motivated by the First World Congress on Tourette Syndrome and Tic Disorders and is supported by the Tourette Association of America. Research reported in this publication was supported by a Conference Grant from the National Institute of Neurological Disorders and Stroke of the National Institutes of Health under Award Number R13NS095344. The content is solely the responsibility of the authors and does not necessarily represent the official views of the National Institutes of Health.

REFERENCES

Abelson, J. F., Kwan, K. Y., O'Roak, B. J., Baek, D. Y., Stillman, A. A., Morgan, T. M., et al. (2005). Sequence variants in SLITRK1 are associated with Tourette's syndrome. *Science* 310, 317–320. doi: 10.1126/science.1116502

Adamczyk, A., Gause, C. D., Sattler, R., Vidensky, S., Rothstein, J. D., Singer, H., et al. (2011). Genetic and functional studies of a missense variant in a glutamate transporter, SLC1A3, in Tourette syndrome. *Psychiatr. Genet.* 21, 90–97. doi: 10.1097/YPG.0b013e328341a307

Barr, C. L., Wigg, K. G., Pakstis, A. J., Kurlan, R., Pauls, D., Kidd, K. K., et al. (1999). Genome scan for linkage to Gilles de la Tourette syndrome. *Am. J. Med. Genet.* 88, 437–445. doi: 10.1002/(SICI)1096-8628(19990820)88:4<437::AID-AJMG24>3.0.CO;2-E
syndrome. *Pediatr. Neurol.* 37, 404–406. doi: 10.1016/j.pediatrneurol.2007.06.017

Church, A. J., Cardoso, F., Dale, R. C., Lees, A. J., Thompson, E. J., Giovannoni, G., et al. (2002). Anti-basal ganglia antibodies in acute and persistent Sydenham's chorea. *Neurology* 59, 227–231. doi: 10.1212/WNL.59.2.227

Comings, D. E., Comings, B. G., Muhleman, D., Dietz, G., Shahbahrami, B., Tast, D., et al. (1991). The dopamine D2 receptor locus as a modifying gene in neuropsychiatric disorders. *JAMA* 266, 1793–1800. doi: 10.1001/jama.1991.03470130073032

Comings, D. E., Wu, S., Chiu, C., Ring, R. H., Gade, R., Ahn, C., et al. (1996). Polygenic inheritance of Tourette syndrome, stuttering, attention deficit hyperactivity, conduct, and oppositional defiant disorder: the additive and subtractive effect of the three dopaminergic genes–DRD2, D beta H, and DAT1. *Am. J. Med. Genet.* 67, 264–288. doi: 10.1002/(SICI)1096-8628(19960531)67:3<264::AID-AJMG4>3.0.CO;2-N

Cruz, C., Camarena, B., King, N., Páez, F., Sidenberg, D., de la Fuente, J. R., et al. (1997). Increased prevalence of the seven-repeat variant of the dopamine D4 receptor gene in patients with obsessive-compulsive disorder with tics. *Neurosci. Lett.* 231, 1–4.

Darrow, S. M., Illmann, C., Gauvin, C., Osiecki, L., Egan, C. A., Greenberg, E., et al. (2015). Web-based phenotyping for Tourette Syndrome: reliability of common co-morbid diagnoses. *Psychiatry Res.* 228, 816–825. doi: 10.1016/j.psychres.2015.05.017

Dehning, S., Müller, N., Matz, J., Bender, A., Kerle, I., Benninghoff, J., et al. (2010). A genetic variant of HTR2C may play a role in the manifestation of Tourette syndrome. *Psychiatr. Genet.* 20, 35–38. doi: 10.1097/YPG.0b013e32833511ce

Deng, H., Gao, K., and Jankovic, J. (2012). The genetics of Tourette syndrome. *Nat. Rev. Neurol.* 8, 203–213. doi: 10.1038/nrneurol.2012.26

Deng, H., Le, W. D., Xie, W. J., and Jankovic, J. (2006). Examination of the SLITRK1 gene in Caucasian patients with Tourette syndrome. *Acta Neurol. Scand.* 114, 400–402. doi: 10.1111/j.1600-0404.2006.00706.x

Díaz-Anzaldúa, A., Joober, R., Rivière, J.-B., Dion, Y., Lespérance, P., Richer, F., et al. (2004). Tourette syndrome and dopaminergic genes: a family-based association study in the French Canadian founder population. *Mol. Psychiatry* 9, 272–277. doi: 10.1038/sj.mp.4001411

Dietrich, A., Fernandez, T. V., King, R. A., State, M. W., Tischfield, J. A., Hoekstra, P. J., et al. (2014). The Tourette International Collaborative Genetics (TIC Genetics) study, finding the genes causing Tourette syndrome: objectives and methods. *Eur. Child Adolesc. Psychiatry* 24, 141–151. doi: 10.1007/s00787-014-0543-x

Egan, C. A., Marakovitz, S. E., O'Rourke, J. A., Osiecki, L., Illmann, C., Barton, L., et al. (2012). Effectiveness of a web-based protocol for the screening and phenotyping of individuals with Tourette syndrome for genetic studies. *Am. J. Med. Genet. B Neuropsychiatr. Genet.* 159B, 987–996. doi: 10.1002/ajmg.b.32107

Elia, J., Gai, X., Xie, H. M., Perin, J. C., Geiger, E., Glessner, J. T., et al. (2010). Rare structural variants found in attention-deficit hyperactivity disorder are preferentially associated with neurodevelopmental genes. *Mol. Psychiatry* 15, 637–646. doi: 10.1038/mp.2009.57

Ercan-Sencicek, A. G., Stillman, A. A., Ghosh, A. K., Bilguvar, K., O'Roak, B. J., Mason, C. E., et al. (2010). L-histidine decarboxylase and Tourette's syndrome. *N. Engl. J. Med.* 362, 1901–1908. doi: 10.1056/NEJMoa0907006

Fernandez, T. V., Sanders, S. J., Yurkiewicz, I. R., Ercan-Sencicek, A. G., Kim, Y.-S. S., Fishman, D. O., et al. (2012). Rare copy number variants in tourette syndrome disrupt genes in histaminergic pathways and overlap with autism. *Biol. Psychiatry* 71, 392–402. doi: 10.1016/j.biopsych.2011.09.034

Gade, R., Muhleman, D., Blake, H., MacMurray, J., Johnson, P., Verde, R., et al. (1998). Correlation of length of VNTR alleles at the X-linked MAOA gene and phenotypic effect in Tourette syndrome and drug abuse. *Mol. Psychiatry* 3, 50–60.

Girirajan, S., Brkanac, Z., Coe, B. P., Baker, C., Vives, L., Vu, T. H., et al. (2011). Relative burden of large CNVs on a range of neurodevelopmental phenotypes. *PLoS Genet.* 7:e1002334. doi: 10.1371/journal.pgen.1002334

Grice, D. E., Leckman, J. F., Pauls, D. L., Kurlan, R., Kidd, K. K., Pakstis, A. J., et al. (1996). Linkage disequilibrium between an allele at the dopamine D4 receptor locus and Tourette syndrome, by the transmission-disequilibrium test. *Am. J. Hum. Genet.* 59, 644–652.

Hartmann, A., and Worbe, Y. (2013). Pharmacological treatment of Gilles de la Tourette syndrome. *Neurosci. Biobehav. Rev.* 37, 1157–1161. doi: 10.1016/j.neubiorev.2012.10.014

Hasstedt, S. J., Leppert, M., Filloux, F., van de Wetering, B. J., and McMahon, W. M. (1995). Intermediate inheritance of Tourette syndrome, assuming assortative mating. *Am. J. Hum. Genet.* 57, 682–689.

Herzberg, I., Valencia-Duarte, A. V., Kay, V. A., White, D. J., Müller, H., Rivas, I. C., et al. (2010). Association of DRD2 variants and Gilles de la Tourette syndrome in a family-based sample from a South American population isolate. *Psychiatr. Genet.* 20, 179–183. doi: 10.1097/YPG.0b013e32833a215a

Hirschtritt, M. E., Lee, P. C., Pauls, D. L., Dion, Y., Grados, M. A., Illmann, C., et al. (2015). Lifetime prevalence, age of risk, and genetic relationships of comorbid psychiatric disorders in Tourette syndrome. *JAMA Psychiatry* 72, 325–333. doi: 10.1001/jamapsychiatry.2014.2650

Hoekstra, P. J., Dietrich, A., Edwards, M. J., Elamin, I., and Martino, D. (2013). Environmental factors in Tourette syndrome. *Neurosci. Biobehav. Rev.* 37, 1040–1049. doi: 10.1016/j.neubiorev.2012.10.010

Kalanithi, P. S. A., Zheng, W., Kataoka, Y., DiFiglia, M., Grantz, H., Saper, C. B., et al. (2005). Altered parvalbumin-positive neuron distribution in basal ganglia of individuals with Tourette syndrome. *Proc. Natl. Acad. Sci. U.S.A.* 102, 13307–13312. doi: 10.1073/pnas.0502624102

Karagiannidis, I., Dehning, S., Sandor, P., Tarnok, Z., Rizzo, R., Wolanczyk, T., et al. (2013). Support of the histaminergic hypothesis in Tourette syndrome: association of the histamine decarboxylase gene in a large sample of families. *J. Med. Genet.* 50, 760–764. doi: 10.1136/jmedgenet-2013-101637

Karagiannidis, I., Rizzo, R., Tarnok, Z., Wolanczyk, T., Hebebrand, J., Nöthen, M. M., et al. (2012). Replication of association between a SLITRK1 haplotype and Tourette Syndrome in a large sample of families. *Mol. Psychiatry* 17, 665–668. doi: 10.1038/mp.2011.151

Katuwawela, I. (2012). Good response to clonidine in tourette syndrome associated with chromosomal translocation involving the IMMP2L gene. *J. Neuropsychiatry Clin. Neurosci.* 24:E17. doi: 10.1176/appi.neuropsych.11010032

Kroisel, P. M., Petek, E., Emberger, W., Windpassinger, C., Wladika, W., Wagner, K., et al. (2001). Candidate region for Gilles de la Tourette syndrome at 7q31. *Am. J. Med. Genet.* 101, 259–261. doi: 10.1002/1096-8628(20010701)101:3<259::AID-AJMG1374>3.0.CO;2-#

Kurlan, R., Eapen, V., Stern, J., McDermott, M. P., and Robertson, M. M. (1994). Bilineal transmission in Tourette's syndrome families. *Neurology* 44, 2336–2342.

Lam, S., Shen, Y., Nguyen, T., Messier, T. L., Brann, M., Comings, D., et al. (1996). A serotonin receptor gene (5HT1A) variant found in a Tourette's syndrome patient. *Biochem. Biophys. Res. Commun.* 219, 853–858.

Lawson-Yuen, A., Saldivar, J.-S., Sommer, S., and Picker, J. (2008). Familial deletion within NLGN4 associated with autism and Tourette syndrome. *Eur. J. Hum. Genet.* 16, 614–618. doi: 10.1038/sj.ejhg.5202006

Lee, C. C., Chou, I.-C., Tsai, C.-H., Wang, T.-R., Li, T.-C., Tsai, F.-J., et al. (2005). Dopamine receptor D2 gene polymorphisms are associated in Taiwanese children with Tourette syndrome. *Pediatr. Neurol.* 33, 272–276. doi: 10.1016/j.pediatrneurol.2005.05.005

Lei, J., Deng, X., Zhang, J., Su, L., Xu, H., Liang, H., et al. (2012). Mutation screening of the HDC gene in Chinese Han patients with Tourette syndrome. *Am. J. Med. Genet. B Neuropsychiatr. Genet.* 159B, 72–76. doi: 10.1002/ajmg.b.32003

Maestrini, E., Pagnamenta, A. T., Lamb, J. A., Bacchelli, E., Sykes, N. H., Sousa, I., et al. (2010). High-density SNP association study and copy number variation analysis of the AUTS1 and AUTS5 loci implicate the IMMP2L-DOCK4 gene region in autism susceptibility. *Mol. Psychiatry* 15, 954–968. doi: 10.1038/mp.2009.34

Martino, D., Dale, R. C., Gilbert, D. L., Giovannoni, G., and Leckman, J. F. (2009). Immunopathogenic mechanisms in tourette syndrome: a critical review. *Mov. Disord.* 24, 1267–1279. doi: 10.1002/mds.22504

Mathews, C. A., and Grados, M. A. (2011). Familiality of Tourette syndrome, obsessive-compulsive disorder, and attention-deficit/hyperactivity disorder: heritability analysis in a large sib-pair sample. *J. Am. Acad. Child Adolesc. Psychiatry* 50, 46–54. doi: 10.1016/j.jaac.2010.10.004

Mathews, C. A., Scharf, J. M., Miller, L. L., Macdonald-Wallis, C., Lawlor, D. A., and Ben-Shlomo, Y. (2014). Association between pre- and perinatal exposures and Tourette syndrome or chronic tic disorder in the ALSPAC cohort. *Br. J. Psychiatry* 204, 40–45. doi: 10.1192/bjp.bp.112.125468

McGrath, L. M., Yu, D., Marshall, C., Davis, L. K., Thiruvahindrapuram, B., Li, B., et al. (2014). Copy number variation in obsessive-compulsive disorder and tourette syndrome: a cross-disorder study. *J. Am. Acad. Child Adolesc. Psychiatry* 53, 910–919. doi: 10.1016/j.jaac.2014.04.022

Miranda, D. M., Wigg, K., Kabia, E. M., Feng, Y., Sandor, P., Barr, C. L., et al. (2009). Association of SLITRK1 to Gilles de la Tourette Syndrome. *Am. J. Med. Genet. B Neuropsychiatr. Genet.* 150B, 483–486. doi: 10.1002/ajmg.b.30840

Mössner, R., Müller-Vahl, K. R., Döring, N., and Stuhrmann, M. (2007). Role of the novel tryptophan hydroxylase-2 gene in Tourette syndrome. *Mol. Psychiatry* 12, 617–619. doi: 10.1038/sj.mp.4002004

Moya, P. R., Dodman, N. H., Timpano, K. R., Rubenstein, L. M., Rana, Z., Fried, R. L., et al. (2013). Rare missense neuronal cadherin gene (CDH2) variants in specific obsessive-compulsive disorder and Tourette disorder phenotypes. *Eur. J. Hum. Genet.* 21, 850–854. doi: 10.1038/ejhg.2012.245

Murphy, T. K., Kurlan, R., and Leckman, J. (2010). The immunobiology of Tourette's disorder, pediatric autoimmune neuropsychiatric disorders associated with Streptococcus, and related disorders: a way forward. *J. Child Adolesc. Psychopharmacol.* 20, 317–331. doi: 10.1089/cap.2010.0043

Nag, A., Bochukova, E. G., Kremeyer, B., Campbell, D. D., Muller, H., Valencia-Duarte, A. V., et al. (2013). CNV analysis in Tourette syndrome implicates large genomic rearrangements in COL8A1 and NRXN1. *PLoS ONE* 8:e59061. doi: 10.1371/journal.pone.0059061

O'Rourke, J., Scharf, J., Yu, D., and Pauls, D. (2009). The genetics of Tourette syndrome: a review. *J. Psychosom. Res.* 67, 533–545. doi: 10.1016/j.jpsychores.2009.06.006

Pagnamenta, A. T., Bacchelli, E., de Jonge, M. V., Mirza, G., Scerri, T. S., Minopoli, F., et al. (2010). Characterization of a family with rare deletions in CNTNAP5 and DOCK4 suggests novel risk loci for autism and dyslexia. *Biol. Psychiatry* 68, 320–328. doi: 10.1016/j.biopsych.2010.02.002

Pakstis, A. J., Heutink, P., Pauls, D. L., Kurlan, R., van de Wetering, B. J., Leckman, J. F., et al. (1991). Progress in the search for genetic linkage with Tourette syndrome: an exclusion map covering more than 50% of the autosomal genome. *Am. J. Hum. Genet.* 48, 281–294.

Paschou, P. (2013). The genetic basis of gilles de la Tourette syndrome. *Neurosci. Biobehav. Rev.* 37, 1026–1039. doi: 10.1016/j.neubiorev.2013.01.016

Paschou, P., Yu, D., Gerber, G., Evans, P., Tsetsos, F., Davis, L. K., et al. (2014). Genetic association signal near NTN4 in Tourette syndrome. *Ann. Neurol.* 76, 310–315. doi: 10.1002/ana.24215

Patel, C., Cooper-Charles, L., McMullan, D. J., Walker, J. M., Davison, V., Morton, J., et al. (2011). Translocation breakpoint at 7q31 associated with tics: further evidence for IMMP2L as a candidate gene for Tourette syndrome. *Eur. J. Hum. Genet.* 19, 634–639. doi: 10.1038/ejhg.2010.238

Pauls, D. L., Fernandez, T. V., Mathews, C., State, M. W., and Scharf, J. M. (2014). The inheritance of Tourette disorder: a review. *J. Obsessive Compuls. Relat. Disord.* 3, 380–385. doi: 10.1016/j.jocrd.2014.06.003

Petek, E., Schwarzbraun, T., Noor, A., Patel, M., Nakabayashi, K., Choufani, S., et al. (2007). Molecular and genomic studies of IMMP2L and mutation screening in autism and Tourette syndrome. *Mol. Genet. Genomics* 277, 71–81. doi: 10.1007/s00438-006-0173-1

Petek, E., Windpassinger, C., Vincent, J. B., Cheung, J., Boright, A. P., Scherer, S. W., et al. (2001). Disruption of a novel gene (IMMP2L) by a breakpoint in 7q31 associated with Tourette syndrome. *Am. J. Hum. Genet.* 68, 848–858. doi: 10.1086/319523

Peterson, B. S., Thomas, P., Kane, M. J., Scahill, L., Zhang, H., Bronen, R., et al. (2003). Basal Ganglia volumes in patients with Gilles de la Tourette syndrome. *Arch. Gen. Psychiatry* 60, 415–424. doi: 10.1001/archpsyc.60.4.415

Poot, M., Beyer, V., Schwaab, I., Damatova, N., Van'T Slot, R., Prothero, J., et al. (2010). Disruption of CNTNAP2 and additional structural genome changes in a boy with speech delay and autism spectrum disorder. *Neurogenetics* 11, 81–89. doi: 10.1007/s10048-009-0205-1

Rapanelli, M., Frick, L. R., Pogorelov, V., Ota, K. T., Abbasi, E., Ohtsu, H., et al. (2014). Dysregulated intracellular signaling in the striatum in a pathophysiologically grounded model of Tourette syndrome. *Eur. Neuropsychopharmacol.* 24, 1896–1906. doi: 10.1016/j.euroneuro.2014.10.007

Robertson, M. M. (2008). The prevalence and epidemiology of Gilles de la Tourette syndrome. Part 1: the epidemiological and prevalence studies. *J. Psychosom. Res.* 65, 461–472. doi: 10.1016/j.jpsychores.2008.03.006

Sanders, S. J., He, X., Willsey, A. J., Ercan-Sencicek, A. G., Samocha, K. E., Cicek, A. E., et al. (2015). Insights into autism spectrum disorder genomic architecture and biology from 71 risk loci. *Neuron* 87, 1215–1233. doi: 10.1016/j.neuron.2015.09.016

Scharf, J. M., Miller, L. L., Gauvin, C. A., Alabiso, J., and Mathews, C. A. (2015). Population prevalence of Tourette syndrome : a systematic review and meta-analysis. *Mov. Disord.* 30, 221–228. doi: 10.1002/mds.26089

Scharf, J. M., Moorjani, P., Fagerness, J., Platko, J. V., Illmann, C., Galloway, B., et al. (2008). Lack of association between SLITRK1var321 and Tourette syndrome in a large family-based sample. *Neurology* 70, 1495–1496. doi: 10.1212/01.wnl.0000296833.25484.bb

Scharf, J. M., Yu, D., Mathews, C. A., Neale, B. M., Stewart, S. E., Fagerness, J. A., et al. (2013). Genome-wide association study of Tourette's syndrome. *Mol. Psychiatry* 18, 721–728. doi: 10.1038/mp.2012.69

State, M. W. (2011). The genetics of Tourette disorder. *Curr. Opin. Genet. Dev.* 21, 302–309. doi: 10.1016/j.gde.2011.01.007

Sun, N., Tischfield, J. A., King, R. A., and Heiman, G. A. (2016). Functional evaluations of genes disrupted in patients with Tourette's disorder. *Front. psychiatry* 7:11. doi: 10.3389/fpsyt.2016.00011

Sundaram, S. K., Huq, A. M., Wilson, B. J., and Chugani, H. T. (2010). Tourette syndrome is associated with recurrent exonic copy number variants. *Neurology* 74, 1583–1590. doi: 10.1212/WNL.0b013e3181e0f147

Swain, J. E., Scahill, L., Lombroso, P. L., King, R. A., and Leckman, J. F. (2007). Tourette syndrome and tic disorders: a decade of progress. *J. Am. Acad. Child Adolesc. Psychiatry* 46, 947–968. doi: 10.1097/chi.0b013e318068fbcc

Swedo, S. E., Leonard, H. L., Garvey, M., Mittleman, B., Allen, A. J., Perlmutter, S., et al. (1998). Pediatric autoimmune neuropsychiatric disorders associated with streptococcal infections: clinical description of the first 50 cases. *Am. J. Psychiatry* 155, 264–271. doi: 10.1176/ajp.155.2.264

Tarnok, Z., Ronai, Z., Gervai, J., Kereszturi, E., Gadoros, J., Sasvari-Szekely, M., et al. (2007). Dopaminergic candidate genes in Tourette syndrome: association between tic severity and 3′ UTR polymorphism of the dopamine transporter gene. *Am. J. Med. Genet. Part B Neuropsychiatr. Genet.* 144, 900–905. doi: 10.1002/ajmg.b.30517

TSAICG (2007). Genome scan for tourette disorder in affected-sibling-pair and multigenerational families. *Am. J. Hum. Genet.* 80, 265–272. doi: 10.1086/511052

Verkerk, A., Mathews, C. A., Joosse, M., Eussen, B. B. H. J., Heutink, P., Oostra, B. B. A., et al. (2003). CNTNAP2 is disrupted in a family with Gilles de la Tourette syndrome and obsessive comulsive disorder. *Genomics* 82, 1–9. doi: 10.1016/S0888-7543(03)00097-1

Willsey, A. J., Sanders, S. J., Li, M., Dong, S., Tebbenkamp, A. T., Muhle, R. A., et al. (2013). Coexpression networks implicate human midfetal deep cortical projection neurons in the pathogenesis of autism. *Cell* 155, 997–1007. doi: 10.1016/j.cell.2013.10.020

Yoon, D. Y., Gause, C. D., Leckman, J. F., and Singer, H. S. (2007). Frontal dopaminergic abnormality in Tourette syndrome: a postmortem analysis. *J. Neurol. Sci.* 255, 50–56. doi: 10.1016/j.jns.2007.01.069

Yu, D., Mathews, C. A., Scharf, J. M., Neale, B. M., Davis, L. K., Gamazon, E. R., et al. (2015). Cross-disorder genome-wide analyses suggest a complex genetic relationship between Tourette's syndrome and OCD. *Am. J. Psychiatry* 172, 82–93. doi: 10.1176/appi.ajp.2014.13101306

Zilhão, N. R., Padmanabhuni, S. S., Pagliaroli, L., Barta, C., Smit, D. J. A., Cath, D., et al. (2015). Epigenome-wide association study of tic disorders. *Twin Res. Hum. Genet.* 18, 699–709. doi: 10.1017/thg.2015.72

Zimprich, A., Hatala, K., Riederer, F., Stogmann, E., Aschauer, H. N., Stamenkovic, M., et al. (2008). Sequence analysis of the complete SLITRK1 gene in Austrian patients with Tourette's disorder. *Psychiatr. Genet.* 18, 308–309. doi: 10.1097/YPG.0b013e3283060f6f

7

Non-Motor Aspects of Tic Disorders—New Developments

Daphna Ruhrman[1,2], Ella Gev[1,2], Noa Benaroya-Milshtein[1,2], Silvana Fennig[1,2], Orit Krispin[1], Alan Apter[1,2] and Tamar Steinberg[1,2]*

[1] The Matta and Harry Freund Neuropsychiatric Tourette Clinic, Schneider Children's Medical Center of Israel, Petach Tikva, Israel, [2] Sackler Faculty of Medicine, Tel Aviv University, Tel Aviv, Israel

Edited by:
Kirsten R. Müller-Vahl, Hannover Medical School, Germany

Reviewed by:
Andreas Hartmann, Assistance Publique des Hopitaux de Paris, France
Judith Katharina Buse, Technische Universität Dresden, Germany

***Correspondence:**
Daphna Ruhrman
daphnaruhrman@gmail.com

The cardinal characteristics of tic-related disorders are stereotyped motor movements and vocalizations. However, they may be accompanied by non-motor features that appear sequentially during the course of the disorder and can sometimes be more disabling than the tics themselves. This review presents our perspectives on several non-motor aspects of Tourette syndrome based on the long experience of the Neuropsychiatric Tourette Clinic of a tertiary pediatric medical center. The effect of premonitory urges, sensory modulation disorder, tic-related cognitions, and environmental conditions on the expression and intensity of tics is elaborated, with suggestions for treatment approaches to each. We also describe the mediatory effect of parental attachment style on the link between maternal stress and ticcing intensity and the need to adjust psychotherapy interventions to account for the importance of this factor in emotion regulation. This review is intended to direct attention to the non-motor aspects of Tourette syndrome. An in-depth understanding of this complex and debilitating disorder will facilitate the formulation of innovative therapeutic protocols.

Keywords: tic disorders, premonitory urge, acceptance, sensory modulation, environmental influences, attachment, emotion dysregulation

BACKGROUND

The stereotyped motor movements and vocalizations that are the cardinal characteristics of tic disorders are often accompanied by non-motor features that appear sequentially during the course of the disorder and can sometimes be more disabling than the tics themselves. The Neuropsychiatric Tourette Clinic of Schneider Children's Medical Center of Israel, a tertiary university-affiliated pediatric hospital, has long experience in treating children with Tourette syndrome and its associated clinical manifestations. The aim of this review is to share our subjective perspectives on the non-motor aspects of Tourette syndrome based on findings and observations in our clinic, as presented at the first World Congress on Tourette Syndrome and Tic Disorders (1). We start with premonitory urges, which play a significant role in tic expression and tic sequence, and the impact of acceptance procedures on decreasing their intensity. This is followed by a discussion of sensory modulation disorder (SMD) as an important component of the reaction to premonitory urges and as a comorbidity of Tourette syndrome, in addition to the development of tic-related cognitions and their influence on tics and tic-related behaviors. The effect of environmental factors on tic expression and their bearing on the development and refinement of behavioral treatment strategies are elaborated. There is also a section on the relevance of attachment theory and the modulatory role of parental attachment style in the relationship between children with Tourette syndrome and their parents.

PREMONITORY URGES

Studies have shown that premonitory urges play a significant role in tic expression (2–6). However, the exact functional relationship between premonitory urges and tics has not been explored.

A premonitory urge is an internal physical sensation that is experienced as a drive to perform a movement, either motor or vocal. Specifically, it is an impulse to tic. In a cross-sectional study of 135 patients aged 8–71 years with tic disorder, Leckman et al. (2) found a 95% prevalence rate of premonitory urges. The exact experience of premonitory urges, however, is extremely diverse. They have been described as an itch, a burn, an energy that must be released, a need to release tension, and a mental will (7). Some individuals fail to discriminate the physical experience of premonitory urges from the tics themselves (5, 7). Studies have repeatedly shown that the premonitory urges and the internal struggle to control them may be even more debilitating than the tics themselves. We have found that psychoeducation may help patients distinguish premonitory urges and reduce their discomfort.

The mean age at which patients with Tourette syndrome first become aware of premonitory urges is 10 years, an average 3.1 years after onset of the tics (2). Our clinical experience has shown that younger children (<10 years) can identify premonitory urges, but older children report them more clearly and consistently (8). Furthermore, urge ratings correlate with tic severity only in older children. These findings may be attributable to the increase in cognitive maturity with age (3, 5).

Several instruments have been developed to help children capture the urge experience using various definitions and descriptions. The well-established Premonitory Urge Scale for Tics (PUTS) (5) was found to facilitate premonitory urge recognition in children as young as 8 years and is widely used to measure the intensity of urges. In addition, therapeutic programs such as exposure and response prevention (ERP), habit reversal therapy (HRT), and comprehensive behavioral intervention for tics (CBIT) can initially assist young children in verbally describing what they feel during tics. Using these tools or similar ones, researchers found that urge frequency and intensity decreased in response to medications such as neuroleptics and relaxation and concentration exercises and increased in states of stress and anxiety (2). Others, including a group from our center, reported that the intensity of premonitory urges increased during tic suppression (6, 9), suggesting that the urges may serve as precipitators of tics (10) and that tic performance is directed at alleviating the premonitory urges (3). This was supported by studies using ERP protocols (11–13). Himle et al. (6) postulated that urges are an aversive experience and tics serve as a response to them and are negatively reinforced by urge removal. Accordingly, tic suppression temporarily increases the salience of the urge. Thus, when a child is allowed to tic freely, the premonitory urge is relatively low in intensity (6). However, whether premonitory urges are a conditioned stimulus for tics remains controversial, as other studies failed to find changes in self-reports of urge intensity during tic suppression (14, 15). As in most instances of mind–body relations, the urge–tic relationship is not linear and clear-cut. Subjects with tics may adopt the belief that the tics are the best solution for the unease caused by premonitory urges. The tics themselves later become aversive themselves because they do not allow the individual to relax or concentrate, and in severe cases, may even result in serious injury. This situation is exacerbated when the environment responds negatively to the tics. Accordingly, Capriotti et al. (16) found that the intensity of the premonitory urge is correlated with the aversive consequences of ticcing. Therefore, clinicians need to address both components of the premonitory urge–tic complex and help children find the most suitable way to deal with each. Our group uses the acceptance-based approach of the acceptance and commitment therapy (ACT) protocol proposed by Hayes and Wilson (17). These researches suggested that attempts to control aversive sensations are not only ineffective, they may even amplify the experience the individual was trying to avoid. However, accepting these experiences, that is, viewing them as only something to be experienced reduces their negative impact (17, 18). To test this hypothesis, we compared urge intensity, frequency, and discomfort with tic frequency under three conditions: ticcing freely, tic suppression, and urge acceptance (using mindfulness techniques and diaphragmatic breathing). The results showed that the frequency and intensity of the urges was significantly reduced in the urge acceptance condition compared to the others. A similar pattern was found for the level of discomfort caused by urges. We also noted a significant reduction in tic expression in the urge acceptance condition compared to the freely ticcing condition, suggesting that accepting urges can help children not only to cope with premonitory urges but also to reduce tic expression (9). This finding was supported by a recent study by Reese et al. (19) showing a correlation between a reduction in tic severity and increased mindfulness. Thus, premonitory urges may be considered a core aspect of Tourette syndrome, and they need to be distinguished from the tics in order to improve our understanding and treatment of the disorder as a whole. The experience of our group suggests that alternative approaches of acceptance aimed specifically at premonitory urges should be incorporated into modern treatment protocols for tics.

SMD

Sensory modulation disorder is an impairment in regulation of the degree, intensity, and nature of responses to sensory input (either over- or under-sensitivity), with an adverse effect on activities and routines of daily living (20). A study from our clinic showed that the prevalence of SMD is considerably higher in children with Tourette syndrome (34.7%) than in healthy children (<5%) (21), suggesting that SMD is a comorbidity of Tourette syndrome. The presence of SMD can directly affect how individuals with Tourette syndrome respond to premonitory urges. That is, if the premonitory urge constitutes an over-reactivity to sensory input (before emergence of the tic), and SMD creates an over-attentiveness to aversive sensory input, then children with Tourette syndrome may feel obligated to tic to rid themselves of the unpleasant inner stimulus.

Children with both SMD and Tourette syndrome also have high rates of other common comorbidities, such as obsessive–compulsive disorder (OCD), depression, and attention-deficit and hyperactivity disorder (ADHD), which significantly impact their quality of life. We speculate that children with SMD and Tourette syndrome undergo a long learning process, beginning at a very young age and continuing toward adulthood, during which they incorporate the intense relationship between sensory inputs and the immediate response to them. As a consequence, a strong link evolves between the two, creating the illusion that they constitute a single entity. The challenge during treatment is to break this link (21).

TIC-RELATED COGNITIONS

Studies of illness-related beliefs have shown that the beliefs and expectations (cognitions) of patients about their illness or somatic symptoms play an important role in the impact of the illness on their life. In individuals with Tourette syndrome, tic-related cognitions develop in childhood along with the experience of tics and premonitory urges. The cognitions include appraisals and beliefs regarding inner (premonitory urges) and outer (environmental) sensory inputs, responses to these inputs (tics), and the ability to express, suppress, or modify one's responses. To investigate the different thoughts of children about the origin and consequences of their tics, we designed a self-report inventory, the Beliefs About Tic Scale (BATS) (22), which we administered to a sample of 56 patients aged 10–18 years with Tourette syndrome. The results showed that patients' negative beliefs about their ability to suppress tics (or to resist premonitory urges) were related to higher perceived urge intensity (measured by PUTS scores). Apparently, the perception of a lack of control increases the adverse emotional consequences of premonitory urges. This illness-related distress can be triggered by cognitive as well as emotional processes (23). Our findings are in line with the study of tinnitus by Sirois et al. (24) showing that among patients with the same symptom severity, those who believed they had control over their condition had lower levels of depression and a better quality of life. Additionally, our group showed that the level of depression was highly correlated with negative beliefs about the ability to suppress (i.e., control) tics, but only in children older than 13 years (22). We also noted several positive correlations between perceived urge intensity (measured by PUTS scores) and psychiatric symptoms. In children with OCD, PUTS scores were correlated with OCD severity, again only in those older than 13 years. There was a correlation between PUTS scores and obsessions, which increased with an increase in age, to almost complete congruence (22). Hence, premonitory urges can be considered a type of "obsession" with bodily sensations. These findings are in agreement with the suggestion of O'Connor (25) that children with Tourette syndrome have excess sensitivity to sensory stimuli and as a result tend to associate negative feelings with perceptions. This in turn leads to exaggerated negative perceptual biases, comparable to the cognitive distortions found in depression and anxiety. It is probable that as the child grows, he/she learns to associate these negative appraisals with the urges and tics. The negativity becomes increasingly more debilitating and bothersome and may take the form of an obsession. The lack of control associated with tics accentuates these negative feelings, and quality of life is diminished (25).

ENVIRONMENTAL FACTORS

Although tics arise from a disturbance in the underlying brain circuitry, there is increasing evidence that tic expression may be either exacerbated and attenuated by environmental and psychological factors (13), such as psychosocial stress (26). In their literature review, Conelea and Woods (27) identified a variety of situations associated with changes in tic frequency, including boredom and passive states, social gatherings, concentration on a task, watching TV, and playing sports. The consequences of tic expression may also influence its appearance. These may be external, such as social attention (teasing, comforting, release from demanding tasks) or internal (subjective feeling of relief of a premonitory urge after tick, shame, or guilt) (28, 29). Studies of the impact of environmental factors on tic expression have improved our understanding of the etiology and maintenance of tics. They have also influenced the strategies used to treat tic disorders. Behavioral treatment approaches, such as HRT, are based on the rationale that despite their biological origin, tics may be worsened, improved, or maintained by environmental events. Treatment is therefore partly directed at systematically identifying and modifying events or experiences that contribute to tic severity (30).

The mechanisms whereby different environmental conditions affect tics have been hardly investigated, apart from those related to learning theories and emotional effects. Therefore, we conducted a study at our clinic in which tic expression was evaluated under five challenging environmental situations: watching television; doing homework; being alone; receiving attention when ticcing; and talking to a stranger study (1). Two measures were used: a subjective measure consisting of a structured interview in which children were asked to describe the level of tics in these situations, and an objective measure consisting of a video recording of the child's response in each situation. The results yielded differential effects of the different environmental situations on tic expression. The objective measure revealed that the highest number of tics appeared in the watching television situation, and the lowest, in the alone situation. Combined with the report on the effect of stress on tic severity by Conelea et al. (31), our findings suggest that highly stimulating environmental conditions can interfere with motor inhibition and thereby exacerbate tic expression. Therefore, the higher the level of stimulation in each of our situations, the greater the number of tics expressed. By contrast to the objective measure, the subjective self-reports of the subjects served only as a moderate–low predictor of the effect of the environment on tics. This points to a low level of patient self-awareness of the impact of the environment on the performance and intensity of tics. It may also indicate a low reliability of subjective reports of tic severity, which form the basis of most clinical and research evaluations. Interestingly, the subjective reports were more in line with the objective measure in the presence of strong premonitory urges. Thus, it is possible that the tic brings the urge to the child's attention, increasing his/her awareness of both the tic and the environmental influences. We suggest that alerting children to environmental factors that affect tic performance may help them acquire better coping skills in situations associated with tic exacerbation.

PARENT–CHILD ATTACHMENT

The parent–child relationship is a basic component of the clinical understanding of children with Tourette syndrome. Our group attempted to investigate this aspect of Tourette syndrome through the prism of attachment theory (32), which has been found to serve as a useful framework for understanding parent–child relationships under conditions of stress (33, 34). As noted above, the psychological dynamic of children with Tourette syndrome is often complicated by comorbidities involving impaired emotion regulation, such as OCD, ADHD, anxiety disorders, depression, and rage attacks (35), which can be a major impediment to normal childhood development (35, 36). We focused on the reciprocal effect of emotion dysregulation in a developmental context and the experience of self between children with Tourette syndrome and their parents and the impact of these interactions on the child's mental health (32). Parents of children with Tourette syndrome are subject to a vicious cycle on a daily basis of the child's emotion dysregulation on the one hand and their own inability to serve as a container on the other. This cycle is dictated by two interrelated factors: the characteristics of the parent–child relationship and the child's self-representation and emotion-regulation abilities. Insights for the study were derived from Bowlby's attachment theory (37), which claims that children tend to seek the protection of the parent or significant other in order to gain security. To survive, they form an array of internal conscious and unconscious representations of the self and related others, and these determine their attachment style: secure or insecure (anxious and/or avoidant). Children with a secure attachment style have internal working models of others as positive and protective. In times of need, they search for comfort and support from the other in order to achieve emotion regulation, a cornerstone of good mental health. Children with an anxious or avoidant attachment style have representations of others as unavailable, rejecting, or even harming, and acquire a lasting fear of rejection and abandonment. Thus, their ability to get comfort and help from others is damaged. The broadening of the theory to apply to adulthood, suggesting that the system that gives rise to the emotional bond between children and parents continues to play a role when the children reach adulthood and confront obstacles of parenting (33, 38). Our study focused on the relationship between parental stress and attachment style and its influence on tic severity and impairment (32). We showed that an increase in the level of maternal stress, as measured by the mother's perception of the child as "difficult" using a subscale of the Parental Stress Index (39), was associated with an increase in the intensity of the child's ticcing. These findings pave the way for designing new clinical interventions for both children with Tourette syndrome and their parents based on the attachment theory. Vulnerable families should be identified by their attachment style, followed by adjustments to the psychotherapy intervention, mainly with a focus on the parents, in order to enhance their ability to identify, adjust to, and fulfill the child's needs in terms of emotion regulation. In this manner, common comorbidities of Tourette syndrome can be better managed and children will derive greater benefit from existing tic-targeted treatments, ensuring their healthier mental development.

CONCLUSION

Tourette syndrome is a complex disorder, comprising both motor and non-motor/emotional components. This review was intended to direct attention to the non-motor aspects of Tourette syndrome and to encourage further research into their role in the underlying mechanism of the disorder. An in-depth understanding of this disabling condition will lead to better and more innovative treatments.

AUTHOR CONTRIBUTIONS

All the authors listed have made substantial, direct, and intellectual contribution to the work and approved it for publication.

REFERENCES

1. Barnea M. Environmental influence on tic expression. *Presented at the 1st World Congress on Tourette Syndrome & Tic Disorders June 24-26*. London (2015).
2. Leckman JF, Walker DE, Cohen DJ. Premonitory urges in Tourette's syndrome. *Am J Psychiatry* (1993) 150:98–102. doi:10.1176/ajp.150.1.98
3. Leckman JF. Tourette's syndrome. *Lancet* (2002) 360:1577–86. doi:10.1016/S0140-6736(02)11526-1
4. Verdellen CWJ, Keijsers GPJ, Cath DC, Hoogduin CAL. Exposure with response prevention versus habit reversal in Tourette's syndrome: a controlled study. *Behav Res Ther* (2004) 42:501–11. doi:10.1016/S0005-7967(03)00154-2
5. Woods DW, Piacentini J, Himle MB, Chang S. Premonitory urge for tics scale (PUTS): initial psychometric results and examination of the premonitory urge phenomenon in youths with tic disorders. *J Dev Behav Pediatr* (2005) 26:397–403. doi:10.1097/00004703-200512000-00001
6. Himle MB, Woods DW, Conelea CA, Bauer CC, Rice KA. Investigating the effects of tic suppression on premonitory urge ratings in children and adolescents with Tourette's syndrome. *Behav Res Ther* (2007) 45:2964–76. doi:10.1016/j.brat.2007.08.007
7. Ganos C, Hummel FC. My urge, my tic–a missing link between urges and tic inhibition. *Cogn Neurosci* (2011) 2(3-4):249–50. doi:10.1080/17588928.2011.618634
8. Steinberg T, Shmuel Baruch S, Harush A, Dar R, Woods DW, Piacentini J, et al. Tic disorders and the premonitory urge. *J Neural Transm (Vienna)* (2010) 117:277–84. doi:10.1007/s00702-009-0353-3
9. Gev E, Pilowsky-Peleg T, Fennig S, Ben-Aroya-Milshtein N, Woods DW, Piacentini J, et al. Acceptance of premonitory urges and tics. *J Obsessive Compuls Relat Disord* (2016) 10:78–83. doi:10.1016/j.jocrd.2016.06.001
10. Kane MJ. Premonitory urges as "attentional tics" in Tourette's syndrome. *J Am Acad Child Adolesc Psychiatry* (1994) 33:805–8. doi:10.1097/00004583-199407000-00005
11. Hoogduin K, Verdellen C, Cath D. Exposure and response prevention in the treatment of Gilles de la Tourette's syndrome: four case studies. *Clin Psychol Psychother* (1997) 4:125–35. doi:10.1002/(SICI)1099-0879(199706)4:2<125::AID-CPP125>3.0.CO;2-Z
12. Verdellen C, Van de Grirndt J, Hartman A, Murphy T. European clinical guidelines for Tourette syndrome and other tic disorders. Part III: behavioral and psychosocial interventions. *Eur Child Adolesc Psychiatry* (2011) 20:197–207. doi:10.1007/s00787-011-0167-3

13. Frank M, Cavanna AE. Behavioural treatments for Tourette syndrome: an evidence-based review. *Behav Neurol* (2013) 27:105–17. doi:10.1155/2013/134863
14. Ganos C, Kahl U, Schunke O, Kuhn S, Haggard P, Gerloff C, et al. Are premonitory urges a prerequisite of tic inhibition in Gilles de la Tourette syndrome? *Neurol Neurosurg Psychiatry* (2012) 83:975–8. doi:10.1136/jnnp-2012-303033
15. Specht MW, Woods DW, Nicorta CM, Kelly LM, Ricketts EJ, Conelea CA, et al. Effects of tic suppression: ability to suppress, rebound, negative reinforcement, and habituation to the premonitory urge. *Behav Res Ther* (2013) 51:24–30. doi:10.1016/j.brat.2012.09.009
16. Capriotti MR, Espil FM, Conelea CA, Woods DW. Environmental factors as potential determinants of premonitory urge severity in youth with Tourette syndrome. *J Obsessive Compuls Relat Disord* (2013) 2:37–42. doi:10.1016/j.jocrd.2012.10.004
17. Hayes SC, Wilson KG. Acceptance and commitment therapy: altering the verbal support for experiential avoidance. *Behav Anal* (1994) 17:289–303.
18. Hayes SC, Strosahl KD, Wilson KG. *Acceptance and Commitment Therapy: An Experiential Approach to Behavior Change.* New York: Guilford Press (1999).
19. Reese HE, Vallejo Z, Rasmussen J, Crowe K, Rosenfield E, Wilhelm S. Mindfulness-based stress reduction for Tourette syndrome and chronic tic disorder: a pilot study. *J Psychosom Res* (2015) 78:293–8. doi:10.1016/j.jpsychores.2014.08.001
20. Miller LJ. *Sensational Kids: Hope and Help for Children with Sensory Processing Disorders.* New York: Putnam Press (2006).
21. Steinberg T. The impact of sensory modulation on tic characteristics, comorbid disorders and quality of life. *Presented at the 1st World Congress on Tourette Syndrome & Tic Disorders June 24-26.* London (2015).
22. Steinberg T, Harush A, Barnea M, Dar R, Piacentini J, Woods D, et al. Tic-related cognition, sensory phenomena, and anxiety in children and adolescents with Tourette syndrome. *Compr Psychiatry* (2013) 54:462–6. doi:10.1016/j.comppsych.2012.12.012
23. Leventhal H, Diefenbach M, Leventhal EA. Illness cognition: using common sense to understand treatment adherence and affect cognition interactions. *Cognit Ther Res* (1992) 16:143–63. doi:10.1007/BF01173486
24. Sirois FM, Davis CG, Morgan MS. "Learning to live with what you can't rise above": control beliefs, symptom control, and adjustment to tinnitus. *Health Psychol* (2006) 25:119–23. doi:10.1037/0278-6133.25.1.119
25. O'Connor K. A cognitive-behavioral/psychophysiological model of tic disorders. *Behav Res Ther* (2002) 40:1113–42. doi:10.1016/S0005-7967(02)00048-7
26. Lin H, Katsovich L, Ghebremichael M, Findley DB, Grantz H, Lombroso PJ, et al. Psychosocial stress predicts future symptom severities in children and adolescents with Tourette syndrome and/or obsessive-compulsive disorder. *J Child Psychol Psychiatry* (2007) 48:157–66. doi:10.1111/j.1469-7610.2006.01687.x
27. Conelea CA, Woods DW. The influence of contextual factors on tic expression in Tourette's syndrome: a review. *J Psychosom Res* (2008) 65:487–96. doi:10.1016/j.jpsychores.2008.04.010
28. Leckman JF, Bloch MH, Sukhodolsky DG, Scahill L, King RA. Phenomenology of tics and sensory urges: the self under siege. In: Martino D, Leckman JF, editors. *Tourette Syndrome.* Oxford: Oxford University Press (2013). p. 3–25.
29. Cohen DJ. The pathology of the self in primary childhood autism and Gilles de la Tourette syndrome. *Psychiatr Clin North Am* (1980) 3:383–402.
30. Piacentini J, Woods DW, Scahill L, Wilhelm S, Peterson AL, Chang S, et al. Behavior therapy for children with Tourette disorder: a randomized controlled trial. *JAMA* (2010) 303(19):1929–37. doi:10.1001/jama.2010.607
31. Conelea CA, Woods DW, Brandt BC. The impact of a stress induction task on tic frequencies in youth with Tourette syndrome. *Behav Res Ther* (2011) 49:492–7. doi:10.1016/j.brat.2011.05.006
32. Ruhrman D, Mikulincer M, Steinberg T, Benaroya-Milshtein N, Apter A. Parenthood and Tourette syndrome: the interface between attachment, stress, emotion regulation and the child's experience of self. Implications for psychological interventions. *9th European Conference on Tourette Syndrome and Tic Disorders, June 8-11.* Warsaw, Poland (2016). [oral presentation]
33. Berant E, Mikulincer M, Shaver PR. Mothers' attachment style, their mental health and their children's emotional vulnerabilities: a 7-year study of children with congenital heart disease. *J Pers* (2008) 76:31–66. doi:10.1111/j.1467-6494.2007.00479.x
34. Oppenheim D, Koren-Karie N, Dolev S, Yirmiya N. Maternal insightfulness and resolution of the diagnosis are associated with secure attachment in preschoolers with autism spectrum disorders. *Child Dev* (2009) 80(2):519–27. doi:10.1111/j.1467-8624.2009.01276.x
35. Hirschtritt ME, Lee PC, Pauls DL, Dion Y, Grados MA, Illmann C, et al. Lifetime prevalence, age of risk, and genetic relationships of comorbid psychiatric disorders in Tourette syndrome. *JAMA Psychiatry* (2015) 72:325–33. doi:10.1001/jamapsychiatry.2014.2650
36. Robertson MM. A personal 35 year perspective on Gilles de la Tourette syndrome: prevalence, phenomenology, comorbidities, and coexistent psychopathologies. *Lancet Psychiatry* (2015) 2:68–87. doi:10.1016/S2215-0366(14)00132-1
37. Bowlby J. *Attachment and Loss, Vol.1, Attachment.* London: Hogarth Press and the Institute of Psycho-Analysis (1982/1969).
38. Mikulincer M, Shaver PR. *Attachment in Adulthood: Structure, Dynamics, and Change.* New York: Guilford Press (2007).
39. Abidin RR. *Parenting Stress Index: Manual.* Odessa, FL: Psychology Assessment Resources (1983).

8

Pediatric Autoimmune Disorders Associated with Streptococcal Infections and Tourette's Syndrome in Preclinical Studies

Chiara Spinello, Giovanni Laviola and Simone Macrì *

Section of Behavioural Neuroscience, Department of Cell Biology and Neuroscience, Istituto Superiore di Sanità, Roma, Italy

Edited by:
Kirsten R. Müller-Vahl,
Medical Doctor, Germany

Reviewed by:
Yang Xu,
Washington University, USA
James Leckman,
Yale University, USA
Kurt-Wolfram Sühs,
Hannover Medical School, Germany

***Correspondence:**
Simone Macrì
simone.macri@iss.it

Accumulating evidence suggests that Tourette's Syndrome (TS) – a multifactorial pediatric disorder characterized by the recurrent exhibition of motor tics and/or vocal utterances – can partly depend on immune dysregulation provoked by early repeated streptococcal infections. The natural and adaptive antibody-mediated reaction to streptococcus has been proposed to potentially turn into a pathological autoimmune response in vulnerable individuals. Specifically, in conditions of increased permeability of the blood brain barrier (BBB), streptococcus-induced antibodies have been proposed to: (i) reach neuronal targets located in brain areas responsible for motion control; and (ii) contribute to the exhibition of symptoms. This theoretical framework is supported by indirect evidence indicating that a subset of TS patients exhibit elevated streptococcal antibody titers upon tic relapses. A systematic evaluation of this hypothesis entails preclinical studies providing a proof of concept of the aforementioned pathological sequelae. These studies shall rest upon individuals characterized by a vulnerable immune system, repeatedly exposed to streptococcus, and carefully screened for phenotypes isomorphic to the pathological signs of TS observed in patients. Preclinical animal models may thus constitute an informative, useful tool upon which conducting targeted, hypothesis-driven experiments. In the present review we discuss the available evidence in preclinical models in support of the link between TS and pediatric autoimmune neuropsychiatric disorders associated with streptococcus infections (PANDAS), and the existing gaps that future research shall bridge. Specifically, we report recent preclinical evidence indicating that the immune responses to repeated streptococcal immunizations relate to the occurrence of behavioral and neurological phenotypes reminiscent of TS. By the same token, we discuss the limitations of these studies: limited evidence of behavioral phenotypes isomorphic to tics and scarce knowledge about the immunological phenomena favoring the transition from natural adaptive immunity to pathological outcomes.

Keywords: PANDAS, Tourette's Syndrome, animal models, group A-beta hemolytic streptococcus, autoimmunity

INTRODUCTION

Neuropsychiatric and neurological disorders are among the leading causes of disability worldwide (Silberberg et al., 2015). Several studies reported that people affected by neuropsychiatric illnesses show a set of psychosocial disturbances, ranging from difficulties in social interactions to emotional instability (Hartley et al., 2014; Cieza et al., 2015), ultimately resulting in difficulties in routine activities (Coenen et al., 2016). Since neuropsychiatric illnesses have a strong impact on the well-being of affected individuals, understanding the etiology of these diseases may beget remarkable heuristic advancements. Within this framework, epidemiological, clinical, and preclinical studies reveal that different determinants contribute to the pathogenesis of neuropsychiatric diseases. Among them, genetic factors (Hyman, 2008) and several environmental risk factors, such as prenatal and perinatal injuries or stressors (Bronson and Bale, 2016) and infectious phenomena (John et al., 2015), play a key role.

Autoimmunity, defined by Davison as "the failure of an organism to recognize its own part as self, resulting in a series of immunological responses to its own cells and tissues" (Davison, 2012) has emerged as a potential pathogenic factor in different types of neuropsychiatric illnesses, including autoimmune encephalitis (Höftberger, 2015), systemic lupus erythematosus (SLE; Podolska et al., 2015), or schizophrenia (Margari et al., 2013). Infectious phenomena constitute a vulnerability factor in the onset of autoimmune disorders. In particular, infections may trigger the onset of autoimmune diseases in the presence of vulnerability conditions. With respect to neuropsychiatric disorders, these vulnerability conditions are represented, for example, by an abnormal permeability of the blood brain barrier (BBB; Almutairi et al., 2016). Hornig (2013) proposed that microbes may contribute to the etiology of autoimmune neurological and neuropsychiatric disorders by triggering the production of autoantibodies that directly bind brain targets. In susceptible individuals, these phenomena can result in the appearance of behavioral and neurochemical abnormalities (Hornig, 2013).

Within this framework, streptococcal infections have been linked to a series of neuropsychiatric and movement disorders (Swedo et al., 1998). For example, different studies documented that the onset of Sydenham Chorea (SC), a variant of rheumatic fever, is linked to group A β-hemolitic streptococcus infections (Swedo et al., 1993; Cardoso et al., 1999). SC is characterized by choreiform movements that typically involve face and extremities and, in some cases, by behavioral difficulties and emotional liability (Swedo et al., 1989; Marques-Dias et al., 1997). Besides SC, several authors proposed that streptococcus infections may constitute an etiological factor also in a series of illnesses that typically arise during childhood. In particular, Swedo and colleagues proposed the acronym PANDAS (Pediatric Autoimmune Neuropsychiatric Disorder Associated with Streptococcal infections) to define a series of neurological and psychiatric disorders characterized by the presence of antibodies produced in response to group A β-hemolytic streptococcus infections (Swedo et al., 1998). The diagnostic criteria for PANDAS include: prepubertal onset; obsessive compulsive disorder (OCD) or chronic tic disorder; relapsing-remitting course of the disease; motor hyperactivity or reduced fine motor coordination; onset of the disease or symptoms exacerbation temporally related to streptococcal infection (Swedo et al., 1998).

In PANDAS and SC, antibodies produced in response to streptococcus have been proposed to be pathogenic in CNS in the context of an increased BBB permeability. Since the BBB is the primary protective barrier for neurons in central nervous system (CNS), BBB dysfunctions may contribute to the etiology of several neuropsychiatric disorders (Almutairi et al., 2016). In particular, in PANDAS and SC, after crossing the damaged BBB, cross-reactive antibodies may bind specific brain targets at the level of Basal Ganglia (BG), a brain structure involved in motor control (Martino et al., 2009; Murphy et al., 2010; Cutforth et al., 2016).

Streptococcal infections have also been suggested to relate to Tourette's Syndrome (TS), a multifactorial and complex disorder that may, in some cases, match the criteria for PANDAS (Hoekstra et al., 2013). TS is a childhood-onset disorder, in which chronic motor or phonic tics are the main symptoms. Tics are considered chronic if persist over a period longer than 12 months (Lombroso and Scahill, 2008). Tic, according to the DSM-5, is defined as "a sudden, rapid, recurrent, non-rhythmic motor movement or vocalization" (APA, 2013). TS is more frequent in males than females, with a ratio of 4:1. Typically, symptoms occur during prepubertal age, between 5 and 7 years, and have a waxing and waning course (Lombroso and Scahill, 2008). A gradual increase in tic frequency and severity is generally shown until 8–12 years, while a relevant reduction occurs in most patients at the end of adolescence (Leckman et al., 2010). Co-morbid conditions are typical in TS. In particular, obsessive-compulsive disorder (OCD) and attention-deficit/hyperactivity disorder (ADHD) are the most common comorbidities (Leckman et al., 2010). The pathogenesis of TS is multifactorial, and include genetic vulnerability (Deng et al., 2012), and several environmental risk factors such as prenatal and perinatal stressors or injuries and bacterial and viral infections (Leckman et al., 1987, 1990; Leckman and Peterson, 1993). With respect to precocious vulnerability, maternal factors (genetic or environmental) have been shown to increase individual vulnerability to TS. For example, Dalsgaard et al. (2015) recently reported that maternal autoimmune diseases significantly increase vulnerability to TS in the progeny (Dalsgaard et al., 2015).

While maternal autoimmunity can influence vulnerability to TS, it is yet to be determined whether these effects are genetic or environmental. With respect to genetic predispositions, several authors identified a series of genes for which a direct contribution to TS can be reasonably proposed. Thus, genetic linkage, cytogenetics and molecular genetic studies allowed identifying a set of genes potentially involved in TS (State, 2011). Among them, contactin-associated protein-like 2 (CNTNAP2), SLIT and NTRK-like 1 (SLITRK1) or membrane peptidase 2 like (IMMP2L) have been proposed as vulnerability genes. The proteic product of IMMP2L gene is a peptide with a catalytic function that, in the dysfunctional form, may cause the activation of the cell apoptotic mechanism through an aberrant mithocondrial functionality (Ma et al., 2011). Several authors reported in some members of a family with TS the presence of a translocation between chromosome 7 and 18 that causes the disruption of IMMP2L gene (Boghosian-Sell et al., 1996; Petek et al., 2001). However, the role of this gene in TS etiology remains unclear. CNTNAP2 is a transmembrane protein of the family of neurexin, abundantly expressed at the level of the axonal nodes of Ranvier, where it plays a crucial role in the cell-cell interaction. Poliak et al. (1999), hypothesized that this peptide may be involved in the positioning of K^+ voltage-gated channel at the level of juxtaparanode region (Poliak et al., 1999). Verkerk et al. (2003) observed a chromosomal translocation between chromosome 2 and 7, in the region encoding CNTNAP2 protein, in a family of TS patients (Verkerk et al., 2003). The disruption of this region has been proposed to affect brain areas involved in motor control, thereby being responsible for the onset of tics (Verkerk et al., 2003). SLTRK1 is a member of a gene family that encodes a series of transmembrane proteins. The proteic product of SLTRK1 gene is a peptide that contains two leucine-rich repeat (LRR) motive and an intracellular C terminus having similarities with the tropomyosin-related kinase (Trk) neurotrophin's receptor (Aruga and Mikoshiba, 2003). SLTRK1 favors the formation of synapses, neuritic outgrowth and neuronal survival (Kajiwara et al., 2009). SLTRK1 transcription is regionally regulated in CNS; the pattern of expression is conserved among different mammalian species, such as mouse, rhesus monkey and human, and shows a preferential expression in brain areas involved in motor control, such as cortex, thalamus and basal ganglia (Stillman et al., 2009). In particular, SLRTK1 is expressed in the body compartment of cortex pyramidal projection neurons during adult life, and is preferentially associated, in the striatum, with neurons of the direct circuit expressing substance P and dopamine receptor D1, that project to substantia nigra (SN) and to globus pallidus (GP; Stillman et al., 2009). Some TS patients showed a missense mutation at the level of 3′ UTR of the SLTRK1 gene; this mutation leads to the production of a protein with an altered capacity of binding the microRNA 189 (Abelson et al., 2005). Moreover, an inversion in chromosome 13 in proximity of the region of the gene has been reported in patients with TS and ADHD (Proenca et al., 2011). Recently, Ercan-Sencicek et al. (2010) proposed that a mutation of the gene encoding for histidine decarboxylase (HDC) constitutes a rare genetic cause in TS (Ercan-Sencicek et al., 2010). In particular, the authors identified, through a study of a 2-generation pedigree in a family with a high incidence of TS, a rare segregating non-sense mutation in the *l-hystidine decarboxylase (hdc)* gene (Ercan-Sencicek et al., 2010). HDC is an enzyme necessary for the synthesis of histamine (HA) which, in turn, has been hypothesized to modulate DA level in CNS (Haas et al., 2008). Subsequently, a reduced concentration of HA in CNS (caused by the non-sense *hdc* gene mutation) may result in an altered dopaminergic regulation at the level of the basal ganglia circuitry, thereby resulting in TS symptomatology (Castellan Baldan et al., 2014). In the same study, Castellan Baldan and collaborators translated this evidence in an experimental model (*hdc* knock-out mice, see discussion for additional details). Moreover, an analysis of rare copy number variants in TS conducted on 460 patients, revealed the presence of a significant enrichment of genes involved in histaminergic pathways (Fernandez et al., 2012). In particular, the authors reported an enrichment in striatum and cortex of HA coupled G receptors H2 and H3. Those receptors are located both presinaptically and postsinaptically: presynaptic HA receptors are involved in the regulation not only of HA transmission, but also of dopamine (Fernandez et al., 2012). It is thus tenable to propose that dysfunctions in histaminergic pathway may contribute to the onset of TS through the modulation of dopaminergic transmission.

GAS infections, occurring after TS onset, have been proposed as a vulnerability factor potentially exacerbating symptoms (Martino et al., 2009; Landau et al., 2012). Additionally, in line with the possibility that altered immune capability constitutes a predisposing factor, clinical data support an increased vulnerability of the immune system in TS patients. For example, whilst Bos-Veneman et al. (2011) observed that TS children were characterized by decreased levels of IgG3 (Bos-Veneman et al., 2011), Kawikova et al. (2007) observed reduced concentrations of regulatory T cells in TS patients compared to controls (Kawikova et al., 2007). Moreover, during tic exacerbations, TS patients showed increased concentrations of cytokines, interleukin 12 (IL-12) and tumor necrosis factor alpha (TFN-α) in serum (Leckman et al., 2005; Martino et al., 2015). Several authors reported the presence of peripheral anti-streptococcal antibodies and anti-BG antibodies in patients affected by TS. For example, Cardona and Orefici observed that a large cohort of TS patients showed significantly higher levels of anti-streptococcal antibodies compared to control subjects; moreover, they reported that those patients had previously been exposed to streptococcal infections (Cardona and Orefici, 2001). Similarly, Rizzo and colleagues reported remarkably higher concentrations of anti-streptococcal antibody titers and a significantly higher presence of anti-BG antibodies in TS patients compared to control subjects (Rizzo et al., 2006). Martino and colleagues reported a similar increase in anti-BG antibodies in TS patients compared to controls (Martino et al., 2011).

Although these studies support the existence of a link between streptococcal infections and TS, several other studies failed to identify a direct link between immunization and TS symptoms (Singer et al., 2005a; Dale et al., 2006; Morris et al., 2009; Brilot et al., 2011). In particular, Singer et al. (2005a) performed ELISA and Western blot analyses against several epitopes present in the CNS (e.g., human postmortem caudate, putamen, prefrontal cortex) with sera obtained from PANDAS and TS patients, and controls. The authors did not detect differences in serum autoantibodies among groups (Singer et al., 2005a). Similarly, Morris et al. (2009), using a different experimental approach (immunofluorescence), failed to observe any difference among PANDAS and TS patients, and controls in terms of serum anti-striatal antibody reactivity (Morris et al., 2009). Finally, Brilot et al. (2011) reported the presence of serum autoantibodies capable of binding neuronal cell surface in SC patients, but not in PANDAS or TS patients (Brilot et al., 2011). These results demonstrate that the presence of autoimmune phenomena is neither a necessary nor a sufficient condition in the etiology of TS. However, the evidence discussed above indicates that a subset of TS cases may be dependent on autoimmune phenomena. Moreover, as already discussed, some cases of TS match criteria for PANDAS, suggesting that these two disorders may share — in specific circumstances — analogous etiopathological mechanisms.

Preclinical experimental models may constitute a valuable complement to clinical studies whereby they can aid the comprehension of the fundamental mechanisms favoring disease onset. Animal models may allow testing different hypotheses regarding the role exerted by variable factors in the onset and course of a given disease, and to design innovative therapeutic approaches (Rickard, 2004; van der Staay, 2006; van der Staay et al., 2009). Within this framework, several aspects of TS (symptomatology, genetic predisposition and environmental risk factors) have been translated into preclinical animal models (Hallett et al., 2000; Yaddanapudi et al., 2010; Brimberg et al., 2012; Macrì et al., 2015; see Macrì et al., 2013 for a detailed review).

Here, we will review preclinical data suggesting a link between autoimmunity and neurological diseases. In particular, we will discuss empirical evidence supporting the connection between TS and PANDAS, and the gaps of these studies that shall be filled in the future. Finally, in the light of the role of immunity in the onset of psychiatric disturbance, we discuss the possibility that peripheral autoantibodies may constitute an innovative biomarker of diagnostic use (Giana et al., 2015).

PRECLINICAL ANIMAL MODELS AND AUTOIMMUNITY

Animal models constitute an important tool to aid the understanding of a given pathology and to potentially inform innovative therapeutic avenues. Thus, preclinical experimental models allow dissecting a given phenomenon into its fundamental determinants (e.g., genetic vs. environmental predisposing factors) and addressing the role that each of them plays, either in isolation or in combination with each other. The development of disease-related animal models rests upon several stages: the generation of a disease model based on a theoretical construct, the identification of abnormalities isomorphic to the symptoms observed in the patient population and the study of the efficacy of pharmacological treatments. The validity of each of these stages can be systematically scrutinized. Willner proposed three validity criteria: *construct, face,* and *predictive validity* (Willner, 1984).

Construct validity can be defined as the etiological similarity between the disease in human population and the experimental approach attempting to model such disease.

Face validity relates to the degree of similarity between the symptoms identified in the disorder examined and the phenotype (e.g., behavioral, physiological, immunological, neurobiological) in the experimental model (Willner and Mitchell, 2002). To fulfill this criterion, a valid animal model shall resemble the symptomatology observed in humans (van der Staay et al., 2009).

Predictive validity pertains to the therapeutic efficacy of available treatments. Specifically, to possess an elevated degree of predictive validity, a given experimental disease model shall be sensitive to the same available therapeutic approaches adopted in the patients (Willner, 1984).

Within this framework, the use of preclinical models has been extensively applied to the study of autoimmune neurological disorders (see Levite, 2014 and Hornig and Lipkin, 2013 for detailed reviews). Several preclinical animal models have been developed to address the link between circulating natural antibodies (directed against specific brain targets), and behavioral and neurochemical abnormalities. For example, mice immunized with GluR1 peptide fragments (a subunit of glutamate AMPA receptors) showed a significant elevation in circulating anti-GluR1 antibodies, marked hyperactivity, and increased self-grooming (Capone et al., 2008), the latter being associated with repetitive behavior (Kalueff et al., 2016). Also, mice immunized with dopamine transporter (DAT) fragments, displayed spontaneous hyperactivity, reduced cognitive flexibility and impulse control in operant behavioral paradigms. Moreover, the immunization protocol caused, as expected, an elevation in antibodies targeting dopamine transporter and a variation in brain striatal concentrations of dopamine and its metabolites (Adriani et al., 2012).

Glutamate is the main excitatory neurotransmitter in CNS (Platt, 2007) and is crucial for several neuronal functions. Abnormalities in glutamatergic neurotransmission have been shown to directly contribute to CNS disorders (Scoriels et al., 2015). The overactivation of glutamate receptors (excitotoxicity), induced by the excess of glutamate, may result in brain damage and neuronal death (Meldrum, 2000). Besides excitotoxicity, several types of anti-glutamate receptors antibodies are capable of inducing pathological effects in CNS (Levite, 2014). These autoantibodies emerged as one of the most widespread and dangerous pathogenic agents in CNS, causing impaired neuronal signaling and brain damages and contributing to the onset of a series of neuropsychiatric disorders (Levite, 2014). For example, patients affected by epilepsy and SLE, showed antibodies directed to different types of glutamate receptors, anti AMPA-GluR3B (Ganor et al., 2004, 2005a,b,c; Goldberg-Stern et al., 2014) and anti NMDA-NR2 (Borchers et al., 2005; Asano et al., 2013; Fanouriakis et al., 2013). From a translational perspective, antibodies against the same glutamate receptors have been shown to favor the onset of behavioral and neurochemical alterations also in preclinical models (see Levite, 2014 for a detailed review). These results have been observed in conditions of an increased permeability of the BBB (Kowal and Diamond, 2012). Several authors reported increased levels of anti-GluR3B antibodies in different mouse strains (specifically directed against peptide B of subunit R3 of glutamate AMPA receptors) after immunization with GluR3B peptide (Levite et al., 1999; Levite and Hermelin, 1999; Ganor et al., 2014). Specifically, Ganor et al. (2014) reported that DBA/2J mice (genetically epilepsy-prone mice) developed elevated titers of GluR3B antibodies after immunization with GluR3B peptide emulsified in Complete Freund's adjuvant

(CFA). The presence of these antibodies aggravated seizures induced by the administration of a chemoconvulsant agent, and caused abnormal behaviors in mice. With respect to behavioral alterations, the authors observed, in mice positive to GluR3B antibodies, increased anxiety-like behaviors and motor impairments (problems in balance, motor coordination and muscle strength) compared to mice that did not show GluR3B antibodies in serum (Ganor et al., 2014).

Kowal and colleagues developed an immune-mediated mouse model of SLE (Kowal et al., 2004). These authors reported that the immunization of BALB/C mice with DNA peptide mimotope, arrayed as an octamer on a polylysine backbone (MAP peptide), induced the production of antibodies against subunit NR2 of NMDA glutamate receptor, associated with neuronal damages and cognitive impairments. In particular, following the administration of lipopolysaccharide (LPS, a procedure known to increase the permeability of the BBB) to immunized mice, NR2 antibodies bound neurons preferentially in hippocampus, inducing neuronal death and impaired memory (Kowal et al., 2004). NMDA-NR2 receptors are expressed throughout the brain, but at highest density within hippocampus, hypothalamus, and amygdala. When the BBB damage was induced in mice by epinephrine administration, Huerta et al. (2006) showed that anti-NR2 antibodies bound preferentially amygdala's neurons. Accordingly, immunized mice showed alteration in emotional behavior whereby they responded deficiently to fear-conditioning paradigms (Huerta et al., 2006). The latter has been shown to depend on an intact functionality of the amygdala (Sengupta et al., 2016).

Beside glutamate receptors, autoimmune phenomena in CNS involve other receptors, such as leucine-rich glioma inactivated 1 (LGI1), acquaporin-4 (AQP4), Gamma-Amino Butyric Acid ($GABA_B$), or myelin oligodendrocyte protein (MOG; see Irani et al., 2014 for a detailed review). In preclinical studies, immunization with MOG has been shown, in susceptible animals, to trigger the onset of a series of inflammatory diseases and thereafter named experimental autoimmune encephalomyelitis (EAE). EAE, considered as a valid animal model of multiple sclerosis (MS), are a group of pathologies characterized by neurodegeneration, extensive inflammation and demyelination in CNS. These neurochemical alterations cause severe progressive motor impairments that ultimately result in flaccid paralysis of hind limbs (see Kipp et al., 2012 for a detailed review). Beside MOG (Amor et al., 1994, 1996), other myelin antigens are capable of triggering the onset of EAE in rodents, such as myelin basic protein (MBP, see Swanborg, 2001 and Amor et al., 1996), proteolipid protein (PLP, see Amor et al., 1993 and Amor et al., 1996) in presence of increased BBB permeability (Rabchevsky et al., 1999). Several preclinical studies showed that EAE are associated not only with severe motor deficits, but also with behavioral and cognitive impairments (Mandolesi et al., 2010; Acharjee et al., 2013; Olechowski et al., 2013). For example, Mandolesi et al. (2010) reported that EAE mice, compared to controls, showed hippocampal-dependent deficit in learning and memory (Mandolesi et al., 2010). Similarly, Acharjee and colleagues observed that EAE mice exhibited cognitive and behavioral impairments in a precocious phase of the disease (Acharjee et al., 2013). In particular, EAE mice exhibited reduction in the time spent in the target quadrant of Morris Water maze and impaired memory extinction in a fear-conditioning paradigm (Acharjee et al., 2013). Regarding behavioral impairments, authors observed in EAE mice increased anxiety-like behaviors. EAE mice showed, compared to controls, more time in the marginal zone of the apparatus during open field test and increased time in the closed arm of plus maze test (Acharjee et al., 2013). Finally, Olechowski et al. (2013) observed impairments in cognitive processes (assessed with a novel object recognition test) in a precocious phase of the disease (Olechowski et al., 2013).

The experimental evidence described above suggests that autoimmune phenomena against CNS targets may trigger, in vulnerability conditions, the development of remarkable phenotypic abnormalities. The appearance of different behavioral and neurochemical impairments depends on the brain target affected by the autoimmune phenomena and, in some instances, by the tools adopted to modulate BBB integrity. As reported above (see Introduction), analogous mechanisms have been proposed to contribute to the onset and exacerbation of streptococcal-related motor disturbances in clinical populations. Specifically, several authors (Martino et al., 2009; Murphy et al., 2010) proposed that antibodies produced in response to streptococcal infections (STREP) may, in presence of an increased vulnerability of the BBB, induce a pathological phenotype. In particular, these authors proposed that STREP-related antibodies may cross the damaged BBB and bind specific brain targets at the level of Basal Ganglia (BG), a brain structure involved in motor control. This cascade of events may ultimately provoke a symptomatology typical of streptococcal-related motor disturbances. In the next section we will describe some specific animal models developed with the aim of dissecting the mechanisms bridging the immunologic responses to streptococcal infections to the onset of neurological and behavioral dysfunctions.

A Potential Link between Streptococcal Infections and TS

Passive Transfer of Sera from TS Patients

Different approaches have been used to develop animal models addressing the role of streptococcal infections in immune-mediated neuropsychiatric disorders (**Table 1**). The first line of studies entailed direct intracerebral administration, in rats, of anti-neuronal antibodies sampled from TS patients (Hallett et al., 2000; Taylor et al., 2002; Loiselle et al., 2004; Singer et al., 2005b; Ben-Pazi et al., 2012; Yeh et al., 2012). Hallett et al. (2000) showed that brain intra-striatal microinfusions of TS sera induced behavioral stereotypies and episodic utterances (EU, repetitive, medium pitched sound of short duration) in male Fischer 344 rats. Stereotypies and EUs are considered analogous to involuntary movements observed in TS patients. In particular, the authors performed two separate studies, microinfusing either sera obtained from TS children or Gamma Immunoglobulin (IgG) isolated from these sera. In the first study, compared to facility-reared controls, rats microinfused with TS-sera showed exacerbated licking behavior, forepaw shaking and EU. Those abnormal behaviors were present during microinfusion, and on

TABLE 1 | Summary of the main findings in TS/PANDAS animal models.

References	Passive transfer (PT) or direct immunization (DI)	Reference pathology	Neurochemical/Neuroanatomical abnormalities	Behavioral outcome
Hallett et al., 2000	PT of sera or purified IgG from TS patients	TS	IgG deposits in striatum	(↑) Licking (↑) Forepaw shacking (↑) Episodic utterances
Taylor et al., 2002	PT of sera from TS patients	TS	–	(↑) Oral stereotypies
Yeh et al., 2012	PT of sera or purified anti-HCN4 from TS patients	TS	–	(↑) Stereotyped tic behavior
Hoffman et al., 2004	DI	TS/PANDAS	IgG deposits in deep cerebellar nuclei (DCN)	(↑) Rearing behavior
Yaddanapudi et al., 2010	DI	TS/PANDAS	IgG deposits in cerebellum and striatum	(↓) Social activities and social investigation (↓) Ability in olfactory discrimination (↓) Motor coordination (↓) Aggressive behavior (↑) Rearing behavior
	PT of sera from immunized mice	TS/PANDAS	IgG deposits in hippocampus and paraventricular area	(↑) Rearing behavior (↓) Social interaction
Macrì et al., 2015	DI	TS/PANDAS	Inflammation in rostral diencephalon	(↓) Pre-pulse inhibition (↑) Perseveration
Brimberg et al., 2012	DI	TS/PANDAS	IgG deposits in striatum, thalamus and frontal cortex	(↓) Motor capacity (↑) Compulsive behavior
Lotan et al., 2014	DI	TS/PANDAS	–	(↑) Rearing behavior (↓) Food manipulation (↓) Fine motor coordination
	PT of purified IgG from immunized rats	TS/PANDAS	Co-localized IgG deposits with D1/D2 receptor and SERT in striatum	(↓) Food manipulation (↓) Fine motor coordination

Summary of the main articles in which an autoimmune hypothesis of motor disturbances has been addressed. We report the immunization method, the reference pathology, the neuroanatomical, neurochemical, and behavioral alterations identified.

days 8–10 after the end of microinfusion, when behavior was assessed. EUs were particularly interesting, since rats usually do not emit audible vocalizations in non-threatening environment (Kaltwasser, 1990), as the one adopted in this study. The authors proposed that sudden and involuntary contraction of respiratory muscles (resulting from the effect of serum on rats' striatal functionality) may provoke EU. Furthermore, these sudden and audible vocalizations occurred in association with head or oral stereotypies, suggesting that contraction of respiratory muscles could be involved in their occurrence (Ebrahimi et al. 1992). In the second study, IgG was isolated from both control and TS sera and microinfused into rats' striatum. Compared to control individuals, rats microinfused with TS-IgG exhibited a much higher level of licking activity. Moreover, immunohistochemical analyses of brain sections showed that TS-IgG selectively bind striatal neurons in rats microinfused with TS-IgG. These results supported the hypothesis that IgG recognize specific neuronal antigens within the striatum and interfere with its normal functioning, inducing abnormalities in motor control (Hallett et al., 2000). Similarly, Taylor et al. (2002) observed an increase in oral stereotypies after infusions of TS sera into the ventrolateral striatum of male Sprague-Dawley rats. In this study, the authors performed 5 days of microinfusions and conducted systematic behavioral observations throughout the entire treatment period. Specifically, the authors assessed the behavior of three groups of rats, with different sera received during microinfusion: TS-sera containing high levels of autoantibodies, TS-sera containing low levels of autoantibodies and control sera. Rats microinfused with TS-sera characterized by highest antibody titers exhibited remarkably elevated oral stereotypies compared to the other groups (Taylor et al., 2002). Finally, Yeh et al. (2012) showed that TS sera were immunoreactive against a 120 kDa protein, identified as hyperpolarization-activated nucleotide channel 4 (HCN4) protein. Male Sprague-Dawley rats received microinfusion in striatum of purified anti-HCN4 antibodies and of TS-sera. Behavioral observation after infusion revealed that both TS sera and purified anti-HCN4 antibodies induced the increase of behavioral stereotypies in rats in a dose-dependent manner (Yeh et al., 2012). Additionally, several studies reported that passive transfer, in striatum of naïve animals, of anti-streptococcal sera or of purified IgG from animals exposed to GABHS, leads to the onset of behavioral and neurochemical abnormalities that resemble PANDAS symptomatology (Yaddanapudi et al.,

2010; Lotan et al., 2014). These studies are detailed in the next section.

Although these results support the existence of a link between autoimmune phenomena and behavioral stereotypies, analogous subsequent studies failed to replicate these findings (Loiselle et al., 2004; Singer et al., 2005b; Ben-Pazi et al., 2012). In particular, Loiselle et al. (2004) performed microstriatal infusions of serum from TS and PANDAS patients in Fischer rats' striatum. In this study, rats received bilateral microinfusions of sera in ventral and ventrolateral striatum. As in the experimental protocol described in Hallett et al. (2000), sera were microinfused for 3 days, and animal behavior was assessed during microinfusions and for 10 days after the end of microinfusions. Unlike the two studies previously described (Hallett et al., 2000; Taylor et al., 2002), rats microinfused with TS sera or PANDAS sera did not show a significant increase in terms of motor or vocal stereotypies (Loiselle et al., 2004). Similarly, Singer et al. (2005b) observed that infusions of sera from patients with TS in ventrolateral striatum of Sprague-Dawley rats, did not significantly increase stereotypies (Singer et al., 2005b). A total of 16 rats received (for 4 days) sera containing elevated or low levels of antineural antibodies (ANAb), while eight control rats were infused with phosphate buffered saline (PBS). Behavioral observations were performed for 3 days before infusions, on days 2–4 during infusions, and for 3 days after the end of infusions. Stereotypies resulted significantly increased after serum infusion, but authors did not observe significant differences between control group and groups treated with low or elevated ANAb sera. Moreover, in contrast with Taylor et al. (2002), this study suggests that the level of antibodies in blood may have no influence on their pathogenicity; low or elevated titers of antineural antibodies in sera did not induce a differential behavioral response in terms of stereotypies (Singer et al., 2005b). Finally, Ben-Pazi et al. (2012), did not observe motor behavioral changes in rats after the injections of sera from Sydenhams's Chorea (SC) patients (Ben-Pazi et al., 2012). In particular, authors injected stereotaxically 6 μl of the IgG fraction of serum in rats' left striatum, and induced rotational behavior administering amphetamine and apomorphine (after 10 and 17 days from injections respectively). Authors observed that the injections of SC-IgG in rats brain striatum did not induce a significant increase in rotational behavior. Moreover, immunohistology staining, specific for dopaminergic or GABA-ergic markers, did not reveal cellular changes in rats injected with SDC-IgG compared to controls (Ben-Pazi et al., 2012). Although the reason for failure to detect stereotypies is unclear, Loiselle et al. (2004), proposed that methodological variations may constitute a possible explanation for the variable results obtained among different studies. These variations comprise different methods to quantify antineural antibodies in sera, strain of rodents, timing of microinfusion, timing of observation, and concentrations of microinfused sera (Loiselle et al., 2004).

Active Immunization with Group A Beta–Hemolytic Streptococcus Homogenate

Other experimental studies, using a different approach based on active immunization, reported that streptococcal infections may trigger, in the presence of a vulnerable BBB, basal ganglia dysfunctions (Swerdlow and Sutherland, 2005). These studies show that streptococcus exposure may favor the onset of behavioral disturbances and neurochemical alterations, thereby providing additional information regarding PANDAS etiology (Hoffman et al., 2004; Yaddanapudi et al., 2010; Brimberg et al., 2012; Macrì et al., 2015). These results may support the hypothesis that antibodies produced in response to streptococcus infections may bind, in a context of BBB permeability, brain targets at the level of basal ganglia, causing the onset of behavioral and motor disturbances and neurochemical alterations (Martino et al., 2009).

For example, SJL/J mice (a mouse strain prone to the induction of autoimmune encephalitis, see Korngold et al., 1986) repeatedly immunized with a group A beta—hemolytic streptococcus (GABHS) homogenate emulsified in Freund's adjuvant (FA), showed increased behavioral abnormalities compared to control subjects immunized with FA alone (Hoffman et al., 2004). Mice were screened in several behavioral tests to assess anxiety-like behavior, general behavioral responses, and exploratory behavior. Moreover, sera from all mice were tested for immunoreactivity to mouse brain, while the presence of IgG deposits has been assessed performing immunohistochemistry on cerebral tissues. The authors reported that a subset of sera collected after the second boost from GABHS mice were immunoreactive to several brain regions. In particular, GABHS sera labeled neurons in deep cerebellar nuclei (DCN), globus pallidus, and thalamus. GABHS immunized mice, characterized by serum immunoreactivity to DCN, showed also IgG deposits in the same brain area. Mice that showed serum immunoreactivity to DCN exhibited also increased rearing behavior (considered as repetitive behavior) compared to control mice and to GABHS subjects that did not show sera immunoreactivity to DCN. Moreover, the increase in rearing behavior correlated with DCN IgG deposits, and with serum IgG immunoreactivity to GABHS proteins. These results partially fulfill the criteria for PANDAS proposed by Swedo et al. (1998). In particular, the animal model described meets two criteria: the presence of chronic tic disorder and/or OCD; and the onset and exacerbation of symptoms associated with GABHS infections. Mice exposed to GABHS showed abnormal repetitive behavior, partially reproducing OCD symptomatology in humans. Moreover, the exhibition of repetitive behavior was temporally related with the exposure to GABHS (Hoffman et al., 2004).

In a subsequent study, Yaddanapudi et al. (2010) showed that humoral immunity is necessary and sufficient to induce PANDAS related symptoms. The authors passively immunized SJL mice by exposing them to serum obtained from donor mice immunized with GABHS homogenate, and observed an abnormal behavioral phenotype (Yaddanapudi et al., 2010). Direct exposure to GABHS homogenate resulted in diminished motor coordination, increased rearing behavior, reduced social activities and social investigation, inhibition of aggressive behavior and impaired ability in olfactory discrimination. Passive transfer of GABHS sera reproduced the increment in rearing behavior and the alteration in social interaction, while did not have effects on motor coordination. To demonstrate that the effects were due to the immune response to the streptococcus immunization, the authors also performed a passive transfer study in which sera of donor mice was depleted from Immunoglobulin G. IgG emerged as the active component of GABHS donor sera whereby its depletion abolished the behavioral abnormalities observed in mice injected with non-depleted IgG GABHS sera. Consistently with what emerged regarding behavioral observations, donor GABHS mice showed brain IgG deposits in cerebellum and striatum and mice injected with non-depleted IgG GABHS sera showed brain IgG deposits in hippocampus and paraventricular area. Conversely, IgG-depleted GABHS mice did not show brain deposits, confirming that IgG is the active component of GABHS sera. The different localization of brain IgG deposits in donor mice and in mice that received non-depleted sera, may depend on the different approaches used to increase the permeability of BBB (Freund's adjuvant and LPS respectively). These results, together with what observed in experimental studies involving animal models of SLE (see Kowal et al., 2004 and Huerta et al., 2006), suggest that BBB permeability is crucial in mediating the involvement of peripheral immunity in PANDAS and, in general, in neuropsychiatric and neurological disorders (Almutairi et al., 2016). Recently, Dileepan et al. (2016), proposed a mechanism that allows antibodies produced in response to streptococcal infections to cross the BBB and trigger autoimmune diseases of the CNS (Dileepan et al., 2016). In particular, they reported the presence of group A streptococcal specific Th17 lymphocytes in tonsils of humans previously exposed to natural GABHS infections (Dileepan et al., 2016). Repeated intranasal (i.n.) inoculations of GABHS in mice triggered the expansion of Th17 cells and the production of interleukin 17 (IL17), as shown in a previous study (Dileepan et al., 2011). IL17 causes the damaging of BBB barrier through the production of reactive oxygen species (ROS) in endothelial cells (Kebir et al., 2007; Huppert et al., 2010). Dileepan et al. (2016) repeatedly inoculated mice i.n. with GABHS to investigate if exposure to streptococcus induces Th17 GABHS-specific cells enter the mice brain. They reported that group A streptococcal infections trigger in mice a lymphocyte Th17 response together with the production of IL-17A in nasal-associated lymphoid tissue (NALT). NALT is a tissue located in proximity of cribriform plate and has an equivalent functionality of palatine tonsils in humans (Park et al., 2003). Moreover, they reported the presence of GABHS-specific Th17 cells associated with damaged BBB; the damaged BBB allowed the deposition of serum IgG. Finally they reported the presence of activated microglia (neuroinflammation) and impaired synaptic transmission. The authors suggested that the abnormal production of cytokine induced by infections may disrupt the BBB, permitting autoantibodies to access the brain and bind neural targets, ultimately causing the onset of pathological phenotypes (Dileepan et al., 2016).

Recently, we repeatedly exposed developing male SJL/J mice to a GABHS homogenate, showing that a single exposure to streptococcus is not sufficient to trigger behavioral abnormalities related to PANDAS (Macrì et al., 2015). In particular, we exposed mice to a primary immunization (GABHS homogenate emulsified in CFA), followed by three boosts (GABHS homogenate emulsified in incomplete Freund's adjuvant). We screened mice in two different behavioral test batteries performed between the primary immunization and the first boost, and after the second boost. Mice exposed to a single GABHS immunization did not show a differential phenotype compared to controls. Conversely, after the second boost, GABHS mice showed increased repetitive and perseverative behaviors and impaired sensorimotor gating. To evaluate sensorimotor gating, we measured their motor response in the Prepulse Inhibition of the startle reflex (PPI) task. PPI is an experimental measure in which the startle reflex (response to sudden and intense stimulus) is inhibited by a weak stimulus. This task is of common use in human laboratory and holds an elevated translational value (Swerdlow, 2013). In rodents, whole-body startle is measured by assessing the force resulting from the contraction of skeletal muscles (Swerdlow, 2013). PPI results impaired in a series of neuropsychiatric disorders, including schizophrenia (Swerdlow et al., 2006), Huntington disease (Swerdlow et al., 1995; Valls-Sole et al., 2004), OCD (Swerdlow et al., 1993; Hoenig et al., 2005; Ahmari et al., 2012), as well as TS (Castellanos et al., 1996; Swerdlow et al., 2001a,b; Zebardast et al., 2013). Preclinical evidence showed that in rodents experimental lesions of striatal circuits significantly reduced PPI (Baldan Ramsey et al., 2011), and that the administration of dopaminergic drugs modulated its expression (Mansbach et al., 1988; Russig et al., 2004). Therefore, impaired PPI observed in GABHS mice supports the hypothesis that repeated exposures to streptococcus may cause dysfunctions in cortico-striatal-thalamocortical (CSTC) circuits, involved in TS (Swerdlow, 2013). A dysfunctional regulation of the CSTC has been proposed to constitute a common factor among TS and comorbid problems, such OCD (Berardelli et al., 2003; Leckman et al., 2010). This hypothesis is supported by clinical evidence suggesting the involvement of the central dopaminergic system in TS: tics frequency is increased by dopamine (DA) D2 receptor agonists (Shprecher and Kurlan, 2009), and reduced by D2 antagonists (Scahill et al., 2006).

The increased perseverative behavior observed in GABHS mice constitutes an additional evidence supporting the hypothesis that repeated exposure to streptococcus may cause dysfunctions in brain areas considered involved in TS. In particular, we assessed perseverative behavior in T-maze test to measure spontaneous alternation, considered as a natural tendency to explore the environment (Deacon and Rawlins, 2006). Lalonde (2002) showed that the exhibition of spontaneous alternation depends on the integrity of several brain areas, including prefrontal cortex and dorsal striatum (Lalonde, 2002). Moreover, the administration of dopaminergic and serotoninergic drugs modulates spontaneous alternation behavior (Irwin et al., 1983; Jaffard et al., 1991).

The fact that behavioral abnormalities have been observed after repeated exposures to GABHS supports the hypothesis that a single immunization with streptococcus is not sufficient to trigger a pathological phenotype. The exhibition of symptoms may require a prolonged exposure, associated with the development of a high level of peripheral anti-GABHS antibodies. This hypothesis is supported by the fact that we found elevated concentrations of antibodies in GABHS-mice sera after repeated injections, but not after the primary immunization. Mice repeatedly exposed to streptococcus showed also neurochemical alterations (reduced serotonin and increased lactate) in prefrontal cortex, a brain structure involved in the control of the behavioral domains addressed in the study. Moreover, GABHS mice exhibited inflammatory processes (presence of infiltrates and active microglia) in the rostral diencephalon. Thus, our study supports the hypothesis that exposure to streptococcus is a vulnerability factor in the onset of behavioral and neurochemical phenotypes homologous to symptoms observed in PANDAS.

Brimberg et al. (2012) reported that male Lewis rats exposed to GABHS antigens, showed behavioral, immunological, and neural characteristics resembling symptoms observed in PANDAS patients (Brimberg et al., 2012). Rats exposed to GABHS exhibit impaired motor capacity and compulsive behavior. The administration of haloperidol and paroxetine, both used to treat motor symptoms and compulsion in PANDAS, alleviated symptoms observed in GABHS mice. Importantly, this study was the first reporting the presence of peripheral autoantibodies against D1 and D2 receptors following active immunization with GABHS homogenate. Moreover, GABHS-exposed rats showed IgG deposits in striatum, thalamus and frontal cortex. This study supports the link between GABHS exposure and the development of anti-brain antibodies (in rats sera), specifically directed against dopamine receptors. This evidence supports the idea that dopaminergic system has an important role in the onset of symptoms related to PANDAS (including TS). Finally, Lotan et al. (2014) extended these results by the identification of the serotonergic system as an additional mediator of the onset of PANDAS related symptoms. Specifically, beside replicating the presence of antibodies against D1 and D2 receptors, they observed peripheral antibodies against serotonin (5HT-2A and 5HT-2C) receptors in rats previously exposed to GABHS (Lotan et al., 2014). Furthermore, the active immunization of male Lewis rats resulted in a series of phenotypic abnormalities associated with compulsive behavior and motor impairments: increased grooming; impairments in food manipulation; and impairments in fine motor activity tested through walking on a narrow beam (Lotan et al., 2014). These observations are in line with pharmacological evidence indicating that several serotonergic agonists may constitute an effective treatment for the GABHS-dependent psychiatric symptoms (Swedo and Grant, 2005; Murphy et al., 2010). Additionally, these results parallel our study in which we showed that active streptococcal immunization throughout development may alter serotonergic transmission in the adult brain (Macrì et al., 2015). In the same study, Lotan et al. (2014) addressed whether the antibodies produced in response to GABHS were sufficient to induce an abnormal phenotype. To investigate this aspect, the authors performed a passive transfer experiment in which they injected purified IgG from immunized and control rats directly in the striatum of naïve rats (Lotan et al., 2014). In accordance with the predictions, microinfusion of IgG from immunized rats partially reproduced the phenotype of rats exposed to the direct immunization: impairments in food manipulation and in beam walking test (Lotan et al., 2014). Finally, immunoistochemical analysis of IgG deposits in striatum revealed the presence of IgG clusters in striatum of rats passively exposed to GABHS; moreover, the authors observed that these clusters co-localized with D1 and D2 receptors and with serotonin transporter (SERT; Lotan et al., 2014).

LIMITATIONS OF THE STUDIES AND FUTURE PERSPECTIVES

In the present manuscript, we aimed at describing animal models developed to investigate the link between streptococcus infections and the onset of autoimmune-mediated neuropsychiatric disorder. Within this framework, animal models developed using active immunization constitute a valid tool to investigate the etiological mechanisms of PANDAS and other related disorders, such as TS. Yet, these animal models present a series of limitations that need to be addressed in future experimental studies. Specifically, current experimental models are limited in terms of the timing of symptoms observation (prepubertal onset in humans in spite of the fact that abnormalities in rodents are generally addressed in already adult subjects) and in the limited exploitation of gene × environment interactions. In the following section, we discuss these limitations and propose an approach to overcome them in the future (these aspects are summarized in **Table 2**). As briefly mentioned, one of the core limitations is represented by the timing of the onset of PANDAS-like phenotype in preclinical models. PANDAS, as already discussed, are a series of streptococcal-related disorders that occur specifically in the pediatric population. Most of the PANDAS-related symptoms observed in animals (stereotypies, repetitive and perseverative behavior, impaired sensorimotor gating) have instead been addressed in late adolescent/adult individuals. Such limitation is predominantly related to technical constraints associated with the immunization protocol. In all the studies analyzed, the first immunization of a repeated protocol has been performed at four (Hoffman et al., 2004; Yaddanapudi et al., 2010; Macrì et al., 2015), five (Brimberg et al., 2012), or 6 weeks (Hoffman et al., 2004; Yaddanapudi et al., 2010) of age, corresponding, in rodents, to puberty and adolescence. Moreover, the subsequent injections (performed to simulate a repeated exposure to streptococcus) were always interspaced by 3 weeks. Thus, the consequences of the repeated exposure to streptococcus have been evaluated in fully adult mice. To assess the effects of streptococcus in younger individuals and come closer to the specific characteristic of the pediatric population, future studies shall entail an earlier timing of the primary injection, and much shorter intervals between boosts.

Animal Models and Gene × Environment Interactions

With particular attention to TS, the utility of autoimmune models should be extended to investigate the role gene × environment interactions. Considering the multifactorial and complex etiology of TS (entailing also genetic vulnerability), several experimental models leveraged the use of genetically-engineered animals. For example, SLITRK knockout (ko) mice, have been developed

TABLE 2 | Experimental models of PANDAS and TS.

Pandas and TS	Experimental models of pandas and TS	Future perspectives
Chronic tic disorders and/or OCD[1]	**OCD-like behaviors: increased repetitive behaviors, stereotypies, perseverative behavior and fine motor coordination[4–11]**	Extension of the behavioral phenotype to incorporate patterns analogous to tics
Association with streptococcal infections[1]	**Association with streptococcal infections through active immunization[7–11] or passive transfer of sera from TS patients[4–6]**	Design of complex experimental protocols entailing a double hit hypothesis (e.g., stress during pregnancy x streptococcal immunization early in puberty)
Motor hyperactivity[1]	Motor hyperactivity	Prolongation of the analysis of motor behavior (e.g., continuous monitoring of behavior through automated systems)
Prepubertal onset[1]	Prepubertal onset	Earlier administration of streptococcal antigens
Relapsing and remitting course of the disease[1]	Relapsing and remitting course of the disease	–
Impaired PPI[2]	**Impaired PPI[9]**	–
Autoantibodies developed following streptococcal infections, cross the BBB and bind specific target at the level of BG, causing morphological alteration in CNS[3]	**IgG deposits in cerebellum, striatum, hippocampus and paraventricular area[7, 8] inflammation in rostral diencephalon[9]**	Investigation of the role of microglia and astrocytes in the autoimmune sequelae in preclinical models[12]

Bold, Scientific evidence; Italics, hypothesis; Normal text, Clinical evidence not reproduced in animal models.
Numbers indicate the references in which the corresponding information has been described. (1) Swedo et al., 1998; (2) Swerdlow et al., 2001b; (3) Martino et al., 2009; (4) Hallett et al., 2000; (5) Taylor et al., 2002; (6) Yeh et al., 2012; (7) Hoffman et al., 2004; (8) Yaddanapudi et al., 2010; (9) Macrì et al., 2015; (10) Brimberg et al., 2012; (11) Lotan et al., 2014; (12) Benedek et al., 2016.

following the identification of mutations in SLITRK genes in TS patients (Katayama et al., 2010). Although Slitrk1-deficient mice possess a great degree of construct validity, this model does not resemble TS symptomatology, thereby possessing a limited degree of face validity. In particular, Sltrk1 ko mice did not show tic-like symptoms or neurochemical abnormalities typical of TS. Other genetic models have been developed based on the link between TS and glutamatergic hyperactivity inside the CSTC. In particular, Nordstrom and colleagues developed a D1 receptor transgenic animal model (D1CT-7), expressing hyperactivity in two groups of neural populations located (expressing D1 receptors) in the insular and piriform cortices and in the amygdala (Nordstrom and Burton, 2002). These mice exhibit features that are analogous to the tics observed in TS patients (very brief isolated head or body *jerk* or *shake*); moreover, these symptoms are alleviated by the administration of drugs that have analogous effects in humans. Despite the good degree of face and predictive validity of this model, D1CT-7 mice exhibit also features that are not typical of TS (see Macrì et al., 2013 for a detailed review). Recently, Castellan Baldan et al. (2014) developed an animal model resting upon the observation that the *hdc* gene may be involved in TS (Ercan-Sencicek et al., 2010). Within this framework, the authors developed a line of mice (*hdc* ko) lacking histidine decarboxylase, which is necessary to synthesize histamine (Castellan Baldan et al., 2014). These mice exhibited a significant increase in behavioral stereotypies after D-amphetamine injection and a deficit in sensorimotor gating, reflected in impairments in PPI. Haloperidol pretreatment mitigated behavioral stereotypies. Moreover, while in the brain of wild type mice HA concentration increased during the dark-active phase of the diurnal cycle (Haas et al., 2008) HA concentration was significantly reduced in left hypothalamus, striatum and right neocortex of ko mice (Castellan Baldan et al., 2014). Although daytime striatal DA concentration did not differ between genotypes, *hdc* ko mice showed a significant increase in DA concentration during the active phase of the diurnal cycle, when HA was increased in wild type mice (Castellan Baldan et al., 2014). This result further supports the hypothesis that HA negatively regulates DA (Haas et al., 2008). Finally, ko mice showed a reduction of D2 + D3 receptor density in striatum, and an increase of D2 + D3 receptor density in substantia nigra, suggesting a cellular response to the persistent elevation of DA (Stanwood et al., 2000). Thus, in the light of the theoretical framework in which it has been developed (clinical evidence indicating the importance of HA in TS; Ercan-Sencicek et al., 2010), the phenotypic alterations observed (motor abnormalities and impaired sensorimotor gating), and the pharmacological efficacy of haloperidol (one of the treatments of choice in TS, Bornstein et al., 1990), this experimental model seems to possess an elevated degree of construct, face and predictive validity.

Given the limitations of both autoimmune and genetic models, future attempts should be focused on combining some of the models previously described, aiming at investigating gene × environment interactions.

Neonatal Environmental Factors and Individual Vulnerability to PANDAS

Future efforts should be focused also on investigating the possibility that neonatal environmental factors may calibrate, and eventually suppress, individual vulnerability to PANDAS. Several studies reported that precocious experiences affect the individual resilience toward future challenges (Heim et al., 2004, 2008; Lyons and Macrì, 2011). In particular, while traumatic precocious experiences result in increased individual vulnerability to future challenges (Heim et al., 2004, 2008), stimulating early conditions have been proposed to favor individual resilience (Lyons and Macrì, 2011). The immune system is particularly sensitive to early experiences (Roque et al., 2014). For example, several studies conducted in rodents showed that maternal separation (daily 3–6 h mother-offspring separations during the first 2 weeks of life) or exposure to early physiological stressors result in increased susceptibility toward viral infections (Meagher et al., 2010) or vulnerability toward autoimmune phenomena (Bakker et al., 2000). Individual reactivity to immune challenge has been proposed to depend on the functionality of hypothalamic-pituitary-adrenocortical (HPA) axis (Bakker et al., 2000; Meagher et al., 2010). In particular, the differential response to immune challenge depends on the modulation of the functionality of immune system exerted by elevations in levels of corticosterone (Laban et al., 1995). Several studies showed that circulating corticosteroids have a direct effect on T-cell, suppressing immune responses (Wick et al., 1993). Thus, it is tenable to propose that the modulation of corticosterone reactivity through experimental stressors, may calibrate individual susceptibility toward phenomena that relate to immunity (immune and autoimmune phenomena). Within this framework, Levine and Saltzman (1987) reported that experimental stressors favoring an upregulation of the HPA-axis alter individual vulnerability to EAE (Levine and Saltzman, 1987). Moreover, Levine and colleagues showed that stress reduces (Levine et al., 1962a) and adrenalectomy enhances (Levine et al., 1962b) vulnerability to EAE. Thus, a persistent upregulation of HPA axis induced by neonatal stressor may consistently prevent some of the consequences of experimental models of autoimmunity, such as PANDAS. Beside analyzing the role of environmental factors in modulating the functionality of the immune system, future studies shall thoroughly detail which portions of the immune system are involved in the autoimmune sequelae (Benedek et al., 2016). An interesting target to be contemplated in future studies is the activation of microglia and the role exerted by astrocytes (Benedek et al., 2016; Lécuyer et al., 2016). These targets appear particularly relevant whereby their involvement has already been demonstrated in experimental models of autoimmunity (Correale, 2014; Shemer and Jung, 2015; Benedek et al., 2016; Lécuyer et al., 2016). While these studies addressed the role of astrocytes and microglia in experimental models of MS, it may be important to evaluate whether these outcomes translate to experimental models of PANDAS or TS. This need is also corroborated by clinical evidence indicating that microglia can be activated in TS and PANDAS patients (Kumar et al., 2015), see below for a detailed description.

Peripheral Autoantibodies As Diagnostic Biomarker in TS

Finally, we emphasize the value of the detection of peripheral autoantibodies as a reliable method potentially aiding the diagnosis of neurological disorders. The search of biological markers measurable and detectable using non-invasive approaches constitutes an important tool in the diagnosis of these diseases (Damoiseaux et al., 2015). With particular attention to autoimmune disorders, the measurement of autoantibodies has been proposed as a valuable tool not only in the diagnosis, but also in the prediction and in the prognosis of autoimmune diseases (Harel and Shoenfeld, 2006; Shepshelovich and Shoenfeld, 2006; Bizzaro et al., 2007; see Damoiseaux et al., 2015 for a detailed review). Within this framework, several peripheral autoantibodies emerged as clinically relevant in several neurological and neuropsychiatric disorders, such as multiple sclerosis (Comabella and Montalban, 2014), limbic encephalitis (Beck et al., 2009; Schlumberger et al., 2014), myasthenia gravis (Verschuuren et al., 2013), or ADHD (Giana et al., 2015). However, the debate on the efficacy of serum autoantibodies as diagnostic markers is still open. For example Höftberger (2015) reported that in the case of autoimmune encephalitis (AIE), serum did not contain antineural antibodies in the 14% of patients, while autoantibodies were always detected in patients' cerebrospinal fluid (CSF). Thus, the absence of autoantibodies in serum may not be sufficient to exclude AIE (Höftberger, 2015). With respect to TS, as already discussed (see Introduction), several clinical studies reported the presence of anti-BG antibodies in sera of TS patients (Rizzo et al., 2006; Martino et al., 2011). Moreover, the injections of TS sera (containing autoantibodies) directly into rodents' striatum, result, in some cases, in behavioral and neurochemical alterations that partially resemble PANDAS symptomatology (Hallett et al., 2000; Yeh et al., 2012). In addition, autoantibodies in TS sera seem to induce PANDAS-like behavioral phenotypes in a concentration-dependent manner (high or low level of autoantibodies titers, see Taylor et al., 2002). These results seem to support the hypothesis that anti-BG antibodies may constitute a valid biomarker in the diagnosis of some cases of TS. However, results reported in subsequent studies, where the passive transfer of TS sera in rodents' striatum failed to induce PANDAS-like phenotypes (Loiselle et al., 2004; Ben-Pazi et al., 2012), suggest that additional studies are necessary to investigate the diagnostic value of the detection of peripheral BG-antigens in TS. Further efforts may be focused, for example, on the standardization of the assays used to quantify antineural antibodies in sera (Jacobs et al., 2015). In particular, further studies should be focused on investigating the use of immunohistochemistry as a method for the detection of anti-neuronal autoantibodies in CNS disorders. Hachiya et al. (2013) showed, in a recent study, that immunohistochemistry may constitute a reliable method for the detection of autoantibodies in serum of patients affected by CNS disorders associated with GABHS infections (Hachiya et al., 2013). In particular, they assessed immunoreactivity of sera (obtained during the acute phase of disease or during remission or convalescence) from patients affected by three CNS disorders linked to GABHS infections (acute disseminated encephalomyelitis, PANDAS and subacute encephalitis). The authors performed immunohistochemistry on brain sections of hippocampus, basal ganglia, cerebellar cortex and midbrain obtained from male controls (aged 5 and 9 years) that did not present CNS alterations. Sera obtained from patients affected by acute disseminated encephalomyelitis and PANDAS showed immunoreactivity in globus pallidus neurons, while sera obtained from patients affected by subacute encephalitis showed immunoreactivity in the extra pyramidal cell layers in the temporal cortex. Conversely, sera obtained during remission or convalescence did not show immunoreactivity

(Hachiya et al., 2013). With particular attention to PANDAS and TS, future efforts should be focused, for example, on analyzing immunoreactivity of sera from patients toward dopamine D2 receptors. In the context of the identification of immune-related diagnostic biomarkers, Kumar et al. (2015) recently evaluated neuroinflammation in TS and PANDAS children. Specifically, the authors performed a Positron Emission Tomographic (PET) study to identify markers of activated microglia (Kumar et al., 2015). Activated microglia has been proposed to constitute a valid indicator of the presence of neuroinflammation (Kreutzberg, 1996). To address this aspect, the authors exploited the capacity of activated microglia to express the translocator protein receptor (TSPO). TSPO, in turn, can be selectively identified through the radioactive tracer ^{11}C-[R]-PK11195 (PK) (Cagnin et al., 2007). Using this approach, the authors analyzed neuroinflammation in basal ganglia and thalamus and observed increased binding potential in bilateral caudate and bilateral lentiform nucleus in PANDAS patients. TS children exhibited neuroinflammation in bilateral lentiform nucleus only, suggesting possible neuroanatomical differences between PANDAS and TS diseases (Kumar et al., 2015). Thus, the monitoring of neuroinflammation through PET may constitute a potential method to clarify pathophysiological mechanisms in TS and PANDAS.

AUTHOR CONTRIBUTIONS

CS and SM wrote the first draft of the manuscript; CS, SM, and GL worked on the subsequent versions of the manuscript.

ACKNOWLEDGMENTS

The authors of this manuscript received funding from the European Community's Seventh Framework Programme (FP7/2007-2013) under grant agreements n° 278367 (Project EMTICS) and n° 603016 (Project MATRICS). This paper reflects only the authors' views and the European Union is not liable for any use that may be made of the information contained therein. We sincerely thank Prof. Francesco Cardona for critical reading of a previous version of this manuscript, and Prof. Graziella Orefici for constant and constructive feedback on the topic of the present manuscript.

REFERENCES

Abelson, J. F., Kwan, K. Y., O'Roak, B. J., Baek, D. Y., Stillman, A. A., Morgan, T. M., et al. (2005). Sequence variants in SLITRK1 are associated with Tourette's syndrome. *Science* 310, 317–320. doi: 10.1126/science.1116502

Acharjee, S., Nayani, N., Tsutsui, M., Hill, M. N., Ousman, S. S., and Pittman, Q. J. (2013). Altered cognitive-emotional behavior in early experimental autoimmune encephalitis–cytokine and hormonal correlates. *Brain Behav. Immun.* 33, 164–172. doi: 10.1016/j.bbi.2013.07.003

Adriani, W., Koot, S., Columba-Cabezas, S., Romano, E., Travaglini, D., van den Bos, R., et al. (2012). Immunization with DAT fragments is associated with long-term striatal impairment, hyperactivity and reduced cognitive flexibility in mice. *Behav. Brain Funct.* 8:54. doi: 10.1186/1744-9081-8-54

Ahmari, S. E., Risbrough, V. B., Geyer, M. A., and Simpson, H. B. (2012). Impaired sensorimotor gating in unmedicated adults with obsessive-compulsive disorder. *Neuropsychopharmacology* 37, 1216–1223. doi: 10.1038/npp.2011.308

Almutairi, M. M., Gong, C., Xu, Y. G., Chang, Y., and Shi, H. (2016). Factors controlling permeability of the blood-brain barrier. *Cell. Mol. Life Sci.* 73, 57–77. doi: 10.1007/s00018-015-2050-8

Amor, S., Baker, D., Groome, N., and Turk, J. L. (1993). Identification of a major encephalitogenic epitope of proteolipid protein (residues 56–70) for the induction of experimental allergic encephalomyelitis in Biozzi AB/H and nonobese diabetic mice. *J. Immunol.* 150, 5666–5672.

Amor, S., Groome, N., Linington, C., Morris, M. M., Dornmair, K., Gardinier, M. V., et al. (1994). Identification of epitopes of myelin oligodendrocyte glycoprotein for the induction of experimental allergic encephalomyelitis in SJL and Biozzi AB/H mice. *J. Immunol.* 153, 4349–4356.

Amor, S., O'Neill, J. K., Morris, M. M., Smith, R. M., Wraith, D. C., Groome, N., et al. (1996). Encephalitogenic epitopes of myelin basic protein, proteolipid protein, myelin oligodendrocyte glycoprotein for experimental allergic encephalomyelitis induction in Biozzi ABH (H-2Ag7) mice share an amino acid motif. *J. Immunol.* 156, 3000–3008.

APA (2013). *Diagnostic and Statistical Manual of Mental Disorders*. Arlington, VA: American Psychiatric Association.

Aruga, J., and Mikoshiba, K. (2003). Identification and characterization of Slitrk, a novel neuronal transmembrane protein family controlling neurite outgrowth. *Mol. Cell. Neurosci.* 24, 117–129. doi: 10.1016/S1044-7431(03)00129-5

Asano, N. M., Coriolano, M., Asano, B. J., and Lins, O. G. (2013). Psychiatric comorbidities in patients with systemic lupus erythematosus: a systematic review of the last 10 years. *Rev. Bras. Reumatol.* 53, 431–437. doi: 10.1016/S2255-5021(13)70114-7

Bakker, J. M., Kavelaars, A., Kamphuis, P. J., Cobelens, P. M., van Vugt, H. H., van Bel, F., et al. (2000). Neonatal dexamethasone treatment increases susceptibility to experimental autoimmune disease in adult rats. *J. Immunol.* 165, 5932–5937. doi: 10.4049/jimmunol.165.10.5932

Baldan Ramsey, L. C., Xu, M., Wood, N., and Pittenger, C. (2011). Lesions of the dorsomedial striatum disrupt prepulse inhibition. *Neuroscience* 180, 222–228. doi: 10.1016/j.neuroscience.2011.01.041

Beck, L. H. Jr., Bonegio, R. G., Lambeau, G., Beck, D. M., Powell, D. W., Cummins, T. D., et al. (2009). M-type phospholipase A2 receptor as target antigen in idiopathic membranous nephropathy. *N. Engl. J. Med.* 361, 11–21. doi: 10.1056/NEJMoa0810457

Benedek, G., Zhang, J., Bodhankar, S., Nguyen, H., Kent, G., Jordan, K., et al. (2016). Estrogen induces multiple regulatory B cell subtypes and promotes M2 microglia and neuroprotection during experimental autoimmune encephalomyelitis. *J. Neuroimmunol.* 293, 45–53. doi: 10.1016/j.jneuroim.2016.02.009

Ben-Pazi, H., Sadan, O., and Offen, D. (2012). Striatal microinjection of Sydenham chorea antibodies: using a rat model to examine the dopamine hypothesis. *J. Mol. Neurosci.* 46, 162–166. doi: 10.1007/s12031-011-9559-6

Berardelli, A., Currà, A., Fabbrini, G., Gilio, F., and Manfredi, M. (2003). Pathophysiology of tics and Tourette syndrome. *J. Neurol.* 250, 781–787. doi: 10.1007/s00415-003-1102-4

Bizzaro, N., Tonutti, E., Visentini, D., Alessio, M. G., Platzgummer, S., Morozzi, G., et al. (2007). Antibodies to the lens and cornea in anti-DFS70-positive subjects. *Ann. N.Y. Acad. Sci.* 1107, 174–183. doi: 10.1196/annals.1381.019

Boghosian-Sell, L., Comings, D. E., and Overhauser, J. (1996). Tourette syndrome in a pedigree with a 7;18 translocation: identification of a YAC spanning the translocation breakpoint at 18q22.3. *Am. J. Hum. Genet.* 59, 999–1005.

Borchers, A. T., Aoki, C. A., Naguwa, S. M., Keen, C. L., Shoenfeld, Y., and Gershwin, M. E. (2005). Neuropsychiatric features of systemic lupus erythematosus. *Autoimmun. Rev.* 4, 329–344. doi: 10.1016/j.autrev.2005.01.008

Bornstein, R. A., Stefl, M. E., and Hammond, L. (1990). A survey of Tourette syndrome patients and their families: the 1987 Ohio Tourette Survey. *J. Neuropsychiatry Clin. Neurosci.* 2, 275–281.

Bos-Veneman, N. G., Olieman, R., Tobiasova, Z., Hoekstra, P. J., Katsovich, L., Bothwell, A. L., et al. (2011). Altered immunoglobulin profiles in children with Tourette syndrome. *Brain Behav. Immun.* 25, 532–538. doi: 10.1016/j.bbi.2010.12.003

Brilot, F., Merheb, V., Ding, A., Murphy, T., and Dale, R. C. (2011). Antibody binding to neuronal surface in Sydenham chorea, but not in PANDAS or Tourette syndrome. *Neurology* 76, 1508–1513. doi: 10.1212/WNL.0b013e3182181090

Brimberg, L., Benhar, I., Mascaro-Blanco, A., Alvarez, K., Lotan, D., Winter, C., et al. (2012). Behavioral, pharmacological, and immunological abnormalities after streptococcal exposure: a novel rat model of Sydenham chorea and related neuropsychiatric disorders. *Neuropsychopharmacology* 37, 2076–2087. doi: 10.1038/npp.2012.56

Bronson, S. L., and Bale, T. L. (2016). The Placenta as a mediator of stress effects on neurodevelopmental reprogramming. *Neuropsychopharmacology* 41, 207–218. doi: 10.1038/npp.2015.231

Cagnin, A., Kassiou, M., Meikle, S. R., and Banati, R. B. (2007). Positron emission tomography imaging of neuroinflammation. *Neurotherapeutics* 4, 443–452. doi: 10.1016/j.nurt.2007.04.006

Capone, F., Adriani, W., Shumilina, M., Izykenova, G., Granstrem, O., Dambinova, S., et al. (2008). Autoantibodies against opioid or glutamate receptors are associated with changes in morphine reward and physical dependence in mice. *Psychopharmacology* 197, 535–548. doi: 10.1007/s00213-007-1062-y

Cardona, F., and Orefici, G. (2001). Group A streptococcal infections and tic disorders in an Italian pediatric population. *J. Pediatr.* 138, 71–75. doi: 10.1067/mpd.2001.110325

Cardoso, F., Vargas, A. P., Oliveira, L. D., Guerra, A. A., and Amaral, S. V. (1999). Persistent Sydenham's chorea. *Mov. Disord.* 14, 805–807.

Castellan Baldan, L., Williams, K. A., Gallezot, J. D., Pogorelov, V., Rapanelli, M., Crowley, M., et al. (2014). Histidine decarboxylase deficiency causes tourette syndrome: parallel findings in humans and mice. *Neuron* 81, 77–90. doi: 10.1016/j.neuron.2013.10.052

Castellanos, F. X., Fine, E. J., Kaysen, D., Marsh, W. L., Rapoport, J. L., and Hallett, M. (1996). Sensorimotor gating in boys with Tourette's syndrome and ADHD: preliminary results. *Biol. Psychiatry* 39, 33–41. doi: 10.1016/0006-3223(95)00101-8

Cieza, A., Anczewska, M., Ayuso-Mateos, J. L., Baker, M., Bickenbach, J., Chatterji, S., et al. (2015). Understanding the impact of brain disorders: towards a 'horizontal epidemiology' of psychosocial difficulties and their determinants. *PLoS ONE* 10:e0136271. doi: 10.1371/journal.pone.0136271

Coenen, M., Cabello, M., Umlauf, S., Ayuso-Mateos, J. L., Anczewska, M., Tourunen, J., et al. (2016). Psychosocial difficulties from the perspective of persons with neuropsychiatric disorders. *Disabil. Rehabil.* 38, 1134–1145. doi: 10.3109/09638288.2015.1074729

Comabella, M., and Montalban, X. (2014). Body fluid biomarkers in multiple sclerosis. *Lancet Neurol.* 13, 113–126. doi: 10.1016/S1474-4422(13)70233-3

Correale, J. (2014). The role of microglial activation in disease progression. *Mult. Scler.* 20, 1288–1295. doi: 10.1177/1352458514533230

Cutforth, T., DeMille, M. M., Agalliu, I., and Agalliu, D. (2016). CNS autoimmune disease after infections: animal models, cellular mechanisms and genetic factors. *Future Neurol.* 11, 63–76. doi: 10.2217/fnl.16.4

Dale, R. C., Church, A. J., Candler, P. M., Chapman, M., Martino, D., and Giovannoni, G. (2006). Serum autoantibodies do not differentiate PANDAS and Tourette syndrome from controls. *Neurology* 66:1612. doi: 10.1212/01.wnl.0000226832.36908.4c

Dalsgaard, S., Waltoft, B. L., Leckman, J. F., and Mortensen, P. B. (2015). Maternal history of autoimmune disease and later development of tourette syndrome in offspring. *J. Am. Acad. Child Adolesc. Psychiatry* 54, 495–501.e1. doi: 10.1016/j.jaac.2015.03.008

Damoiseaux, J., Andrade, L. E., Fritzler, M. J., and Shoenfeld, Y. (2015). Autoantibodies 2015: from diagnostic biomarkers toward prediction, prognosis and prevention. *Autoimmun. Rev.* 14, 555–563. doi: 10.1016/j.autrev.2015.01.017

Davison, K. (2012). Autoimmunity in psychiatry. *Br. J. Psychiatry* 200, 353–355. doi: 10.1192/bjp.bp.111.104471

Deacon, R. M., and Rawlins, J. N. (2006). T-maze alternation in the rodent. *Nat. Protoc.* 1, 7–12. doi: 10.1038/nprot.2006.2

Deng, H., Gao, K., and Jankovic, J. (2012). The genetics of Tourette syndrome. *Nat. Rev. Neurol.* 8, 203–213. doi: 10.1038/nrneurol.2012.26

Dileepan, T., Linehan, J. L., Moon, J. J., Pepper, M., Jenkins, M. K., and Cleary, P. P. (2011). Robust antigen specific th17 T cell response to group A Streptococcus is dependent on IL-6 and intranasal route of infection. *PLoS Pathog.* 7:e1002252. doi: 10.1371/journal.ppat.1002252

Dileepan, T., Smith, E. D., Knowland, D., Hsu, M., Platt, M., Bittner-Eddy, P., et al. (2016). Group A Streptococcus intranasal infection promotes CNS infiltration by streptococcal-specific Th17 cells. *J. Clin. Invest.* 126, 303–317. doi: 10.1172/JCI80792

Ebrahimi, A., Pochet, R., and Roger, M. (1992). Topographical organization of the projections from physiologically identified areas of the motor cortex to the striatum in the rat. *Neurosci. Res.* 14, 39–60.

Ercan-Sencicek, A. G., Stillman, A. A., Ghosh, A. K., Bilguvar, K., O'Roak, B. J., Mason, C. E., et al. (2010). L-histidine decarboxylase and Tourette's syndrome. *N. Engl. J. Med.* 362, 1901–1908. doi: 10.1056/NEJMoa0907006

Fanouriakis, A., Boumpas, D. T., and Bertsias, G. K. (2013). Pathogenesis and treatment of CNS lupus. *Curr. Opin. Rheumatol.* 25, 577–583. doi: 10.1097/BOR.0b013e328363eaf1

Fernandez, T. V., Sanders, S. J., Yurkiewicz, I. R., Ercan-Sencicek, A. G., Kim, Y. S., Fishman, D. O., et al. (2012). Rare copy number variants in tourette syndrome disrupt genes in histaminergic pathways and overlap with autism. *Biol. Psychiatry* 71, 392–402. doi: 10.1016/j.biopsych.2011.09.034

Ganor, Y., Freilinger, M., Dulac, O., and Levite, M. (2005a). Monozygotic twins discordant for epilepsy differ in the levels of potentially pathogenic autoantibodies and cytokines. *Autoimmunity* 38, 139–150. doi: 10.1080/08916930500100825

Ganor, Y., Goldberg-Stern, H., Amrom, D., Lerman-Sagie, T., Teichberg, V. I., Pelled, D., et al. (2004). Autoimmune epilepsy: some epilepsy patients harbor autoantibodies to glutamate receptors and dsDNA on both sides of the blood-brain barrier, which may kill neurons and decrease in brain fluids after hemispherotomy. *Clin. Dev. Immunol.* 11, 241–252. doi: 10.1080/17402520400001736

Ganor, Y., Goldberg-Stern, H., Blank, M., Shoenfeld, Y., Dobrynina, L. A., Kalashnikova, L., et al. (2005c). Antibodies to glutamate receptor subtype 3 (GluR3) are found in some patients suffering from epilepsy as the main disease, but not in patients whose epilepsy accompanies antiphospholipid syndrome or Sneddon's syndrome. *Autoimmunity* 38, 417–424. doi: 10.1080/08916930500246339

Ganor, Y., Goldberg-Stern, H., Cohen, R., Teichberg, V., and Levite, M. (2014). Glutamate receptor antibodies directed against AMPA receptors subunit 3 peptide B (GluR3B) can be produced in DBA/2J mice, lower seizure threshold and induce abnormal behavior. *Psychoneuroendocrinology* 42, 106–117. doi: 10.1016/j.psyneuen.2014.01.005

Ganor, Y., Goldberg-Stern, H., Lerman-Sagie, T., Teichberg, V. I., and Levite, M. (2005b). Autoimmune epilepsy: distinct subpopulations of epilepsy patients harbor serum autoantibodies to either glutamate/AMPA receptor GluR3, glutamate/NMDA receptor subunit NR2A or double-stranded DNA. *Epilepsy Res.* 65, 11–22. doi: 10.1016/j.eplepsyres.2005.03.011

Giana, G., Romano, E., Porfirio, M. C., D'Ambrosio, R., Giovinazzo, S., Troianiello, M., et al. (2015). Detection of auto-antibodies to DAT in the serum: interactions with DAT genotype and psycho-stimulant therapy for ADHD. *J. Neuroimmunol.* 278, 212–222. doi: 10.1016/j.jneuroim.2014.11.008

Goldberg-Stern, H., Ganor, Y., Cohen, R., Pollak, L., Teichberg, V., and Levite, M. (2014). Glutamate receptor antibodies directed against AMPA receptors subunit 3 peptide B (GluR3B) associate with some cognitive/psychiatric/behavioral abnormalities in epilepsy patients. *Psychoneuroendocrinology* 40, 221–231. doi: 10.1016/j.psyneuen.2013.11.007

Haas, H. L., Sergeeva, O. A., and Selbach, O. (2008). Histamine in the nervous system. *Physiol. Rev.* 88, 1183–1241. doi: 10.1152/physrev.00043.2007

Hachiya, Y., Miyata, R., Tanuma, N., Hongou, K., Tanaka, K., Shimoda, K., et al. (2013). Autoimmune neurological disorders associated with group-A beta-hemolytic streptococcal infection. *Brain Dev.* 35, 670–674. doi: 10.1016/j.braindev.2012.10.003

Hallett, J. J., Harling-Berg, C. J., Knopf, P. M., Stopa, E. G., and Kiessling, L. S. (2000). Anti-striatal antibodies in Tourette syndrome cause neuronal dysfunction. *J. Neuroimmunol.* 111, 195–202. doi: 10.1016/S0165-5728(00)00320-9

Harel, M., and Shoenfeld, Y. (2006). Predicting and preventing autoimmunity, myth or reality? *Ann. N.Y. Acad. Sci.* 1069, 322–345. doi: 10.1196/annals.1351.031

Hartley, S., McArthur, M., Coenen, M., Cabello, M., Covelli, V., Roszczynska-Michta, J., et al. (2014). Narratives reflecting the lived experiences of people with brain disorders: common psychosocial difficulties and determinants. *PLoS ONE* 9:e96890. doi: 10.1371/journal.pone.0096890

Heim, C., Newport, D. J., Mletzko, T., Miller, A. H., and Nemeroff, C. B. (2008). The link between childhood trauma and depression: insights from HPA axis studies in humans. *Psychoneuroendocrinology* 33, 693–710. doi: 10.1016/j.psyneuen.2008.03.008

Heim, C., Plotsky, P. M., and Nemeroff, C. B. (2004). Importance of studying the contributions of early adverse experience to neurobiological findings in depression. *Neuropsychopharmacology* 29, 641–648. doi: 10.1038/sj.npp.1300397

Hoekstra, P. J., Dietrich, A., Edwards, M. J., Elamin, I., and Martino, D. (2013). Environmental factors in Tourette syndrome. *Neurosci. Biobehav. Rev.* 37, 1040–1049. doi: 10.1016/j.neubiorev.2012.10.010

Hoenig, K., Hochrein, A., Quednow, B. B., Maier, W., and Wagner, M. (2005). Impaired prepulse inhibition of acoustic startle in obsessive-compulsive disorder. *Biol. Psychiatry* 57, 1153–1158. doi: 10.1016/j.biopsych.2005.01.040

Hoffman, K. L., Hornig, M., Yaddanapudi, K., Jabado, O., and Lipkin, W. I. (2004). A murine model for neuropsychiatric disorders associated with group A beta-hemolytic streptococcal infection. *J. Neurosci.* 24, 1780–1791. doi: 10.1523/JNEUROSCI.0887-03.2004

Höftberger, R. (2015). Neuroimmunology: an expanding frontier in autoimmunity. *Front. Immunol.* 6:206. doi: 10.3389/fimmu.2015.00206

Hornig, M. (2013). The role of microbes and autoimmunity in the pathogenesis of neuropsychiatric illness. *Curr. Opin. Rheumatol.* 25, 488–795. doi: 10.1097/BOR.0b013e32836208de

Hornig, M., and Lipkin, W. I. (2013). Immune-mediated animal models of Tourette syndrome. *Neurosci. Biobehav. Rev.* 37, 1120–1138. doi: 10.1016/j.neubiorev.2013.01.007

Huerta, P. T., Kowal, C., DeGiorgio, L. A., Volpe, B. T., and Diamond, B. (2006). Immunity and behavior: antibodies alter emotion. *Proc. Natl. Acad. Sci. U.S.A.* 103, 678–683. doi: 10.1073/pnas.0510055103

Huppert, J., Closhen, D., Croxford, A., White, R., Kulig, P., Pietrowski, E., et al. (2010). Cellular mechanisms of IL-17-induced blood-brain barrier disruption. *FASEB J.* 24, 1023–1034. doi: 10.1096/fj.09-141978

Hyman, S. E. (2008). A glimmer of light for neuropsychiatric disorders. *Nature* 455, 890–893. doi: 10.1038/nature07454

Irani, S. R., Gelfand, J. M., Al-Diwani, A., and Vincent, A. (2014). Cell-surface central nervous system autoantibodies: clinical relevance and emerging paradigms. *Ann. Neurol.* 76, 168–184. doi: 10.1002/ana.24200

Irwin, J., Tombaugh, T. N., Zacharko, R. M., and Anisman, H. (1983). Alteration of exploration and the response to food associated cues after treatment with pimozide. *Pharmacol. Biochem. Behav.* 18, 235–246.

Jacobs, J. F., van der Molen, R. G., Bossuyt, X., and Damoiseaux, J. (2015). Antigen excess in modern immunoassays: to anticipate on the unexpected. *Autoimmun. Rev.* 14, 160–167. doi: 10.1016/j.autrev.2014.10.018

Jaffard, R., Mocaer, E., Poignant, J. C., Micheau, J., Marighetto, A., Meunier, M., et al. (1991). Effects of tianeptine on spontaneous alternation, simple and concurrent spatial discrimination learning and on alcohol-induced alternation deficits in mice. *Behav. Pharmacol.* 2, 37–46.

John, C. C., Carabin, H., Montano, S. M., Bangirana, P., Zunt, J. R., and Peterson, P. K. (2015). Global research priorities for infections that affect the nervous system. *Nature* 527, S178–S186. doi: 10.1038/nature16033

Kajiwara, Y., Buxbaum, J. D., and Grice, D. E. (2009). SLITRK1 binds 14-3-3 and regulates neurite outgrowth in a phosphorylation-dependent manner. *Biol. Psychiatry* 66, 918–925. doi: 10.1016/j.biopsych.2009.05.033

Kaltwasser, M. T. (1990). Acoustic signaling in the black rat (*Rattus rattus*). *J. Comp. Psychol.* 104, 227–232.

Kalueff, A. V., Stewart, A. M., Song, C., Berridge, K. C., Graybiel, A. M., and Fentress, J. C. (2016). Neurobiology of rodent self-grooming and its value for translational neuroscience. *Nat. Rev. Neurosci.* 17, 45–59. doi: 10.1038/nrn.2015.8

Katayama, K., Yamada, K., Ornthanalai, V. G., Inoue, T., Ota, M., Murphy, N. P., et al. (2010). Slitrk1-deficient mice display elevated anxiety-like behavior and noradrenergic abnormalities. *Mol. Psychiatry* 15, 177–184. doi: 10.1038/mp.2008.97

Kawikova, I., Leckman, J. F., Kronig, H., Katsovich, L., Bessen, D. E., Ghebremichael, M., et al. (2007). Decreased numbers of regulatory T cells suggest impaired immune tolerance in children with tourette syndrome: a preliminary study. *Biol. Psychiatry* 61, 273–278. doi: 10.1016/j.biopsych.2006.06.012

Kebir, H., Kreymborg, K., Ifergan, I., Dodelet-Devillers, A., Cayrol, R., Bernard, M., et al. (2007). Human TH17 lymphocytes promote blood-brain barrier disruption and central nervous system inflammation. *Nat. Med.* 13, 1173–1175. doi: 10.1038/nm1651

Kipp, M., van der Star, B., Vogel, D. Y., Puentes, F., van der Valk, P., Baker, D., et al. (2012). Experimental *in vivo* and *in vitro* models of multiple sclerosis: EAE and beyond. *Mult. Scler. Relat. Disord.* 1, 15–28. doi: 10.1016/j.msard.2011.09.002

Korngold, R., Feldman, A., Rorke, L. B., Lublin, F. D., and Doherty, P. C. (1986). Acute experimental allergic encephalomyelitis in radiation bone marrow chimeras between high and low susceptible strains of mice. *Immunogenetics* 24, 309–315.

Kowal, C., and Diamond, B. (2012). Aspects of CNS lupus: mouse models of anti-NMDA receptor antibody mediated reactivity. *Methods Mol. Biol.* 900, 181–206. doi: 10.1007/978-1-60761-720-4_9

Kowal, C., DeGiorgio, L. A., Nakaoka, T., Hetherington, H., Huerta, P. T., Diamond, B., et al. (2004). Cognition and immunity; antibody impairs memory. *Immunity* 21, 179–188. doi: 10.1016/j.immuni.2004.07.011

Kreutzberg, G. W. (1996). Microglia: a sensor for pathological events in the CNS. *Trends Neurosci.* 19, 312–318.

Kumar, A., Williams, M. T., and Chugani, H. T. (2015). Evaluation of basal ganglia and thalamic inflammation in children with pediatric autoimmune neuropsychiatric disorders associated with streptococcal infection and tourette syndrome: a positron emission tomographic (PET) study using 11C-[R]-PK11195. *J. Child Neurol.* 30, 749–756. doi: 10.1177/0883073814543303

Laban, O., Dimitrijevic, M., von Hoersten, S., Markovic, B. M., and Jankovic, B. D. (1995). Experimental allergic encephalomyelitis in adult DA rats subjected to neonatal handling or gentling. *Brain Res.* 676, 133–140.

Lalonde, R. (2002). The neurobiological basis of spontaneous alternation. *Neurosci. Biobehav. Rev.* 26, 91–104. doi: 10.1016/S0149-7634(01)00041-0

Landau, Y. E., Steinberg, T., Richmand, B., Leckman, J. F., and Apter, A. (2012). Involvement of immunologic and biochemical mechanisms in the pathogenesis of Tourette's syndrome. *J. Neural Transm.* 119, 621–626. doi: 10.1007/s00702-011-0739-x

Leckman, J. F., and Peterson, B. S. (1993). The pathogenesis of Tourette's syndrome: epigenetic factors active in early CNS development. *Biol. Psychiatry* 34, 425–427.

Leckman, J. F., Bloch, M. H., Smith, M. E., Larabi, D., and Hampson, M. (2010). Neurobiological substrates of Tourette's disorder. *J. Child Adolesc. Psychopharmacol.* 20, 237–247. doi: 10.1089/cap.2009.0118

Leckman, J. F., Dolnansky, E. S., Hardin, M. T., Clubb, M., Walkup, J. T., Stevenson, J., et al. (1990). Perinatal factors in the expression of Tourette's syndrome: an exploratory study. *J. Am. Acad. Child Adolesc. Psychiatry* 29, 220–226. doi: 10.1097/00004583-199003000-00010

Leckman, J. F., Katsovich, L., Kawikova, I., Lin, H., Zhang, H., Krönig, H., et al. (2005). Increased serum levels of interleukin-12 and tumor necrosis factor-alpha in Tourette's syndrome. *Biol. Psychiatry* 57, 667–673. doi: 10.1016/j.biopsych.2004.12.004

Leckman, J. F., Price, R. A., Walkup, J. T., Ort, S., Pauls, D. L., and Cohen, D. J. (1987). Nongenetic factors in Gilles de la Tourette's syndrome. *Arch. Gen. Psychiatry* 44:100.

Lécuyer, M. A., Kebir, H., and Prat, A. (2016). Glial influences on BBB functions and molecular players in immune cell trafficking. *Biochim. Biophys. Acta* 1862, 472–482. doi: 10.1016/j.bbadis.2015.10.004

Levine, S., and Saltzman, A. (1987). Nonspecific stress prevents relapses of experimental allergic encephalomyelitis in rats. *Brain Behav. Immun.* 1, 336–341.

Levine, S., Strebel, R., Wenk, E. J., and Harman, P. J. (1962a). Suppression of experimental allergic encephalomyelitis by stress. *Proc. Soc. Exp. Biol. Med.* 109, 294–298.

Levine, S., Wenk, E. J., Muldoon, T. N., and Cohen, S. G. (1962b). Enhancement of experimental allergic encephalomyelitis by adrenalectomy. *Proc. Soc. Exp. Biol. Med.* 111, 383–385.

Levite, M. (2014). Glutamate receptor antibodies in neurological diseases: anti-AMPA-GluR3 antibodies, anti-NMDA-NR1 antibodies, anti-NMDA-NR2A/B antibodies, anti-mGluR1 antibodies or anti-mGluR5 antibodies are present in subpopulations of patients with either: epilepsy, encephalitis, cerebellar ataxia, systemic lupus erythematosus (SLE) and neuropsychiatric SLE, Sjogren's syndrome, schizophrenia, mania or stroke. These autoimmune anti-glutamate receptor antibodies can bind neurons in few brain regions, activate glutamate receptors, decrease glutamate receptor's expression, impair glutamate-induced signaling and function, activate blood brain barrier endothelial cells, kill neurons, damage the brain, induce behavioral/psychiatric/cognitive abnormalities and ataxia in animal models, and can be removed or silenced in some patients by immunotherapy. *J. Neural Transm.* 121, 1029–1075. doi: 10.1007/s00702-014-1193-3

Levite, M., and Hermelin, A. (1999). Autoimmunity to the glutamate receptor in mice–a model for Rasmussen's encephalitis? *J. Autoimmun.* 13, 73–82. doi: 10.1006/jaut.1999.0297

Levite, M., Fleidervish, I. A., Schwarz, A., Pelled, D., and Futerman, A. H. (1999). Autoantibodies to the glutamate receptor kill neurons via activation of the receptor ion channel. *J. Autoimmun.* 13, 61–72. doi: 10.1006/jaut.1999.0301

Loiselle, C. R., Lee, O., Moran, T. H., and Singer, H. S. (2004). Striatal microinfusion of Tourette syndrome and PANDAS sera: failure to induce behavioral changes. *Mov. Disord.* 19, 390–396. doi: 10.1002/mds.10522

Lombroso, P. J., and Scahill, L. (2008). Tourette syndrome and obsessive-compulsive disorder. *Brain Dev.* 30, 231–237. doi: 10.1016/j.braindev.2007.09.001

Lotan, D., Benhar, I., Alvarez, K., Mascaro-Blanco, A., Brimberg, L., Frenkel, D., et al. (2014). Behavioral and neural effects of intra-striatal infusion of anti-streptococcal antibodies in rats. *Brain Behav. Immun.* 38, 249–262. doi: 10.1016/j.bbi.2014.02.009

Lyons, D. M., and Macrì, S. (2011). Resilience and adaptive aspects of stress in neurobehavioral development. *Neurosci. Biobehav. Rev.* 35:1451. doi: 10.1016/j.neubiorev.2010.09.004

Ma, Y., Mehta, S. L., Lu, B., and Li, P. A. (2011). Deficiency in the inner mitochondrial membrane peptidase 2-like (Immp21) gene increases ischemic brain damage and impairs mitochondrial function. *Neurobiol. Dis.* 44, 270–276. doi: 10.1016/j.nbd.2011.06.019

Macrì, S., Ceci, C., Onori, M. P., Invernizzi, R. W., Bartolini, E., Altabella, L., et al. (2015). Mice repeatedly exposed to Group-A beta-Haemolytic Streptococcus show perseverative behaviors, impaired sensorimotor gating, and immune activation in rostral diencephalon. *Sci. Rep.* 5:13257. doi: 10.1038/srep13257

Macrì, S., Proietti Onori, M., and Laviola, G. (2013). Theoretical and practical considerations behind the use of laboratory animals for the study of Tourette syndrome. *Neurosci. Biobehav. Rev.* 37, 1085–1100. doi: 10.1016/j.neubiorev.2013.03.014

Mandolesi, G., Grasselli, G., Musumeci, G., and Centonze, D. (2010). Cognitive deficits in experimental autoimmune encephalomyelitis: neuroinflammation and synaptic degeneration. *Neurol. Sci.* 31(Suppl. 2), S255–S259. doi: 10.1007/s10072-010-0369-3

Mansbach, R. S., Geyer, M. A., and Braff, D. L. (1988). Dopaminergic stimulation disrupts sensorimotor gating in the rat. *Psychopharmacology* 94, 507–514.

Margari, F., Petruzzelli, M. G., Mianulli, R., Toto, M., Pastore, A., Bizzaro, N., et al. (2013). Anti-brain autoantibodies in the serum of schizophrenic patients: a case-control study. *Psychiatry Res.* 210, 800–805. doi: 10.1016/j.psychres.2013.09.006

Marques-Dias, M. J., Mercadante, M. T., Tucker, D., and Lombroso, P. (1997). Sydenham's chorea. *Psychiatr. Clin. North Am.* 20, 809–820.

Martino, D., Chiarotti, F., Buttiglione, M., Cardona, F., Creti, R., Nardocci, N., et al. (2011). The relationship between group A streptococcal infections and Tourette syndrome: a study on a large service-based cohort. *Dev. Med. Child Neurol.* 53, 951–957. doi: 10.1111/j.1469-8749.2011.04018.x

Martino, D., Dale, R. C., Gilbert, D. L., Giovannoni, G., and Leckman, J. F. (2009). Immunopathogenic mechanisms in tourette syndrome: a critical review. *Mov. Disord.* 24, 1267–1279. doi: 10.1002/mds.22504

Martino, D., Zis, P., and Buttiglione, M. (2015). The role of immune mechanisms in Tourette syndrome. *Brain Res.* 1617, 126–143. doi: 10.1016/j.brainres.2014.04.027

Meagher, M. W., Sieve, A. N., Johnson, R. R., Satterlee, D., Belyavskyi, M., Mi, W., et al. (2010). Neonatal maternal separation alters immune, endocrine, and behavioral responses to acute Theiler's virus infection in adult mice. *Behav. Genet.* 40, 233–249. doi: 10.1007/s10519-010-9333-5

Meldrum, B. S. (2000). Glutamate as a neurotransmitter in the brain: review of physiology and pathology. *J. Nutr.* 130(4S Suppl), 1007S–1015S.

Morris, C. M., Pardo-Villamizar, C., Gause, C. D., and Singer, H. S. (2009). Serum autoantibodies measured by immunofluorescence confirm a failure to differentiate PANDAS and Tourette syndrome from controls. *J. Neurol. Sci.* 276, 45–48. doi: 10.1016/j.jns.2008.08.032

Murphy, T. K., Kurlan, R., and Leckman, J. (2010). The immunobiology of Tourette's disorder, pediatric autoimmune neuropsychiatric disorders associated with Streptococcus, and related disorders: a way forward. *J. Child Adolesc. Psychopharmacol.* 20, 317–331. doi: 10.1089/cap.2010.0043

Nordstrom, E. J., and Burton, F. H. (2002). A transgenic model of comorbid Tourette's syndrome and obsessive-compulsive disorder circuitry. *Mol. Psychiatry* 7, 617–625, 524. doi: 10.1038/sj.mp.4001144

Olechowski, C. J., Tenorio, G., Sauve, Y., and Kerr, B. J. (2013). Changes in nociceptive sensitivity and object recognition in experimental autoimmune encephalomyelitis (EAE). *Exp. Neurol.* 241, 113–121. doi: 10.1016/j.expneurol.2012.12.012

Park, H. S., Francis, K. P., Yu, J., and Cleary, P. P. (2003). Membranous cells in nasal-associated lymphoid tissue: a portal of entry for the respiratory mucosal pathogen group A streptococcus. *J. Immunol.* 171, 2532–2537. doi: 10.4049/jimmunol.171.5.2532

Petek, E., Windpassinger, C., Vincent, J. B., Cheung, J., Boright, A. P., Scherer, S. W., et al. (2001). Disruption of a novel gene (IMMP2L) by a breakpoint in 7q31 associated with Tourette syndrome. *Am. J. Hum. Genet.* 68, 848–858. doi: 10.1086/319523

Platt, S. R. (2007). The role of glutamate in central nervous system health and disease–a review. *Vet. J.* 173, 278–286. doi: 10.1016/j.tvjl.2005.11.007

Podolska, M. J., Biermann, M. H., Maueröder, C., Hahn, J., and Herrmann, M. (2015). Inflammatory etiopathogenesis of systemic lupus erythematosus: an update. *J. Inflamm. Res.* 8, 161–171. doi: 10.2147/JIR.S70325

Poliak, S., Gollan, L., Martinez, R., Custer, A., Einheber, S., Salzer, J. L., et al. (1999). Caspr2, a new member of the neurexin superfamily, is localized at the juxtaparanodes of myelinated axons and associates with K+ channels. *Neuron* 24, 1037–1047.

Proenca, C. C., Gao, K. P., Shmelkov, S. V., Rafii, S., and Lee, F. S. (2011). Slitrks as emerging candidate genes involved in neuropsychiatric disorders. *Trends Neurosci.* 34, 143–153. doi: 10.1016/j.tins.2011.01.001

Rabchevsky, A. G., Degos, J. D., and Dreyfus, P. A. (1999). Peripheral injections of Freund's adjuvant in mice provoke leakage of serum proteins through the blood-brain barrier without inducing reactive gliosis. *Brain Res.* 832, 84–96.

Rickard, M. D. (2004). The use of animals for research on animal diseases: its impact on the harm-benefit analysis. *Altern. Lab. Anim.* 32(Suppl. 1A), 225–227.

Rizzo, R., Gulisano, M., Pavone, P., Fogliani, F., and Robertson, M. M. (2006). Increased antistreptococcal antibody titers and anti-basal ganglia antibodies in patients with Tourette syndrome: controlled cross-sectional study. *J. Child Neurol.* 21, 747–753. doi: 10.1177/08830738060210091001

Roque, S., Mesquita, A. R., Palha, J. A., Sousa, N., and Correia-Neves, M. (2014). The behavioral and immunological impact of maternal separation: a matter of timing. *Front. Behav. Neurosci.* 8:192. doi: 10.3389/fnbeh.2014.00192

Russig, H., Spooren, W., Durkin, S., Feldon, J., and Yee, B. K. (2004). Apomorphine-induced disruption of prepulse inhibition that can be normalised by systemic haloperidol is insensitive to clozapine pretreatment. *Psychopharmacology* 175, 143–147. doi: 10.1007/s00213-004-1810-1

Scahill, L., Erenberg, G., Berlin, C. M. Jr., Budman, C., Coffey, B. J., Jankovic, J., et al. (2006). Contemporary assessment and pharmacotherapy of Tourette syndrome. *NeuroRx* 3, 192–206. doi: 10.1016/j.nurx.2006.01.009

Schlumberger, W., Hornig, N., Lange, S., Probst, C., Komorowski, L., Fechner, K., et al. (2014). Differential diagnosis of membranous nephropathy with autoantibodies to phospholipase A2 receptor 1. *Autoimmun. Rev.* 13, 108–113. doi: 10.1016/j.autrev.2013.09.005

Scoriels, L., Salek, R. M., Goodby, E., Grainger, D., Dean, A. M., West, J. A., et al. (2015). Behavioural and molecular endophenotypes in psychotic disorders reveal heritable abnormalities in glutamatergic neurotransmission. *Transl. Psychiatry* 5:e540. doi: 10.1038/tp.2015.26

Sengupta, A., Winters, B., Bagley, E. E., and McNally, G. P. (2016). Disrupted prediction error links excessive amygdala activation to excessive fear. *J. Neurosci.* 36, 385–395. doi: 10.1523/JNEUROSCI.3670-15.2016

Shemer, A., and Jung, S. (2015). Differential roles of resident microglia and infiltrating monocytes in murine CNS autoimmunity. *Semin. Immunopathol.* 37, 613–623. doi: 10.1007/s00281-015-0519-z

Shepshelovich, D., and Shoenfeld, Y. (2006). Prediction and prevention of autoimmune diseases: additional aspects of the mosaic of autoimmunity. *Lupus* 15, 183–190. doi: 10.1191/0961203306lu2274rr

Shprecher, D., and Kurlan, R. (2009). The management of tics. *Mov. Disord.* 24, 15–24. doi: 10.1002/mds.22378

Silberberg, D., Anand, N. P., Michels, K., and Kalaria, R. N. (2015). Brain and other nervous system disorders across the lifespan - global challenges and opportunities. *Nature* 527, S151–S154. doi: 10.1038/nature16028

Singer, H. S., Hong, J. J., Yoon, D. Y., and Williams, P. N. (2005a). Serum autoantibodies do not differentiate PANDAS and Tourette syndrome from controls. *Neurology* 65, 1701–1707. doi: 10.1212/01.wnl.0000183223.69946.f1

Singer, H. S., Mink, J. W., Loiselle, C. R., Burke, K. A., Ruchkina, I., Morshed, S., et al. (2005b). Microinfusion of antineuronal antibodies into rodent striatum: failure to differentiate between elevated and low titers. *J. Neuroimmunol.* 163, 8–14. doi: 10.1016/j.jneuroim.2005.02.018

Stanwood, G. D., Lucki, I., and McGonigle, P. (2000). Differential regulation of dopamine D2 and D3 receptors by chronic drug treatments. *J. Pharmacol. Exp. Ther.* 295, 1232–1240.

State, M. W. (2011). The genetics of Tourette disorder. *Curr. Opin. Genet. Dev.* 21, 302–309. doi: 10.1016/j.gde.2011.01.007

Stillman, A. A., Krsnik, Z., Sun, J., Rasin, M. R., State, M. W., Sestan, N., et al. (2009). Developmentally regulated and evolutionarily conserved expression of SLITRK1 in brain circuits implicated in Tourette syndrome. *J. Comp. Neurol.* 513, 21–37. doi: 10.1002/cne.21919

Swanborg, R. H. (2001). Experimental autoimmune encephalomyelitis in the rat: lessons in T-cell immunology and autoreactivity. *Immunol. Rev.* 184, 129–135. doi: 10.1034/j.1600-065x.2001.1840112.x

Swedo, S. E., and Grant, P. J. (2005). Annotation: PANDAS: a model for human autoimmune disease. *J. Child Psychol. Psychiatry* 46, 227–234. doi: 10.1111/j.1469-7610.2004.00386.x

Swedo, S. E., Leonard, H. L., Garvey, M., Mittleman, B., Allen, A. J., Perlmutter, S., et al. (1998). Pediatric autoimmune neuropsychiatric disorders associated with streptococcal infections: clinical description of the first 50 cases. *Am. J. Psychiatry* 155, 264–271.

Swedo, S. E., Leonard, H. L., Schapiro, M. B., Casey, B. J., Mannheim, G. B., Lenane, M. C., et al. (1993). Sydenham's chorea: physical and psychological symptoms of St Vitus dance. *Pediatrics* 91, 706–713.

Swedo, S. E., Rapoport, J. L., Cheslow, D. L., Leonard, H. L., Ayoub, E. M., Hosier, D. M., et al. (1989). High prevalence of obsessive-compulsive symptoms in patients with Sydenham's chorea. *Am. J. Psychiatry* 146, 246–249. doi: 10.1176/ajp.146.2.246

Swerdlow, N. R. (2013). Update: studies of prepulse inhibition of startle, with particular relevance to the pathophysiology or treatment of Tourette Syndrome. *Neurosci. Biobehav. Rev.* 37, 1150–1156. doi: 10.1016/j.neubiorev.2012. 09.002

Swerdlow, N. R., and Sutherland, A. N. (2005). Using animal models to develop therapeutics for Tourette Syndrome. *Pharmacol. Ther.* 108, 281–293. doi: 10.1016/j.pharmthera.2005.05.003

Swerdlow, N. R., Benbow, C. H., Zisook, S., Geyer, M. A., and Braff, D. L. (1993). A preliminary assessment of sensorimotor gating in patients with obsessive compulsive disorder. *Biol. Psychiatry* 33, 298–301.

Swerdlow, N. R., Geyer, M. A., and Braff, D. L. (2001a). Neural circuit regulation of prepulse inhibition of startle in the rat: current knowledge and future challenges. *Psychopharmacology* 156, 194–215. doi: 10.1007/s002130100799

Swerdlow, N. R., Karban, B., Ploum, Y., Sharp, R., Geyer, M. A., and Eastvold, A. (2001b). Tactile prepuff inhibition of startle in children with Tourette's syndrome: in search of an "fMRI-friendly" startle paradigm. *Biol. Psychiatry* 50, 578–585. doi: 10.1016/S0006-3223(01)01164-7

Swerdlow, N. R., Light, G. A., Cadenhead, K. S., Sprock, J., Hsieh, M. H., and Braff, D. L. (2006). Startle gating deficits in a large cohort of patients with schizophrenia: relationship to medications, symptoms, neurocognition, and level of function. *Arch. Gen. Psychiatry* 63, 1325–1335. doi: 10.1001/archpsyc.63.12.1325

Swerdlow, N. R., Paulsen, J., Braff, D. L., Butters, N., Geyer, M. A., and Swenson, M. R. (1995). Impaired prepulse inhibition of acoustic and tactile startle response in patients with Huntington's disease. *J. Neurol. Neurosurg. Psychiatr.* 58, 192–200.

Taylor, J. R., Morshed, S. A., Parveen, S., Mercadante, M. T., Scahill, L., Peterson, B. S., et al. (2002). An animal model of Tourette's syndrome. *Am. J. Psychiatry* 159, 657–660. doi: 10.1176/appi.ajp.159.4.657

Valls-Sole, J., Munoz, J. E., and Valldeoriola, F. (2004). Abnormalities of prepulse inhibition do not depend on blink reflex excitability: a study in Parkinson's disease and Huntington's disease. *Clin. Neurophysiol.* 115, 1527–1536. doi: 10.1016/j.clinph.2004.02.014

van der Staay, F. J. (2006). Animal models of behavioral dysfunctions: basic concepts and classifications, and an evaluation strategy. *Brain Res. Rev.* 52, 131–159. doi: 10.1016/j.brainresrev.2006.01.006

van der Staay, F. J., Arndt, S. S., and Nordquist, R. E. (2009). Evaluation of animal models of neurobehavioral disorders. *Behav. Brain Funct.* 5:11. doi: 10.1186/1744-9081-5-11

Verkerk, A. J., Mathews, C. A., Joosse, M., Eussen, B. H., Heutink, P., Oostra, B. A., et al. (2003). CNTNAP2 is disrupted in a family with Gilles de la Tourette syndrome and obsessive compulsive disorder. *Genomics* 82, 1–9. doi: 10.1016/S0888-7543(03)00097-1

Verschuuren, J. J., Huijbers, M. G., Plomp, J. J., Niks, E. H., Molenaar, P. C., Martinez-Martinez, P., et al. (2013). Pathophysiology of myasthenia gravis with antibodies to the acetylcholine receptor, muscle-specific kinase and low-density lipoprotein receptor-related protein 4. *Autoimmun. Rev.* 12, 918–923. doi: 10.1016/j.autrev.2013.03.001

Wick, G., Hu, Y., Schwarz, S., and Kroemer, G. (1993). Immunoendocrine communication via the hypothalamo-pituitary-adrenal axis in autoimmune diseases. *Endocr. Rev.* 14, 539–563. doi: 10.1210/edrv-14-5-539

Willner, P. (1984). The validity of animal models of depression. *Psychopharmacology* 83, 1–16.

Willner, P., and Mitchell, P. J. (2002). The validity of animal models of predisposition to depression. *Behav. Pharmacol.* 13, 169–188. doi: 10.1097/00008877-200205000-00001

Yaddanapudi, K., Hornig, M., Serge, R., De Miranda, J., Baghban, A., Villar, G., et al. (2010). Passive transfer of streptococcus-induced antibodies reproduces behavioral disturbances in a mouse model of pediatric autoimmune neuropsychiatric disorders associated with streptococcal infection. *Mol. Psychiatry* 15, 712–726. doi: 10.1038/mp.2009.77

Yeh, C. B., Shui, H. A., Chu, T. H., Chen, Y. A., Tsung, H. C., and Shyu, J. F. (2012). Hyperpolarisation-activated cyclic nucleotide channel 4 (HCN4) involvement in Tourette's syndrome autoimmunity. *J. Neuroimmunol.* 250, 18–26. doi: 10.1016/j.jneuroim.2012.05.009

Zebardast, N., Crowley, M. J., Bloch, M. H., Mayes, L. C., Wyk, B. V., Leckman, J. F., et al. (2013). Brain mechanisms for prepulse inhibition in adults with Tourette syndrome: initial findings. *Psychiatry Res.* 214, 33–41. doi: 10.1016/j.pscychresns.2013.05.009

9

The International Deep Brain Stimulation Registry and Database for Gilles de la Tourette Syndrome: How Does It Work?

Wissam Deeb[1], Peter J. Rossi[1], Mauro Porta[2], Veerle Visser-Vandewalle[3], Domenico Servello[4], Peter Silburn[5,6], Terry Coyne[6,7], James F. Leckman[8], Thomas Foltynie[9], Marwan Hariz[9], Eileen M. Joyce[9], Ludvic Zrinzo[9], Zinovia Kefalopoulou[9], Marie-Laure Welter[10], Carine Karachi[11,12], Luc Mallet[11,13,14], Jean-Luc Houeto[15], Joohi Shahed-Jimenez[16], Fan-Gang Meng[17], Bryan T. Klassen[18], Alon Y. Mogilner[19], Michael H. Pourfar[19], Jens Kuhn[20], L. Ackermans[21], Takanobu Kaido[22], Yasin Temel[23,24], Robert E. Gross[25], Harrison C. Walker[26], Andres M. Lozano[27], Suketu M. Khandhar[28], Benjamin L. Walter[29], Ellen Walter[30], Zoltan Mari[31], Barbara K. Changizi[32], Elena Moro[33], Juan C. Baldermann[34], Daniel Huys[34], S. Elizabeth Zauber[35], Lauren E. Schrock[36], Jian-Guo Zhang[37], Wei Hu[1], Kelly D. Foote[1,38], Kyle Rizer[1], Jonathan W. Mink[39], Douglas W. Woods[40], Aysegul Gunduz[1,41] and Michael S. Okun[1]*

[1] Department of Neurology, University of Florida and Center for Movement Disorders and Neurorestoration, Gainesville, FL, USA, [2] Tourette's Syndrome and Movement Disorders Center, Galeazzi Hospital, Milan, Italy, [3] Department of Stereotactic and Functional Neurosurgery, University of Cologne, Cologne, Germany, [4] Neusurgical Department, IRCCS Galeazzi, Milan, Italy, [5] Asia-Pacific Centre for Neuromodulation, Queensland Brain Institute, Brisbane, Queensland, Australia, [6] University of Queensland Centre for Clinical Research, The University of Queensland, Brisbane, Queensland, Australia, [7] BrizBrain&Spine, Brisbane, QLD, Australia, [8] Departments of Psychiatry, Pediatrics and Psychology, Child Study Center, Yale University, New Haven, CT, USA, [9] Sobell Department of Motor Neuroscience, University College London Institute of Neurology, London, UK, [10] Assistance Publique – Hôpitaux de Paris, Institut du Cerveau et de la Moelle Epiniere, Institut National de la Santé et de la Recherche Médicale 1127, Pitié-Salpêtrière Hospital, Sorbonne Universités, UPMC Univ Paris 06, Unité Mixte de Recherche 1127, Centre National de la Recherche Scientifique, Unité Mixte de Recherche 7225, Paris, France, [11] Institut National de la Santé et de la Recherche Médicale U 1127, Centre National de la Recherche Scientifique UMR 7225, Sorbonne Universités, UPMC Univ Paris 06 UMR S 1127, Institut du Cerveau et de la Moelle épinière, Paris, France, [12] Department of Neurosurgery, Assistance Publique – Hôpitaux de Paris, Hôpital de la Pitié-Salpêtrière, Paris, France, [13] Assistance Publique – Hôpitaux de Paris, DHU Pe-PSY, Pôle de Psychiatrie et d'addictologie des Hôpitaux Universitaires H Mondor, Université Paris Est Créteil, Créteil, France, [14] Department of Mental Health and Psychiatry, Geneva University Hospital, Geneva, Switzerland, [15] Service de Neurologie, Institut National de la Santé et de la Recherche Médicale-Centres d'Investigation Clinique 1402, Centre Hospitalier Universitaire de Grenoble de Poitiers, Université de Poitiers, Poitiers, France, [16] Parkinson's Disease Center and Movement Disorders Clinic, Baylor College of Medicine, Houston, TX, USA, [17] Beijing Neurosurgical Institute, Capital Medical University, Beijing, China, [18] Department of Neurology, Mayo Clinic College of Medicine, Rochester, MN, USA, [19] Department of Neurosurgery, Center for Neuromodulation, NYU Langone Medical Center, New York, NY, USA, [20] Department of Psychiatry and Psychotherapy, University of Cologne, Cologne, Germany, [21] Department of Neurosurgery, Maastricht University Medical Centre, Maastricht, Netherlands, [22] Department of Neurosurgery, National Center Hospital, National Center of Neurology and Psychiatry, Kodaira, Japan, [23] Department of Neurosurgery, Maastricht University Medical Center, Maastricht, Netherlands, [24] Faculty of Health, Medicine and Life Sciences, School for Mental Health and Neuroscience, Maastricht University, Maastricht, Netherlands, [25] Department of Neurosurgery, Emory University, Atlanta, GA, USA, [26] Department of Neurology, Department of Biomedical Engineering, University of Alabama at Birmingham, Birmingham, AL, USA, [27] Division of Neurosurgery, University of Toronto, Toronto, Canada, [28] Department of Neurology, The Permanente Medical Group (Tidewater Physicians Multispecialty Group), Movement Disorders Program, Sacramento, CA, USA, [29] University Hospitals, Case Western Reserve University School of Medicine, Cleveland, OH, USA, [30] Department of Neurology, University Hospitals Case Medical Center, Neurological Institute, Cleveland, OH, USA, [31] Parkinson's & Movement Disorder Center/Division, Johns Hopkins University, School of Medicine, Baltimore, MD, USA, [32] Department of Neurology, The Ohio State University Wexner Medical Center, Columbus, OH, USA , [33] Division of Neurology, Centre Hospitalier Universitaire de Grenoble, Grenoble Alpes University, Grenoble, France, [34] Department of Psychiatry and Psychotherapy, Universitätsklinikum Köln, Köln, Germany, [35] Department of Neurology, Indiana University School of Medicine, Indianapolis, IN, USA, [36] Department of Neurology, University of Utah, Salt Lake City, UT, USA, [37] Department of Functional Neurosurgery, Beijing Tiantan Hospital, Capital Medical University, Beijing, China, [38] Department of Neurological Surgery, University of Florida, Gainesville, FL, USA, [39] Department of Neurology, University of Rochester Medical Center, Rochester, NY, USA, [40] Department of Psychology, Marquette University, Milwaukee, WI, USA, [41] J. Crayton Pruitt Family Department of Biomedical Engineering, University of Florida, Gainesville, FL, USA

Edited by:
Peristera Paschou,
Democritus University of Thrace, Greece

Reviewed by:
Jeremy Samuel Stern,
St George's University of London, UK
Pieter J. Hoekstra,
University Medical Center Groningen, Netherlands

***Correspondence:**
Wissam Deeb
wissam.deeb@neurology.ufl.edu

Tourette Syndrome (TS) is a neuropsychiatric disease characterized by a combination of motor and vocal tics. Deep brain stimulation (DBS), already widely utilized for Parkinson's disease and other movement disorders, is an emerging therapy for select and severe cases of TS that are resistant to medication and behavioral therapy. Over the last two decades, DBS has been used experimentally to manage severe TS cases. The results of case reports and small case series have been variable but in general positive. The reported interventions have, however, been variable, and there remain non-standardized selection criteria, various brain targets, differences in hardware, as well as variability in the programming parameters utilized. DBS centers perform only a handful of TS DBS cases each year, making large-scale outcomes difficult to study and to interpret. These limitations, coupled with the variable effect of surgery, and the overall small numbers of TS patients with DBS worldwide, have delayed regulatory agency approval (e.g., FDA and equivalent agencies around the world). The Tourette Association of America, in response to the worldwide need for a more organized and collaborative effort, launched an international TS DBS registry and database. The main goal of the project has been to share data, uncover best practices, improve outcomes, and to provide critical information to regulatory agencies. The international registry and database has improved the communication and collaboration among TS DBS centers worldwide. In this paper we will review some of the key operation details for the international TS DBS database and registry.

Keywords: Tourette syndrome, deep brain stimulation, database, registry, tics, regulatory agencies

INTRODUCTION

Gilles de la Tourette Syndrome (TS) is a neuropsychiatric disorder characterized by motor and vocal tics. In a subset of cases, these tics can be severely debilitating (Freeman et al., 2000; Malaty and Akbar, 2014; Shprecher et al., 2014). The pathophysiology of TS has been increasingly linked to dysfunction in a complex basal ganglia thalamo-cortical circuit (BGTCC) (Da Cunha et al., 2015). Deep brain stimulation (DBS)—effective for movement disorders including Parkinson's disease, dystonia, and tremor—has been explored since 1999 as a potential therapy for select cases of severe, medication-resistant TS (Müller-Vahl et al., 2011). However, DBS use in TS is still considered investigational and has not received regulatory agency approval.

Initial stereotactic surgical treatment with thalamotomy for TS was introduced by Rolf Hassler in 1970 (Hassler and Dieckmann, 1970). Cooper, Hassler, and Dieckmann were part of surgical teams performing this procedure for few TS patients. Hassler initially targeted the centromedian-parafascicular complex. Thus, the selection of the thalamic target for DBS was motivated by the relative successes of Hassler and other clinicians applying the thalamotomy procedure in this brain region.

Despite the initial successes, thalamotomy was never widely adopted as a treatment for TS. The invasiveness of the procedure, the issues with accuracy using early stereotaxic equipment, and the risk of speech, swallowing, and cognitive side effects due to the large size of the lesions all limited its widespread use. Three decades later in 1999 Vandewalle and colleagues implanted DBS electrodes bilaterally in the nucleus ventro-oralis internus/centromedian-parafascicular complex (Voi/CM/Pf) of the thalamus (Vandewalle et al., 1999). The Vandewalle group was able to demonstrate the relative safety and potential effectiveness in a small series of patients published over the next several years. This initial experience sparked the interest of other groups and led to a dialogue about the possibility of applying DBS in various brain targets along the BGTCC.

This interest has been supported by a growing number of studies in the peer-reviewed literature (Ackermans et al., 2011; Massano et al., 2013; Jimenez-Shahed, 2015; Kefalopoulou et al., 2015). These studies reveal generally positive results with occasional side effects (e.g., hemorrhage, stimulation-induced), however it should be kept in mind that most studies have been small and uncontrolled (Duits et al., 2012; Sachdev et al., 2012; Savica et al., 2012; Ackermans et al., 2013; Dehning et al., 2014; Kim and Pouratian, 2014; Malaty and Akbar, 2014; Zhang et al., 2014; Kefalopoulou et al., 2015). Additionally, there were other important differences in the DBS intervention such as the brain target (Martínez-Fernández et al., 2011; Viswanathan et al., 2012), the surgical targeting methods, the type(s) of devices implanted, the stimulation paradigm (Rotsides and Mammis, 2013), and the baseline disease characteristics (Okun et al., 2008).

Teams performing DBS have in the past decade explored at least eight possible brain targets for TS cases (Cavanna et al., 2011; Porta et al., 2012). These targets have included the thalamic CM/Pf (Visser-Vandewalle et al., 2003; Maciunas et al., 2007;

Ackermans et al., 2010, 2011), the subthalamic nucleus, the posterolateral globus pallidus internus, the anteromedial globus pallidus internus (Dehning et al., 2008; Massano et al., 2013; Dong et al., 2014), the globus pallidus externus (Piedimonte et al., 2013), the nucleus accumbens (Kuhn et al., 2007; Sachdev et al., 2012), the dorsomedial nucleus of the thalamus, and the anterior limb of the internal capsule (Flaherty et al., 2005).

Academic medical centers with specialized TS clinics have collectively reported only a handful of appropriate DBS candidates presenting for a surgical intervention each year, rendering it nearly impossible to achieve the statistical power necessary to draw critical conclusions about DBS therapy in this population. We therefore aimed to develop an International DBS Registry and Database for TS with the idea that the statistical power necessary to refine and improve this procedure could only be achieved through the collection of a large worldwide community of cases.

Questions to be answered include best targets, best phenotypical indications, most appropriate surgical and programming approaches, efficacy, and other outcomes. There are many obstacles for investigator initiated device studies as noted recently by Foote et al (Kelly et al., 2014). This is most problematic in less common disorders such as TS. Limited funding and lack of insurance coverage for devices in clinical trials have created a vicious cycle discouraging investigator-initiated device trials (Kelly et al., 2014; Rossi et al., 2014). The TS registry and database has the potential to facilitate a paradigm shift by collecting important information about TS DBS that cannot be obtained by using standard clinical trial design. One important goal of this project is to obtain approval for the procedure from appropriate regulatory agencies.

REVIEW OF THE LITERATURE

A review of the English language literature was performed through PUBMED using the medical subheading database with the keywords "deep brain stimulation" AND "Tourette syndrome." The review was focused on original articles and excluded review articles.

A large number of reports were available, however most were case reports or small series. A relatively recent article by Motlagh et al. (2013) reviewed the available published cases. In **Table 1**, we summarize the studies reporting a minimum of four TS DBS patients. We excluded reports with less than four patients.

The most recent TS DBS study appeared in the Lancet Neurology in June 2015 (Kefalopoulou et al., 2015). It was a randomized double-blind crossover trial conducted in 15 patients. The target for most patients was the anteromedial GPi (two were targeted in the posteroventral GPi) and all subjects were randomly assigned 1:1 to either 3 months of on-stimulation or 3 months off stimulation. All subjects switched to the alternative condition. Only 13 of 15 patients completed the two-blinded assessments. There was a small benefit in tic reduction as noted by a mean improvement of 12.4 points (equivalent to 15.3%) on the Yale Global Tic Severity Scale (YGTSS).

Three other randomized double-blind trials have also been published. The target was CM/Pf and these studies had smaller numbers. Maciunas et al. (2007) randomized five patients to receive bilateral DBS electrode implantation in a single operative session. There was a standardized follow-up at 17–21 days following implantation. The first outcome was measured at 7 days, and patients were randomized to stimulation in one of four combinations (right on, left off; right off, left on; right on, left on; right off, left off). Each 7 days during a 28-day follow-up period another randomized outcome was implemented until all potential conditions were tested. This study procedure was then followed by 3 months of open label DBS. Tics were assessed by standardized rating scales and also by independent video analysis. Unilateral stimulation proved not as effective as bilateral DBS, and overall there were positive benefits in tic reduction reported in three of the five patients.

Ackermans et al. (2011) randomized six patients to receive bilateral DBS electrodes in the Voi/CM/Pf complex of the thalamus. Patients were assigned to 3 months on stimulation followed by 3 months off stimulation (group A) or vice-versa (group B). This crossover period was followed by 6 months of open label on stimulation. Only one patient was randomized to group B. There was a significant improvement of 37% in tics when comparing on vs. off states as well as at comparing baseline to final outcome. Assessments were performed using the Yale Global Tic Severity Scale. The authors noted that at 1 year, patients required more time to finish a selective attention and response inhibition test (Stroop Color Word Card Test).

Okun et al. (2013) randomized five patients who received bilateral DBS electrodes in the centromedian complex of the thalamus. A scheduled stimulation paradigm was used instead of the conventional continuous stimulation paradigm. Two patients were randomized to start stimulation at 30 days from implantation and the remaining three patients to start stimulation at 60 days from implantation. There was a statistically significant improvement in YGTSS total score (by 19%) and in the modified Rush Tic Rating Scale Score. The authors reported that tic suppression was most effective at deep contacts on the lead.

All of the studies published reported limitations and concerns regarding individual variability in outcome, the level of stimulation required, the effect of tolerance, battery life, electrical current spread, small sample size, and difficulty in maintaining the patient blinding.

THE INTERNATIONAL TS DBS REGISTRY AND DATABASE: GOALS AND DESIGN

The international community collectively responded to the critical need in the DBS field by collaborating with the Tourette Syndrome Association (since renamed to the Tourette Association of America TAA) in 2012 and by launching an International TS DBS registry and database. The project sought to consolidate all of the information available for TS DBS cases worldwide. This effort aimed to shift the field from small case series and reports to an international large-scale collaborative

TABLE 1 | This table summarizes the published literature about DBS in Tourette Syndrome with number of subjects ≥ 4.

References	*n*	Age (years)	Gender	Target	Laterality of stimulation	Follow-up time	High frequency stimulation	Continuous stimulation	Tic improvement	Study country	Year published	Double blind randomized trial
Servello et al., 2008	18	17–47	15 m, 3 f	Centromedian-parafascicular and ventralis oralis complex of the thalamus	Bilateral	3–18 months	Yes	Yes	YGTSS decreased from 33–48 to 7–22	Italy	2008	No
Motlagh et al., 2013	8	16–48	8 m, 0 f	Thalamus (5) and Globus pallidus internus (3—two in the sensorimotor portion and one in limbic portion)	Bilateral	6–107 months	Yes	Yes	YGTSS decreased by 0–72%	USA	2013	No
Maciunas et al., 2007	5	18–34	NA	Centromedian-parafascicular and ventralis oralis complex of the thalamus	Blinded off-off, off-on, on-off, on-on combinations of 1 week each, then open-label bilateral	3 months	Yes	Yes	three of five patients showed improvement, mean preop YGTSS 37.2, 3-month score 28.2	USA	2007	Yes (cross-over design)
Servello et al., 2009	4	25–47	3 m, 1 f	Internal capsule/nucleus accumbens in patients with centromedian-parafascicular and ventralis oralis complex of the thalamus (except one patient with only internal capsule/nucleus accumbens leads)	Bilateral	8–51 months	Yes	Yes	two patients showed at best mild improvement in OCD and tic scores, two showed more clinically significant improvement in OCD scores and functionality, with limited effect on tics	Italy	2009	No (case-series)
Porta et al., 2009	15	17–47	12 m, 3 f	Centromedian-parafascicular and ventralis oralis complex of the thalamus	Bilateral	24 months	Yes	Yes	Persistent improvement in tic scores. No deleterious effect on cognition, improvement in behavioral ratings	Italy	2009	No
Ackermans et al., 2010	6	28–42	6 m, 0 f	Centromedian-parafascicular and ventralis oralis complex of the thalamus	Bilateral, 3 months of either on or off, then 6 months on	12 months	Yes	Yes	YGTSS decreased from a mean of 42.3 prior to surgery to 21.5 on 1 year follow-up, $p = 0.028$	Netherlands	2010	Yes (cross-over design)
Martínez-Fernández et al., 2011	5	21–60	5 m, 0 f	Globus pallidus internus (two patients with anteromedial location, two patients with posterolateral location, one patient initially with posterolateral switched after 18 months to antermedial location	Bilateral	3–24 months	Yes	Yes	Mean YGTSS was 77.8 at baseline and 54.2 at last follow up, mean MRVRS was 28.3 at baseline and 15.7 at last follow up, TSQOL was 61.7 at baseline and 28.5 at last follow up	UK	2011	No (case-series)
Dehning et al., 2011	4	25–44	1 m, 3 f	Globus pallidus internus (posteroventrolateral location)	Bilateral	5–48 months	Yes	Yes	two patients responded with > 80% reduction in tics, two patients were non-responders	Germany	2011	No (case-series)

(Continued)

TABLE 1 | Continued

References	*n*	Age (years)	Gender	Target	Laterality of stimulation	Follow-up time	High frequency stimulation	Continuous stimulation	Tic improvement	Study country	Year published	Double blind randomized trial
Cannon et al., 2012	11	18–50	8 m, 3 f	Globus pallidus internus (anteromedial location)	Bilateral	4–30 months	Yes	Yes	one patient was a non-responder; mean YGTSS was 84.45 before surgery and 42.55 at 3 months, mean TSQOL was 39.09 before surgery and 79.09 at 3 months	Australia	2012	No
Porta et al., 2012	18	17–47	15 m, 3 f	Centromedian-parafascicular and ventralis oralis complex of the thalamus	Bilateral	5–6 years	Yes	Yes	Mean YGTSS was 80.83 prior to surgery and 22.11 at the extended follow up ($p < 0.001$)	Italy	2012	No
Maling et al., 2012	5	28–39	2 m, 3 f	Centromedian-parafascicular and ventralis oralis complex of the thalamus	Bilateral	6 months	Yes	Yes	YGTSS decreased by 1–41%; noted correlation between gamma band activity change and YGTSS change after DBS	USA	2012	No
Okun et al., 2013	5	28–39	2 m, 3 f	Centromedian-parafascicular and ventralis oralis complex of the thalamus	Bilateral	6 months	Yes	No	YGTSS decreased by 17.8 points ($p = 0.01$), MRVRS decreased by 5.8 points ($p = 0.01$)	USA	2013	No
Dehning et al., 2014	6	19–39	3 m, 3 f	Globus pallidus internus (posteroventrolateral location)	Bilateral	12–60 months	Yes	Yes	two patients were non-responders, mean YGTSS was 90.2 prior to surgery and 29.5 at last follow up ($p = 0.001$), TSQOL was 88.75 prior to surgery and 7.75 at last follow up (one person did not fill TSQOL)	Germany	2013	No
Zhang et al., 2014	13	16–34	12 m, 1 f	Globus pallidus internus (posterolateral location)	Bilateral	13–80 months	Yes	Yes	Mean YGTSS decreased by 52.1% at last follow up, mean TSQOL improved by 45.7% at last follow up	China	2014	No
Huys et al., 2014	8	19–56	5 m, 3 f	Ventral anterior and ventrolateral motor parts of the thalamus	Bilateral except in two patients unilateral	12 months	Yes	Yes	YGTSS motor, impairment and total scores decreased by 51, 60, and 58% respectively compared to baseline. MRVRS score decreased by 58%. Significant improvement in quality of life and global functioning measures were noted	Germany	2014	No
Kefalopoulou et al., 2015	15	24–55	11 m, 4 f	Globus pallidus internus (anteromedial location)	Bilateral, 3 months on or off, then open label on stimulation	6 months blinded and then 8–36 months unblinded	Yes	Yes	YGTSS decreased by 12.4 between on and off states in the blinded phase ($p = 0.048$), YGTSS decreased by 23.8–48.9 points ($p < 0.0001$) between baseline and open label phase	UK	2015	Yes (cross-over design)

effort. The elements included in the database are summarized in **Figure 1**.

This multi-center effort has resulted in the formation of a registry and a database. There is no restriction on investigators or groups wishing to join the project, and there is no limitation to the maximum data necessary to register a case. However, in order for the case to qualify for database status and outcome measurement, there must be a minimal amount of information available to facilitate a group analysis of all of the participating centers. Additionally, groups with negative as well as positive experiences with DBS cases are strongly encouraged to participate. Enrolling all subjects regardless of the quality of the outcome is mandatory and is an important factor to better understand the current state of the field.

The database and registry have facilitated networking of clinician-researchers and have led to the generation of new hypotheses for both research and care. The database and registry will provide a repository of valuable information for patient advocacy groups (e.g., TAA), device manufacturers, as well as third party payers who are keenly focused on the potential benefits, burdens, risks, and harms of the therapy.

The registry and database were constructed to collect information on each case (refer to **Figure 1**). Currently supported data have been divided into six categories: (1) demographic information and disease characteristics, (2) pre-operative clinical scales (i.e., Yale-Brown obsessive compulsive scale (YBOCS), YGTSS, Hamilton depression scale, etc.), (3), surgical procedure data (including brain target, targeting procedure, lead location, device type, and imaging data), (4) DBS programming parameters, (5), regular follow-up clinical assessment and scales, and (6) surgical as well as stimulation-related adverse events. Electrophysiological data from the DBS procedure is not currently being collected; however, efforts are underway to enable for those interested and familiar with the techniques, intraoperative single cell recordings, and local field potential (LFP) data extracted from next generation devices capable of chronic LFP recordings. As these devices become more widely used, these data will become more available and, importantly, could add to the insights into the physiology of tic and the mechanisms underlying DBS-related improvements in tic behaviors.

CURRENT STATUS OF THE REGISTRY

Participants involved in the database include investigators who have been implanting TS DBS patients with and without the intent to publish.

To date 157 patients are registered from 10 different countries. 126 of the patients (80%) are male. The targets used include the thalamus (92 cases), anteromedial and posteroventral GPi (61 cases), and the anterior limb of the internal capsule/nucleus accumbens (2 cases).

The following are the most commonly submitted data:

1. Demographic data
   a. Patient identifier
   b. Gender

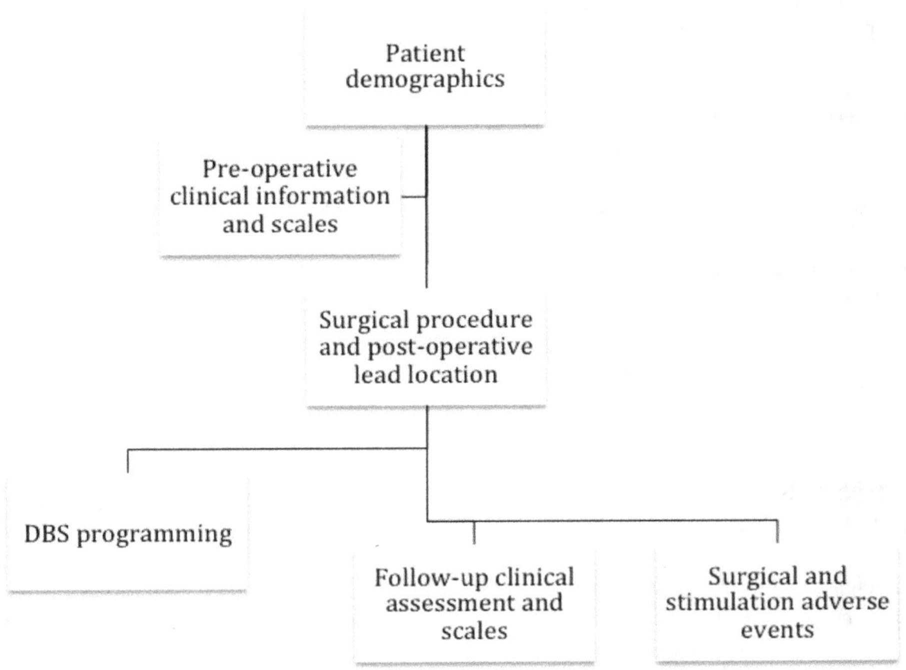

FIGURE 1 | The flowchart reveals the collaborative group's information collected on each TS DBS case.

c. Country
d. Age at onset
e. Age at surgery
f. Co-morbidities with a specific focus on obsessive compulsive disorder (OCD)
g. List of medications tried and at the time of surgery

2. Pre-operative clinical scales

a. YGTSS at baseline

i. Total score
ii. Motor tic subcomponent (less commonly available)
iii. Vocal tic subcomponent (less commonly available)
iv. Impairment subcomponent (less commonly available)

b. YBOCS at baseline

3. Surgical procedure data

a. Lead location and target
b. Device used

4. DBS programming parameters (limited data available at this point)
5. Follow up clinical assessment and scales

a. YGTSS at 1 year

i. Total score

b. YBOCS at 1 year

6. Adverse events

Another important objective of the database is to track safety. Many outcomes are collected and these outcomes have been aligned to the variables potentially necessary for a future humanitarian device exemption approval by regulatory agencies in different countries and regions. An adverse event form is available to participants in the database and was modeled after requirements from the American Food and Drug Administration (FDA). Participants have been asked to report all adverse events. The patient identifier has been used to link the adverse event to the patient. The following information has been collected: start date of adverse event, end date of adverse event, weight of patient at onset of event, outcome of adverse event (resolution, disability, hospitalization, death), description of the adverse event and associated relevant history, needed workup and laboratory studies, DBS hardware information (device name, serial number, implant date, explant date), and any therapies/surgeries needed as a result of the adverse event.

UNIQUE CHALLENGES FACING THE TS REGISTRY AND DATABASE

There are many challenges facing an ambitious initiative, particularly of this size. One major challenge will be to assure data quality, particularly given the large number of participating centers. This challenge has been addressed by process refinement and feedback of data to the participating centers and sites. Frequent meetings of participating centers have been a critical element to improving data quality and also for informing sites about the minimum data necessary to move from a registration status to a full database status (submitting data about their own DBS in TS cases). Additionally, the database has fully dedicated support for data collection that is headquartered at the University of Florida Center for Movement Disorders and Neurorestoration. The central data repository has a full-time principal investigator (Professor Michael Okun) and a database manager who together are focused on the mission and objectives, defining policies and procedures, and assigning responsibilities for each participant. Additionally, the coordinating center has defined a clear communication plan, compliance monitoring, and data policy enforcement.

A more substantial challenge facing this international DBS registry will be to achieve data uniformity. Several scales exist to measure tics and each has advantages and limitations. Scales may assess one or more disease features (i.e., motor tics, vocal tics, OCD symptoms, and quality of life). There has been variability among groups in preferences for outcome measures and in time frames for assessment; standardization of submitted measures and clinical scales would allow more cases for analysis.

Another important issue facing TS DBS will be to ensure the database is highly accessible to its contributors and to promote transparency among investigators. This process if executed properly has the potential to instill confidence in contributors and to encourage programs to invest the resources necessary to obtain the critical measurements necessary for the success of the project.

STRATEGIES TO ACHIEVE SUCCESS

Several measures have been implemented to counteract potential database-related problems. One of the cornerstones of success will be continuous education of the investigators on data collection. The database has been purposely designed to draw in as many TS centers in the world participating in DBS operations. This large-scale effort will increase the number of patients and expand the potential for multiple data points for later analysis. Additionally, as centers enroll more patients the hope is that they will adapt and begin to collect more appropriate and relevant data-points.

An important strategy is scheduling regular meetings of the collaborating centers to foster cooperation and to provide updates on their progress and the obstacles faced. In June 2015, the second annual meeting was convened to discuss the Tourette database effort and was held at the World Congress on Tourette Syndrome and Tic Disorders (London, UK). Most TSA DBS contributors were in attendance and there were presenters from each country. An image registration initiative was launched to identify DBS lead locations within the cohort. The hope was that this initiative would substantially add to the lead localization images analyzed in conjunction with already collected information about DBS lead coordinates and programming parameters. This data may aid in the identification of the volumes of tissue activation across the targets and would facilitate the correlation to outcome. Another initiative was to locate a health economist to determine what information would be meaningful to collect across centers. One example of an immediate use of the data was a question raised at the annual investigator meeting. The group sought to answer whether there was an outcome difference between earlier vs. later DBS implantation. This type of collaborative meetings will be an important cornerstone for an international database, and the meetings will continue to create improvement opportunities and to answer new questions facing the field.

TS REGISTRY AND DATABASE ROLE IN REGULATORY AGENCY APPROVAL PROCESSES

Another important goal of the database will be to facilitate applications to appropriate regulatory agencies worldwide for approval of TS DBS. This includes regulatory agencies worldwide such as FDA (USA), CE (European Union), PMDS (Japan), SFDA (China), TGA (Australia), and many other national and regional regulatory bodies. In the USA, the most likely approval would be through a FDA humanitarian device exemption given the small number of patients currently requiring therapy. DBS approval on a humanitarian basis for obsessive compulsive disorder was obtained using pooled data from several small n studies. The use of a database for TS will facilitate an analysis of a larger number of patients. It will facilitate the collection of important safety data, a crucial step needed for regulatory agency approval. The multi-center data collection will encourage a shift to a more uniform data collection and analysis.

CONCLUSIONS

The international registry and database has been designed to overcome the severe limitations of *small-n* studies for TS DBS. The project has made considerable progress toward a truly global database. We have now demonstrated proof of principle that reliable and comprehensive data can be collected. This data will be used to address fundamental questions facing the TS DBS field, including identification of optimal brain target(s) for each patient based on individual symptom profiles, as well as stimulation parameters for each brain target and/or symptom. Additionally, a robust dataset will facilitate analysis of important questions that may potentially inform outcomes such as the relationship between baseline disease characteristics and the short and long-term clinical outcome. As data expand we will be able to move toward more advanced queries that can be used to address complex questions such as the relationship between electrode placement and clinical outcomes, as well as the correlation of lead location to adverse events. These basic, yet critical questions remain unanswered (Rotsides and Mammis, 2013; Jimenez-Shahed, 2015). Importantly, the systematic conglomeration of TS DBS datasets will generate the "higher n" critical to design clinical trials, power meaningful analyses, and generate recommendations for patient, target, and stimulation parameter selection. Finally, the database will be instrumental in applying for regulatory device exemptions.

AUTHOR CONTRIBUTIONS

AM, AL, AG, BC, BW, BK, CK, DH, DS, DW, EJ, EM, EW, FM, HW, JL, JK, JZ, JH, JM, JS, JB, KF, LS, LA, LM, LZ, MW, MH, MP, MHP, PS, RG, SZ, SK, TK, TC, TF, VV, WH, YT, ZK, and ZM fulfilled the authorship criteria by substantial contributions to the conception of the work, revisiting it critically for important intellectual content, approving the final version, and agreeing to be accountable for all aspects of the work in ensuring that questions related to the accuracy or integrity of any part of the work are appropriately investigated and resolved. WD, PR, KR, and MO fulfilled the authorship criteria by substantial contributions to the design of the work and the acquisition, analysis, and interpretation of data for the work, drafting the work and revising it critically for important intellectual content, approving the final version to be published and agreeing to be accountable for all aspects of the work in ensuring that questions related to the accuracy or integrity of any part of the work are appropriately investigated and resolved.

ACKNOWLEDGMENTS

We thank all the different members of the multiple teams around the world that collaborated to create the International Tourette Syndrome DBS Registry and Database. We thank the Tourette Association of America for the continued support. This manuscript was motivated by the 1st World Congress on Tourette Syndrome and Tic Disorders (London, June 24-26, 2015) and is supported by the Tourette Association of America.

REFERENCES

Ackermans, L., Duits, A., Temel, Y., Winogrodzka, A., Peeters, F., Beuls, E. A., et al. (2010). Long-term outcome of thalamic deep brain stimulation in two patients with Tourette syndrome. *J. Neurol. Neurosurg. Psychiatry* 81, 1068–1072. doi: 10.1136/jnnp.2009.176859

Ackermans, L., Duits A., van der Linden, C., Tijssen, M., Schruers, K., Temel, Y., et al. (2011). Double-blind clinical trial of thalamic stimulation in patients with Tourette syndrome. *Brain* 134(Pt 3), 832–844. doi: 10.1093/brain/awq380

Ackermans, L., Neuner, I., Temel, Y., Duits, A., Kuhn, J., and Visser-Vandewalle, V. (2013). Thalamic deep brain stimulation for Tourette syndrome. *Behav. Neurol.* 27, 133–138. doi: 10.1155/2013/835253

Cannon, E., Silburn, P., Coyne, T., O'Maley, K., Crawford, J. D., and Sachdev, P. S. (2012). Deep brain stimulation of anteromedial globus pallidus interna for severe Tourette's syndrome. *Am. J. Psychiatry* 169, 860–866. doi: 10.1176/appi.ajp.2012.11101583

Cavanna, A. E., Eddy, C. M., Mitchell, R., Pall, H., Mitchell, I., Zrinzo, L., et al. (2011). An approach to deep brain stimulation for severe treatment-refractory Tourette syndrome: the UK perspective. *Br. J. Neurosurg.* 25, 38–44. doi: 10.3109/02688697.2010.534200

Da Cunha, C., Boschen, S. L., Goómez, A. A., Ross, E. K., Gibson, W. S., Min, H. K., et al. (2015). Toward sophisticated basal ganglia neuromodulation: Review on basal ganglia deep brain stimulation. *Neurosci. Biobehav. Rev.* 58, 186–210. doi: 10.1016/j.neubiorev.2015.02.003

Dehning, S., Feddersen, B., Cerovecki, A., Botzel, K., Muller, N., and Mehrkens, J. H. (2011). Globus pallidus internus-deep brain stimulation in Tourette's syndrome: can clinical symptoms predict response? *Mov. Disord.* 26, 2440–2441. doi: 10.1002/mds.23892

Dehning, S., Leitner, B., Schennach, R., Muller, N., Botzel, K., Obermeier, M., et al. (2014). Functional outcome and quality of life in Tourette's syndrome after deep brain stimulation of the posteroventrolateral globus pallidus internus: long-term follow-up. *World J. Biol. Psychiatry* 15, 66–75. doi: 10.3109/15622975.2013.849004

Dehning, S., Mehrkens, J. H., Müller, N., and Bötzel, K. (2008). Therapy-refractory Tourette syndrome: beneficial outcome with globus pallidus internus deep brain stimulation. *Mov. Disord.* 23, 1300–1302. doi: 10.1002/mds.21930

Dong, S., Zhang, X., Li, J., and Li, Y. (2014). The benefits of low-frequency pallidal deep brain stimulation in a patient with Tourette syndrome. *Parkinsonism Relat. Disord.* 20, 1438–1439. doi: 10.1016/j.parkreldis.2014.09.028

Duits, A., Ackermans, L., Cath, D., and Visser-Vandewalle, V. (2012). Unfavourable outcome of deep brain stimulation in a Tourette patient with severe comorbidity. *Eur. Child Adolesc. Psychiatry* 21, 529–531. doi: 10.1007/s00787-012-0285-6

Flaherty, A. W., Williams, Z. M., Amirnovin, R., Kasper, E., Rauch, S. L., Cosgrove, G. R., et al. (2005). Deep brain stimulation of the anterior internal capsule for the treatment of Tourette syndrome: technical case report. *Neurosurgery* 57(4 Suppl.):E403. discussion: E403. doi: 10.1227/01.neu.0000176854.24694.95

Freeman, R. D., Fast, D. K., Burd, L., Kerbeshian, J., Robertson, M. M., and Sandor, P. (2000). An international perspective on Tourette syndrome: selected findings from 3,500 individuals in 22 countries. *Dev. Med. Child Neurol.* 42, 436–447. doi: 10.1017/S0012162200000839

Hassler, R., and Dieckmann, G. (1970). Stereotaxic treatment of tics and inarticulate cries or coprolalia considered as motor obsessional phenomena in Gilles de la Tourette's disease. *Rev. Neurol. (Paris)* 123, 89–100.

Huys, D., Bartsch, C., Koester, P., Lenartz, D., Maarouf, M., Daumann, J., et al. (2014). Motor improvement and emotional stabilization in patients with tourette syndrome after deep brain stimulation of the ventral anterior and ventrolateral motor part of the thalamus. *Biol. Psychiatry.* 79, 392–401. doi: 10.1016/j.biopsych.2014.05.014

Jimenez-Shahed, J. (2015). Design challenges for stimulation trials of Tourette's syndrome. *Lancet Neurol.* 14, 563–565. doi: 10.1016/S1474-4422(15)00043-5

Kefalopoulou, Z., Zrinzo, L., Jahanshahi, M., Candelario, J., Milabo, C., Beigi, M., et al. (2015). Bilateral globus pallidus stimulation for severe Tourette's syndrome: a double-blind, randomised crossover trial. *Lancet Neurol.* 14, 595–605. doi: 10.1016/S1474-4422(15)00008-3

Kelly, M. L., Malone, D., Okun, M. S., Booth, J., and Machado, A. G. (2014). Barriers to investigator-initiated deep brain stimulation and device research. *Neurology.* 82, 1465–1473. doi: 10.1212/WNL.0000000000000345

Kim, W., and Pouratian, N. (2014). Deep brain stimulation for Tourette syndrome. *Neurosurg. Clin N. Am.* 25, 117–135. doi: 10.1016/j.nec.2013.08.009

Kuhn, J., Lenartz, D., Mai, J. K., Huff, W., Lee, S. H., Koulousakis, A., et al. (2007). Deep brain stimulation of the nucleus accumbens and the internal capsule in therapeutically refractory Tourette-syndrome. *J Neurol.* 254, 963–965. doi: 10.1007/s00415-006-0404-8

Maciunas, R. J., Maddux, B. N., Riley, D. E., Whitney, C. M., Schoenberg, M. R., Ogrocki, P. J., et al. (2007). Prospective randomized double-blind trial of bilateral thalamic deep brain stimulation in adults with Tourette syndrome. *J. Neurosurg.* 107, 1004–1014. doi: 10.3171/JNS-07/11/1004

Malaty, I. A., and Akbar, U. (2014). Updates in medical and surgical therapies for Tourette syndrome. *Curr. Neurol. Neurosci. Rep.* 14:458. doi: 10.1007/s11910-014-0458-4

Maling, N., Hashemiyoon, R., Foote, K. D., Okun, M. S., and Sanchez, J. C. (2012). Increased thalamic gamma band activity correlates with symptom relief following deep brain stimulation in humans with Tourette's syndrome. *PLoS ONE* 7:e44215. doi: 10.1371/journal.pone.0044215

Martínez-Fernández, R., Zrinzo, L., Aviles-Olmos, I., Hariz, M., Martinez-Torres, I., Joyce, E., et al. (2011). Deep brain stimulation for Gilles de la Tourette syndrome: a case series targeting subregions of the globus pallidus internus. *Mov. Disord.* 26, 1922–1930. doi: 10.1002/mds.23734

Massano, J., Sousa, C., Foltynie, T., Zrinzo, L., Hariz, M., and Vaz, R. (2013). Successful pallidal deep brain stimulation in 15-year-old with Tourette syndrome: 2-year follow-up. *J. Neurol.* 260, 2417–2419. doi: 10.1007/s00415-013-7049-1

Motlagh, M. G., Smith, M. E., Landeros-Weisenberger, A., Kobets, A. J., King, R. A., Miravite, J., et al. (2013). Lessons learned from open-label deep brain stimulation for tourette syndrome: eight cases over 7 years. *Tremor Other Hyperkinet. Mov. (N.Y.)* 3:tre-03-170-4428-1. doi: 10.7916/D8M32TGM

Müller-Vahl, K. R., Cath, D. C., Cavanna, A. E., Dehning, S., Porta, M., Robertson, M. M., et al. (2011). European clinical guidelines for Tourette syndrome and other tic disorders. Part IV: deep brain stimulation. *Eur. Child Adolesc. Psychiatry* 20, 209–217. doi: 10.1007/s00787-011-0166-4

Okun, M. S., Fernandez, H. H., Foote, K. D., Murphy, T. K., and Goodman, W. K. (2008). Avoiding deep brain stimulation failures in Tourette syndrome. *J. Neurol. Neurosurg. Psychiatry* 79, 111–112. doi: 10.1136/jnnp.2007.135715

Okun, M. S., Foote, K. D., Wu, S. S., Ward, H. E., Bowers, D., Rodriguez, R. L., et al. (2013). A trial of scheduled deep brain stimulation for Tourette syndrome: moving away from continuous deep brain stimulation paradigms. *JAMA Neurol.* 70, 85–94. doi: 10.1001/jamaneurol.2013.580

Piedimonte, F., Andreani, J. C., Piedimonte, L., Graff, P., Bacaro, V., Micheli, F., et al. (2013). Behavioral and motor improvement after deep brain stimulation of the globus pallidus externus in a case of Tourette's syndrome. *Neuromodulation* 16, 55–58. discussion: 8. doi: 10.1111/j.1525-1403.2012.00526.x

Porta, M., Brambilla, A., Cavanna, A. E., Servello, D., Sassi, M., Rickards, H., et al. (2009). Thalamic deep brain stimulation for treatment-refractory Tourette syndrome: two-year outcome. *Neurology* 73, 1375–1380. doi: 10.1212/WNL.0b013e3181bd809b

Porta, M., Servello, D., Zanaboni, C., Anasetti, F., Menghetti, C., Sassi, M., et al. (2012). Deep brain stimulation for treatment of refractory Tourette syndrome: long-term follow-up. *Acta Neurochir. (Wien)* 154, 2029–2041. doi: 10.1007/s00701-012-1497-8

Rossi, P. J., Machado, A., and Okun, M. S. (2014). Medicare coverage of investigational devices: the troubled path forward for deep brain stimulation. *JAMA Neurol.* 71, 535–536. doi: 10.1001/jamaneurol.2013.6042

Rotsides, J., and Mammis, A. (2013). The use of deep brain stimulation in Tourette's syndrome. *Neurosurg. Focus* 35:E4. doi: 10.3171/2013.8.FOCUS13292

Sachdev, P. S., Cannon, E., Coyne, T. J., and Silburn, P. (2012). Bilateral deep brain stimulation of the nucleus accumbens for comorbid obsessive compulsive disorder and Tourette's syndrome. *BMJ Case Rep.* 2012:bcr2012006579. doi: 10.1136/bcr-2012-006579

Savica, R., Stead, M., Mack, K. J., Lee, K. H., and Klassen, B. T. (2012). Deep brain stimulation in tourette syndrome: a description of 3 patients with excellent outcome. *Mayo Clin. Proc.* 87, 59–62. doi: 10.1016/j.mayocp.2011.08.005

Servello, D., Porta, M., Sassi, M., Brambilla, A., and Robertson, M. M. (2008). Deep brain stimulation in 18 patients with severe Gilles de la Tourette syndrome refractory to treatment: the surgery and stimulation. *J. Neurol. Neurosurg. Psychiatry* 79, 136–142. doi: 10.1136/jnnp.2006.104067

Servello, D., Sassi, M., Brambilla, A., Porta, M., Haq, I., Foote, K. D., et al. (2009). *De novo* and rescue DBS leads for refractory Tourette syndrome patients with severe comorbid OCD: a multiple case report. *J. Neurol.* 256, 1533–1539. doi: 10.1007/s00415-009-5159-6

Shprecher, D. R., Schrock, L., and Himle, M. (2014). Neurobehavioral aspects, pathophysiology, and management of Tourette syndrome. *Curr. Opin. Neurol.* 27, 484–492. doi: 10.1097/WCO.0000000000000119

Vandewalle, V., van der Linden, C., Groenewegen, H. J., and Caemaert, J. (1999). Stereotactic treatment of Gilles de la Tourette syndrome by high frequency stimulation of thalamus. *Lancet* 353:724. doi: 10.1016/S0140-6736(98)05 964-9

Visser-Vandewalle, V., Temel, Y., Boon, P., Vreeling, F., Colle, H., Hoogland, G., et al. (2003). Chronic bilateral thalamic stimulation: a new therapeutic approach in intractable Tourette syndrome. Report of three cases. *J. Neurosurg.* 99, 1094–1100. doi: 10.3171/jns.2003.99.6.1094

Viswanathan, A., Jimenez-Shahed, J., Baizabal Carvallo, J. F., and Jankovic, J. (2012). Deep brain stimulation for Tourette syndrome: target selection. *Stereotact. Funct. Neurosurg.* 90, 213–224. doi: 10.1159/000337776

Zhang, J. G., Ge, Y., Stead, M., Zhang, K., Yan, S. S., Hu, W., et al. (2014). Long-term outcome of globus pallidus internus deep brain stimulation in patients with Tourette syndrome. *Mayo Clin. Proc.* 89, 1506–1514. doi: 10.1016/j.mayocp.2014.05.019

10

Addressing the Complexity of Tourette's Syndrome through the Use of Animal Models

Ester Nespoli[1,2*†], *Francesca Rizzo*[2,3*†], *Tobias M. Boeckers*[3], *Bastian Hengerer*[1] and *Andrea G. Ludolph*[2]

[1] Competence in Neuro Spine Department, Boehringer Ingelheim Pharma GmbH & Co. KG, Biberach an der Riss, Germany, [2] Department of Child and Adolescence Psychiatry/Psychotherapy, University of Ulm, Ulm, Germany, [3] Institute of Anatomy and Cell Biology, University of Ulm, Ulm, Germany

Edited by:
Peristera Paschou, Democritus University of Thrace, Greece

Reviewed by:
Izhar Bar-Gad, Bar-Ilan University, Israel
Kirsten R. Müller-Vahl, Medical School of Hannover, Germany

***Correspondence:**
Ester Nespoli
ester.nespoli@uni-ulm.de;
Francesca Rizzo
francesca.rizzo@uni-ulm.de

† These authors have contributed equally to this work.

Tourette's syndrome (TS) is a neurodevelopmental disorder characterized by fluctuating motor and vocal tics, usually preceded by sensory premonitions, called premonitory urges. Besides tics, the vast majority—up to 90%—of TS patients suffer from psychiatric comorbidities, mainly attention deficit/hyperactivity disorder (ADHD) and obsessive-compulsive disorder (OCD). The etiology of TS remains elusive. Genetics is believed to play an important role, but it is clear that other factors contribute to TS, possibly altering brain functioning and architecture during a sensitive phase of neural development. Clinical brain imaging and genetic studies have contributed to elucidate TS pathophysiology and disease mechanisms; however, TS disease etiology still is poorly understood. Findings from genetic studies led to the development of genetic animal models, but they poorly reflect the pathophysiology of TS. Addressing the role of neurotransmission, brain regions, and brain circuits in TS disease pathomechanisms is another focus area for preclinical TS model development. We are now in an interesting moment in time when numerous innovative animal models are continuously brought to the attention of the public. Due to the diverse and largely unknown etiology of TS, there is no single preclinical model featuring all different aspects of TS symptomatology. TS has been dissected into its key symptomst hat have been investigated separately, in line with the Research Domain Criteria concept. The different rationales used to develop the respective animal models are critically reviewed, to discuss the potential of the contribution of animal models to elucidate TS disease mechanisms.

Keywords: tics, repetitive behavior, genetics, environment, PPI, TS comorbidities

INTRODUCTION

TS Definition, Epidemiology, Symptoms, and Natural Course

Tourette's Syndrome (TS) was named after Georges Gilles de la Tourette (1857–1904) who first described it as a "tic syndrome" in 1885 and whose observations are still considered mostly valid today. Tics are involuntary movements or vocalizations that can involve different parts of the body changing in frequency, intensity and duration. A diagnose of TS requires the presence of both

---

Abbreviations: ADHD, Attention Deficit/Hyperactivity Disorder; CSTC, Cortico-striato-thalamo-cortical circuit; DA, Dopamine; DOI, 2,5-Dymethoxy-4-iodoamphetamine; DR, Dopaminergic Receptor; DSM-5, Diagnostic and Statistical Manual of Mental Disorders, Fifth Edition; GABA, Gamma-Aminobutyric acid; GPe, Globus pallidus externus; HDC, Histidine decarboxylase; KO, Knock-out; NTs, Neurotransmitters; OCD, Obsessive-Compulsive Disorder; PPI, Pre-Pulse Inhibition; PU, Premonitory Urge; TS, Tourette's Syndrome.

multiple motor and one or more vocal tics with an onset before age 18 years and a persistence for at least 1 year (DSM-5).

But TS is not only about tics: up to 90% of all TS patients experience psychiatric comorbidities, mainly Attention Deficit/Hyperactivity Disorder (ADHD) and obsessive compulsive disorder (OCD), but also depression, anxiety disorders, conduct disorders, personality disorders, and self-injurious behaviors (Khalifa and Knorring, 2007; Cavanna et al., 2009; Pallanti et al., 2011).

TS has long been considered to be rare, as it was reported to affect only 1 in 2000 (Bruun, 1984). Nowadays the prevalence of TS in the general population has been re-evaluated, and is estimated to be 0.4–1% (Robertson et al., 2009), but could be even higher since, especially in childhood, tics are often so mild that are hardly perceived and easily overlooked. In many cases only an expert eye is able to identify tics in patients presented to the clinician as a consequence of behavioral problems or ADHD.

Role of CSTC Circuitry in TS Pathophysiology

The exact neurobiological background of TS remains still unclear, but a central role of the cortico-striato-thalamo-cortical (CSTC) circuit appears uncontroversial, as numerous anatomical and functional imaging studies were able to detect morphological and functional alterations in CSTC components of TS patients compared to controls (Singer et al., 1993; Peterson et al., 2003; Sowell et al., 2008).

The pre-motor and motor cortices, the striatum, composed of caudate and putamen, the globus pallidus internus (GPi) and externus (GPe), the subthalamic nucleus (STN), the thalamus, and the substantia nigra (SN) are connected in the CSTC circuit. Under physiological circumstances, an activation of this circuit physiologically results in voluntary movements, while involuntary movements are repressed.

Movements occur as the motor cortex is activated by the thalamus, which is controlled by the STN-GPe-GPi microcircuit. When the pre-motor cortex activates the putamen, the inhibitory striatal projection neurons release the thalamus from inhibition held by the STN-GPe-GPi, and eventually the motor cortex can be activated, leading to movement (Obeso and Lanciego, 2011).

Tics are supposed to be caused by a deregulated activity of the basal ganglia, which consequentially leads to disinhibition of the thalamus and a hyperexcitability of the motor cortex (Albin and Mink, 2006; Wang et al., 2011).

When the beneficial effect of dopaminergic modulators such as haloperidol and pimozide on tic management was observed, a dysfunction in the dopaminergic system was seen as the main responsible of TS neuropathology (for review see Buse et al., 2013). Nowadays the use of haloperidol and pimozide has been gradually left aside in favor of the better tolerable atypical antipsychotics and atypical neuroleptics, such as aripiprazole or risperidone, acting on dopamine and serotonin. In general, there is growing evidence indicating that TS is not a pure DA-related disorder, and the interplay of other neurotransmitters is strongly supported to contribute or cause the disease (for review see Udvardi et al., 2013; **Figure 1**).

Importance of a TS Animal Model

In vivo animal models are important tools to challenge and validate pathophysiological hypotheses and test new therapeutic options. An animal model is constructed to fulfill one or more of the following parameters: *face validity* (ability to show similar symptoms to the patients' ones), *construct validity* (model developed according to a rationale matching the pathological hypothesis), and *predictive validity* (model responds to a treatment similarly to patients). The ideal model is able to show all these three features, but in most cases the main focus remains on one of the three aspects. The use of animal models could help the major means of investigations of TS thanks to their ability to verify pathophysiological hypotheses and test pharmacological compounds.

METHODS

This article is a review about the *"now-in-use"* preclinical models of TS, extracted from the literature of the last decade. As a perfect model for TS has not yet been produced, we aim at showing the different successful methods used by researchers to independently model all major aspects involved in TS pathology, that we separately describe and analyze. Strengths and limitations of animal models are explained with a focus on recent research findings. The aim is to provide up-to-date information on TS animal models for students, researchers, and clinicians, and hints to be used by preclinical experimenter in developing new TS animal models.

Electronic literature search via MEDLINE/PubMed has been conducted for articles that had been published in English since year 2000. Combinations of keywords were used to identify relevant articles, including: "Tourette Syndrome," "TS animal model," "TS *in vivo*," "motor tic," "stereotype," "premonitory urge," "PPI," "genetic TS," "environment TS," "immune TS," "ADHD," "TS neurobiology," "OCD." Systematic and narrative reviews, as well as original research articles were included. The last search was conducted on November 2015. The literature search was also supplemented with key publications and book chapters known to the authors.

TS PHENOMENOLOGY

Genetics

TS has a strong genetic basis. Family studies in children with TS reveal that 8–57% of their parents had a history of tics, and first-degree relatives had a significant increased risk of developing the disorder (Pauls et al., 1991). Twin studies also report a 53–56% concordance rate for TS in monozygotic twins, compared with only 8% in dizygotic twins (Price et al., 1985; Hyde et al., 1992).

The initial idea of TS being a monogenic Mendelian disorder has been quickly revised and TS is now considered a complex disorder with many open questions regarding its overall genomic architecture. The identification of TS-related genes through linkage and association studies is hindered by the unclear mode of inheritance, the genetic heterogeneity of the disease and its apparently incomplete penetrance (Pauls, 2003).

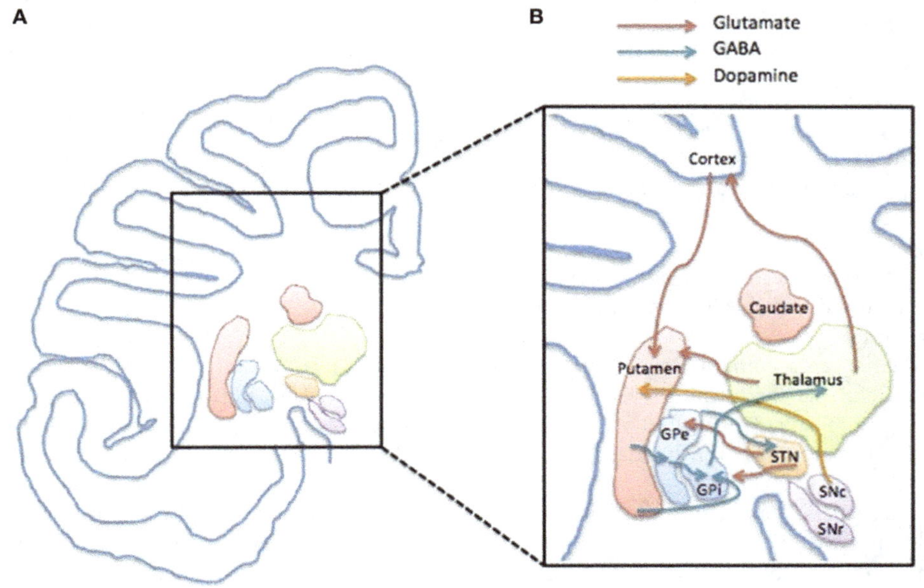

FIGURE 1 | Structure and compartments of CSTC circuit. (A) Representation of a left side of human brain coronal section depicting the anatomical localization of the basal ganglia components and the cerebral cortex. **(B)** Schematic illustration of the CSTC internal network within the circuit depicting the glutamatergic (red arrow), GABAergic (blue arrow) and the dopaminergic connection (yellow arrow). Abbreviations: GPe, Globus Pallidus pars externa; GPi, Globus Pallidus pars interna; STN, Nucleus Subtalamicus; SNc, Substantia Nigra pars compacta; SNr, Substantia Nigra pars reticulata.

Specific genetic abnormalities have so far been identified in less than 1% of patients, including polymorphisms and copy number variation. Many of these findings also parallel those of other common neuropsychiatric and neurodevelopmental disorders, unveiling previously unknown disease mechanisms, but their specific role for TS has rarely been elucidated (Sundaram et al., 2010; Crane et al., 2011; Scharf et al., 2013; Bertelsen et al., 2015).

Modeling TS Genetics

Animal genetic manipulation has widely been a key starting point to model numerous diseases.

Sequence variants in *Slirtk 1* were found in TS patients and associated to loss of function in supporting dendritic growth during development of numerous components of CSTC circuit (Abelson et al., 2005). *Slitrk1* KO mice exhibit elevated anxiety- and depression-like behaviors, symptoms which have also been associated withTS-spectrum disorder (Katayama et al., 2010).

The discovery of a mutation in the histidine decarboxylase (*Hdc*) gene in a unique family with marked history of tic disorders lead to the investigation of the disruption of histaminergic pathway in animal models. The core phenomenology of TS, tic-like behaviors, are not observed in *Hdc* KO mice at baseline, but stereotypies as repetitive sniffing and orofacial movements can be elicited by activating the dopamine system with D-amphetamine and are ameliorated after intracerebral administration of dopamine antagonist haloperidol. Fear conditioning significantly increased grooming in these animals (Castellan Baldan et al., 2014)[1].

Furthermore, significant pre-pulse inhibition (PPI) deficits and striatal dopamine dysregulation have also been observed in *Hdc* KO mice, aligning human findings and supporting the interplay between histamine and dopamine, the major known player in TS (Rapanelli et al., 2014; Xu et al., 2015a).

Another recent genetic TS animal model has been developed based onthe observation that cholinergic interneurons are reduced by 50% in TS patient's striatum (Kataoka et al., 2010; Lennington et al., 2014): region-specific knockout of choline acetyltransferase in the dorsolateral striatum led to stress-induced increase in grooming. D-amphetamine administration did not increase the amount of grooming activity, but the animals performed more repetitive stereotyped actions (Xu et al., 2015b)[2].

A main regulator of striatal activity is dopaminergic system whose alterations have been correlated with TS severity and the development of comorbidities. Genetic manipulation has been used as tool to address dopaminergic contribution to the pathology, even though genetic evidence for dopaminergic dysfunction has not been found in TS patients yet. Dopamine transporter (*DAT*) KO mice (Berridge et al., 2005) and dopamine receptor 3 (*DR3*) KO mice (Garner and Mason, 2002) are characterized by a hyperdopaminergic condition and show stereotypies, consolidating their role in repetitive behavior. Furthermore, *DAT* KO mice show a more complex and rigid sequence of actions during grooming, which is in between tics of TS and compulsions of OCD.

The lack of a clear, spontaneous "ticcing" phenotype in these genetic animal models raises the question of further

[1] http://www.ncbi.nlm.nih.gov/pmc/articles/PMC3894588/.

[2] http://www.pnas.org/content/suppl/2015/01/02/1419533112.DCSupplemental.

neurotransmitters, synaptic, or developmental mechanisms that need to be evaluated (**Table 1**).

Tics

A tic is a sudden, rapid, recurrent, non-rhythmic, jerk-like movement, or vocalization that can vary in frequency, intensity, duration and anatomical localization. Tics are classified as simple or complex according to the number of groups of muscles involved, and as motor or vocal tics.

Simple tics usually last few milliseconds engage one or a group of muscles like those involved in eye blinking (simple motor tic) or throat clearing (simple vocal tics). Complex tics last few seconds and can be defined as a combination of simple tics. They can appear purposeful like performing obscene gesture (copropraxia) or uttering racial slurs (coprolalia) or may consist in the imitation of someone elses' actions (echopraxia) or words (echolalia).

Three different tic disorders are included in the DSM-5: provisional tic disorder, persistent motor, or vocal tic disorder and TS. The difference between these disorders relies on the type of tics observed (motor, vocal, or both), and how long the symptoms have lasted. The presence of both motor and vocal tics for a period longer then 1 year since first onset (before 18 years of age) and their "waxing and waning" course differentiate TS. Indeed, they may show a pattern in which old and new tics overcome and fluctuate in frequency and intensity over time.

Other hyperkinetic movements can occur in TS patients and can be easily misdiagnosed and lead to a wrong treatment approach (Kompoliti and Goetz, 1998). This is the case of stereotypies that are fixed, prolonged and rhythmic repetitive behaviors and present an average age of onset of 3 years (DSM-5). Unlike stereotypies, tics are tipically preceded by an uncomfortable phenomenon called "premonitory urge" (PU) and can be voluntarily suppressed by most patients for a short period of time.

In general, tics are intensified by stress, anxiety, excitement, anger, fatigue, or infections (Lombroso et al., 1991; Nelson, 1993; Lin et al., 2007) while their reduction is reported in patients performing focused and effortful activities (Conelea and Woods, 2008).

Modeling Tics

The clear terminology available for clinicians to identify motor disorders is not easily applicable by *in vivo* experimenters, as any parallelism between human and animal condition must be taken carefully.

Literature testifies the lack homogeneity employed to name motor phenotypes in animal models of TS, ranging from "tic," to "tic-like movement," or "repetitive movements" and "stereotypies."

Several animal models of tics have been obtained through systemic or focal administration of active substances, which give a transient but easy to replicate phenotype. Importantly, different compounds with diverse effects were proven to be effective in the induction of tic-like behavior.

The intracerebral infusion of GABAergic antagonists is becoming a more and more appealing strategy of tic-like movement induction and has led to the formulation of the

TABLE 1 | Genetic animal models of TS.

Transgenic Model	Gene target	Association to TS	Phenotype	References
Slitrk1 KO mouse	SLIT and NTRK-like protein1	Slitrk1 mutated variants	Anxiety-like and depression-like behavioral abnormalities attenuated by clonidine (α2 adrenergic agonist) treatment	Katayama et al., 2010
HDC-KO mouse	Histidine Decarboxylase	HDC nonsense mutation	Increased grooming after D- amphetamine (5-HTR agonist) administration or stress. Stereotypies in HDC KO mice are mitigated by haloperidol (DA agonist) pretreatment	Castellan Baldan et al., 2014
ChAT-ablated mouse	Choline acetyltransferase	Reduced cholinergic interneurons in striatum of TS patients	No tic-like stereotypies and PPI deficit at baseline; increased and fragmented grooming after acoustic startle stimuli; increased stereotypies after amphetamine (5-HTR agonist) administration	Xu et al., 2015b
DAT-KO mouse	Dopamine transporter	–	Hyperdopaminergia in striatum and supestereotypies.	Berridge et al., 2005
			DA/5-HT imbalance in basal ganglia	Pogorelov et al., 2005
			PPI deficits and perseverative motor patterns	Ralph et al., 2001
DRD3-KO mouse	Dopamine receptor D3	–	Increase in spontaneous stereotypies	Garner and Mason, 2002
			Hyperlocomotor activity after amphetamine (5-HTR agonist) treatment	McNamara et al., 2006
DRD3-KO rat		–	Hyperactivity and rotational behaviors	

List of TS animal models obtained through genetic manipulation. Note that not all human genetic mutations known to have a role in TS have been used to create a valid TS preclinical model. On the other hand, several transgenic animal models have shown a TS-related phenotype but no correlation with a known TS mutation has been found so far. Abbreviations: 5HT2c-KO, Serotonin receptor knock out; CNTNAP2, Contactin-associated protein-like2; COL27A1, Type XXVII collagen alpha chain gene; CRL, controls; DAT-KO, Dopamine transporter knock out; DAT-KD, Dopamine transporter knock down; DRD1-KD, Dopamine receptor D1 knock down; DRD3-KO, Dopamine receptor D3 knock out; GABRB3, GABA A-receptor beta-3; HDC, Histidine decarboxylase; IMMP2L, Inner mitochondrial membrane peptidase; NLGN4X, Neuroligin-4 protein; POLR3B, polymerase (RNA) III (DNA directed) polypeptide B; PPI, Pre-pulse Inhibition; SLITRK1, SLIT and NTRK-like protein1; 5-HTR, serotonin receptor.

hypothesis that disequilibrium between cortical glutamatergic output and striatal GABAergic metabolism plays an important role in tic induction. The GPe was one of the first basal ganglia components to be investigated with this approach (Grabli et al., 2004), but is now the functional disruption of the striatum to be the major target of investigation.

Striatal injections of the GABAergic antagonist bicuculline in primates cause simple tic-like movements, hyperactivity and stereotyped behaviors (McCairn et al., 2009). These three phenotypes are independent processes and appear to be associated with different brain regions: the sensorimotor network, the prefrontal cortex and associative territories and the orbitofrontal cortex and limbic part of the basal ganglia respectively (Worbe et al., 2013). Electrophysiological data also suggest a role for the cerebellum in tic expression in this model (McCairn et al., 2013). The application of the same approach in adult rats results in an acute tic session that varies in intensity and body parts involved and is characterized by additional hyperactivity (Bronfeld et al., 2013)[3]. In mice, tics were also evoked by striatal picrotoxin injections, while cortical injections induce seizures (Pogorelov et al., 2015)[4].

Systemic administration of hallucinogens acting on serotonin receptors (Tizabi et al., 2001; Fantegrossi et al., 2005, 2006; Halberstadt and Geyer, 2014; Ceci et al., 2015) induce head-twitches responses, while the use of monoamines modulators, induces stereotypies (Lv et al., 2009; Taylor et al., 2010). Stereotypic behaviors were also observed after administration of 3,3′-iminodipropionitrile (IDPN) (Wang et al., 2013) and *Catha edulis extract* (Oyungu et al., 2007).

The D1CT-7 transgenic mouse, originally proposed for OCD, shows head twitching and abnormal movements of limbs and trunk with juvenile onset and sexual dimorphism (Nordstrom and Burton, 2002). These animals display PPI deficits and tic-like manifestations that are increased in presence of spatial confinement-induced. This model appears to show higher hyperactive stress reduced by antipsychotics and clonidine (Nordstrom et al., 2015), making it the first model to show *face validity* for tics and feature also common TS-related phenotypes (**Table 2**).

Premonitory Urge

Since pediatric age, TS patients become aware of an uncomfortable sensation that precedes tics known as premonitory urge (PU) that, for about 57% of cases, is more bothersome then tics themselves (Cohen and Leckman, 1992; Reese et al., 2014).

From a therapeutic point of view, the understanding of PU might help tic management since it could enhance the patient's own ability to suppress it (Leckman et al., 1993; Frank and Cavanna, 2013).

In adult TS patients the neurophysiological system of urge and tic generation appears to be distinct from the one implied in tic control (Ganos et al., 2012): the urge would include both voluntary motor circuits and somatic sensation circuits (anterior cingulate cortex and supplementary motor area), while tic generation is known to take place in prefrontal structures involved in the primary inhibition of the motor control, as confirmed by neuroimaging studies (Peterson et al., 1998).

The genesis of PU is still unknown but some evidence led to the hypothesis that this feeling might reflect abnormalities of sensorimotor gating, i.e., the neurological process able to filter out redundant or unnecessary environmental stimuli that constantly reach our brain (Braff et al., 2001; Biermann-Ruben et al., 2012).

Modeling TS Sensorimotor Gating Deficit

Tics are, to a certain extent, an easy-to-detect phenomenon; PU is more complicated to be translated into a preclinical model but can be investigated through the study of sensorimotor gating deficit.

To assess sensorimotor gating functions, the pre-pulse inhibition (PPI) of the startle response is used in both humans and laboratory animals. PPI is a behavioral phenomenon in which a weak pre-stimulus (i.e., prepulse) diminishes the reaction to a subsequent stronger stimulus (i.e., pulse) that could otherwise trigger a strong startle response. In presence of acoustic, visual or tactile stimuli, TS patients show PPI deficits manifesting the inability to filter unnecessary information (Castellanos et al., 1996; Zebardast et al., 2013).

Due to its conformity to the validity criteria, this animal model of sensorimotor gating deficits has now reasonably been extended from the single research of schizophrenia (Wan and Swerdlow, 1996) to the study of TS and its comorbidities (Swerdlow and Sutherland, 2005). In rodents, PPI appears to be regulated by the nucleus accumbens and its dopaminergic activation. Similar to tics, PPI abnormalities develop in rats treated with dopaminergic agonists (Alsene et al., 2010; Mosher et al., 2015), hallucinogens (Swerdlow et al., 2003; Chen et al., 2012) and glutamate antagonists (Swerdlow et al., 2007; Pietraszek et al., 2009). PPI deficit could also be detected in spontaneous hypertensive rats (SHR), the model of choice for ADHD (Van Den Buuse, 2004; **Table 3**).

Environmental Risk Factors

Similar to other developmental neuropsychiatric disorders, TS perfectly fits in a so-called "multistrike model" of etiology. In this model the first hit is represented by the genetic vulnerability to the disease that is likely to be translated in structural and functional neurological changes. If these changes disturb regions with physiological self-regulatory functions -second hit- tic expression is evoked. In addition, various environmental factors (neuroendocrine, infectious, autoimmune, toxic, and psychosocial influences), representing a third strike, further increase the risk of tic expression (Spessot et al., 2004).

Numerous studies have investigated environmental factors that might contribute to the onset and severity of TS and associated comorbidities. Chao et al. (2014) systematically reviewed studies investigating the contribution of pre- and perinatal adverse events on onset and severity of TS and its comorbidities, if present.

Maternal smoking appears to be consistently implicated to TS pathology (Mathews et al., 2006; Motlagh et al., 2010).

[3]http://www.frontiersin.org/Systems_Neuroscience/10.3389/fnsys.2013.00050/abstract.

[4]http://www.sciencedirect.com/science/article/pii/S0014488615000035.

TABLE 2 | Animal models of tics.

Approach	Method		Compound	Phenotype	References
Pharmacological	Systemic injection	Hallucinogens (5HTR agonists)	DOI in mice	Head twitch response. Reduced by donepezil (acetylcholinesterase inhibitor), nicotine (nAChR agonist) and haloperidol (DA antagonist) chronic or acute treatment	Hayslett and Tizabi, 2003; Tizabi et al., 2001
			DOI in ABH, C57BL/6N, SJL/J, and CD-1 mice	Head twitch response and skin jerk responses. URB597 (FAAH inhibitor) reduced head twitch in all strains	Ceci et al., 2015
			2C-I in mice	Head twitch response. Blocked by M100907 (5-HTR antagonist) administration	Halberstadt and Geyer, 2014
			2C-T-7 in mice	Head twitch response. Antagonized by M100907 (5-HTR antagonist)	Fantegrossi et al., 2005
			5-MeO-DIPT in mice	Head twitch response. Antagonized by M100907 (5-HTR antagonist) pretreatment	Fantegrossi et al., 2006
			Metamphetamine-induced hyperactive mice	Motor tics and hyperactivity. Reduced by hispidulin (plant extract with antiepileptic activity) pretreatment	Huang et al., 2015
		Dopamine modulators	Apomorphine in rats	Stereotyped actions. Inhibited by ningdong (biological extract) and haloperidol (DA antagonist) treatment	Lv et al., 2009
			SKF38393 in rats	Super-stereotyped syntactic grooming chain. Ameliorated by haloperidol (DA antagonist)	Taylor et al., 2010
		Others	IDPN (neurotoxin) in mice	Stereotypies ecresaed by tiapride (DA antagonist) and by Jian-Pi-Zhi-Dong Decoction (plants extracts)	Wang et al., 2013
			Khat cathinone (*Catha edulis extract*) in rats	Seizures, stereotyped behaviors	Oyungu et al., 2007
	Focal and systemic injection	Hallucinogens in frontal cortex of wild type and B-arr2 KO mice		Head twitch response	Schmid and Bohn, 2010
	Focal injection	GABA antagonists	Picrotoxin injections in DLS and SMC of mice	Injections in DLS induced tic-like movement attenuated or abrogated by PMPA (NMDAR antagonist) and muscimol (GABA agonist) pretreatment; injecitons in SMC produced tic-like movements and hyperactivity abrogated by muscimol pretreatment	Pogorelov et al., 2015
			BIM injections in rat GPe	Stereotypies, attention deficits and hyperactivity	Grabli et al., 2004
			BIM injections in rat striatum	Tic movements somatotopically organized and hyperbehavioral abnormalities	Bronfeld et al., 2013
			BIM injections in primate striatum	Periodic orofacial tics and forelimb tics, hyperactivity and stereotypic behaviors. Tics did not interfere with overall normal behavior	McCairn et al., 2009; Worbe et al., 2013

(Continued)

TABLE 2 | Continued

Approach	Method	Compound	Phenotype	References
Genetic	D1CT-7 transgenic mice	–	Seizures, tics and compulsive behaviors increased by pentylenetetrazol (convulsivant)	Campbell et al., 2000
		–	Repetitive climbing and leaping. Dizocilpine (non-competitive NMDAR antagonist) aggravated the phenotype and induced seizures; NBQX (AMPAR blocker) reduced stereotypies and seizures.	McGrath et al., 2000
		–	Tic-like movements; sensorimotor gating deficit in response to spatial confinement	Godar et al., 2015

List of animal models that show a motor phenotype that can be related to tic spectrum as predominant and relative drugs treatment approaches. Phenotypes are indicated as reported in literature. Abbreviations: BIM, bicuculline methiotide; DLS, dorsolateral striatum; DOI, 2,5-Dimethoxy-4-iodoamphetamine; FAAH, fatty acid amide hydrolase; IDPN, 3,3′-iminodipropionitrile; M100907, (R)-(+)-α-(2,3-dimethoxyphenyl)-1-[2-(4-fluorophenyl)ethyl]-4-piperidinemethanol; NBQX, (2,3-dihydroxy-6-nitro-7-sulfamoyl-benzo[f]quinoxaline-2,3-dione); nAChR, nicotinic acetylcholine receptor; PMPA, (RS)-4-(phosphonomethyl)piperazine-2-carboxylic acid; SMC, sensorimotor cortex; URB597, fatty acid amide hydrolase; 2C-I, 2; C-I (2,5-dimethoxy]]-4-iodophenethylamine; 2C-T-7, 4-propylthio-2,5-dimethoxyphenethylamine; 5-MeO-DIPT, 5-Methoxy-diisopropyltryptamine; 5-HTR, serotonin receptor; 5-HTTP, 5-hydroxy-L-tryptophan.

Infections, and particularly Pediatric Autoimmune Neuropsychiatric Disorders Associated with Streptococcal Infections (PANDAS) were associated to worsening or causing TS (Kurlan, 2004; Kirkman et al., 2008; Singer et al., 2012; Swedo et al., 2012), however, a causal relationship between streptococcal infections and TS is still under investigation (Hoekstra and Minderaa, 2005; Krause et al., 2010).

Finally, only a few clinical studies were conducted investigating the extent to which stressors affect TS patients' life (Silva et al., 1995) but TS patients report a strong link between stress and tics exacerbation. The hypothalamic-pituitary-adrenal axis is supported to have an enhanced responsivity in children with TS (Corbett et al., 2008) and tic severity seems to correlate to cortisol levels (Conelea and Woods, 2008).

Modeling TS Environmental Risk Factors

Several immune-mediated models have been developed according to different strategies.

Passive exposure to immunomediators (Ponzio et al., 2007; Smith et al., 2007; Depino et al., 2011; Patel et al., 2012; Zalcman et al., 2012) or to immunogenic microbial components (Hoffman et al., 2004; De Miranda et al., 2010; Yaddanapudi et al., 2010; Brimberg et al., 2012; Kirsten et al., 2012; Malkova et al., 2012) led to increased stereotypies and locomotion. However, additional deficits in motor coordination, learning/memory and social interaction, and the presence of immune deposits in the brain severely hamper their *face validity* for TS (Yaddanapudi et al., 2010).

Transplantation into naïve animals of antibodies derived from animals actively immunized with patients' sera (Taylor et al., 2002; Singer et al., 2005; Martin et al., 2008; Zhang et al., 2012) led to a similar phenotype and episodic vocalizations were reported (Hallett et al., 2000).

The importance of stress as a factor able to exacerbate tics has for long been referred by patients. Stress paradigms have proven capable of worsening the phenotype in animal models and have been recently introduced as a way to improve their validity (Xu et al., 2015a,b).

Stress paradigms can also be used to evaluate the ability of different stressors to predispose to abnormal behavioral development (Hall, 1998; Pryce and Feldon, 2003). For istance, maternal deprivation affects the social, emotional and attention domain of primates leading often to stereotypies or other dysfunctional motor activities (Márquez-Arias et al., 2010; Rommeck et al., 2011; **Table 4**).

Related Psychiatric Conditions

ADHD

Attention-deficit/hyperactivity disorder (ADHD) is the most common comorbidity in TS.

ADHD is a neurodevelopmental disorder with an onset before age 12 (DSM-5). It affects about 5% of children, with 2–4:1 boys/girls prevalence (Polanczyk and Rohde, 2007). The three core symptoms of ADHD are inattention, motor hyperactivity, and increased impulsivity. Inattention refers to disorganization and difficulty in sustaining focus; hyperactivity manifests as excessive motor activity or talking activeness in inappropriate

TABLE 3 | Animal models of PPI deficit: List of animal models that show a PPI deficit.

Approach	Method	Compound	Phenotype	References
Pharmacological	Systemic administration	Metamphetamine (5-HTR agonist), ketamine, and dizocilpine (non-competitive NMDAR antagonists) in mice	PPI deficits alleviated by *Clerodendrum inerme* ethanol extract treatment	Chen et al., 2012
		Apomorphine (DA agonits), amphetamine (5-HTR agonist), and DOI (5-HTR agonist) in parental Sprague Dawley and Long Evans rats, and offspring	Strain related heritable PPI changes	Swerdlow et al., 2003
		Dizocilpine (non-competitive NMDAR antagonists) in rat	Locomotor hyperactivity, PPI disruption, working memory deficit not alleviated by 1MeTIQ (NMDAR antagonistic)	Pietraszek et al., 2009
		Amphetamine (5-HTR agonist) in rat	PPI deficit and hyperactivity. Blocked by prazosin (α1 adrenergic receptor blocker) and partially by terazosin (α1 adrenergic receptor antagonist) focal administration in nucleus accumbens	Alsene et al., 2010
		Dizocilpine (non-competitive NMDAR antagonists) or apomorphine (DA agonits) in rat	PPI deficit. Abolished by GTS-21 (AChR partial agonist) clozapine (5-HTR partial agonist) and haloperidol (DA antagonist)	Callahan et al., 2014
		SKF82958 (DA full agonist) in Sprague-Dawley, Wistar, and Long Evans rats	Strain-specific PPI deficits.	Mosher et al., 2015
	Focal administration	p-Hydroxyamphetamine (TAAR1 agonist) in mice	PPI deficit attenuated by pretreatment with 5,7-DHT (serotonin-containing neurons neurotoxin), PCPA (serotonin synthesis inhibitor), ketanserin (5-HTR antagonist), and MDL100,907 (5-HTR antagonist)	Onogi et al., 2011
		Granulocyte-Macrophage Colony-Stimulating Factor in rat	Hyperlocomotion; social interaction and PPI deficits. Alleviated by minocycline (antibiotic)	Zhu et al., 2014
	Systemic and focal administration	Apomorphine (DA agonits) in Sprague Dawley and Long Evand rats	PPI distrupted in Sprague-Dawley	Swerdlow et al., 2007
		Apomorphine (DA agonits) and amphetamine (5-HTR agonist) in rats	PPI deficit. Prevented by finasteride (5α-reductase inhibitor)	Devoto et al., 2012
Genetic	–	BTBR mice	Spontaneous stereotypic behavior	Pearson et al., 2011
	–	Wistar and SHR rat	SHR PPI lower then Wistar rats. Reversed by WIN55212,2 (CBR agonist) and cannabidiol (CBR indirect antagonist)	Levin et al., 2014
	–	HET mice	Behavioral and PPI deficits	Chohan et al., 2014
Environmental	Prolonged maternal deprivation in rats	–	PPI reduction and impaired spatial learning in adulthood	Garner et al., 2007
	Social isolation in rats	–	Increased self-grooming and locomotor activity, PPI deficit	Strauss et al., 2014
	Pre- and post- weaning maternal separation and social isolation in rats	–	PPI changes in the adults following maternal separation and not social isolation	Weiss et al., 2011

Abbreviations: CBR, Cannabinoid receptor; DA, Dopamine; DOI, 2,5-Dimethoxy-4-iodoamphetamine; GTS-21, α7-nAChR agonists (also known as DMXB-A); HET, head tilt gene; KO, knock out; PPI, Pre Pulse Inhibition; PCPA, p-chlorophenylalanine; SHR, Spontanueous Hypertensive Rat; TAAR1, Trace amine-associated receptor 1; 1MeTIQ, 1-Methyl-1,2,3,4-tetrahydroisoquinoline; 5,7-DHT, 5,7-dihydroxytryptamine.

TABLE 4 | Animal model of environmental factors influencing TS.

Approach	Method	Compound	Phenotype	References
Immuno-mediation	Overexpression of brain immunemediators levels	Peripheral injection of IL-2 in rats during mid gestation	Stereotypic behaviors and decreased conditioned eye response	Ponzio et al., 2007
		Peripheral injection of IL-6 in mice during mid-gestation	PPI deficit	Smith et al., 2007
		Focal injection of TGFbeta-1 in mice hippocampus	Early: stereotypy behaviors, depression. Adult: decreased stereotypies and depression	Depino et al., 2011
		Peripheral injection of sIL-2R alfa/beta	Increased rearing, turning, grooming, head obbing, and jumping	Zalcman et al., 2012
		Focal injection of sIL-6R alfa	Hyper locomotor activity and stereotypic behaviors	Patel et al., 2012
	Auto-antibodies injections	Focal injection of IgG positive for antineuronal abs in rat striatum	Increased motor stereotypies and episodic vocalizations	Hallett et al., 2000
		Focal injection of anti-strep IgM mAb in mice.	Increased stereotypies, head bobbing, and grooming.	Zhang et al., 2012
		Focal injection of TS sera in rat striatum	Increased oral stereotypies and genital grooming	Taylor et al., 2002; Singer et al., 2005
		Peripheral injection of IgG from mothers of ASD children in the first trimester of pregnancy in primates	Increased stereotypies and hyperactivity	Martin et al., 2008
	Exposure to microbial immunogen or mimics.	Focal injection of GAS (M6-type) homogenate in mice	Stereotypic behavior, anxiety, and depression	Hoffman et al., 2004; Yaddanapudi et al., 2010
		Peripheral injection of GAS (M18 type) cell wall components in rats	Motor abnormalities and obsessive-compulsive behaviors. Alleviated by haloperidol (D_2R antagonist) and paroxetine (SSRI), respectively	Brimberg et al., 2012
		Peripheral Poly I:C injection in mice during mid gestation	Increased grooming	Malkova et al., 2012
		Peripheral Poly I:C injection in mice during late gestation	Poor early motor coordination, PPI deficit, increased locomotor activity. Behavioral deficits reversed by carprofen (COX-2 inhibitor)	De Miranda et al., 2010
		Peripheral LPS injection in rats during mid gestation	Increased repetitive behaviors in male offspring	Kirsten et al., 2012
Stress	Differential raising conditions in primates	–	Stereotypies and SIB in nursery-raised group more than mother-raised and in the indoor raised group more then outdoor raised groups	Rommeck et al., 2011
	Environmen-tal enrichment Captive primates	–	Repetitive movements without paying attention to the surroundings, such as pulling one's hair, cheek pinching and swinging the body Stereotypies. Environmental enrichment reduces stereotypies, aggression and coprophilia and enhances exploration	Márquez-Arias et al., 2010

List of animal models in which the TS-related phenotype is reached using environmental factor modification. Abbreviations: Ab, antibody; GAS, group A streptococcus; COX, cyclooxygenase; Ig, immunoglobulin; IL, interleukine; LPS, Lipopolysaccharide; mAb, monoclonal antibody; PPI, Pre-Pulse Inhibition; SIB, self-injury behavior; SSRI, selective serotonin re-uptake inhibitors; TGF, tumor growth factor; TS, Tourette's syndrome.

situations; impulsivity refers to the tendency to perform, without adequate forethought.

The cause of ADHD still remains elusive but it most likely results from a combination of cofactors that can be genetic, developmental, and/or environmental. The observation that the most effective drugs for ADHD treatment are psychostimulants (Sagvolden et al., 2005), implicates a role for catecholamines in the development of the disease. Indeed, the dopaminergic D1, D4, and D5 receptor genes, the α2-adrenoceptor gene, and both dopamine and norepinephrine transporters (DAT1, NET1) genes show polymorphisms in ADHD patients (Cook et al., 1995; Manor et al., 2004; Bobb et al., 2005; Park et al., 2005; Kickler et al., 2009). Serotonin has also been indicated to play a role in ADHD, as suggested by polymorphisms in genes that encode the serotonin transporter and the serotonin 1B receptor (Kent et al., 2002).

Since ADHD affects 60–80% of children with TS (Khalifa and Knorring, 2007), a common pathophysiological link between these two disorders seems evident. A debate is going on whether the two pathologies are independent (additive model), combined (interactive model), or a phenotype subgroup of one of the two major clinical forms (phenotype model) (Cavanna et al., 2009; Greimel et al., 2011; Schlander et al., 2011), however, there is increasing evidence for an additive model (Lebowitz et al., 2012; Roessner et al., 2007).

Modeling ADHD

Inattention, motor hyperactivity, and increased impulsivity are the three core features of ADHD. They have been differently modeled using (i) genetic manipulation, for instance in DAT-KO mice, coloboma mutant mice, nicotinic receptor mutant mice, human thyroid receptor expressing mice, GAT1-KO mice, ACC mice, and mutant tachinin-1 mice (Gainetdinov and Caron, 2000; Granon and Changeux, 2006; Siesser et al., 2006; Bruno et al., 2007; Yan et al., 2009; Zimmermann et al., 2014), (ii) selective breeding, as in SHR rats and Naples high excitability rats (Sadile et al., 1993; Sagvolden, 2000) (iii) insulting events during early developmental stages through 6-hydroxydopamine lesion and prenatal nicotine exposure (Stead et al., 2006; Schneider et al., 2011; Zhu et al., 2012; Freund et al., 2014) (iv) social isolation (Ouchi et al., 2013).

To validate these models, sustained attention deficits should be shown when stimuli are widely spaced in time, hyperactivity should be absent in novel situations and develop gradually over time and impulsivity should be sensitive to reinforcers (for review see Sagvolden et al., 2005).

SHR rats have been the most extensively used model of ADHD and feature all core aspects of this disorders. However, in SHR rats and in all previously listed ADHD models tic-like behaviors have not been documented.

Animal models of TS showing comorbid full ADHD spectrum have not been reported so far, but some validity for the single features were documented: hyperactivity was associated to specific bicuculline injections sites in the dorsal striatum and dorsal GPe of primates (Grabli et al., 2004; Worbe et al., 2009) and attention deficit occurred after injections in associative regions of the GPe (Grabli et al., 2004).

OCD

OCD is a neuropsychiatric disease that is frequently found as comorbidity in adult TS patients. It is a chronic disorder, which affects approximately 1–3% of the population (Pallanti et al., 2011).

According to DSM-5, obsessions, compulsions, or both, have to be present for an OCD diagnosis. Obsessions are defined as recurrent and persistent thoughts (e.g., fear of contamination), urges (e.g., need to wash hands), or images (e.g., of a violent or horrific scene) that are experienced as intrusive and unwanted, and cause marked anxiety and distress. The individual will try to suppress or to neutralize obsessions with some other thoughts or actions, for instance by performing a compulsion. Compulsions are defined as repetitive mental acts (e.g., counting) or behaviors (e.g., washing hands) performed in response to an obsession or according to rules that must be applied rigidly to a clearly excessive point when they become disruptive for daily living. OCD patients are able to recognize their obsessions and compulsions, but are unable to avoid them (Koran et al., 1996; Okasha et al., 2000).

The etiology of OCD is not completely understood.

Serotonin was the first neurotransmitter to be associated with OCD pathophysiology when selective serotonin re-uptake inhibitors (SSRIs) were shown to be efficacious in treating OCD (Barr et al., 1992). However, many patients do not respond to SSRIs treatment suggesting the additional involvement of other NTs such as dopamine (Carey et al., 2005; Taj et al., 2013), GABA (Simpson et al., 2012; Russo and Pietsch, 2013; Russo et al., 2014) and particularly glutamate (Arnold et al., 2006; Alonso et al., 2012; Porton et al., 2013). Growing evidence indicates the latter as a putative central player in OCD pathophysiology, strengthening the glutamate hypothesis of OCD and opening a new window for the development of novel treatment strategies (Coric et al., 2005; Grant et al., 2007; Bakhla et al., 2013).

Dopamine, GABA, and glutamate are commonly associated to CSTC circuit malfunction, implicating a role for this circuit in OCD pathophysiology (Stahl, 1988; Insel and Winslow, 1992; Graybiel and Rauch, 2000; Welch et al., 2007). Such alterations are also thought to be causative of tics, which 30% of OCD patients develop (Bloch et al., 2006; Pallanti et al., 2011). Tics and compulsions are now considered to be two different sides of the same coin that may be grouped under the general term of "tic-like" activities (Lombroso and Scahill, 2008; Worbe et al., 2010; Cath et al., 2011; Martino et al., 2013).

Modeling OCD

In animal models reported to have validity for OCD the presence of obsessions has been reasonably left aside and the focus was on the presence of behavioral compulsivity, intended as the performance of repetitive, and perseverating actions and stereotypies (for review see Alonso et al., 2015).

It is interesting to underline the existence of an analog to OCD in dogs: the Canine Compulsive Disorder (CCD), which leads to excessive tail chasing, light/shadow chasing, and flank sucking. These behaviors are attenuated with the same treatments used for OCD, indicating that its study may help elucidate the etiology of compulsive disorders (Ogata et al., 2013).

Numerous validated approaches have been developed aiming to evaluate and quantify compulsive-like behaviors. Examples are the schedule-induced polydipsia (Woods et al., 1993), the marble burying test (Ichimaru et al., 1995), the signal attenuation test (Joel et al., 2005) the nest building test (Hoffman and Rueda Morales, 2012) and the nestlet shredding test (Angoa-Pérez et al., 2012). These models provide the greatest ease of use and do not require any pharmacological or genetic intervention but on the other hand they do not offer any pathophysiological information.

Based on the clinical evidence for an involvement of serotonin in OCD, OCD-like behaviors are induced in animals by treatments with serotonergic agonists 8-hydroxy-2-(di-n-propylamino) tetralin (8-OH-DPAT) (Carli et al., 2006; Arora et al., 2013) and m-chlorophenylpiperazine (mCPP) (Kreiss et al., 2013), as well as with the serotonin releasing agent compound 48–80 (Wald et al., 2009). Mice lacking TPH2, the rate-limiting enzyme of serotonin synthesis in the brain, display highly repetitive and compulsive behaviors (Kane et al., 2012).

The glutamatergic hypothesis of OCD finds also a strong support in animal models. In mice lacking the AMPA receptor trafficking protein SAPAP3, glutamate signaling dysfunction is accompanied by compulsive grooming behavior (Welch et al., 2007; Wu et al., 2012).

Astrocyte-specific glutamate transporter (GLT1) inducible knockout mice exhibit OCD/TS-like behavioral spectrum, with marked increased self-injurious grooming behavior (Aida et al., 2015). Interestigly, this is the first hint of a role for non-neuronal cells in this brain disorder. Lastly, transmembrane protein *Slitrk5* KO mice show OCD-like behavioral abnormalities that seem to be associated to a deficient corticostriatal neurotransmission (Abelson et al., 2005; Shmelkov et al., 2010). *Slitrk5* belongs to the same family of *Slitrk1*, a protein associated to TS.

Dopamine, that has been largely associated to TS and ADHD, is supported by animal models findings to play a role in compulsive behaviors. The treatment with the DR2 agonist quinpirole in mice marks the expression of the behavioral repertoire and long-term exposure to this drug leads to hyperactivity in A/J mice (De Haas et al., 2012). In rats, chronic administration of the same compound causes compulsive checking (Szechtman et al., 1998; Alkhatib et al., 2013).

In the D1CT-7 transgenic mouse, the modulation of the glutamatergic cortical output on the striatal circuits obtained through the chronic potentiation of cortical and limbic D1-expressing neurons leads to the development not only of compulsive behaviors, but also of tics. This makes it the only model of comorbid tics and OCD proposed so far (Smicun et al., 1999; Nordstrom and Burton, 2002).

CONCLUSIONS

Animal models are gaining an important role in understanding TS pathophysiology and in investigating new treatment options. In the recent years numerous models have been developed, many of which summarize more than a single aspect of the syndrome.

Through animal models the idea of a major role for the striatum in tics generation, already suggested by imaging and *post mortem* studies, was importantly strengthened. In fact, independent approaches used to model TS succeeded in showing increased grooming and tic-like phenotype following striatal structural and functional alterations. This indicates the striatum as a research target worth investing more efforts.

Reproducing tics, the core feature of TS, is the actual greatest challenge for animal models. A TS diagnosis requires the coexistence of multiple motor and at least a vocal tic, but so far researchers focused on motor tics while the presence and cause of vocal tics has been poorly investigated and require further attention.

The difference between tics and other movement disorders can be detected in humans but it is subtler in animals that physiologically account a wide range of species-specific repetitive movements in their repertoire. In patients, tics have the peculiar features of being preceded by a PU, have a waxing and waning pattern and can be voluntarily repressed. These distinctive features of tics are difficult to observe in animals and result severely biased by the approach used. Stereotypies, which are fixed, prolonged, and rhythmic repetitive behaviors with an early onset and a fixed presentation pattern (DSM-5), can be confused with tics in animal models, though they are separated clinical entities. A discriminative method between these two motor phenotypes in animal models could increase *face validity* and help the development of more targeted therapeutic strategies. To achieve this point, a better understanding of the animals' behavioral spectrum along with a beter knowledge of tics' generating mechanisms are needed.

Finally, TS is classified as a neurodevelopmental syndrome, as it is typically diagnosed in childhood or adolescence, and tics show spontaneous and substantial reduction toward the end of the second decade of life in more than half of patients. However, so far, animal model research lacked the investigation of the way development affects the phenotype. Juvenile animal models could elucidate the impact of developmental mechanisms and importantly help the study of more effective and safer therapies for young patients.

AUTHOR CONTRIBUTIONS

FR and EN equally contributed to the design, drafting, writing and revising of the work. AL contributed to the design, drafting, and critical revision under a clinical point of view. BH and TB contributed to the drafting, critical revision under a pre-clinical point of view, and final approval of the work.

FUNDING

This work was supported by the European Commission Seventh Framework Programme (FP7-PEOPLE-2012-ITN), under the grant agreement n°316978.

ACKNOWLEDGMENTS

We dedicate this work to our dear colleague and mentor AL who sadly passed away during the preparation of this manuscript.

REFERENCES

Abelson, J. F., Kenneth, K. Y., O'Roak, B. J., Baek, D. Y., Stillman, A. A., Morgan, T. M., et al. (2005). Sequence Variants in SLITRK1 Are Associated with Tourette's Syndrome. *Science* 310, 317–320. doi: 10.1126/science.1116502

Aida, T., Yoshida, J., Nomura, M., Tanimura, A., Iino, Y., Soma, M., et al. (2015). Astroglial glutamate transporter deficiency increases synaptic excitability and leads to pathological repetitive behaviors in mice. *Neuropsychopharmacology* 40, 1569–1579. doi: 10.1038/npp.2015.26

Albin, R. L., and Mink, J. W. (2006). Recent advances in Tourette syndrome research. *Trends Neurosci.* 29, 175–182. doi: 10.1016/j.tins.2006.01.001

Alkhatib, A. H., Dvorkin-Gheva, A., and Szechtman, H. (2013). Quinpirole and 8-OH-DPAT induce compulsive checking behavior in male rats by acting on different functional parts of an OCD neurocircuit. *Behav. Pharmacol.* 24, 65–73. doi: 10.1097/FBP.0b013e32835d5b7a

Alonso, P., Gratacós, M., Segalàs, C., Escaramís, G., Real, E., Bayés, M., et al. (2012). Association between the NMDA Glutamate Receptor GRIN2B Gene and Obsessive-Compulsive Disorder. *J. Psychiatry Neurosci.* 37, 273–281. doi: 10.1503/jpn.110109

Alonso, P., López-Solà, C., Real, E., Segalàs, C., and Menchón, J. M. (2015). Animal models of obsessive-compulsive disorder: utility and limitations. *Neuropsychiatr. Dis. Treat.* 11, 1939–1955. doi: 10.2147/NDT.S62785

Alsene, K. M., Fallace, K., and Bakshi, V. P. (2010). Ventral striatal noradrenergic mechanisms contribute to sensorimotor gating deficits induced by amphetamine. *Neuropsychopharmacology* 35, 2346–2356. doi: 10.1038/npp.2010.106

Angoa-Pérez, M., Kane, M. J., Briggs, D. I., Sykes, C. E., Shah, M. M., Francescutti, D. M., et al. (2012). Genetic depletion of brain 5HT reveals a common molecular pathway mediating compulsivity and impulsivity. *J. Neurochem.* 121, 974–984. doi: 10.1111/j.1471-4159.2012.07739.x

Arnold, P. D., Sicard, T., Burroughs, E., Richter, M. A., and Kennedy, J. L. (2006). Glutamate transporter gene SLC1A1 associated with obsessive-compulsive disorder. *Arch. Gen. Psychiatry* 63, 769–776. doi: 10.1001/archpsyc.63.7.769

Arora, T., Bhowmik, M., Khanam, R., and Vohora, D. (2013). Oxcarbazepine and fluoxetine protect against mouse models of obsessive compulsive disorder through modulation of cortical serotonin and CREB pathway. *Behav. Brain Res.* 247, 146–152. doi: 10.1016/j.bbr.2013.02.038

Bakhla, A. K., Verma, V., Soren, S., Sarkhel, S., and Chaudhury, S. (2013). An open-label trial of memantine in treatment-resistant obsessive-compulsive disorder. *Ind. Psychiatry J.* 22, 149–152. doi: 10.4103/0972-6748.132930

Barr, L. C., Goodman, W. K., Price, L. H., McDougle, C. J., and Charney, D. S. (1992). The serotonin hypothesis of obsessive compulsive disorder: implications of pharmacologic challenge studies. *J. Clin. Psychiatry* 53(Suppl.), 17–28.

Berridge, K. C., Aldridge, J. W., Houchard, K. R., and Zhuang, X. (2005). Sequential super-stereotypy of an instinctive fixed action pattern in hyper-dopaminergic mutant mice: a model of obsessive compulsive disorder and Tourette's. *BMC Biol.* 3:4. doi: 10.1186/1741-7007-3-4

Bertelsen, B., Stefánsson, H., Rif Jensen, L., Melchior, L., Mol Debes, N., Groth, C., et al. (2015). Association of AADAC deletion and Gilles de La Tourette Syndrome in a large European Cohort. *Biol. Psychiatry* 79, 383–391. doi: 10.1016/j.biopsych.2015.08.027

Biermann-Ruben, K., Miller, A., Franzkowiak, S., Finis, J., Pollok, B., Wach, C., et al. (2012). Increased sensory feedback in Tourette syndrome. *Neuroimage* 63, 119–125. doi: 10.1016/j.neuroimage.2012.06.059

Bloch, M. H., Sukhodolsky, D. G., Leckman, J. F., and Schultz, R. T. (2006). Fine-motor skill deficits in childhood predict adulthood tic severity and global psychosocial functioning in Tourette's syndrome. *J. Child Psychol. Psychiatry* 47, 551–559. doi: 10.1111/j.1469-7610.2005.01561.x

Bobb, A. J., Addington, A. M., Sidransky, E., Gornick, M. C., Lerch, J. P., Greenstein, D. K., et al. (2005). Support for association between ADHD and two candidate genes: NET1 and DRD1. *Am. J. Med. Genet. B Neuropsychiatr. Genet.* 134B, 67–72. doi: 10.1002/ajmg.b.30142

Braff, D. L., Geyer, M. A., and Swerdlow, N. R. (2001). Human studies of prepulse inhibition of startle: normal subjects, patient groups, and pharmacological studies. *Psychopharmacology* 156, 234–258. doi: 10.1007/s002130100810

Brimberg, L., Benhar, I., Mascaro-Blanco, A., Alvarez, K., Lotan, D., Winter, C., et al. (2012). Behavioral, pharmacological, and immunological abnormalities after streptococcal exposure: a novel rat model of Sydenham Chorea and related neuropsychiatric disorders. *Neuropsychopharmacology* 37, 2076–2087. doi: 10.1038/npp.2012.56

Bronfeld, M., Yael, D., Belelovsky, K., and Bar-Gad, I. (2013). Motor tics evoked by striatal disinhibition in the rat. *Front. Syst. Neurosci.* 7:50. doi: 10.3389/fnsys.2013.00050

Bruno, K. J., Freet, C. S., Twining, R. C., Egami, K., Grigson, P. S., and Hess, E. J. (2007). Abnormal latent inhibition and impulsivity in coloboma mice, a model of ADHD. *Neurobiol. Dis.* 25, 206–216. doi: 10.1016/j.nbd.2006.09.009

Bruun, R. D. (1984). Gilles de La Tourette's syndrome. An overview of clinical experience. *J. Am. Acad. Child Psychiatry* 23, 126–133. doi: 10.1097/00004583-198403000-00002

Buse, J., Schoenefeld, K., Münchau, A., and Roessner, V. (2013). Neuromodulation in Tourette syndrome: dopamine and beyond. *Neurosci. Biobehav. Rev.* 37, 1069–1084. doi: 10.1016/j.neubiorev.2012.10.004

Callahan, P. M., Terry, A. V., and Tehim, A. (2014). Effects of the nicotinic α7 receptor partial agonist GTS-21 on NMDA-glutamatergic receptor related deficits in sensorimotor gating and recognition memory in rats. *Psychopharmacology* 231, 3695–3706. doi: 10.1007/s00213-014-3509-2

Campbell, K. M., Veldman, M. B., McGrath, M. J., and Burton, F. H. (2000). TS+OCD-like neuropotentiated mice are supersensitive to seizure induction. *Neuroreport* 11, 2335–2338. doi: 10.1097/00001756-200007140-00053

Carey, P. D., Vythilingum, B., Seedat, S., Muller, J. E., van Ameringen, M., and Stein, D. J. (2005). Quetiapine augmentation of SRIs in treatment refractory obsessive-compulsive disorder: a double-blind, randomised, placebo-controlled study [ISRCTN83050762]. *BMC Psychiatry* 5:5 doi: 10.1186/1471-244X-5-5

Carli, M., Baviera, M., Invernizzi, R. W., and Balducci, C. (2006). Dissociable contribution of 5-HT1A and 5-HT2A receptors in the medial prefrontal cortex to different aspects of executive control such as impulsivity and compulsive perseveration in rats. *Neuropsychopharmacology* 31, 757–767. doi: 10.1038/sj.npp.1300893

Castellan Baldan, L., Williams, K. A., Gallezot, J. D., Pogorelov, V., Rapanelli, M., Crowley, M., et al. (2014). Histidine decarboxylase deficiency causes Tourette syndrome: parallel findings in humans and mice. *Neuron* 81, 77–90. doi: 10.1016/j.neuron.2013.10.052

Castellanos, F. X., Fine, E. J., Kaysen, D., Marsh, W. L., Rapoport, J. L., and Hallett, M. (1996). Sensorimotor gating in boys with Tourette's syndrome and ADHD: preliminary results. *Biol. Psychiatry* 39, 33–41. doi: 10.1016/0006-3223(95)00101-8

Cath, D. C., Hedderly, T., Ludolph, A. G., Stern, J. S., Murphy, T., Hartmann, A., et al. (2011). European clinical guidelines for Tourette syndrome and other tic disorders. Part I: Assessment. *Eur. Child Adolesc. Psychiatry* 20, 155–171. doi: 10.1007/s00787-011-0164-6

Cavanna, A. E., Servo, S., Monaco, F., and Robertson, M. M. (2009). The behavioral spectrum of Gilles de La Tourette syndrome. *J. Neuropsychiatry Clin. Neurosci.* 21, 13–23. doi: 10.1176/jnp.2009.21.1.13

Ceci, C., Proietti Onori, M., Macrì, S., and Laviola, G. (2015). Interaction between the endocannabinoid and serotonergic system in the exhibition of head twitch response in four mouse strains. *Neurotox. Res.* 27, 275–283. doi: 10.1007/s12640-014-9510-z

Chao, T. K., Hu, J., and Pringsheim, T. (2014). Prenatal risk factors for Tourette syndrome: a systematic review. *BMC Pregnancy Childbirth* 14:53. doi: 10.1186/1471-2393-14-53

Chen, H.-L., Lee, H.-J., Huang, W.-J., Chou, J.-F., Fan, P.-C., Du, J.-C., et al. (2012). Clerodendrum inerme leaf extract alleviates animal behaviors, hyperlocomotion, and prepulse inhibition disruptions, mimicking Tourette syndrome and Schizophrenia. *Evid. Based Complement. Alternat. Med.* 2012:284301. doi: 10.1155/2012/284301

Chohan, T. W., Boucher, A. A., Spencer, J. R., Kassem, M. S., Hamdi, A. A., Karl, T., et al. (2014). Partial genetic deletion of neuregulin 1 modulates the effects of stress on sensorimotor gating, dendritic morphology, and HPA axis activity in adolescent mice. *Schizophr. Bull.* 40, 1272–1284. doi: 10.1093/schbul/sbt193

Cohen, A. J., and Leckman, J. F. (1992). Sensory phenomena associated with Gilles de La Tourette's syndrome. *J. Clin. Psychiatry* 53, 319–23.

Conelea, C. A., and Woods, D. W. (2008). Examining the impact of distraction on tic suppression in children and adolescents with Tourette syndrome. *Behav. Res. Ther.* 46, 1193–1200. doi: 10.1016/j.brat.2008.07.005

Cook, E. H., Stein, M. A., Krasowski, M. D., Cox, N. J., Olkon, D. M., Kieffer, J. E., et al. (1995). Association of attention-deficit disorder and the dopamine transporter gene. *Am. J. Hum. Genet.* 56, 993–998.

Corbett, B. A., Mendoza, S. P., Baym, C. L., Bunge, S. A., and Levine, S. (2008). Examining cortisol rhythmicity and responsivity to stress in children with Tourette syndrome. *Psychoneuroendocrinology* 33, 810–820. doi: 10.1016/j.psyneuen.2008.03.014

Coric, V., Taskiran, S., Pittenger, C., Wasylink, S., Mathalon, D. H., Valentine, G., et al. (2005). Riluzole augmentation in treatment-resistant obsessive-compulsive disorder: an open-label trial. *Biol. Psychiatry* 58, 424–428. doi: 10.1016/j.biopsych.2005.04.043

Crane, J., Fagerness, J., Osiecki, L., Gunnell, B., Stewart, S. E., Pauls, D. L., et al. (2011). Family-based genetic association study of DLGAP3 in Tourette Syndrome. *Am. J. Med. Genet. B Neuropsychiatr. Genet.* 156B, 108–114. doi: 10.1002/ajmg.b.31134

De Haas, R., Seddik, A., Oppelaar, H., Westenberg, H. G. M., and Kas, M. J. H. (2012). Marked inbred mouse strain difference in the expression of quinpirole induced compulsive like behavior based on behavioral pattern analysis. *Eur. Neuropsychopharmacol.* 22, 657–663. doi: 10.1016/j.euroneuro.2012.01.003

De Miranda, J., Yaddanapudi, K., Hornig, M., Villar, G., Serge, R., and Lipkin, W. I. (2010). Induction of toll-like receptor 3-mediated immunity during gestation inhibits cortical neurogenesis and causes behavioral disturbances. *MBio* 1:e00176-10. doi: 10.1128/mbio.00176-10

Depino, A. M., Lucchina, L., and Pitossi, F. (2011). Early and adult hippocampal TGF-β1 overexpression have opposite effects on behavior. *Brain Behav. Immun.* 25, 1582–1591. doi: 10.1016/j.bbi.2011.05.007

Devoto, P., Frau, R., Bini, V., Pillolla, G., Saba, P., Flore, G., et al. (2012). Inhibition of 5α-reductase in the nucleus accumbens counters sensorimotor gating deficits induced by dopaminergic activation. *Psychoneuroendocrinology* 37, 1630–1645. doi: 10.1016/j.psyneuen.2011.09.018

Fantegrossi, W. E., Harrington, A. W., Eckler, J. R., Arshad, S., Rabin, R. A., Winter, J. C., et al. (2005). Hallucinogen-like Actions of 2,5-Dimethoxy-4-(n)-Propylthiophenethylamine (2C-T-7) in mice and rats. *Psychopharmacology* 181, 496–503. doi: 10.1007/s00213-005-0009-4

Fantegrossi, W. E., Harrington, A. W., Kiessel, C. L., Eckler, J. R., Rabin, R. A., Winter, J. C, et al. (2006). Hallucinogen-like Actions of 5-Methoxy-N,N-Diisopropyltryptamine in mice and rats. *Pharmacol. Biochem. Behav.* 83, 122–129. doi: 10.1016/j.pbb.2005.12.015

Frank, M., and Cavanna, A. E. (2013). Behavioural treatments for tourette syndrome: an evidence-based review. *Behav. Neurol.* 27, 105–117. doi: 10.1155/2013/134863

Freund, N., MacGillivilray, H. T., Thompson, B. S., Lukkes, J. L., Stanis, J. J., Brenhouse, H. C., et al. (2014). Sex-dependent changes in ADHD-like behaviors in juvenile rats following cortical dopamine depletion. *Behav. Brain Res.* 270, 357–363. doi: 10.1016/j.bbr.2014.05.024

Gainetdinov, R. R., and Caron, M. G. (2000). An animal model of attention deficit hyperactivity disorder. *Mol. Med. Today* 6, 43–44. doi: 10.1016/S1357-4310(99)01616-0

Ganos, C., Kahl, U., Schunke, O., Kühn, S., Haggard, P., Gerloff, C., et al. (2012). Are premonitory urges a prerequisite of tic inhibition in Gilles de La Tourette syndrome? *J. Neurol. Neurosurg. Psychiatr.* 83, 975–978. doi: 10.1136/jnnp-2012-303033

Garner, B., Wood, S. J., Pantelis, C., and van den Buuse, M. (2007). Early maternal deprivation reduces prepulse inhibition and impairs spatial learning ability in adulthood: no further effect of post-pubertal chronic corticosterone treatment. *Behav. Brain Res.* 176, 323–332. doi: 10.1016/j.bbr.2006.10.020

Garner, J. P., and Mason, G. J. (2002). Evidence for a relationship between cage stereotypies and behavioural disinhibition in laboratory rodents. *Behav. Brain Res.* 136, 83–92. doi: 10.1016/S0166-4328(02)00111-0

Godar, S. C., Mosher, L. J., Strathman, H. J., Gochi, A. M., Jones, C. M., Fowler, S. C., et al. (2015). The D1CT-7 mouse model of Tourette syndrome displays sensorimotor gating deficits in response to spatial confinement. *Br. J. Pharmacol.* doi: 10.1111/bph.13243. [Epub ahead of print].

Grabli, D., McCairn, K., Hirsch, E. C., Agid, Y., Féger, J., François, C., et al. (2004). Behavioural disorders induced by external globus pallidus dysfunction in primates: I. Behavioural study. *Brain* 127(Pt 9), 2039–2054. doi: 10.1093/brain/awh220

Granon, S., and Changeux, J.-P. (2006). Attention-deficit/hyperactivity disorder: a plausible mouse model? *Acta Paediatr.* 95, 645–649. doi: 10.1080/08035250600719747

Grant, P., Lougee, L., Hirschtritt, M., and Swedo, S. E. (2007). An open-label trial of riluzole, a glutamate antagonist, in children with treatment-resistant obsessive-compulsive disorder. *J. Child Adolesc. Psychopharmacol.* 17, 761–67. doi: 10.1089/cap.2007.0021

Graybiel, A. M., and Rauch, S. L. (2000). Toward a neurobiology of obsessive-compulsive disorder. *Neuron* 28, 343–347. doi: 10.1016/S0896-6273(00)00113-6

Greimel, E., Schulte-Rüther, M., Kamp-Becker, I., Remschmidt, H., Herpertz-Dahlmann, B., and Konrad, K. (2011). Self-report and parental report of empathy in adolescents with autism. *Z. Kinder Jugendpsychiatr. Psychother.* 39, 113–121. doi: 10.1024/1422-4917/a000097

Halberstadt, A. L., and Geyer, M. A. (2014). Effects of the Hallucinogen 2,5-Dimethoxy-4-Iodophenethylamine (2C-I) and Superpotent N-Benzyl derivatives on the head twitch response. *Neuropharmacology* 77, 200–207. doi: 10.1016/j.neuropharm.2013.08.025

Hall, F. S. (1998). Social deprivation of neonatal, adolescent, and adult rats has distinct neurochemical and behavioral consequences. *Critic. Rev. Neurobiol.* 12, 129–162. doi: 10.1615/CritRevNeurobiol.v12.i1-2.50

Hallett, J. J., Harling-Berg, C. J., Knopf, P. M., Stopa, E. G., and Kiessling, L. S. (2000). Anti-striatal antibodies in Tourette syndrome cause neuronal dysfunction. *J. Neuroimmunol.* 111, 195–202. doi: 10.1016/S0165-5728(00)00320-9

Hayslett, R. L., and Tizabi, Y. (2003). Effects of Donepezil on DOI-induced head twitch response in mice: implications for Tourette syndrome. *Pharmacol. Biochem. Behav.* 76, 409–415. doi: 10.1016/j.pbb.2003.08.015

Hoekstra, P. J., and Minderaa, R. B. (2005). Tic disorders and obsessive-compulsive disorder: is autoimmunity involved? *Int. Rev. Psychiatry* 17, 497–502. doi: 10.1080/02646830500382003

Hoffman, K. L., Hornig, M., Yaddanapudi, K., Jabado, O., and Lipkin, W. I. (2004). A murine model for neuropsychiatric disorders associated with group A beta-hemolytic streptococcal infection. *J. Neurosci.* 24, 1780–1791. doi: 10.1523/JNEUROSCI.0887-03.2004

Hoffman, K. L., and Rueda Morales, R. I. (2012). D1 and D2 dopamine receptor antagonists decrease behavioral Bout duration, without altering the Bout's repeated behavioral components, in a naturalistic model of repetitive and compulsive behavior. *Behav. Brain Res.* 230, 1–10. doi: 10.1016/j.bbr.2012.01.041

Huang, W. J., Lee, H. J., Chen, H. L., Fan, P. C., Ku, Y. L., and Chiou, L. C. (2015). Hispidulin, a constituent of clerodendrum inerme that remitted motor tics, alleviated methamphetamine-induced hyperlocomotion without motor impairment in mice. *J. Ethnopharmacol.* 166, 18–22. doi: 10.1016/j.jep.2015.03.001

Hyde, T. M., Aaronson, B. A., Randolph, C., Rickler, K. C., and Weinberger, D. R. (1992). Relationship of birth weight to the phenotypic expression of Gilles de La Tourette's syndrome in monozygotic twins. *Neurology* 42, 652–658. doi: 10.1212/WNL.42.3.652

Ichimaru, Y., Egawa, T., and Sawa, A. (1995). 5-HT1A-receptor subtype mediates the effect of fluvoxamine, a selective serotonin reuptake inhibitor, on marble-burying behavior in mice. *Jpn. J. Pharmacol.* 68, 65–70. doi: 10.1254/jjp.68.65

Insel, T. R., and Winslow, J. T. (1992). Neurobiology of obsessive compulsive disorder. *Psychiatr. Clin. North Am.* 15, 813–824. doi: 10.1097/00004850-199206001-00008

Joel, D., Doljansky, J., and Schiller, D. (2005). 'Compulsive' lever pressing in rats is enhanced following lesions to the orbital cortex, but not to the basolateral nucleus of the amygdala or to the dorsal medial prefrontal cortex. *Eur. J. Neurosci.* 21, 2252–2262. doi: 10.1111/j.1460-9568.2005.04042.x

Kane, M. J., Angoa-Peréz, M., Briggs, D. I., Sykes, C. E., Francescutti, D. M., Rosenberg, D. R., et al. (2012). Mice genetically depleted of brain serotonin display social impairments, communication deficits and repetitive behaviors: possible relevance to autism. *PLoS ONE* 7:e48975. doi: 10.1371/journal.pone.0048975

Kataoka, Y., Kalanithi, P. S., Grantz, H., Schwartz, M. L., Saper, C., Leckman, J. F., et al. (2010). Decreased number of parvalbumin and cholinergic interneurons in the striatum of individuals with Tourette syndrome. *J. Comp. Neurol.* 518, 277–291. doi: 10.1002/cne.22206

Katayama, K., Yamada, K., Ornthanalai, V. G., Inoue, T., Ota, M., Murphy, N. P., et al. (2010). Slitrk1-deficient mice display elevated anxiety-like behavior and noradrenergic abnormalities. *Mol. Psychiatry* 15, 177–184. doi: 10.1038/mp.2008.97

Kent, L., Doerry, U., Hardy, E., Parmar, R., Gingell, K., Hawi, Z., et al. (2002). Evidence that variation at the serotonin transporter gene influences susceptibility to Attention Deficit Hyperactivity Disorder (ADHD): analysis and pooled analysis. *Mol. Psychiatry* 7, 908–912. doi: 10.1038/sj.mp.4001100

Khalifa, N., and Knorring, A.-L. (2007). Tourette syndrome and other tic disorders in a total population of children: clinical assessment and background. *Acta Paediatr.* 94, 1608–1614. doi: 10.1111/j.1651-2227.2005.tb01837.x

Kickler, N., Lacombe, E., Chassain, C., Durif, F., Krainik, A., Farion, R., et al. (2009). Assessment of metabolic changes in the striatum of a rat model of parkinsonism: an *in vivo* 1 H MRS study. *NMR Biomed.* 22, 207–212. doi: 10.1002/nbm.1305

Kirkman, N. J., Libbey, J. E., Sweeten, T. L., Coon, H. H., Miller, J. N., Stevenson, E. K., et al. (2008). How relevant are GFAP autoantibodies in autism and Tourette syndrome? *J. Autism Dev. Disorders* 38, 333–341. doi: 10.1007/s10803-007-0398-9

Kirsten, T. B., Chaves-Kirsten, G. P., Chaible, L. M., Silva, A. C., Martins, D. O., Britto, L. R., et al. (2012). Hypoactivity of the central dopaminergic system and autistic-like behavior induced by a single early prenatal exposure to lipopolysaccharide. *J. Neurosci. Res.* 90, 1903–1912. doi: 10.1002/jnr.23089

Kompoliti, K., and Goetz, C. G. (1998). Hyperkinetic movement disorders misdiagnosed as tics in Gilles de la Tourette syndrome. *Mov. Disord.* 13, 477–480. doi: 10.1002/mds.870130317

Koran, L. M., Thienemann, M. L., and Davenport, R. (1996). Quality of life for patients with obsessive-compulsive disorder. *Am. J. Psychiatry* 153, 783–788. doi: 10.1176/ajp.153.6.783

Krause, D., Matz, J., Weidinger, E., Wagner, J., Wildenauer, A., Obermeier, M., et al. (2010). Association between intracellular infectious agents and Tourette's syndrome. *Eur. Archiv. Psychiatry Clin. Neurosci.* 260, 359–363. doi: 10.1007/s00406-009-0084-3

Kreiss, D. S., Coffman, C. F., Fiacco, N. R., Granger, J. C., Helton, B. M., Jackson, J. C., et al. (2013). Ritualistic chewing behavior induced by mCPP in the rat is an animal model of obsessive compulsive disorder. *Pharmacol. Biochem. Behav.* 104, 119–124. doi: 10.1016/j.pbb.2013.01.006

Kurlan, R. (2004). The PANDAS hypothesis: losing its bite? *Mov. Disord.* 19, 371–374. doi: 10.1002/mds.20107

Lebowitz, E. R., Motlagh, M. G., Katsovich, L., King, R. A., Lombroso, P. J., Grantz, H., et al. (2012). Tourette syndrome in youth with and without obsessive compulsive disorder and attention deficit hyperactivity disorder. *Eur. Child Adolesc. Psychiatry* 21, 451–57. doi: 10.1007/s00787-012-0278-5

Leckman, J. F., Walker, D. E., and Cohen, D. J. (1993). Premonitory urges in Tourette's syndrome. *Am. J. Psychiatry* 150, 98–102. doi: 10.1176/ajp.150.1.98

Lennington, J. B., Coppola, G., Kataoka-Sasaki, Y., Fernandez, T. V., Palejev, D., Li, Y., et al. (2014). Transcriptome analysis of the human striatum in Tourette syndrome. Biol. *Psychiatry* 79, 372–382. doi: 10.1016/j.biopsych.2014.07.018

Levin, R., Peres, F. F., Almeida, V., Calzavara, M. B., Zuardi, A. W., Hallak, J. E. C., et al. (2014). Effects of cannabinoid drugs on the deficit of prepulse inhibition of startle in an animal model of Schizophrenia: the SHR strain. *Front. Pharmacol.* 5:10. doi: 10.3389/fphar.2014.00010

Lin, H., Katsovich, L., Ghebremichael, M., Findley, D. B., Grantz, H., Lombroso, P. J., et al. (2007). Psychosocial stress predicts future symptom severities in children and adolescents with Tourette syndrome and/or obsessive-compulsive disorder. *J. Child Psychol. Psychiatry* 48, 157–166. doi: 10.1111/j.1469-7610.2006.01687.x

Lombroso, P. J., Mack, G., Scahill, L., King, R. A., and Leckman, J. F. (1991). Exacerbation of Gilles de La Tourette's syndrome associated with thermal stress: a family study. *Neurology* 41, 1984–1987. doi: 10.1212/wnl.41.12.1984

Lombroso, P. J., and Scahill, L. (2008). Tourette syndrome and obsessive-compulsive disorder. *Brain Dev.* 30, 231–237. doi: 10.1016/j.braindev.2007.09.001

Lv, H., Li, A., Ma, H., Liu, F., and Xu, H. (2009). Effects of Ningdong Granule on the dopamine system of Tourette's syndrome rat models. *J. Ethnopharmacol.* 124, 488–492. doi: 10.1016/j.jep.2009.05.015

Malkova, N. V., Yu, C. Z., Hsiao, E. Y., Moore, M. J., and Patterson, P. H. (2012). Maternal immune activation yields offspring displaying mouse versions of the three core symptoms of autism. *Brain Behav. Immun.* 26, 607–616. doi: 10.1016/j.bbi.2012.01.011

Manor, I., Corbex, M., Eisenberg, J., Gritsenkso, I., Bachner-Melman, R., Tyano, S., et al. (2004). Association of the dopamine D5 receptor with Attention Deficit Hyperactivity Disorder (ADHD) and scores on a continuous performance test (TOVA). *Am. J. Med. Genet.* 127B, 73–77. doi: 10.1002/ajmg.b.30020

Márquez-Arias, A., Santillán-Doherty, A. M., Arenas-Rosas, R. V., Gasca-Matías, M. P., and Muñoz-Delgado, J. (2010). Environmental enrichment for captive stumptail Macaques (*Macaca Arctoides*). *J. Med. Primatol.* 39, 32–40. doi: 10.1111/j.1600-0684.2009.00392.x

Martin, L. A., Ashwood, P., Braunschweig, D., Cabanlit, M., Van de Water, J., and Amaral, D. G. (2008). Stereotypies and hyperactivity in Rhesus monkeys exposed to IgG from mothers of children with autism. *Brain Behav. Immun.* 22, 806–816. doi: 10.1016/j.bbi.2007.12.007

Martino, D., Macerollo, A., and Leckman, J. F. (2013). Neuroendocrine aspects of Tourette syndrome. *Int. Rev. Neurobiol.* 112, 239–279. doi: 10.1093/med/9780199796267.001.0001

Mathews, C. A., Bimson, B., Lowe, T. L., Herrera, L. D., Budman, C. L., Erenberg, G., et al. (2006). Association between maternal smoking and increased symptom severity in Tourette's syndrome. *Am. J. Psychiatry* 163, 1066–1073. doi: 10.1176/ajp.2006.163.6.1066

McCairn, K. W., Iriki, A., and Isoda, M. (2013). Global dysrhythmia of cerebro-basal ganglia-cerebellar networks underlies motor tics following striatal disinhibition. *J. Neurosci.* 33, 697–708. doi: 10.1523/jneurosci.4018-12.2013

McCairn, K. W., Bronfeld, M., Belelovsky, K., and, Bar-Gad, I. (2009). The neurophysiological correlates of motor tics following focal striatal disinhibition. Brain 132(Pt 8), 2125–2138. doi: 10.1093/brain/awp142

McGrath, M. J., Campbell, K. M., Parks, C. R., and Burton, F. H. (2000). Glutamatergic drugs exacerbate symptomatic behavior in a transgenic model of comorbid Tourette's syndrome and obsessive-compulsive disorder. *Brain Res.* 877, 23–30. doi: 10.1016/S0006-8993(00)02646-9

McNamara, R. K., Logue, A., Stanford, K., Xu, M., Zhang, J., and Richtand, N. M. (2006). Dose-response analysis of locomotor activity and stereotypy in dopamine D3 receptor mutant mice following acute amphetamine. *Synapse* 60, 399–405. doi: 10.1002/syn.20315

Mosher, L. J., Frau, R., Pardu, A., Pes, R., Devoto, P., and Bortolato, M. (2015). Selective activation of D1 dopamine receptors impairs sensorimotor gating in long-evans rats. *Br. J. Pharmacol.* doi: 10.1111/bph.13232. [Epub ahead of print].

Motlagh, M. G., Katsovich, L., Thompson, N., Lin, H., Kim, Y. S., Scahill, L., et al. (2010). Severe psychosocial stress and heavy cigarette smoking during pregnancy: an examination of the pre- and perinatal risk factors associated with ADHD and Tourette syndrome. *Eur. Child Adolesc. Psychiatry* 19, 755–764. doi: 10.1007/s00787-010-0115-7

Nelson, D. A. (1993). Tourette's and stress. *Neurology* 43, 237–239. doi: 10.1212/WNL.43.1_Part_1.237-b

Nordstrom, E. J., Bittner, K. C., McGrath, M. J., Parks, C. R. III, and Burton, F. H. (2015). 'Hyperglutamatergic Cortico-Striato-Thalamo-Cortical Circuit' breaker drugs alleviate tics in a transgenic circuit model of Tourette's syndrome. *Brain Res.* 1629, 38–53. doi: 10.1016/j.brainres.2015.09.032

Nordstrom, E. J., and Burton, F. H. (2002). A transgenic model of comorbid Tourette's syndrome and obsessive-compulsive disorder circuitry. *Mol. Psychiatry* 7, 617–625. doi: 10.1038/sj.mp.4001144

Obeso, J. A., and Lanciego, J. L. (2011). Past, present, and future of the pathophysiological model of the Basal Ganglia. *Front. Neuroanat.* 5:39. doi: 10.3389/fnana.2011.00039

Ogata, N., Gillis, T. E., Liu, X., Cunningham, S. M., Lowen, S. B., Adams, B. L., et al. (2013). Brain structural abnormalities in doberman pinschers with canine compulsive disorder. *Prog. Neuro Psychopharmacol. Biol. Psychiatry* 45, 1–6. doi: 10.1016/j.pnpbp.2013.04.002

Okasha, A., Lotaief, F., Ashour, A. M., el Mahalawy, N., Seif el Dawla, A., and el-Kholy, G. (2000). The prevalence of obsessive compulsive symptoms in a sample of Egyptian psychiatric patients. *L'Encéphale* 26, 1–10.

Onogi, H., Nakagawasai, O., Sato, A., Mitazaki, S., Nakaya, K., Watanabe, K., et al. (2011). P-Hydroxyamphetamine causes prepulse inhibition disruption in mice: contribution of serotonin neurotransmission. *Behav. Brain Res.* 224, 159–165. doi: 10.1016/j.bbr.2011.06.002

Ouchi, H., Ono, K., Murakami, Y., and Matsumoto, K. (2013). Social isolation induces deficit of latent learning performance in mice: a putative animal model of attention deficit/hyperactivity disorder. *Behav. Brain Res.* 238, 146–153. doi: 10.1016/j.bbr.2012.10.029

Oyungu, E., Kioy, P. G., and Patel, N. B. (2007). Effect of Catha Edulis (khat) on behaviour and its potential to induce seizures in Sprague Dawley rats. *East Afr. Med. J.* 84, 219–225.

Pallanti, S., Grassi, G., Sarrecchia, E. D., Cantisani, A., and Pellegrini, M. (2011). Obsessive–compulsive disorder comorbidity: clinical assessment and therapeutic implications. *Front. Psychiatry* 2:70. doi: 10.3389/fpsyt.2011.00070

Park, L., Nigg, J. T., Waldman, I. D., Nummy, K. A., Huang-Pollock, C., Rappley, M., et al. (2005). Association and linkage of alpha-2A adrenergic receptor gene polymorphisms with childhood ADHD. *Mol. Psychiatry* 10, 572–580. doi: 10.1038/sj.mp.4001605

Patel, A., Zhu, Y., Kuzhikandathil, E. V., Banks, W. A., Siegel, A., and Zalcman, S. S. (2012). Soluble Interleukin-6 receptor induces motor stereotypies and co-localizes with gp130 in regions linked to cortico-striato-thalamo-cortical circuits. *PLoS ONE* 7:e41623. doi: 10.1371/journal.pone.0041623

Pauls, D. L. (2003). An update on the genetics of Gilles de La Tourette syndrome. *J. Psychosomat. Res.* 55, 7–12. doi: 10.1016/S0022-3999(02)00586-X

Pauls, D. L., Raymond, C. L., Stevenson, J. M., and Leckman, J. F. (1991). A family study of Gilles de La Tourette syndrome. *Am. J. Hum.* Genet. 48, 154–163.

Pearson, B. L., Pobbe, R. L., Defensor, E. B., Oasay, L., Bolivar, V. J., Blanchard, D. C., et al. (2011). Motor and cognitive stereotypies in the BTBR T+tf/J mouse model of autism. *Genes Brain Behav.* 10, 228–235. doi: 10.1111/j.1601-183X.2010.00659.x

Peterson, B. S., Skudlarski, P., Anderson, A. W., Zhang, H., Gatenby, J. C., Lacadie, C. M., et al. (1998). A functional magnetic resonance imaging study of tic suppression in Tourette syndrome. *Archiv. Gen. Psychiatry* 55, 326–333. doi: 10.1001/archpsyc.55.4.326

Peterson, B. S., Thomas, P., Kane, M. J., Scahill, L., Zhang, H., Bronen, R., et al. (2003). Basal Ganglia volumes in patients with Gilles de La Tourette syndrome. *Archiv. Gen. Psychiatry* 60, 415–424. doi: 10.1001/archpsyc.60.4.415

Pietraszek, M., Michaluk, J., Romańska, I., Wasik, A., Gołembiowska, K., and Antkiewicz-Michaluk, L. (2009). 1-Methyl-1,2,3,4-tetrahydroisoquinoline antagonizes a rise in brain dopamine metabolism, glutamate release in frontal cortex and locomotor hyperactivity produced by MK-801 but not the disruptions of prepulse inhibition, and impairment of working memory in rat. *Neurotoxic. Res.* 16, 390–407. doi: 10.1007/s12640-009-9097-y

Pogorelov, V., Xu, M., Smith, H. R., Buchanan, G. F., and Pittenger, C. (2015). Corticostriatal interactions in the generation of tic-like behaviors after local striatal disinhibition. *Exp. Neurol.* 265, 122–128. doi: 10.1016/j.expneurol.2015.01.001

Pogorelov, V. M., Rodriguiz, R. M., Insco, M. L., Caron, M. G., and Wetsel, W. C. (2005). Novelty seeking and stereotypic activation of behavior in mice with disruption of the Dat1 gene. *Neuropsychopharmacology* 30, 1818–1831. doi: 10.1038/sj.npp.1300724

Polanczyk, G., and Rohde, L. A. (2007). Epidemiology of attention-deficit/hyperactivity disorder across the lifespan. *Curr. Opin. Psychiatry* 20, 386–392. doi: 10.1097/YCO.0b013e3281568d7a

Ponzio, N. M., Servatius, R., Beck, K., Marzouk, A., and Kreider, T. (2007). Cytokine levels during pregnancy influence immunological profiles and neurobehavioral patterns of the offspring. *Ann. N.Y. Acad. Sci.* 1107, 118–128. doi: 10.1196/annals.1381.013

Porton, B., Greenberg, B. D., Askland, K., Serra, L. M., Gesmonde, J., Rudnick, G., et al. (2013). Isoforms of the Neuronal Glutamate Transporter Gene, SLC1A1/EAAC1, Negatively Modulate Glutamate Uptake: Relevance to Obsessive-Compulsive Disorder. *Transl. Psychiatry* 3:e259. doi: 10.1038/tp.2013.35

Price, R. A., Kidd, K. K., Cohen, D. J., Pauls, D. L., and Leckman, J. F. (1985). A twin study of Tourette syndrome. *Arch. Gen. Psychiatry* 42, 815–820. doi: 10.1001/archpsyc.1985.01790310077011

Pryce, C. R., and Feldon, J. (2003). Long-term neurobehavioural impact of the postnatal environment in rats: manipulations, effects and mediating mechanisms. *Neurosci. Biobehav. Rev.* 27, 57–71. doi: 10.1016/S0149-7634(03)00009-5

Ralph, R. J., Paulus, M. P., Fumagalli, F., Caron, M. G., and Geyer, M. A. (2001). Prepulse inhibition deficits and perseverative motor patterns in dopamine transporter knock-out mice: differential effects of D1 and D2 receptor antagonists. *J. Neurosci.* 21, 305–313.

Rapanelli, M., Frick, L. R., Pogorelov, V., Ota, K. T., Abbasi, E., Ohtsu, H., et al. (2014). Dysregulated intracellular signaling in the striatum in a pathophysiologically grounded model of Tourette syndrome. *Eur. Neuropsychopharmacol.* 24, 1896–1906. doi: 10.1016/j.euroneuro.2014.10.007

Reese, H. E., Scahill, L., Peterson, A. L., Crowe, K., Woods, D. W., Piacentini, J., et al. (2014). The premonitory urge to tic: measurement, characteristics, and correlates in older adolescents and adults. *Behav. Ther.* 45, 177–186. doi: 10.1016/j.beth.2013.09.002

Robertson, M. M., Eapen, V., and Cavanna, A. E. (2009). The international prevalence, epidemiology, and clinical phenomenology of Tourette syndrome: a cross-cultural perspective. *J. Psychosomat. Res.* 67, 475–483. doi: 10.1016/j.jpsychores.2009.07.010

Roessner, V., Becker, A., Banaschewski, T., and Rothenberger, A. (2007). Psychopathological profile in children with chronic tic disorder and co-existing ADHD: additive effects. *J. Abnorm. Child Psychol.* 35, 79–85. doi: 10.1007/s10802-006-9086-z

Rommeck, I., Capitanio, J. P., Strand, S. C., and McCowan, B. (2011). Early social experience affects behavioral and physiological responsiveness to stressful conditions in infant Rhesus Macaques (*Macaca Mulatta*). *Am. J. Primatol.* 73, 692–701. doi: 10.1002/ajp.20953

Russo, A. J., and Pietsch, S. C. (2013). Decreased Hepatocyte Growth Factor (HGF) and Gamma Aminobutyric Acid (GABA) in individuals with Obsessive-Compulsive Disorder (OCD). *Biomarker Insights* 8, 107–114. doi: 10.4137/BMI.S11931

Russo, M., Naro, A., Mastroeni, C., Morgante, F., Terranova, C., Muscatello, M. R., et al. (2014). Obsessive-compulsive disorder: a 'Sensory-Motor' problem? *Int. J. Psychophysiol.* 92, 74–78. doi: 10.1016/j.ijpsycho.2014.02.007

Sadile, A. G., Lamberti, C., Siegfried, B., and Welzl, H. (1993). Circadian activity, nociceptive thresholds, nigrostriatal and mesolimbic dopaminergic activity in the Naples High- and Low-Excitability rat lines. *Behav. Brain Res.* 55, 17–27. doi: 10.1016/0166-4328(93)90003-9

Sagvolden, T. (2000). Behavioral validation of the spontaneously hypertensive rat (SHR) as an animal model of attention-deficit/hyperactivity disorder (AD/HD). *Neurosci. Biobehav. Rev.* 24, 31–39. doi: 10.1016/S0149-7634(99)00058-5

Sagvolden, T., Russell, V. A., Aase, H., Johansen, E. B., and Farshbaf, M. (2005). Rodent models of attention-deficit/hyperactivity disorder. *Biol. Psychiatry* 57, 1239–1247. doi: 10.1016/j.biopsych.2005.02.002

Scharf, J. M., Yu, D., Mathews, C. A., Neale, B. M., Stewart, S. E., Fagerness, J. A., et al. (2013). Genome-wide association study of Tourette's syndrome. *Mol. Psychiatry* 18, 721–728. doi: 10.1038/mp.2012.69

Schlander, M., Schwarz, O., Rothenberger, A., and Roessner, V. (2011). Tic disorders: administrative prevalence and co-occurrence with attention-deficit/hyperactivity disorder in a German community sample. *Eur. Psychiatry* 26, 370–374. doi: 10.1016/j.eurpsy.2009.10.003

Schmid, C. L., and Bohn, L. M. (2010). Serotonin, but Not N-Methyltryptamines, Activates the Serotonin 2A Receptor via a ß-arrestin2/Src/Akt signaling complex *in vivo*. *J. Neurosci.* 30, 13513–13524. doi: 10.1523/JNEUROSCI.1665-10.2010

Schneider, T., Ilott, N., Brolese, G., Bizarro, L., Asherson, P. J., and Stolerman, I. P. (2011). Prenatal exposure to nicotine impairs performance of the 5-choice serial reaction time task in adult rats. *Neuropsychopharmacology* 36, 1114–1125. doi: 10.1038/npp.2010.249

Shmelkov, S. V., Hormigo, A., Jing, D., Proenca, C. C., Bath, K. G., Milde, T., et al. (2010). Slitrk5 deficiency impairs corticostriatal circuitry and leads to obsessive-compulsive-like behaviors in mice. *Nat. Med.* 16, 598–602. doi: 10.1038/nm.2125

Siesser, W. B., Zhao, J., Miller, L. R., Cheng, S. Y., and McDonald, M. P. (2006). Transgenic mice expressing a human mutant beta1 thyroid receptor are hyperactive, impulsive, and inattentive. *Genes Brain Behav.* 5, 282–297. doi: 10.1111/j.1601-183X.2005.00161.x

Silva, R. R., Munoz, D. M., Barickman, J., and Friedhoff, A. J. (1995). Environmental factors and related fluctuation of symptoms in children and adolescents with Tourette's disorder. *J. Child Psychol. Psychiatry* 36, 305–312. doi: 10.1111/j.1469-7610.1995.tb01826.x

Simpson, H. B., Shungu, D. C., Bender, J. Jr., Mao, X., Xu, X., Slifstein, M., et al. (2012). Investigation of cortical glutamate-glutamine and γ-aminobutyric acid in obsessive-compulsive disorder by proton magnetic resonance spectroscopy. *Neuropsychopharmacology* 37, 2684–2692. doi: 10.1038/npp.2012.132

Singer, H. S., Gilbert, D. L., Wolf, D. S., Mink, J. W., and Kurlan, R. (2012). Moving from PANDAS to CANS. *J. Pediatrics* 160, 725–731. doi: 10.1016/j.jpeds.2011.11.040

Singer, H. S., Mink, J. W., Loiselle, C. R., Burke, K. A., Ruchkina, I., Morshed, S., et al. (2005). Microinfusion of antineuronal antibodies into rodent striatum: failure to differentiate between elevated and low titers. *J. Neuroimmunol.* 163, 8–14. doi: 10.1016/j.jneuroim.2005.02.018

Singer, H. S., Reiss, A. L., Brown, J. E., Aylward, E. H., Shih, B., Chee, E., et al. (1993). Volumetric MRI changes in Basal Ganglia of children with Tourette's syndrome. *Neurology* 43, 950–956. doi: 10.1212/WNL.43.5.950

Smicun, Y., Campbell, S. D., Chen, M. A., Gu, H., and Rudnick, G. (1999). The role of external loop regions in serotonin transport. Loop scanning mutagenesis of the serotonin transporter external domain. *J. Biol. Chem.* 274, 36058–36064. doi: 10.1074/jbc.274.51.36058

Smith, S. E., Li, J., Garbett, K., Mirnics, K., and Patterson, P. H. (2007). Maternal immune activation alters fetal brain development through interleukin-6. *J. Neurosci.* 27, 10695–10702. doi: 10.1523/jneurosci.2178-07.2007

Sowell, E. R., Kan, E., Yoshii, J., Thompson, P. M., Bansal, R., Xu, D., et al. (2008). Thinning of sensorimotor cortices in children with Tourette syndrome. *Nat. Neurosci.* 11, 637–639. doi: 10.1038/nn.2121

Spessot, A. L., Plessen, K. J., and Peterson, B. S. (2004). Neuroimaging of developmental psychopathologies: the importance of self-regulatory and neuroplastic processes in adolescence. *Ann. N.Y. Acad. Sci.* 1021, 86–104. doi: 10.1196/annals.1308.010

Stahl, S. M. (1988). Basal Ganglia neuropharmacology and obsessive-compulsive disorder: the obsessive-compulsive disorder hypothesis of Basal Ganglia dysfunction. *Psychopharmacol. Bull.* 24, 370–374.

Stead, J. D., Clinton, S., Neal, C., Schneider, J., Jama, A., Miller, S., et al. (2006). Selective breeding for divergence in novelty-seeking traits: heritability and enrichment in spontaneous anxiety-related behaviors. Behav. Genet. 36, 697–712. doi: 10.1007/s10519-006-9058-7

Strauss, L., Brink, C. B., Möller, M., Stein, D. J., and Harvey, B. H. (2014). Late-life effects of chronic methamphetamine exposure during puberty on behaviour and corticostriatal mono-amines in social isolation-reared rats. *Dev. Neurosci.* 36, 18–28. doi: 10.1159/000357495

Sundaram, S. K., Huq, A. M., Wilson, B. J., and Chugani, H. T. (2010). Tourette syndrome is associated with recurrent exonic copy number variants. *Neurology* 74, 1583–1590. doi: 10.1212/WNL.0b013e3181e0f147

Swedo, S. E., Baird, G., Cook, E. H. Jr., Happé, F. G., Harris, J. C., Kaufmann, W. E., et al. (2012). Commentary from the DSM-5 workgroup on neurodevelopmental disorders. *J. Am. Acad. Child Adolesc. Psychiatry* 51, 347–349. doi: 10.1016/j.jaac.2012.02.013

Swerdlow, N. R., Shoemaker, J. M., Bongiovanni, M. J., Neary, A. C., Tochen, L. S., and Saint Marie, R. L. (2007). Strain differences in the disruption of prepulse inhibition of startle after systemic and intra-accumbens amphetamine administration. *Pharmacol. Biochem. Behav.* 87, 1–10. doi: 10.1016/j.pbb.2007.03.014

Swerdlow, N. R., Shoemaker, J. M., Platten, A., Pitcher, L., Goins, J., and Crain, S. (2003). Heritable differences in the effects of amphetamine but not DOI on startle gating in albino and hooded outbred rat strains. *Pharmacol. Biochem. Behav.* 75, 191–197. doi: 10.1016/S0091-3057(03)00078-9

Swerdlow, N. R., and Sutherland, A. N. (2005). Using animal models to develop therapeutics for Tourette syndrome. *Pharmacol. Ther.* 108, 281–293. doi: 10.1016/j.pharmthera.2005.05.003

Szechtman, H., Sulis, W., and Eilam, D. (1998). Quinpirole induces compulsive checking behavior in rats: a potential animal model of obsessive-compulsive disorder (OCD). *Behav. Neurosci.* 112, 1475–1485.

Taj, M. J. R. J., Viswanath, B., Purushottam, M., Kandavel, T., Janardhan Reddy, Y. C., and Jain, S. (2013). DRD4 gene and obsessive compulsive disorder: do symptom dimensions have specific genetic correlates? *Prog. Neuro-Psychopharmacol. Biol. Psychiatry* 41, 18–23. doi: 10.1016/j.pnpbp.2012.10.023

Taylor, J. L., Rajbhandari, A. K., Berridge, K. C., and Aldridge, J. W. (2010). Dopamine receptor modulation of repetitive grooming actions in the rat: potential relevance for Tourette syndrome. *Brain Res.* 1322, 92–101. doi: 10.1016/j.brainres.2010.01.052

Taylor, J. R., Morshed, S. A., Parveen, S., Mercadante, M. T., Scahill, L., Peterson, B. S., et al. (2002). An animal model of Tourette's syndrome. *Am. J. Psychiatry* 159, 657–660. doi: 10.1176/appi.ajp.159.4.657

Tizabi, Y., Russell, L. T., Johnson, M., and Darmani, N. A. (2001). Nicotine attenuates DOI-induced head-twitch response in mice: implications for Tourette syndrome. *Prog. Neuro-Psychopharmacol. Biol. Psychiatry* 25, 1445–1457. doi: 10.1016/S0278-5846(01)00194-4

Udvardi, P. T., Nespoli, E., Rizzo, F., Hengerer, B., and Ludolph, A. G. (2013). Nondopaminergic neurotransmission in the pathophysiology of Tourette syndrome. *Int. Rev. Neurobiol.* 112, 95–130. doi: 10.1016/B978-0-12-411546-0.00004-4

Van Den Buuse, M. (2004). Prepulse inhibition of acoustic startle in spontaneously hypertensive rats. *Behav. Brain Res.* 154, 331–337. doi: 10.1016/j.bbr.2004.02.021

Wald, R., Dodman, N., and Shuster, L. (2009). The combined effects of memantine and fluoxetine on an animal model of obsessive compulsive disorder. *Exp. Clin. Psychopharmacol.* 17, 191–197. doi: 10.1037/a0016402

Wan, F. J., and Swerdlow, N. R. (1996). Sensorimotor gating in rats is regulated by different dopamine-glutamate interactions in the nucleus accumbens core and shell subregions. *Brain Research* 722, 168–176. doi: 10.1016/0006-8993(96)00209-0

Wang, D. H., Li, W., Liu, X. F., Zhang, J. M., and Wang, S. M. (2013). Chinese medicine formula 'Jian-Pi-Zhi-Dong Decoction' attenuates Tourette syndrome via downregulating the expression of dopamine transporter in mice. *Evid. Based Complement. Alternat. Med.* 2013:385685. doi: 10.1155/2013/385685

Wang, Z., Maia, T. V., Marsh, R., Colibazzi, T., Gerber, A., and Peterson, B. S. (2011). The neural circuits that generate tics in Tourette's syndrome. *Am. J. Psychiatry* 168, 1326–1337. doi: 10.1176/appi.ajp.2011.09111692

Weiss, I. C., Franklin, T. B., Vizi, S., and Mansuy, I. M. (2011). Inheritable effect of unpredictable maternal separation on behavioral responses in mice. *Front. Behav. Neurosci.* 5:3. doi: 10.3389/fnbeh.2011.00003

Welch, J. M., Lu, J., Rodriguiz, R. M., Trotta, N. C., Peca, J., Ding, J. D., et al. (2007). Cortico-striatal synaptic defects and OCD-like behaviours in Sapap3-mutant mice. *Nature* 448, 894–900. doi: 10.1038/nature06104

Woods, A., Smith, C., Szewczak, M., Dunn, R. W., Cornfeldt, M., and Corbett, R. (1993). Selective serotonin re-uptake inhibitors decrease schedule-induced polydipsia in rats: a potential model for obsessive compulsive disorder. *Psychopharmacology* 112, 195–198. doi: 10.1007/BF02244910

Worbe, Y., Baup, N., Grabli, D., Chaigneau, M., Mounayar, S., McCairn, K., et al. (2009). Behavioral and movement disorders induced by local inhibitory dysfunction in primate striatum. *Cereb. Cortex* 19, 1844–1856. doi: 10.1093/cercor/bhn214

Worbe, Y., Mallet, L., Golmard, J. L., Béhar, C., Durif, F., Jalenques, I., Damier, P., et al. (2010). Repetitive behaviours in patients with Gilles de La Tourette syndrome: tics, compulsions, or both? *PLoS ONE* 5:e12959. doi: 10.1371/journal.pone.0012959

Worbe, Y., Sgambato-Faure, V., Epinat, J., Chaigneau, M., Tandé, D., François, C., et al. (2013). Towards a primate model of Gilles de La tourette syndrome: anatomo-behavioural correlation of disorders induced by striatal dysfunction. *Cortex* 49, 1126–1140. doi: 10.1016/j.cortex.2012.08.020

Wu, K., Hanna, G. L., Rosenberg, D. R., and Arnold, P. D. (2012). The role of glutamate signaling in the pathogenesis and treatment of obsessive-compulsive disorder. *Pharmacol. Biochem. Behav.* 100, 726–735. doi: 10.1016/j.pbb.2011.10.007

Xu, M., Kobets, A., Du, J. C., Lennington, J., Li, L., Banasr, M., et al. (2015b). Targeted ablation of cholinergic interneurons in the dorsolateral striatum produces behavioral manifestations of Tourette syndrome. *Proc. Natl. Acad. Sci. U.S.A.* 112, 893–898. doi: 10.1073/pnas.1419533112

Xu, M., Li, L., Ohtsu, H., and Pittenger, C. (2015a). Histidine decarboxylase knockout mice, a genetic model of tourette syndrome, show repetitive grooming after induced fear. *Neurosci. Lett.* 595, 50–53. doi: 10.1016/j.neulet.2015.03.067

Yaddanapudi, K., Hornig, M., Serge, R., De Miranda, J., Baghban, A., Villar, G., et al. (2010). Passive transfer of streptococcus-induced antibodies reproduces behavioral disturbances in a mouse model of pediatric autoimmune neuropsychiatric disorders associated with streptococcal infection. *Mol. Psychiatry* 15, 712–726. doi: 10.1038/mp.2009.77

Yan, T. C., Hunt, S. P., and Stanford, S. C. (2009). Behavioural and neurochemical abnormalities in mice lacking functional tachykinin-1 (NK1) receptors: a model of attention deficit hyperactivity disorder. *Neuropharmacology* 57, 627–635. doi: 10.1016/j.neuropharm.2009.08.021

Zalcman, S. S., Patel, A., Mohla, R., Zhu, Y., and Siegel, A. (2012). Soluble cytokine receptors (sIL-2Rα, sIL-2Rβ) induce subunit-specific behavioral responses and accumulate in the cerebral cortex and basal forebrain. *PLoS ONE* 7:e36316. doi: 10.1371/journal.pone.0036316

Zebardast, N., Crowley, M. J., Bloch, M. H., Mayes, L. C., Wyk, B. V., Leckman, J. F., et al. (2013). Brain mechanisms for prepulse inhibition in adults with tourette syndrome: initial findings. *Psychiatry Res.* 214, 33–41. doi: 10.1016/j.pscychresns.2013.05.009

Zhang, D., Patel, A., Zhu, Y., Siegel, A., and Zalcman, S. S. (2012). Anti-streptococcus IgM antibodies induce repetitive stereotyped movements: cell activation and co-localization with Fcα/μ receptors in the striatum and motor cortex. *Brain Behav. Immun.* 26, 521–533. doi: 10.1016/j.bbi.2012.01.005

Zhu, F., Liu, Y., Zhao, J., and Zheng, Y. (2014). Minocycline alleviates behavioral deficits and inhibits microglial activation induced by intrahippocampal administration of granulocyte-macrophage colony-stimulating factor in adult rats. *Neuroscience* 266, 275–281. doi: 10.1016/j.neuroscience.2014.01.021

Zhu, J., Zhang, X., Xu, Y., Spencer, T. J., Biederman, J., and Bhide, P. G. (2012). Prenatal nicotine exposure mouse model showing hyperactivity, reduced cingulate cortex volume, reduced dopamine turnover, and responsiveness to oral methylphenidate treatment. *J. Neurosci.* 32, 9410–9418. doi: 10.1523/JNEUROSCI.1041-12.2012

Zimmermann, A. M., Jene, T., Wolf, M., Görlich, A., Gurniak, C. B., Sassoè-Pognetto, M., et al. (2014). Attention-deficit/hyperactivity disorder-like phenotype in a mouse model with impaired actin dynamics. *Biol. Psychiatry* 78, 95–106. doi: 10.1016/j.biopsych.2014.03.011

11

TS-EUROTRAIN: A European-Wide Investigation and Training Network on the Etiology and Pathophysiology of Gilles de la Tourette Syndrome

Natalie J. Forde[1,2†], Ahmad S. Kanaan[3,4†], Joanna Widomska[2], Shanmukha S. Padmanabhuni[5], Ester Nespoli[6,7], John Alexander[5], Juan I. Rodriguez Arranz[8], Siyan Fan[9,10,11], Rayan Houssari[8], Muhammad S. Nawaz[12,13], Francesca Rizzo[7,14], Luca Pagliaroli[15,16], Nuno R. Zilhão[9,17], Tamas Aranyi[16,18], Csaba Barta[15], Tobias M. Boeckers[17], Dorret I. Boomsma[14,19], Wim R. Buisman[20], Jan K. Buitelaar[2,21], Danielle Cath[9], Andrea Dietrich[1], Nicole Driessen[2], Petros Drineas[22], Michelle Dunlap[23], Sarah Gerasch[3], Jeffrey Glennon[2], Bastian Hengerer[6], Odile A. van den Heuvel[10,11], Cathrine Jespersgaard[8], Harald E. Möller[4], Kirsten R. Müller-Vahl[3], Thaïra J. C. Openneer[1], Geert Poelmans[2,24,25], Petra J. W. Pouwels[26], Jeremiah M. Scharf[27], Hreinn Stefansson[12], Zeynep Tümer[8], Dick J. Veltman[10], Ysbrand D. van der Werf[11,28], Pieter J. Hoekstra[1], Andrea Ludolph[7] and Peristera Paschou[5]*

[1] Department of Psychiatry, University of Groningen, University Medical Center Groningen, Groningen, Netherlands, [2] Department of Cognitive Neuroscience, Donders Institute for Brain, Cognition and Behaviour, Radboud University Medical Center, Nijmegen, Netherlands, [3] Clinic of Psychiatry, Social Psychiatry and Psychotherapy, Hannover Medical School, Hannover, Germany, [4] Max Planck Institute for Human Cognitive and Brain Sciences, Leipzig, Germany, [5] Department of Molecular Biology and Genetics, Democritus University of Thrace, Alexandropoulos, Greece, [6] Boehringer Ingelheim Pharma GmbH & Co. KG, CNS Research, Biberach an der Riss, Germany, [7] Department of Child and Adolescent Psychiatry, University of Ulm, Ulm, Germany, [8] Department of Clinical Genetics, Applied Human Molecular Genetics, Kennedy Center, Copenhagen University Hospital, Rigshospitalet, Denmark, [9] Department of Clinical and health Psychology, Utrecht University, Utrecht, Netherlands, [10] Department of Psychiatry, VU University Medical Center, Amsterdam, Netherlands, [11] Department of Anatomy and Neurosciences, VU University Medical Center, Amsterdam, Netherlands, [12] deCODE Genetics/Amgen, Reykjavik, Iceland, [13] Faculty of Medicine, University of Iceland, Reykjavik, Iceland, [14] Institute for Anatomy and Cell Biology, Ulm University, Ulm, Germany, [15] Institute of Medical Chemistry, Molecular Biology and Pathobiochemistry, Semmelweis University, Budapest, Hungary, [16] Research Centre for Natural Sciences, Institute of Enzymology, Hungarian Academy of Sciences, Budapest, Hungary, [17] Department of Biological Psychology, VU University, Amsterdam, Netherlands, [18] Université d'Angers, BNMI (Institut national de la santé et de la recherche médicale 1083 / Centre National de la Recherche Scientifique 6214), Angers, France, [19] EMGO+ Institute for Health and Care Research, VU University Medical Centre, Amsterdam, Netherlands, [20] Stichting Gilles de la Tourette, Rhoon, Netherlands, [21] Karakter Child and Adolescent Psychiatry, University Centre, Nijmegen, Netherlands, [22] Rensselaer Polytechnic Institute, Troy, NY, USA, [23] Tourette-Gesellschaft Deutschland e.V., Hannover, Germany, [24] Department of Human Genetics, Radboud University Medical Center, Nijmegen, Netherlands, [25] Department of Molecular Animal Physiology, Donders Institute for Brain, Cognition and Behaviour, Radboud Institute for Molecular Life Sciences, Radboud University, Nijmegen, Netherlands, [26] Department of Physics and Medical Technology, VU University Medical Center, Amsterdam, Netherlands, [27] Psychiatric and Neurodevelopmental Genetics Unit, Departments of Psychiatry and Neurology, Center for Human Genetic Research, Harvard Medical School, Massachusetts General Hospital, Boston, MA, USA, [28] Netherlands Institute for Neuroscience, Amsterdam, Netherlands

Gilles de la Tourette Syndrome (GTS) is characterized by the presence of multiple motor and phonic tics with a fluctuating course of intensity, frequency, and severity. Up to 90% of patients with GTS present with comorbid conditions, most commonly attention-deficit/hyperactivity disorder (ADHD), and obsessive-compulsive disorder (OCD), thus providing an excellent model for the exploration of shared etiology across disorders. TS-EUROTRAIN (FP7-PEOPLE-2012-ITN, Grant Agr.No. 316978) is a Marie Curie Initial Training Network (http://ts-eurotrain.eu) that aims to elucidate the complex

Edited by:
Ahmet O. Caglayan,
Yale University, USA

Reviewed by:
Munis Dundar,
Erciyes University, Turkey
Jessica A. Church-Lang,
University of Texas at Austin, USA
Asif Doja,
Children's Hospital of Eastern Ontario,
Canada
Eric R. Gamazon,
University of Chicago, USA

***Correspondence:**
Peristera Paschou
ppaschou@mbg.duth.gr

†These authors have contributed
equally to this work.

etiology of the onset and clinical course of GTS, investigate the neurobiological underpinnings of GTS and related disorders, translate research findings into clinical applications, and establish a pan-European infrastructure for the study of GTS. This includes the challenges of (i) assembling a large genetic database for the evaluation of the genetic architecture with high statistical power; (ii) exploring the role of gene-environment interactions including the effects of epigenetic phenomena; (iii) employing endophenotype-based approaches to understand the shared etiology between GTS, OCD, and ADHD; (iv) establishing a developmental animal model for GTS; (v) gaining new insights into the neurobiological mechanisms of GTS via cross-sectional and longitudinal neuroimaging studies; and (vi) partaking in outreach activities including the dissemination of scientific knowledge about GTS to the public. Fifteen partners from academia and industry and 12 PhD candidates pursue the project. Here, we aim to share the design of an interdisciplinary project, showcasing the potential of large-scale collaborative efforts in the field of GTS. Our ultimate aims are to elucidate the complex etiology and neurobiological underpinnings of GTS, translate research findings into clinical applications, and establish Pan-European infrastructure for the study of GTS and associated disorders.

Keywords: Initial Training Network, Gilles de la Tourette Syndrome, tourette disorder, etiology, genetics, neuroimaging, animal models

INTRODUCTION

Gilles de la Tourette Syndrome (GTS) is a frequent disorder (0.4–1%; Robertson, 2008, 2015b), characterized by multiple motor and phonic tics and high comorbidity with attention-deficit/hyperactivity disorder (ADHD; 50%) and obsessive-compulsive disorder (OCD; 20–60%) (Leckman et al., 1998; Robertson, 2000; Bloch and Leckman, 2009; Debes et al., 2010; American Psychiatric Association, 2013; Hirschtritt et al., 2015). The need to overcome fragmentation and accelerate research into the etiology of GTS and its related conditions has motivated the establishment of TS-EUROTRAIN (http://ts-eurotrain.eu), a Marie Curie Initial Training Network (ITN, 2012–2016) that focuses on the investigation of the genetic etiology and pathophysiology of GTS while aiming to translate findings into clinical research. The network spans 13 academic and two industrial partners as well as two patient groups. Twelve individual, yet complementary, PhD projects interact to form a comprehensive study of GTS and comorbidities from genetics, and epigenetics through to physiology, brain anatomy, and function. These projects are all currently underway and can roughly be divided into three groups by their main approach; genetic (and epigenetic), animal models, and human neuroimaging, respectively. Research into the neurobiology of GTS stands at the precipice of discovery thanks to collaborative efforts (Georgitsi et al., 2016). With this report, we would like to share our efforts as an example of how, taking advantage of expertise across different disciplines, and resources across the GTS scientific and patient community we aimed to build a project that would achieve goals beyond and above the reach of individual labs. At the same time we provide an overview of some of the largest-scale projects aiming to understand the etiology of GTS. These projects may be expected to impact the field considerably in the coming years.

GENETICS, EPIGENETICS, AND GENE EXPRESSION

The first Genome-wide Association Study (GWAS) to investigate the role of single nucleotide polymorphisms (SNPs) in GTS did not manage to identify SNPs that meet the genome-wide significance level for association to GTS, however, four additional GWAS for GTS are currently underway [coordinated by the Tourette Association International Consortium for Genetics (TSAICG), European Multicentre Tics in Children Studies (EMTICS), Netherlands twin register (NTR) and deCODE] and the future meta-analysis of these datasets is expected to provide important insights into the etiology of the disorder (**Figure 1**; Paschou, 2013; Scharf et al., 2013). Furthermore, in recent years, four independent GTS cohorts have been examined, studying the role of Copy Number Variants (CNVs) in GTS (Sundaram et al., 2010; Fernandez et al., 2012; Nag et al., 2013; McGrath et al., 2014). Regarding gene expression investigations, so far, most studies were carried out on samples of small number (Tang et al., 2005; Lit et al., 2007, 2009; Liao et al., 2010; Tian et al., 2011a,b, 2012; Gunther et al., 2012; Gomez et al., 2014; Lennington et al., 2016) and need to be verified in large GTS cohorts. On the other hand, studies on the epigenetics of GTS (such as DNA methylation, histone modification, and micro-RNA (miRNA) alteration Goldberg et al., 2007; Pagliaroli et al., 2016) remain scarce (Abelson et al., 2005; Delgado et al., 2014) and in fact, the first ever epigenome-wide study for GTS was only recently published through TS-EUROTRAIN

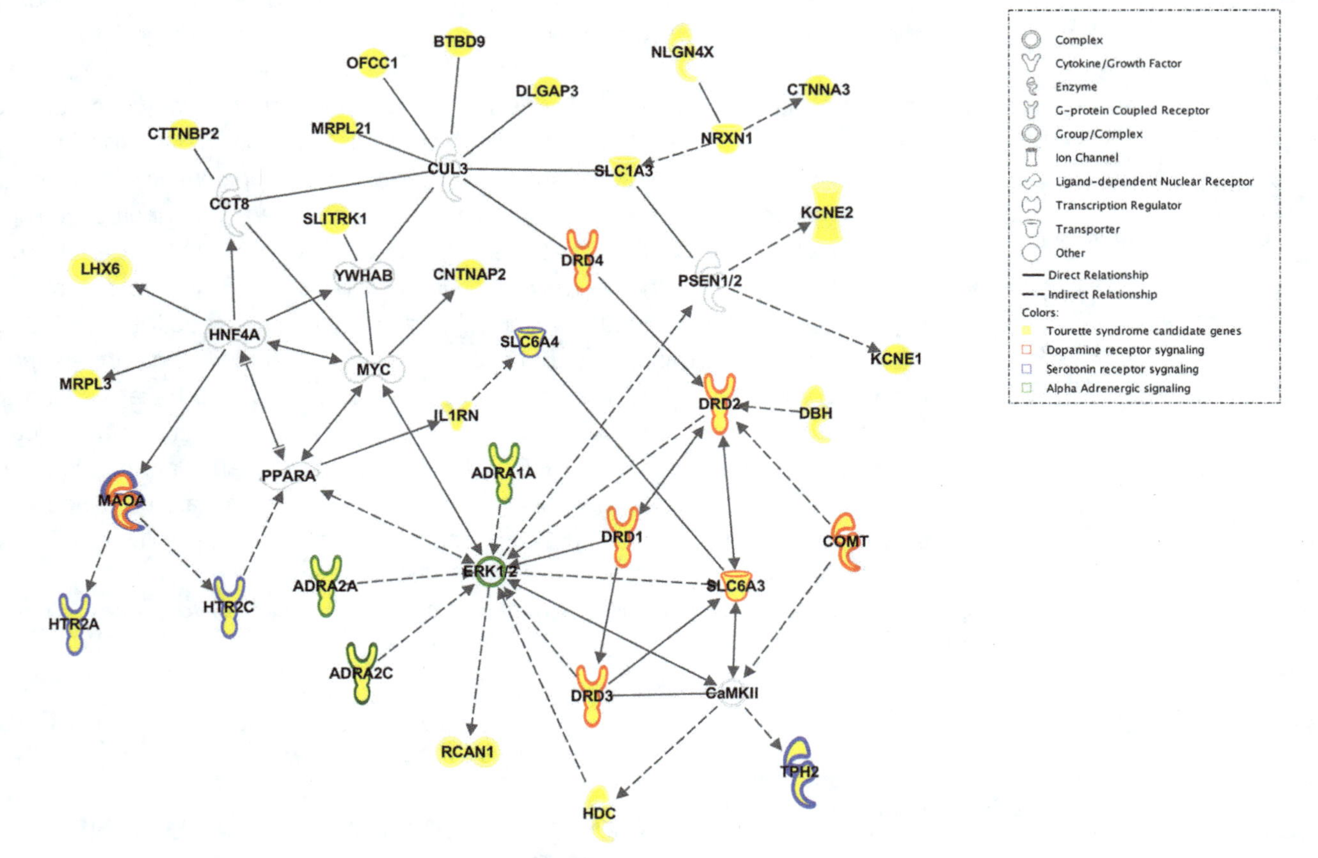

FIGURE 1 | Network of reported candidate genes associated with GTS. This image was produced (by JW) with Ingenuity pathway analysis software and shows how the proteins encoded by the candidate genes reported to be associated with GTS are linked with each other. Please see legend for description of what each symbol and color represents. ADRA1A, adrenoceptor alpha 1A; ADRA2A, adrenoceptor alpha 2A; ADRA2C, adrenoceptor alpha 2C; BTBD9, BTB (POZ) domain containing 9; CaMKII, calcium/calmodulin-dependent protein kinase II; CCT8, chaperonin containing TCP1, subunit 8 (theta); CNTNAP2, contactin-associated protein-like 2; COMT, catechol-O-methyltransferase; CTNNA3, catenin (cadherin-associated protein), alpha 3; CTTNBP2, contactin binding protein 2; CUL3, cullin 3; DBH, dopamine beta-hydroxylase (dopamine beta-monooxygenase); DLGAP3, discs; large (Drosophila) homolog-associated protein 3; DRD1, dopamine receptor D1, DRD2, dopamine receptor D2, DRD3, dopamine receptor D3, DRD4, dopamine receptor D4, ERK 1/2, extracellular signal-regulated kinases 1/2; HDC, histidine decarboxylase, HNF4A, hepatocyte nuclear factor 4 alpha; HTR2A, 5-hydroxytryptamine (serotonin) receptor 2A; G protein-coupled; HTR2C, 5-hydroxytryptamine (serotonin) receptor 2C; G protein-coupled; IL1RN, interleukin 1 receptor antagonist; KCNE1, potassium channel voltage gated subfamily E regulatory beta subunit 1; KCNE2, potassium channel, voltage gated subfamily E regulatory beta subunit 2; LHX6, LIM homeobox 6; MAOA, monoamine oxidase A; MRPL21, mitochondrial ribosomal protein L21; MRPL3, mitochondrial ribosomal protein L3; MYC, v-myc avian myelocytomatosis viral oncogene homolog; NLGN4X, neuroligin 4, X-linked; NRXN1, neurexin 1; OFCC1, orofacial cleft 1 candidate 1; PPARA, peroxisome proliferator-activated receptor alpha; RCAN1, regulator of calcineurin 1; PSEN1/2, presenilin 1/2; SLC1A3, solute carrier family 1 (glial high affinity glutamate transporter), member 3; SLC6A3, solute carrier family 6 (neurotransmitter transporter); member 3; SLC6A4, solute carrier family 6 (neurotransmitter transporter), member 4, SLITRK1, SLIT, and NTRK-like family, member 1; TPH2, tryptophan hydroxylase 2; YWHAB, tyrosine 3-monooxygenase/tryptophan 5-monooxygenase activation protein, beta.

efforts (Zilhão et al., 2015). We address the whole spectrum of GTS genetics from various angles; genetic, epigenetic, gene expression, and their interaction with environmental factors.

Project 1 Genome-Wide Search for Genes Conferring Risk of GTS (Muhammad Sulaman Nawaz and Hreinn Steffanson, Decode Genetics)

This project makes use of the extensive Icelandic population genotyping done by deCODE genetics. Approximately one third of the population (100,000) has been genotyped into which 20,000,000 SNPs from the Icelandic sequencing project have been imputed. Tasks include (i) a genome-wide search for genetic variants conferring risk of GTS. This consists of a search for common and rare variants in more than 500 chip typed subjects diagnosed with GTS, (ii) a genome wide search for CNVs associated with GTS, (iii) a test for association of identified variants with phenotypic measures as well as performance on neuropsychological tests, (iv) an investigation of how implicated variants may lead to alteration of gene-expression pathways through analysis of already generated expression cohorts.

Project 2 Investigation of the Role of CNVs as Genetic Susceptibility Factors Involved in the Pathogenesis of GTS and Co-morbid Disorders (Rayan Houssari, Juan Ignacio Rodriguez Arranz, Mehar Arumilli, and Zeynep Tümer, Kennedy Center, Copenhagen University Hospital, Rigshospitalet)

The aim of this project is to untangle novel molecular genetic mechanisms underlying GTS and related disorders, by using bioinformatic network analysis of CNVs combined with phenotype data of 261 GTS-patients residing in Denmark. All the patients were assessed by experienced clinicians at the Tourette Clinic, Copenhagen University Hospital for GTS, OCD, and ADHD using validated diagnostic instruments (Mol Debes et al., 2008). Furthermore, information about other family members was collected through interviews revealing approximately 77% of the families to be multiplex with at least two family members affected by GTS or one of the common comorbidities. A biobank consisting of cell-lines, DNA, RNA, and serum has been established. All the patients have been screened using the Affymetrix CytoScan HD chromosome microarray platform with more than 2.6 million copy number markers and the bioinformatic data analysis is under way. This study, in collaboration with other members of the network, has already enabled identification of the *AADAC* gene as a susceptibility factor for GTS when deleted (Bertelsen et al., 2016).

Project 3 Gene-Environment Interactions Defining the Onset and Clinical Course of Tics and Obsessive-Compulsive Symptoms (Shanmukha Sampath Padmanabhuni and Peristera Paschou, Democritus University of Thrace)

The aim of this project is to investigate the interaction between genetic and environmental factors that may lead to the onset of tics. Following a systems biology approach information from multiple sources are integrated; including genome-wide genotyping, gene expression patterns, epigenetics, and longitudinal clinical observations. Through collaboration with the FP7-HEALTH project EMTICS, a special focus is placed on group A streptococcal infections and stress as a possible trigger for tic onset. EMTICS also offers us access to genome-wide genotype data of 1000 patients (followed up on a monthly basis for 12 months) as well as gene expression data on 200 GTS patients that are followed up for tic exacerbation and remission in an attempt to correlate with environmental factors. Gene-expression and correlation with environmental triggers is also investigated in a cohort of first degree relatives of patients with GTS that develop tic symptomatology within a 3-year follow-up period. Furthermore, the first ever epigenome-wide association study for tics, analysing data from the NTR, has been carried out [55]. This study comprised the largest epigenetic data collection so far undertaken (411,469 autosomal methylation sites, assessed in 1678 individuals). Although no site reached genomewide significance, the top hits include several genes, and regions previously associated with neurological disorders and warrant further investigation (Zilhão et al., 2015).

Project 4 Epigenetic and Functional Characterization of Proposed Genetic Variants and Regions Implicated in the Pathogenesis of GTS and Related Phenotypes (Luca Pagliaroli and Csaba Barta, Semmelweis University)

The aim of this project is to shed light on the main epigenetic mechanisms, such as DNA methylation, histone modification and miRNA, and their possible role in GTS. Tasks include (i) the study of candidate miRNAs which are predicted to be in the control of tissue-specific gene expression by *in vivo* target validation of *in silico* proposed miRNA target genes, (ii) screening of cell lines and GTS animal models treated with dopaminergic and glutamatergic modulating compounds for epigenetic regulatory markers, (iii) investigation of brain tissue samples from treated and untreated animal models developed within the TS-EUROTRAIN consortium to determine DNA methylation profiles and histone modification changes, and (iv) investigation of blood samples from patients with GTS for whole genome DNA methylation profiling (Zilhão et al., 2015), as mentioned in project 3.

Project 5 Integrated Genetic Networks Underlying Comorbid GTS and OCD (Joanna Widomska, Jan Buitelaar, Geert Poelmans, and Jeffrey Glennon, Radboud University Medical Center, Nijmegen)

The aim of this project is to determine the extent of "genetic overlap" in terms of shared underlying gene pathways and molecular signaling cascades between GTS and OCD and to provide further insights into how aberrant processes underlie these genetically related, clinically overlapping but still distinct neurodevelopmental disorders. Combining literature search approaches with diverse bioinformatics analytic tools (e.g., Ingenuity Pathway Analysis), top candidate genes emerging from GWASs of GTS (Scharf et al., 2013), OCD (Stewart et al., 2013; Mattheisen et al., 2015), and corroborating genetic evidence including data from recurrent and "genome-wide" CNV studies, candidate gene studies, miRNA expression data, animal models, and gene expression studies are selected and evaluated. The genes presenting overlap between GTS and OCD are ranked and used to construct integrated genetic networks that represent the "molecular landscape" of the overlapping traits between GTS and OCD, as well as GTS itself. The molecular landscape of OCD alone has recently been published (van de Vondervoort et al., 2016). This approach will be instrumental to discover unknown causative genes, pathways, and mechanisms and identify common pleiotropic genetic risk variants as possible therapeutic targets.

Project 6 The Genetic Epidemiology of GTS, tics and Related Phenotypes (Nuno Rodrigues Zilhão Nogueira, Dorret i. Boomsma and Danielle Cath, Utrecht University and Vu University Medical Center)

This study uses data that has been gathered by the NTR over the last 25 years, on twins, and family members ($n = 16{,}896$ individuals with SNP, epigenetic and expression data in subsamples), including a range of phenotypic data from questionnaires and genetic data. Structure equation model fitting procedures are used to model the phenotypic resemblance between family members and the relative contribution of genetic and environmental factors to variation and covariation among traits. Also, genome-wide association methodologies are being used to disentangle the genetic architecture underlying the etiology of GTS traits by estimating SNP heritability and polygenic risk scores for example.

Project 7 Developing Algorithmic Prediction Models for GTS and Related Disorders (John Alexander and Peristera Paschou, Democritus University of Thrace)

With the continuous development of state of the art technologies for generating large amounts of genomic data, there is a need to develop new methodologies in order to identify promising SNPs, and candidate genes for further experimental validation. Using genetic data available for GTS and related disorders, this project develops, and applies new methodologies to scan high throughput genomic data (Genome Wide Association data, next generation sequence data, and microarrays). For example, using meta-analysis data comprised of 1285 GTS cases, and 4964 controls ancestry-matched to the GTS sample from the first GWAS (Scharf et al., 2013), we perform pathway, protein-protein interaction and gene-ontology analysis in order to dissect the molecular mechanisms underlying GTS. Furthermore, using novel bioinformatics tools for SNP based and gene based functional analysis, we perform candidate gene prioritization, gene set enrichment, and tissue enrichment analysis. We also construct functional interaction networks using combined information from the enriched functional and pathway results. This project will aid in highlighting pathways involved in the susceptibility of GTS and will bring out susceptibility factors that interact in order to confer risk for GTS.

ANIMAL MODELS

Animal models of disease are an integral part of disease investigation and drug testing. However, ill-suited or inappropriate models are often used for these purposes. While multiple useful animal models for tic disorders exist, not all of these adequately mimic the syndrome, and crucially there is a lack of a juvenile model for GTS, despite it being a childhood onset disorder. Two animal model projects within TS-EUROTRAIN work to remedy these shortcomings, by developing a new juvenile GTS model within which the cortico-striato-thalamo-cortical (CSTC) circuitry and in particular the role of the glutamatergic system are being investigated. Furthermore, the effect of older and newer psychotropic compounds (e.g., riluzole and aripiprazole) are tested and novel targets identified. Similarly to the genetics and human neuroimaging projects a wide field of investigation is taken to include common comorbidities. Furthermore, samples from these projects undergo epigenetic testing as mentioned in project 4.

Project 8 Finding Developmental Aspects and Possible Drug Targets of GTS and OCD: Metabotropic Glutamatergic Mechanisms in a Neurodevelopmental Rat Model of Repetitive Behaviors (Ester Nespoli and Bastian Hengerer, Boehringer Ingelheim pharma GmBH and Co. KG)

The unilaterally lesioned 6-hydroxidopamine (6-OHDA) adult rat is a well-established model used in Levodopa-induced Dyskinesia research. In this model a rapid degeneration of nigrostriatal neurons is chemically induced by the intrastriatal or intranigral administration of 6-OHDA, which selectively targets monoaminergic neurons. Chronic application of L-dopa to 6-OHDA lesioned rats leads to the development of repetitive involuntary movements, mainly involving the forepaw, neck, and mouth (Cenci et al., 1998). This appears as a consequence of the striatal super sensitivity to dopamine, caused by higher surface expression of dopamine receptors, which is a putative pathological mechanism of GTS and is induced in this model via previous dopamine deprivation (Buse et al., 2013). Here this model is translated to juvenile rats, inducing the lesion in postnatal days and monitoring its neurodevelopmental consequences. This provides new insights into the pathological mechanism of tics during development and a new tool to test therapeutic options for this disease.

Project 9 Investigation of the Effect of Classical and New Psychotherapeutic Approach in a Rat Model for GTS—a Magnetic Resonance Spectroscopy (MRS) Study (Francesca Rizzo and Andrea Ludolph, University of ULM)

This study compares the *in vivo* efficacy of a classical and a new therapeutic approach on tic management and their respective neurochemical effect in a rat model of GTS (Bronfeld et al., 2013). Aripiprazole is a second generation antipsychotic drug (classical approach) that has been found to be effective on tic management and to have a well-tolerated side effect profile (Kawohl et al., 2009). It is known that dopamine metabolism is dysfunctional in GTS, but neuroimaging research, and genetic studies also implicate other neurotransmitters in tic generation: histamine, serotonin, noradrenaline, endocannabinoids, glutamate, and GABA (Buse et al., 2013; Udvardi et al., 2013). Since the glutamate and dopamine systems are closely connected, a newly proposed approach for GTS treatment consists of the glutamatergic modulator riluzole, which is known to exert neuroprotection from glutamate excito-toxicity both *in vitro* and *in vivo* (Risterucci et al., 2006). Magnetic resonance spectroscopy (MRS) is used in an animal model to longitudinally analyse glutamate metabolites in the brain over a critical period of time in GTS; childhood through to early adulthood when tics appear and reach their maximum severity. The discovery of new pharmacological targets can provide new direction in drug development for GTS.

NEUROIMAGING

Our three (human) neuroimaging projects are highly complementary with similar techniques used across all sites so as to allow for the cross-comparison of findings with limited methodological confounding factors. Projects 11 and 12 even pool data for certain comparisons. Each project utilizes MRS to evaluate the role of the glutamatergic system; T1-weighted structural magnetic resonance imaging (MRI) to examine structural brain differences; functional MRI (fMRI; resting state and task specific) data to interrogate the functional coupling between cognitive, limbic, and sensory-motor CSTC networks; and diffusion-weighted MRI (dMRI) data to inspect the structural connectivity. Each project does, however, differ in the populations under investigation and aims to address different unknown areas regarding GTS neurobiology. Together these works, along with the animal MRI study, may have implications on future glutamatergic modulatory therapies for tic suppression and could potentially extend the current pathophysiological model of GTS and related circuits beyond CSTC circuitry (**Figure 2**).

Project 10 Structural and Functional Neural Correlates of Pediatric GTS and ADHD (Natalie Forde, Jan Buitelaar, and Pieter Hoekstra, University Medical Center Groningen)

Few neuroimaging studies of GTS have investigated brain structure and function in children with even fewer longitudinal studies tracking the development of GTS (Ganos et al., 2013). Furthermore, the similarities and differences between ADHD and GTS have yet to be explicitly tested (Plessen et al., 2007). For this study structural, functional (resting state and task-dependent stop-signal and reward tasks) and dMRI data are acquired alongside MRS for glutamate and glutamine concentrations, neuropsychological, and phenotypic data from 180 children between 8–12 years of age (60 GTS with or without ADHD, 60 ADHD only, and 60 healthy controls). Common and unique neural correlates of GTS and ADHD are elucidated. Furthermore genetic data is acquired and will be analyzed as part of the EU-funded TACTICs project. Lastly a 3 year follow-up has been granted where the same battery of tests, including MRI, will be undertaken to allow the course of GTS and ADHD to be investigated.

Project 11 Studying the Role of Glutamate in CSTC Circuit Function and Structure in Adult GTS and OCD (Siyan Fan, Dick Veltman, Odile Van Den Heuvel, Petra Pouwels, Ysbrand Van Der Werf, and Danielle Cath, Department of Clinical and Health Psychology, Utrecht University and Vu University Medical Center)

The neural correlates of GTS and OCD have scarcely been compared and contrasted despite the high rate of co-occurrence (Freeman et al., 2000). This project is to investigate how altered glutamatergic function (as measured with MRS) is related to changes in structure (T1- and diffusion- weighted) and function (resting state and task-dependent stop-signal task) of the CSTC circuits in adult patients with GTS and OCD in comparison to healthy individuals. A similar range of neuroimaging, neuropsychological and phenotypic data to the above is acquired from adults with GTS, OCD and healthy controls ($n = 20$ per group). The participants with OCD as well as the controls have been chosen from a previous local OCD study while those with GTS are newly recruited. Genetic data is collected to contribute to genetic analysis within other projects of the network and to perform imaging-genetic analyses.

Project 12 Elemental, Neurochemical, and Network Based Analysis of the Pathophysiological Mechanisms of GTS (Ahmad Seif Kanaan, Harald Möller, and Kirsten Müller-Vahl, Hannover Medical School and Max Planck Institute For Human Cognitive And Brain Sciences)

Neuroimaging and behavioral data are acquired from up to 40 adult patients before and after treatment with the pharmacological agent aripiprazole, an atypical antipsychotic agent which is commonly used to treat GTS. At the elemental level, we use Quantitative Susceptibility Mapping (QSM) techniques to investigate whether patients exhibit an altered distribution of iron concentrations within basal ganglia nuclei in comparison to 40 healthy controls. At the neurochemical level, we investigate the role of the glutamatergic system within cortico-striatal regions using MRS at baseline and following treatment. At the network level, we use resting-state fMRI to investigate the interaction between large scale networks and their relationship to clinical status.

ANTICIPATED OUTCOMES OF TS-EUROTRAIN

TS-EUROTRAIN is a showcase of the potential impact of large-scale interdisciplinary and collaborative efforts aiming to understand GTS. Our basic science research combined with clinical neuroimaging studies will greatly increase our knowledge of the biological underpinnings of GTS

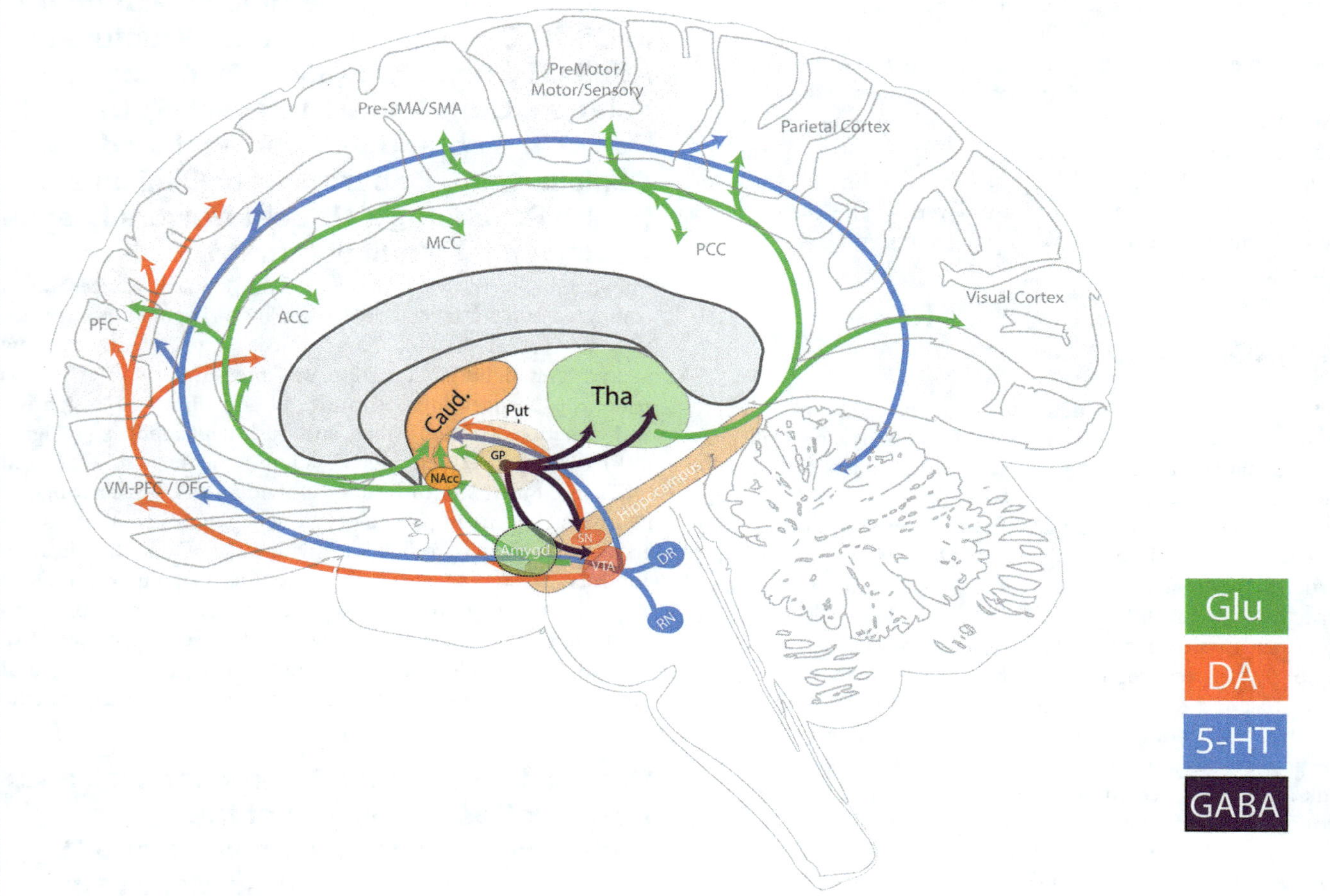

FIGURE 2 | Major neurotransmitter pathways related to GTS pathophysiology. Simplified schematic illustration of the major neurotransmitter systems reported and hypothesized to be involved in GTS pathophysiology. Other neuromodulatory systems that have been implicated include the cholinergic, histaminergic, and endocannabinoid systems. The figure was adapted based on information from Singer (2013) and Schumann et al. (2010). (5-HT, serotonergic; ACC, anterior cingulate cortex; Amygd, amygdala; Caud, Caudate nucleus; DA, dopaminergic; DR, dorsal raphe nucleus; GABA, gamma-aminobutyric acid; Glu, glutamatergic; GP, globus pallidus; MCC, mid cingulate cortex; NAcc, nucleus accumbens; OFC, orbitofrontal cortex; PCC, posterior cingulate cortex; PFC, prefrontal cortex; Put, putamen; RN, raphe nucleus; SMA, supplementary motor area; SN, substantia nigra; Tha, thalamus; VM-PFC, ventromedial prefrontal cortex; VTA: ventral tegmental area).

and related disorders and allow a suitable biological model for these disorders to be established. The benefits of our research will include the potential identification of novel treatment targets and the availability of a suitable animal model on which to test newly developed pharmacotherapies targeting these newly identified biological pathways. This will ultimately lead to improved treatments and consequently increased quality of life for those suffering from GTS and their families. Despite being common, GTS is still considered a rare, unusual disease by the public, and has been associated with symptoms and signs causing social misunderstanding and stigmatization (Roessner et al., 2011; Robertson, 2015a). Undertaking a comprehensive scientific and outreach programme TS-EUROTRAIN has the important aspiration to help raise awareness about GTS, alleviate stigmatization, and transform GTS into a model disorder for the development of European policies for the promotion of childhood mental health.

AUTHOR CONTRIBUTIONS

NF and AK are Joint first authors AL deceased NF and AK wrote the MS. JW, SP, EN, and JA generated/contributed to the figures and contributed to writing along with JR, SF, RH, MN, NZ, LP, and FR. PH and PP reviewed and supervised the writing this MS. TA, CB, TB, DB, JB, DC, AD, PD, JG, BH, OV, CJ, HM, KM, GP, PJWP, JS, HS, ZT, DV, YV, PH, and PP all have roles in setting up and/or supervising the individual projects described in the MS. MD, and WB represent the patient organizations involved in the establishment of the network. ND, SG, and TO also work on the projects.

further acknowledge support by the European Union Seventh Framework Programmes [TACTICS (FP7/2007-2013), Grant Agr.No. 278948 and EMTICS (FP7/2007-2013), Grant Agr.No. 278367]. CB was supported by the Merit-prize scholarship of Semmelweis University and the János Bolyai Research Scholarship of the Hungarian Academy of Sciences BO/00987/16/5.

ACKNOWLEDGMENTS

This paper is dedicated to the memory of Prof Andrea Ludolph whose significant contributions and tireless efforts as a Scientist, Clinician and Educator laid the groundwork for collaborative efforts for the promotion of research and care for GTS in Europe.

REFERENCES

Abelson, J. F., Kwan, K. Y., O'Roak, B. J., Baek, D. Y., Stillman, A. A., Morgan, T. M., et al. (2005). Sequence variants in SLITRK1 are associated with Tourette's syndrome. *Science* 310, 317–320. doi: 10.1126/science.1116502

American Psychiatric Association (2013). "Neurodevelopmental Disorders," in *Diagnostic and Statistical Manual of Mental Disorders DSM Library* (Washington, DC: American Psychiatric Association), 81–82.

Bertelsen, B., Stefánsson, H., Riff Jensen, L., Melchior, L., Mol Debes, N., Groth, C., et al. (2016). Association of *AADAC* deletion and Gilles de la tourette syndrome in a large european cohort. *Biol. Psychiatry* 79, 383–391. doi: 10.1016/j.biopsych.2015.08.027

Bloch, M. H., and Leckman, J. F. (2009). Clinical course of Tourette syndrome. *J. Psychosom. Res* 67, 497–501. doi: 10.1016/j.jpsychores.2009.09.002

Bronfeld, M., Yael, D., Belelovsky, K., and Bar-Gad, I. (2013). Motor tics evoked by striatal disinhibition in the rat. *Front. Syst. Neurosci.* 7:50. doi: 10.3389/fnsys.2013.00050

Buse, J., Schoenefeld, K., Münchau, A., and Roessner, V. (2013). Neuromodulation in Tourette syndrome: dopamine and beyond. *Neurosci. Biobehav. Rev.* 37, 1069–1084. doi: 10.1016/j.neubiorev.2012.10.004

Cenci, M. A., Lee, C. S., and Björklund, A. (1998). L-DOPA-induced dyskinesia in the rat is associated with striatal overexpression of prodynorphin- and glutamic acid decarboxylase mRNA. *Eur. J. Neurosci.* 10, 2694–2706. doi: 10.1046/j.1460-9568.1998.00285.x

Debes, N. M. M. M., Hjalgrim, H., and Skov, L. (2010). Predictive factors for familiarity in a Danish clinical cohort of children with Tourette syndrome. *Eur. J. Med. Genet.* 53, 171–178. doi: 10.1016/j.ejmg.2010.05.001

Delgado, M. S., Camprubí, C., Tümer, Z., Martínez, F., Milà, M., and Monk, D. (2014). Screening individuals with intellectual disability, autism and Tourette's syndrome for KCNK9 mutations and aberrant DNA methylation within the 8q24 imprinted cluster. *Am. J. Med. Genet. Part B Neuropsychiatr. Genet.* 165, 472–478. doi: 10.1002/ajmg.b.32250

Fernandez, T. V., Sanders, S. J., Yurkiewicz, I. R., Ercan-Sencicek, A., G., Kim, Y. S., Fishman, D. O., et al. (2012). Rare copy number variants in tourette syndrome disrupt genes in histaminergic pathways and overlap with autism. *Biol. Psychiatry* 71, 392–402. doi: 10.1016/j.biopsych.2011.09.034

Freeman, R. D., Fast, D. K., Burd, L., Kerbeshian, J., Robertson, M. M., and Sandor, P. (2000). An international perspective on Tourette syndrome: selected findings from 3500 individuals in 22 countries. *Dev. Med. Child Neurol.* 42, 436–447. doi: 10.1111/j.1469-8749.2000.tb00346.x

Ganos, C., Roessner, V., and Münchau, A. (2013). The functional anatomy of Gilles de la Tourette syndrome. *Neurosci. Biobehav. Rev.* 37, 1050–1062. doi: 10.1016/j.neubiorev.2012.11.004

Georgitsi, M., Willsey, J., Mathews, C., State, M., Scharf, J., and Paschou, P. (2016). The genetic etiology of tourette syndrome: large-scale collaborative efforts on the precipice of discovery. *Front. Neurosci.* 10:351. doi: 10.3389/fnins.2016.00351

Goldberg, A. D., Allis, C. D., and Bernstein, E. (2007). Epigenetics: a landscape takes shape. *Cell* 128, 635–638. doi: 10.1016/j.cell.2007.02.006

Gomez, L., Wigg, K., Zhang, K., Lopez, L., Sandor, P., Malone, M., et al. (2014). Association of the KCNJ5 gene with tourette syndrome and attention-deficit/hyperactivity disorder. *Genes Brain Behav.* 13, 535–542. doi: 10.1111/gbb.12141

Gunther, J., Tian, Y., Stamova, B., Lit, L., Corbett, B., Ander, B., et al. (2012). Catecholamine-related gene expression in blood correlates with tic severity in tourette syndrome. *Psychiatry Res.* 200, 593–601. doi: 10.1016/j.psychres.2012.04.034

Hirschtritt, M. E., Lee, P. C., Pauls, D. L., Dion, Y., Grados, M. A., Illmann, C., et al. (2015). Lifetime prevalence, age of risk, and genetic relationships of comorbid psychiatric disorders in tourette syndrome. *JAMA Psychiatry* 72, 325–333. doi: 10.1001/jamapsychiatry.2014.2650

Kawohl, W., Schneider, F., Vernaleken, I., and Neuner, I. (2009). Aripiprazole in the pharmacotherapy of Gilles de la Tourette syndrome in adult patients. *World J. Biol. psychiatry* 10, 827–831. doi: 10.1080/15622970701762544

Leckman, J. F., Zhang, H., Vitale, A., Lahnin, F., Lynch, K., Bondi, C., et al. (1998). Course of tic severity in Tourette syndrome: the first two decades. *Pediatrics* 102, 14–19. doi: 10.1542/peds.102.1.14

Lennington, J. B., Coppola, G., Kataoka-Sasaki, Y., Fernandez, T. V, Palejev, D., Li, Y., et al. (2016). Transcriptome analysis of the human striatum in tourette syndrome. *Biol. Psychiatry* 79, 372–382. doi: 10.1016/j.biopsych.2014.07.018

Liao, I. H., Corbett, B. A., Gilbert, D. L., Bunge, S. A., and Sharp, F. R. (2010). Blood gene expression correlated with tic severity in medicated and unmedicated patients with Tourette Syndrome. *Pharmacogenomics* 11, 1733–1741. doi: 10.2217/pgs.10.160

Lit, L., Enstrom, A., Sharp, F. R., and Gilbert, D. L. (2009). Age-related gene expression in Tourette syndrome. *J. Psychiatr. Res.* 43, 319–330. doi: 10.1016/j.jpsychires.2008.03.012

Lit, L., Gilbert, D. L., Walker, W., and Sharp, F. R. (2007). A subgroup of Tourette's patients overexpress specific natural killer cell genes in blood: a preliminary report. *Am. J. Med. Genet. Part B Neuropsychiatr. Genet.* 144, 958–963. doi: 10.1002/ajmg.b.30550

Mattheisen, M., Samuels, J. F., Wang, Y., Greenberg, B. D., Fyer, A. J., McCracken, J. T., et al. (2015). Genome-wide association study in obsessive-compulsive disorder: results from the OCGAS. *Mol. Psychiatry* 20, 337–344. doi: 10.1038/mp.2014.43

McGrath, L. M., Yu, D., Marshall, C., Davis, L. K., Thiruvahindrapuram, B., Li, B., et al. (2014). Copy number variation in obsessive-compulsive disorder and tourette syndrome: a cross-disorder study. *J. Am. Acad. Child Adolesc. Psychiatry* 53, 910–919. doi: 10.1016/j.jaac.2014.04.022

Mol Debes, N. M. M., Hjalgrim, H., and Skov, L. (2008). Validation of the presence of comorbidities in a danish clinical cohort of children with Tourette Syndrome. *J. Child Neurol.* 23, 1017–1027. doi: 10.1177/0883073808316370

Nag, A., Bochukova, E. G., Kremeyer, B., Campbell, D. D., Muller, H., Valencia-Duarte, A. V., et al. (2013). CNV Analysis in tourette syndrome implicates large genomic rearrangements in COL8A1 and NRXN1. *PLoS ONE* 8:e59061. doi: 10.1371/journal.pone.0059061

Pagliaroli, L., Vető, B., Arányi, T., and Barta, C. (2016). From genetics to epigenetics: new perspectives in tourette syndrome research. *Front. Neurosci.* 10:277. doi: 10.3389/fnins.2016.00277

Paschou, P. (2013). The genetic basis of Gilles de la Tourette Syndrome. *Neurosci. Biobehav. Rev.* 37, 1026–1039. doi: 10.1016/j.neubiorev.2013.01.016

Plessen, K. J., Royal, J. M., and Peterson, B. S. (2007). Neuroimaging of tic disorders with co-existing attention-deficit/hyperactivity disorder. *Eur. Child Adolesc. Psychiatry* 16(Suppl. 1), 60–70. doi: 10.1007/s00787-007-1008-2

Risterucci, C., Coccurello, R., Banasr, M., Stutzmann, J. M., Amalric, M., and Nieoullon, A. (2006). The metabotropic glutamate receptor subtype 5 antagonist MPEP and the Na+ channel blocker riluzole show different neuroprotective profiles in reversing behavioral deficits induced by excitotoxic prefrontal cortex lesions. *Neuroscience* 137, 211–220. doi: 10.1016/j.neuroscience.2005.08.054

Robertson, M. M. (2000). Tourette syndrome, associated conditions and the complexities of treatment. *Brain* 123(Pt 3), 425–462. doi: 10.1093/brain/123.3.425

Robertson, M. M. (2008). The prevalence and epidemiology of Gilles de la Tourette syndrome. Part 1: the epidemiological and prevalence studies. *J. Psychosom. Res.* 65, 461–472. doi: 10.1016/j.jpsychores.2008.03.006

Robertson, M. M. (2015a). A personal 35 year perspective on Gilles de la Tourette syndrome: assessment, investigations, and management. *Lancet Psychiatry* 2, 88–104. doi: 10.1016/S2215-0366(14)00133-3

Robertson, M. M. (2015b). A personal 35 year perspective on Gilles de la Tourette syndrome: prevalence, phenomenology, comorbidities, and coexistent psychopathologies. *Lancet Psychiatry* 2, 68–87. doi: 10.1016/S2215-0366(14)00132-1

Roessner, V., Plessen, K. J., Rothenberger, A., Ludolph, A. G., Rizzo, R., Skov, L., et al. (2011). European clinical guidelines for Tourette syndrome and other tic disorders. Part II: pharmacological treatment. *Eur. Child Adolesc. Psychiatry* 20, 173–196. doi: 10.1007/s00787-011-0163-7

Scharf, J. M., Yu, D., Mathews, C. A., Neale, B. M., Stewart, S. E., Fagerness, J. A., et al. (2013). Genome-wide association study of Tourette's syndrome. *Mol. Psychiatry* 18, 721–728. doi: 10.1038/mp.2012.69

Schumann, G., Loth, E., Banaschewski, T., Barbot, A., Barker, G., Büchel, C., et al. (2010). The IMAGEN study: reinforcement-related behaviour in normal brain function and psychopathology. *Mol. Psychiatry* 15, 1128–1139. doi: 10.1038/mp.2010.4

Singer, H. S. (2013). Motor control, habits, complex motor stereotypies, and Tourette syndrome. *Ann. N.Y. Acad. Sci.* 1304, 22–31. doi: 10.1111/nyas.12281

Stewart, S. E., Yu, D., Scharf, J. M., Neale, B. M., Fagerness, J. A., Mathews, C. A., et al. (2013). Genome-wide association study of obsessive-compulsive disorder. *Mol. Psychiatry* 18, 788–798. doi: 10.1038/mp.2012.85

Sundaram, S. K., Huq, A. M., Wilson, B. J., and Chugani, H. T. (2010). Tourette syndrome is associated with recurrent exonic copy number variants(e-Pub ahead of print)(CME). *Neurology* 74, 1583–1590. doi: 10.1212/WNL.0b013e3181e0f147

Tang, Y., Gilbert, D. L., Glauser, T. A., Hershey, A. D., and Sharp, F. R. (2005). Blood gene expression profiling of neurologic diseases. *Arch. Neurol.* 62, 210–215. doi: 10.1001/archneur.62.2.210

Tian, Y., Gunther, J. R., Liao, I. H., Liu, D., Ander, B. P., Stamova, B. S., et al. (2011a). GABA- and acetylcholine-related gene expression in blood correlate with tic severity and microarray evidence for alternative splicing in Tourette syndrome: a pilot study. *Brain Res.* 1381, 228–236. doi: 10.1016/j.brainres.2011.01.026

Tian, Y., Liao, I. H., Zhan, X., Gunther, J. R., Ander, B. P., Liu, D., et al. (2011b). Exon expression and alternatively spliced genes in tourette syndrome. *Am. J. Med. Genet. Part B Neuropsychiatr. Genet.* 156, 72–78. doi: 10.1002/ajmg.b.31140

Tian, Y., Stamova, B., Ander, B., Jickling, G., Gunther, J., Corbett, B., et al. (2012). Correlations of gene expression with ratings of inattention and hyperactivity/impulsivity in tourette syndrome: a pilot study. *BMC Med. Genomics* 5:49. doi: 10.1186/1755-8794-5-49

Udvardi, P. T., Nespoli, E., Rizzo, F., Hengerer, B., and Ludolph, A. G. (2013). Nondopaminergic neurotransmission in the pathophysiology of tourette syndrome. *Int. Rev. Neurobiol.* 112, 95–130. doi: 10.1016/B978-0-12-411546-0.00004-4

van de Vondervoort, I., Poelmans, G., Aschrafi, A., Pauls, D. L., Buitelaar, J. K., Glennon, J. C., et al. (2016). An integrated molecular landscape implicates the regulation of dendritic spine formation through insulin-related signalling in obsessive-compulsive disorder. *J. Psychiatry Neurosci.* 41, 280–285. doi: 10.1503/jpn.140327

Zilhão, N. R., Padmanabhuni, S. S., Pagliaroli, L., Barta, C., BIOS Consortium, Smit, D. J. A., et al. (2015). Epigenome-wide association study of tic disorders. *Twin Res. Hum. Genet.* 18, 699–709. doi: 10.1017/thg.2015.72

12

Investigation of SNP rs2060546 Immediately Upstream to *NTN4* in a Danish Gilles de la Tourette Syndrome Cohort

Shanmukha S. Padmanabhuni [1]***, Rayan Houssari*** [2]***, Ann-Louise Esserlind*** [3]***, Jes Olesen*** [3]***, Thomas M. Werge*** [4]***, Thomas F. Hansen*** [4]***, Birgitte Bertelsen*** [2]***, Fotis Tsetsos*** [1]***, Peristera Paschou*** [1,5] ***and Zeynep Tümer*** [2]*

[1] *Department of Molecular Biology and Genetics, Democritus University of Thrace, Alexandroupoli, Greece,* [2] *Applied Human Molecular Genetics, Kennedy Center, Department of Clinical Genetics, Copenhagen University Hospital, Rigshospitalet, Glostrup, Denmark,* [3] *Danish Headache Center and Department of Neurology, Faculty of Health Sciences, University of Copenhagen, Glostrup Hospital, Glostrup, Denmark,* [4] *Institute of Biological Psychiatry, Mental Health Center Sct. Hans, Copenhagen University Hospital, Roskilde, Denmark,* [5] *Department of Biological Sciences, Purdue University, West Lafayette, IN, USA*

Edited by:
John Vijay Sagar Kommu, National Institute of Mental Health and Neurosciences, India

Reviewed by:
Munis Dundar, Erciyes University, Turkey
Subhash Chakraborty, Hindustan Aeronautics Limited Hospital, India

****Correspondence:***
Zeynep Tümer
zeynep.tumer@region.dk

Gilles de la Tourette syndrome (GTS) is a neuropsychiatric disorder characterized by multiple motor and vocal tics. GTS is a complex disorder, with environmental factors and several genes involved. Although variations within a few genes such as *AADAC*, *NRXN1*, *SLITRK1*, *HDC*, and *IMMP2L* have been tentatively associated with GTS (in a small number of patients), the causative genes underlying GTS pathophysiology remain unknown. In a previous genome-wide association study (GWAS) a single nucleotide polymorphism (SNP, rs2060546) near the Netrin-4 (*NTN4* - MIM 610401) gene was shown to be associated with GTS [odds ratio (OR) = 1.7; *p*-value = 5.8 × 10-7] thus warranting further investigations. As *NTN4* is one of the axon guidance molecules expressed in the central nervous system and it interacts with the encoded proteins of *SLIT* and *WNT* genes guiding the growth cone toward its target, it is an attractive candidate susceptibility gene for GTS. In this study we attempted to replicate the association of rs2060546 with GTS by genotyping a Danish cohort of 240 GTS patients and 1006 healthy controls. Our results did not reveal an association (OR = 1.363; *p*-value = 0.3329) in the Danish cohort alone, which may be due to the small sample size. However, a meta-analysis including the present cohort and a total of 1316 GTS patients and 5023 controls from the GTS GWAS Replication Initiative (GGRI) and the first GTS-GWAS yielded a significant signal (OR = 3.74; *p*-value = 0.00018) and same direction of effect in the three cohorts. Thus, our study strengthens the evidence of the possible involvement of *NTN4* in GTS etiology, suggesting that further studies in even larger samples and functional studies are warranted to investigate the role of this region in GTS pathogenesis.

Keywords: axon guidance, Gilles de la Tourette syndrome, GTS, Netrin-4, *NTN4*, single nucleotide polymorphism, SNP

INTRODUCTION

Gilles de la Tourette syndrome (GTS) is a complex juvenile-onset neuro-developmental disorder characterized by the occurrence of multiple motor and vocal tics (Nag et al., 2013). Recent epidemiological studies estimated the worldwide prevalence of GTS to be approximately 1% with a male:female ratio of 4:1 (Robertson et al., 2009). GTS is often associated with co-morbidities such as attention-deficit hyperactivity disorder and obsessive-compulsive disorder (Dietrich et al., 2014). Additional co-occurring conditions are behavioral and emotional difficulties (hyperactivity, anxiety, and depression), sleeping disturbances, intellectual disabilities and autism spectrum disorder (Singer and Rosenberg, 1988; Wood et al., 2003). Studies so far conducted on GTS showed that there is a complex interplay of environmental and genetic factors, confirming the notion that GTS is a highly complex disorder (Davis et al., 2013; Dietrich et al., 2014).

To identify the causative genes and the biological pathways involved in GTS several approaches have been pursued, including candidate gene studies, family studies using linkage analysis, analysis of chromosomal abnormalities including copy number variants (CNV) and hypothesis-free genome-wide association studies (GWAS) (Paschou, 2013). For instance, chromosomal abnormalities have proven useful for identifying new candidate genes in GTS affected patients (Bertelsen et al., 2013). Chromosomal abnormalities have probed new candidate regions containing susceptible genes such as Slit- and Ntrk-Like Family, Member 1 (*SLITRK1*—MIM 609678), Neuroligin

TABLE 1 | Summary of the three different cohorts included in the meta-analysis.

Cohort	Cases				Controls			
	Male	Female	Unknown	Total	Male	Female	Unknown	Total
Danish	208	53	0	261	649	403	1	1053
GGRI	498	127	11	636	346	284	11	641
GTS-GWAS	1012	273	0	1285	1931	3033	0	4964

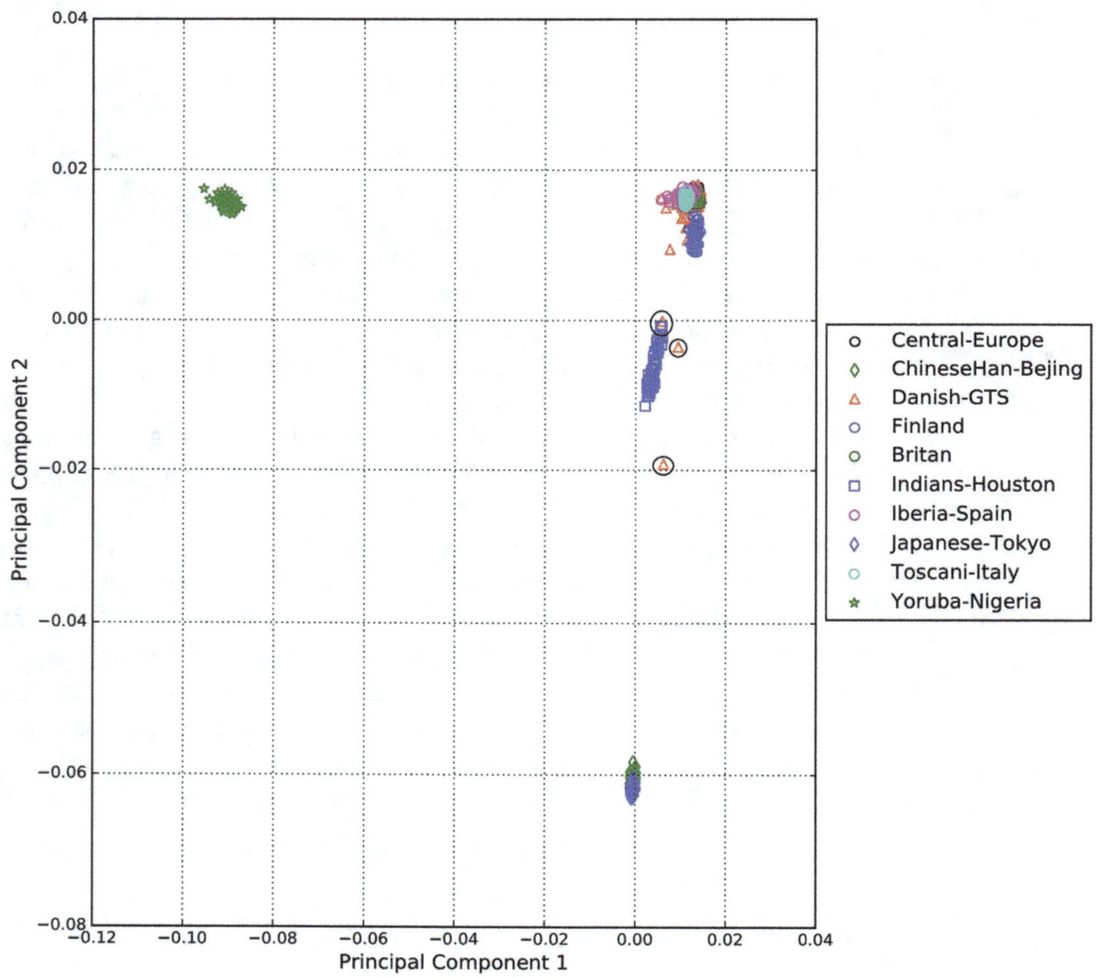

FIGURE 1 | Two dimensional PCA plot of Danish GTS cases with selected populations from 1000genomes cohort.

4 (*NLGN4*—MIM 300427) and Contactin-Associated Protein-Like2 (*CNTNAP2*—MIM 604569) (Verkerk et al., 2003; Abelson et al., 2005; Lawson-Yuen et al., 2008; Patel et al., 2011). Specific CNV analyses have resulted in the identification of several other candidate genes, including Arylacetamide Deacetylase (*AADAC*—MIM 600338), Collagen, Type VIII, Alpha-1 (*COL8A1*—MIM 120251), Neurexin I (*NRXN1*—MIM 00565), Catenin Alpha-3 (*CTNNA3*—MIM 607667) and Inner Mitochondrial Membrane Peptidase, Subunit 2, (*IMMP2L—MIM* 605977) (Sundaram et al., 2010; Nag et al., 2013; Bertelsen et al., 2014, 2015). The first large GWAS for GTS did not identify any genome-wide significance SNP (Scharf et al., 2013). A multinational consortium, GTS GWAS Replication Initiative (GGRI), followed up on the results of the initial GWAS in an independent cohort of 636 cases and 641 controls, showing an association between GTS and rs2060546 (OR = 2.41; p-value = 5.8×10^{-7}) on chromosome 12q23.1, ~32 kb upstream to the transcriptional start site of Netrin-4 (*NTN4*); a gene encoding an axon guidance protein expressed in the central nervous system (Paschou et al., 2014). As *NTN4* is an attractive candidate susceptibility gene, we investigated the association of rs2060546 with GTS in a Danish cohort of 240 GTS patients and 1006 healthy controls.

MATERIALS AND METHODS

Samples

We investigated a Danish cohort and two previously published datasets (GGRI and GTS-GWAS) (**Table 1**). The first cohort (n = 1314) includes 261 deeply phenotyped GTS patients and 1053 healthy controls from Denmark. Danish ancestry was investigated using the genotype information. The second cohort from GGRI includes 1277 individuals (636 GTS cases and 641 healthy controls) from different European populations (Paschou et al., 2014). The third cohort (GTS-GWAS) includes 6249

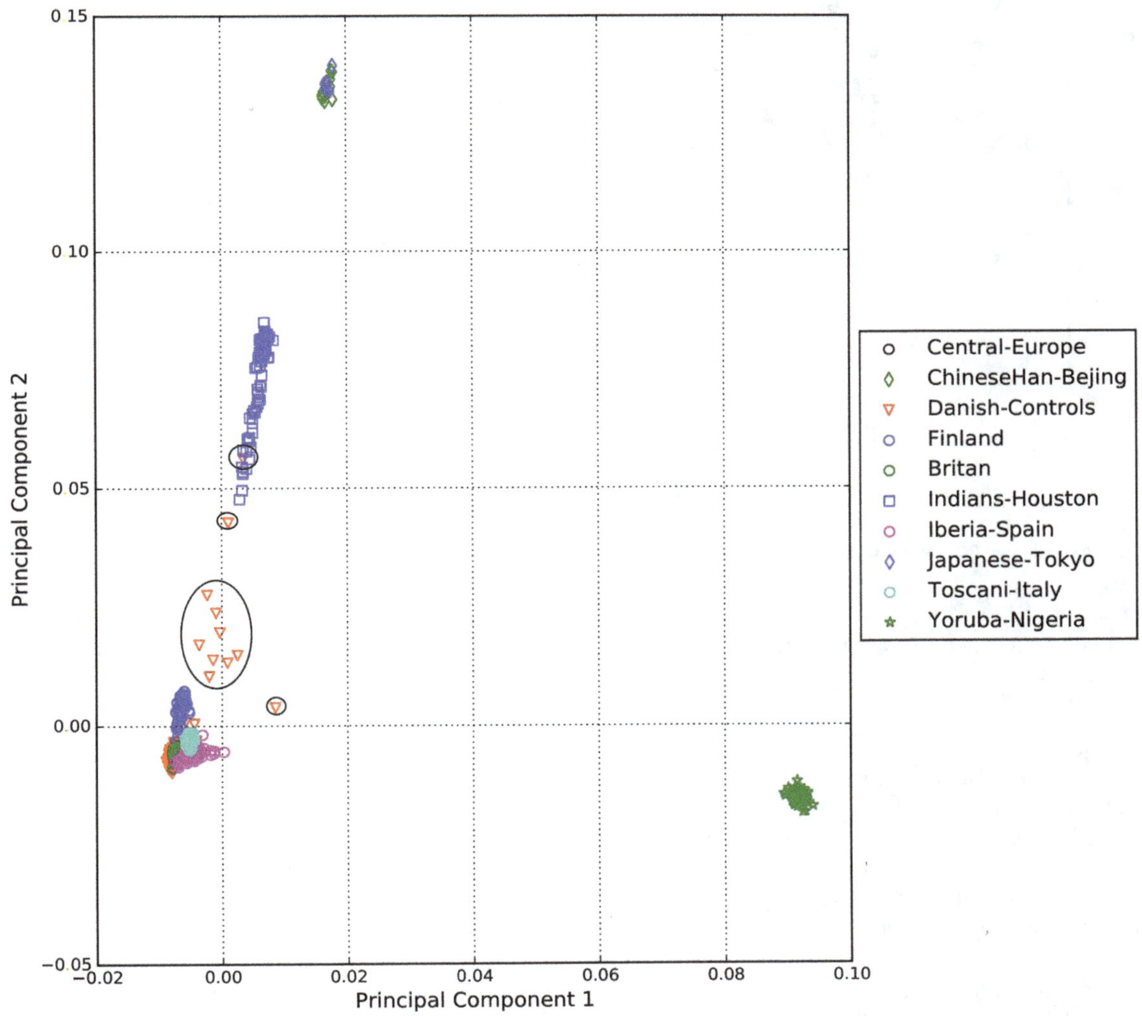

FIGURE 2 | Two dimensional PCA plots of Danish controls and selected populations of 1000genomes cohort.

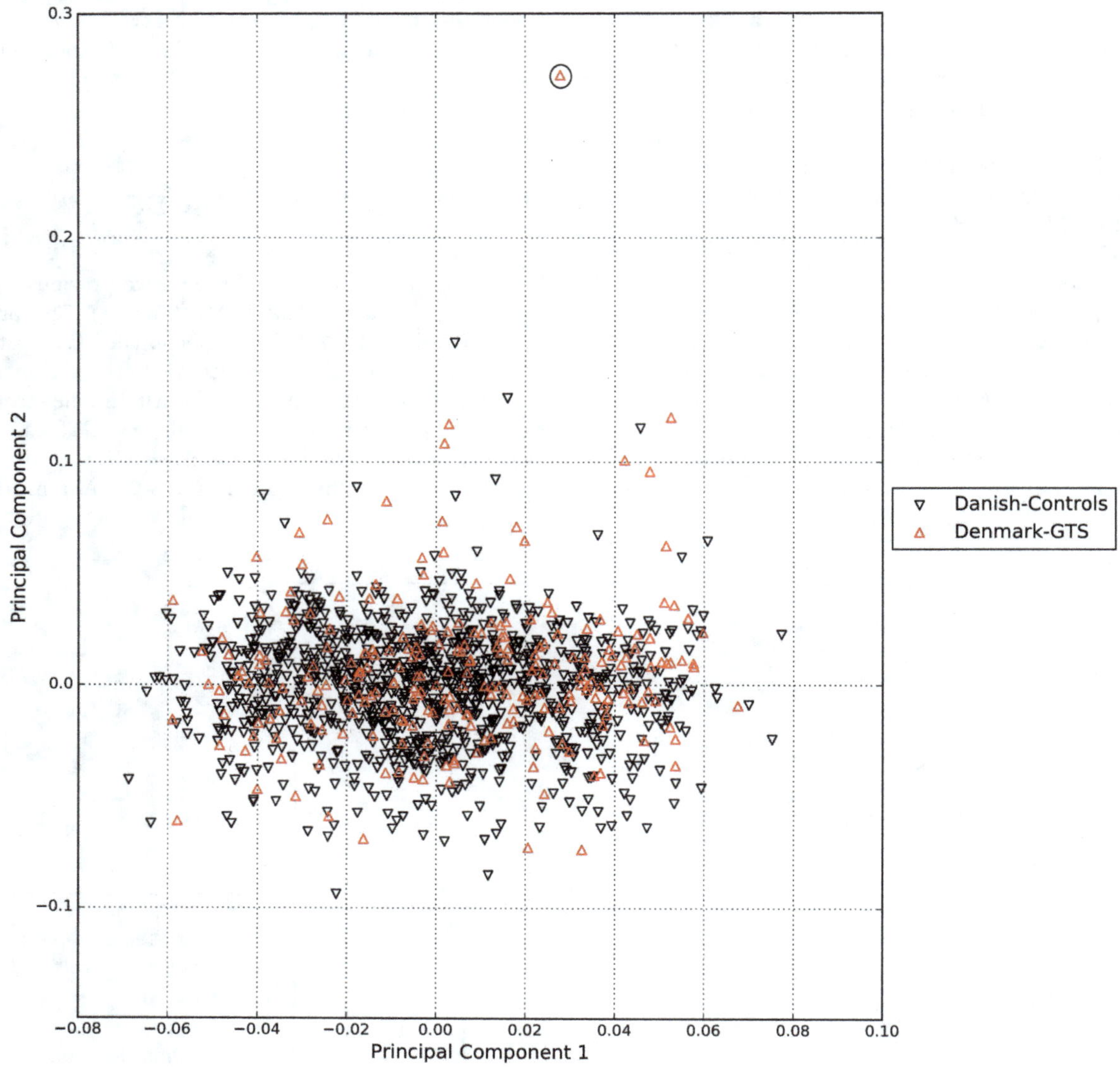

FIGURE 3 | Two dimensional PCA plot of Danish GTS cases and controls to check for population outliers.

individuals (1285 GTS cases and 4964 controls) of European ancestry (Scharf et al., 2013).

Genotyping

261 GTS cases from Denmark were genotyped on the Affymetrix CytoScanHD array (Affymetrix, Santa Clara, CA) covering around 750,000 single nucleotide polymorphisms (SNPs) and ~1.9 million single-locus copy number (CN) markers. 1053 healthy controls were genotyped on Illumina HumanOmniExpress arrays—18 on HumanOmniExpress12v1 and 1034 on HumanOmniExpress12v1-1 covering around 700,000 SNPs each. SNP calling and pre-processing of the raw data for Illumina controls were carried out using Illumina Genomestudio® software. For GTS cases genotyped on Affymetrix CytoScanHD SNP calling a pre-processing was carried out using default parameters for method apt-copynumber-cyto from Affymetrix Power Tools (APT, version 1.16) software.

Quality Control

A standard GWAS quality control measure (Scharf et al., 2013) was applied on both cases and controls from the Danish cohort to filter for population outliers and samples with low call rate; and to remove systematic bias using the software PLINK (Purcell et al., 2007). Quality control at SNP level includes removal of monomorphic SNPs, SNPs with genotyping rate < 98%, SNPs with no information about chromosome location, SNPs with absolute minor allele frequency difference > 0.15, SNPs that fail Hardy-Weinberg Equilibrium and SNPs with AT/CG alleles. To check the quality of the Danish GTS cases metric values for CytoScanHD array recommended by the manufacture was used in the pre-processing step. Sample call rate calculated using PLINK (Purcell et al., 2007) was used to filter out samples that had more than 2% of SNPs missing. F statistic was calculated using SNPs from the X-chromosome. $F < 0.25$ was assigned to female and $F > 0.75$ was assigned to male. Samples with an F-value between 0.25 and 0.75 were discarded due to sex ambiguity. Estimates of pairwise Identity-by-descent from PLINK (Purcell et al., 2007) were used to remove one of the samples from each pair which pass the relatedness metrics either pi-hat > 0.1 or Z1 > 0.2. Samples with high rates of heterozygosity $F_{het} > \pm 0.05$ are more likely to be result of contamination and were removed from the analysis. Principal Component Analysis (PCA) was applied using EIGENSTRAT (Price et al., 2006) and remaining samples were merged with the 1000 genomes cohort to remove European cluster and population outliers. Out of 261 GTS cases, four samples were removed as they did not lie inside the European cluster in **Figure 1**. Eleven healthy controls lied outside of the European cluster in **Figure 2** and were removed from the association analysis. After removing the European outliers, Danish GTS cases and healthy controls were merged for 126,821 common SNPs. The PCA plot in **Figure 3** was made using a LD-pruned set of ~90,000 SNPs to identify Danish outliers. One GTS case was removed as population outlier seen in **Figure 3** which left in total 240 Danish GTS cases and 1006 healthy controls.

Association Analysis

Standard case control association analysis using PLINK (Purcell et al., 2007) was performed using χ^2 test comparing SNP frequency between cases and controls.

TABLE 2 | Quality control steps at sample level with number of samples failed at each step.

Quality Control (QC) Step	Danish GTS Affymetrix CytoScanHD	Danish Controls Illumina OmniExpress
Samples before QC	261	1053
Pre-processing SNP quality	10	0
Sample Call Rate < 98%	0	2
Sex ambiguous samples	0	0
Low level related samples	1	26
Abnormal heterozygosity	5	8
European Outliers	4	11
Danish Outliers	1	0
Final Samples after QC	240	1006

Meta-Analysis

Metal (Willer et al., 2010) was used to perform sample weighted meta-analysis of association results of the SNP rs2060546 from all three cohorts. Association results for the GGRI and GTS-GWAS cohorts were taken from the original studies (Scharf et al., 2013; Paschou et al., 2014).

RESULTS

We attempted to replicate the association of SNP rs2060546 with GTS by investigating quality control passed genotyped data of 240 GTS patients and 1006 healthy controls from Denmark (**Table 2**). We did not find the SNP rs2060546 to be significantly associated in the Danish cohort (OR =1.363, 95% CI 0.7188-2.675; p-value = 0.3329) (**Table 3**). This might be attributed to the small size of the cohort and we proceeded to perform a meta-analysis with previously published data (Paschou et al., 2014). However, meta-analysis of the Danish, the GGRI and the first GTS-GWAS cohorts, showed significant association to the studied SNP (OR = 3.74; p-value = 0.00018) and the same direction of effect in all three cohorts (**Table 3**). Thus, the results supported the involvement of this particular chromosomal region in GTS etiology, and potentially *NTN4*.

DISCUSSION

Involvement of NTN4 in neurodevelopment makes it an attractive candidate protein as a contributing factor to GTS pathology. During the development of the nervous system, numerous dynamic guidance cues direct the trajectory of the migrating developed axon toward its suitable target (Killeen and Sybingco, 2008). Netrins are axon guidance cues which are composed of six members: Netrin 1-4 Netrin-related molecules, Netrin-G1 and G2 (Davis et al., 2013). Netrin-4 functions as guidance cue for axonal growth, neurite elongation, neuronal remodeling and plasticity (Zhang et al., 2004). The neuronal growth cones sense Netrin-4 as either attractant or repellent cues, depending on different receptors expressed on their surface or differences in the cellular signal transduction machinery (Koch et al., 2000; Qin et al., 2007). Netrin-4 might mediate axon outgrowth by attracting actions through deleted in colorectal carcinoma (DCC) or neogenin (Neo 1) receptors and repulsive effects through unc-5 homolog (UNC5A) receptors (Qin et al., 2007; Schubert et al., 2009). Previous imaging studies showed that changes in the thalamus and cerebral cortex volumes play a significant role in regulating the severity of tic symptoms implicated in GTS cases (Rueda et al., 2005; Rickards et al., 2008). Notably, expression of the *NTN4* gene was detected in human

TABLE 3 | The association results for *NTN4*—rs2060546 SNP in the three different cohorts.

Cohort	Minor allele	Mino allele frequency in GTS cases	Minor allele frequency in controls	*p*-value	Odds ratio (OR)
Danish	A	0.03099	0.02293	0.3329	1.363
GGRI	A	0.04844	0.02131	0.00033	2.41
GTS-GWAS	A	0.03834	0.02746	0.02	1.44

brain regions such as cerebellum, thalamus, cerebral cortex and olfactory bulb, thus, supporting the role of this gene in GTS pathogenesis (Zhang et al., 2004; Amat et al., 2006; Lee et al., 2006).

In this study, we could not identify any association between rs2060546 SNP and GTS in a relatively small Danish cohort alone, however, meta-analyses with the GGRI and GTS-GWAS cohorts provides further support for the possible association of this SNP with GTS in European populations. The close localization of rs2060546 to *NTN4* and the abundant expression of Netrin-4 in different brain regions, associated with GTS pathogenesis, rendered further support to the hypothesis that *NTN4* might be a new candidate gene for GTS.

AUTHOR CONTRIBUTIONS

SP, performed data analysis, interpretation, and participated in manuscript writing. ZT and PP supervised the study, interpretation of the results, and participated in manuscript writing. RH participated in biological relevance of result and manuscript writing. FT participated in data analysis and manuscript writing. AE, JO, TW, TH, ZT, BB provided the data and participated in manuscript writing. All authors read and approved the final version to be published and agreed to be accountable for all aspects of the work.

FUNDING

This project was supported by FP7-People-2012-ITN, project: TS-EUROTRAIN, grant number 316978; and Lundbeck Foundation, grant number R24-A2419 and R100-A9332.

ACKNOWLEDGMENTS

We would like to thank all individuals who participated and contributed to this work.

REFERENCES

Abelson, J. F., Kwan, K. Y., Roak, B. J. O., Baek, D. Y., Stillman, A. A., Morgan, T. M., et al. (2005). Sequence Variants in SLITRK1 are associated with Tourette' s Syndrome. *Science* 2126, 317–320. doi: 10.1126/science.1116502

Amat, J. A., Bronen, R. A., Saluja, S., Sato, N., Zhu, H., Gorman, D. A., et al. (2006). Increased number of subcortical hyperintensities on MRI in children and adolescents with Tourette's syndrome, obsessive-compulsive disorder, and attention deficit hyperactivity disorder. *Am. J. Psychiatry* 163, 1106–1108. doi: 10.1176/ajp.2006.163.6.1106

Bertelsen, B., Debes, N. M., Hjermind, L. E., Skov, L., Brøndum-Nielsen, K., and Tümer, Z. (2013). Chromosomal rearrangements in Tourette syndrome: implications for identification of candidate susceptibility genes and review of the literature. *Neurogenetics* 14, 197–203. doi: 10.1007/s10048-013-0372-y

Bertelsen, B., Melchior, L., Jensen, L. R., Groth, C., Glenthøj, B., Rizzo, R., et al. (2014). Intragenic deletions affecting two alternative transcripts of the IMMP2L gene in patients with Tourette syndrome. *Eur. J. Hum. Genet.* 22, 1283–1289. doi: 10.1038/ejhg.2014.24

Bertelsen, B., Stefánsson, H., Riff Jensen, L., Melchior, L., Mol Debes, N., Groth, C., et al. (2015). Association of AADAC Deletion and Gilles de la Tourette Syndrome in a Large European Cohort. *Biol. Psychiatry* 79, 383–391. doi: 10.1016/j.biopsych.2015.08.027

Davis, L. K., Yu, D., Keenan, C. L., Gamazon, E. R., Konkashbaev, A. I., Derks, E. M., et al. (2013). Partitioning the Heritability of Tourette Syndrome and obsessive compulsive disorder reveals differences in Genetic Architecture. *PLoS Genet.* 9:e1003864. doi: 10.1371/journal.pgen.1003864

Dietrich, A., Fernandez, T. V., King, R. A., State, M. W., Tischfield, J. A., Hoekstra, P. J., et al. (2014). The Tourette International Collaborative Genetics (TIC Genetics) study, finding the genes causing Tourette syndrome: objectives and methods. *Eur. Child Adolesc. Psychiatry* 24, 141–151. doi: 10.1007/s00787-014-0543-x

Killeen, M. T., and Sybingco, S. S. (2008). Netrin, Slit and Wnt receptors allow axons to choose the axis of migration. *Dev. Biol.* 323, 143–151. doi: 10.1016/j.ydbio.2008.08.027

Koch, M., Murrell, J. R., Hunter, D. D., Olson, P. F., Jin, W., Keene, D. R., et al. (2000). A novel member of the netrin family, beta-netrin, shares homology with the beta chain of laminin: identification, expression, and functional characterization. *J. Cell Biol.* 151, 221–234. doi: 10.1083/jcb.151.2.221

Lawson-Yuen, A., Saldivar, J.-S., Sommer, S., and Picker, J. (2008). Familial deletion within NLGN4 associated with autism and Tourette syndrome. *Eur. J. Hum. Genet.* 16, 614–618. doi: 10.1038/sj.ejhg.5202006

Lee, J. S., Yoo, S. S., Cho, S. Y., Ock, S. M., Lim, M. K., and Panych, L. P. (2006). Abnormal thalamic volume in treatment-naïve boys with Tourette syndrome. *Acta Psychiatr. Scand.* 113, 64–67. doi: 10.1111/j.1600-0447.2005.00666.x

Nag, A., Bochukova, E. G., Kremeyer, B., Campbell, D. D., Muller, H., Valencia-Duarte, A. V., et al. (2013). CNV analysis in Tourette syndrome implicates large genomic rearrangements in COL8A1 and NRXN1. *PLoS ONE* 8:e59061. doi: 10.1371/journal.pone.0059061

Paschou, P. (2013). The genetic basis of Gilles de la Tourette Syndrome. *Neurosci. Biobehav. Rev.* 37, 1026–1039. doi: 10.1016/j.neubiorev.2013.01.016

Paschou, P., Yu, D., Gerber, G., Evans, P., Tsetsos, F., Davis, L. K., et al. (2014). Genetic association signal near NTN4 in Tourette syndrome. *Ann. Neurol.* 76, 310–315. doi: 10.1002/ana.24215

Patel, C., Cooper-Charles, L., McMullan, D. J., Walker, J. M., Davison, V., and Morton, J. (2011). Translocation breakpoint at 7q31 associated with tics: further evidence for IMMP2L as a candidate gene for Tourette syndrome. *Eur. J. Hum. Genet.* 19, 634–639. doi: 10.1038/ejhg.2010.238

Price, A. L., Patterson, N. J., Plenge, R. M., Weinblatt, M. E., Shadick, N. A., and Reich, D. (2006). Principal components analysis corrects for stratification in genome-wide association studies. *Nat. Genet.* 38, 904–909. doi: 10.1038/ng1847

Purcell, S., Neale, B., Todd-Brown, K., Thomas, L., Ferreira, M. A. R., Bender, D., et al. (2007). PLINK: a tool set for whole-genome association and population-based linkage analyses. *Am. J. Hum. Genet.* 81, 559–575. doi: 10.1086/519795

Qin, S., Yu, L., Gao, Y., Zhou, R., and Zhang, C. (2007). Characterization of the receptors for axon guidance factor netrin-4 and identification of the binding domains. *Mol. Cell. Neurosci.* 34, 243–250. doi: 10.1016/j.mcn.2006.11.002

Rickards, H., Wood, C., and Cavanna, A. E. (2008). Hassler and Dieckmann's seminal paper on stereotactic thalamotomy for Gilles de la Tourette syndrome: Translation and critical reappraisal. *Mov. Disord.* 23, 1966–1972. doi: 10.1002/mds.22238

Robertson, M. M., Eapen, V., and Cavanna, A. E. (2009). The international prevalence, epidemiology, and clinical phenomenology of Tourette syndrome: a cross-cultural perspective. *J. Psychosom. Res.* 67, 475–483. doi: 10.1016/j.jpsychores.2009.07.010

Rueda, M. R., Posner, M. I., and Rothbart, M. K. (2005). The development of executive attention: contributions to the emergence of self-regulation. *Dev. Neuropsychol.* 28, 573–594. doi: 10.1207/s15326942dn2802_2

Scharf, J. M., Yu, D., Mathews, C. A., Neale, B. M., Stewart, S. E., Fagerness, J. A., et al. (2013). Genome-wide association study of Tourette Syndrome. *Mol. Psychiatry* 18, 721–728. doi: 10.1038/mp.2012.69

Schubert, T., Denk, A., Mägdefrau, U., Kaufmann, S., Bastone, P., Lowin, T., et al. (2009). Role of the Netrin system of repellent factors on synovial fibroblasts in rheumatoid arthritis and osteoarthritis. *Int. J. Immunopathol. Pharmacol.* 22, 715–722. doi: 10.1177/039463200902200317

Singer, H. S., and Rosenberg, L. A. (1988). Development of behavioral and emotional problems in Tourette syndrome. *Pediatr. Neurol.* 5, 41–44. doi: 10.1016/0887-8994(89)90008-8

Sundaram, S. K., Huq, A. M., Wilson, B. J., and Chugani, H. T. (2010). Tourette syndrome is associated with recurrent exonic copy number variants. *Neurology* 74, 1583–1590. doi: 10.1212/WNL.0b013e3181e0f147

Verkerk, A. J. M. H., Mathews, C. A., Joosse, M., Eussen, B. H. J., Heutink, P., and Oostra, B. A. (2003). CNTNAP2 is disrupted in a family with Gilles de la Tourette syndrome and obsessive compulsive disorder. *Genomics* 82, 1–9. doi: 10.1016/S0888-7543(03)00097-1

Willer, C. J., Li, Y., and Abecasis, G. R. (2010). METAL: fast and efficient meta-analysis of genomewide association scans. *Bioinformatics* 26, 2190–2191. doi: 10.1093/bioinformatics/btq340

Wood, B. L., Klebba, K., Gbadebo, O., Lichter, D., Kurlan, R., Miller, B., et al. (2003). Pilot study of effect of emotional stimuli on tic severity in children with Tourette's syndrome. *Mov. Disord.* 18, 1392–1395. doi: 10.1002/mds.10552

Zhang, C., Meng, F., Wang, C., Guo, H., Fan, M., Liu, S., et al. (2004). Identification of a novel alternative splicing form of human netrin-4 and analyzing the expression patterns in adult rat brain. *Brain Res. Mol. Brain Res.* 130, 68–80. doi: 10.1016/j.molbrainres.2004.07.009

13

Functional Evaluations of Genes Disrupted in Patients with Tourette's Disorder

Nawei Sun[1,2], *Jay A. Tischfield*[1,2], *Robert A. King*[3] *and Gary A. Heiman*[1,2*]

[1] *Department of Genetics, Rutgers University, Piscataway, NJ, USA,* [2] *Human Genetics Institute of New Jersey, Piscataway, NJ, USA,* [3] *Child Study Center, Yale School of Medicine, New Haven, CT, USA*

Edited by:
Peristera Paschou,
Democritus University of Thrace,
Greece

Reviewed by:
Fotis Tsetsos,
Democritus University of Thrace,
Greece
Marianthi Georgitsi,
Aristotle University of Thessaloniki,
Greece

***Correspondence:**
Gary A. Heiman
heiman@dls.rutgers.edu

Tourette's disorder (TD) is a highly heritable neurodevelopmental disorder with complex genetic architecture and unclear neuropathology. Disruptions of particular genes have been identified in subsets of TD patients. However, none of the findings have been replicated, probably due to the complex and heterogeneous genetic architecture of TD that involves both common and rare variants. To understand the etiology of TD, functional analyses are required to characterize the molecular and cellular consequences caused by mutations in candidate genes. Such molecular and cellular alterations may converge into common biological pathways underlying the heterogeneous genetic etiology of TD patients. Herein, we review specific genes implicated in TD etiology, discuss the functions of these genes in the mammalian central nervous system and the corresponding behavioral anomalies exhibited in animal models, and importantly, review functional analyses that can be performed to evaluate the role(s) that the genetic disruptions might play in TD. Specifically, the functional assays include novel cell culture systems, genome editing techniques, bioinformatics approaches, transcriptomic analyses, and genetically modified animal models applied or developed to study genes associated with TD or with other neurodevelopmental and neuropsychiatric disorders. By describing methods used to study diseases with genetic architecture similar to TD, we hope to develop a systematic framework for investigating the etiology of TD and related disorders.

Keywords: Tourette's disorder, functional studies, genes, neurobiology, induced pluripotent stem cells

INTRODUCTION

Tourette's Disorder (TD) is a childhood-onset neurodevelopment disorder characterized by the presence of both motor and vocal tics. Prevalence ranges from 1–3% and is found across many ethnic groups around the world (1). However, a recent meta-analysis of previous TD prevalence studies re-estimates the population prevalence of TD to be 0.3–0.9% (2). Males are affected three to four times more often than females (3–5). A high percentage of TD patients have comorbid conditions, most commonly attention-deficit/hyperactivity disorder (ADHD) and obsessive–compulsive disorder (OCD) and to a lesser extent autism spectrum disorders (ASDs).

Consistent evidence from family and twin studies suggest a significant genetic contribution to TD, most likely the result of complex and heterogeneous inheritance involving both common and rare variants, though most of specific findings still require replication. The neurobiological basis of TD is not well understood, but appears to involve alterations in the development, structure, and/or functioning of cortico-striato-thalamo-cortical (CSTC) circuits (6). Specific genes have been found to be associated with TD. It is unclear if mutations in these genes cause TD and, if so, how these alterations affect the function or structural development of the nervous system. Our focus is to review the neurobiology of TD, describe the biological functions of those genes previously associated with TD, and discuss the various functional analyses that are required for evaluating and establishing the pathogenicity of these putative genetic causal variants for TD.

NEUROBIOLOGY OF TOURETTE'S DISORDER

Alterations of the CSTC circuits are considered as the neuropathological basis of tic generation (6, 7). These alterations are apparent in functional and structural imaging studies (8), histopathological studies of specific neuronal populations (9), and defective inhibition in various electroneurophysiological experimental paradigms (10, 11). In addition to the male predominance, the developmental features of TD pose an explanatory challenge, with tics usually not appearing till 4–6 years of age and most often, but not always, improving spontaneously by late adolescence.

Neurotransmitter pathways that modulate the activity and the output of the CSTC circuits in the basal ganglia have been the focus of intensive investigation, driven in part by the quest for more effective pharmacological interventions. The most supported neurotransmitter dysregulation hypothesis in TD involves the hyperactivity or imbalance of the dopamine signaling in the striatum (12). Within the basal ganglia, dopamine is released to the striatum by dopaminergic neurons originating from the substantia nigra. In the striatum, the effect of dopamine on subsequent neural signal transmission is modulated by the striatal medium spiny neurons expressing either D1 or D2-like dopamine receptors (13). The dopamine hypothesis is supported by the clinical observation that dopamine D2 receptor antagonists effectively reduced tics in some TD patients (14, 15). Also, dopamine pathway dysregulation was reported in post-mortem TD brain samples (16, 17) and in living TD patients' brain (12, 18).

Due to their excitatory and inhibitory effects within CSTC circuits, glutamatergic and GABAergic pathways have also been studied in TD. In post-mortem samples, lower levels of glutamate in subcortical brain regions were reported (19). However, it is unclear whether TD is associated with hyper- or hypo-glutamate levels (20). For the GABAergic pathway, an altered number and distribution of striatal GABAergic neurons were described in TD post-mortem brain samples (9, 21).

Disrupted serotonin signaling has been implicated in OCD, a common comorbid condition among TD patients. Selective serotonin reuptake inhibitors (SSRIs) have proven effective in reducing OCD symptoms (22) and are also used to treat TD patients with comorbid OCD (23). Interestingly, sequence variants at the serotonin transporter (SERT) gene were found in both OCD and TD patients (24), suggesting alterations in the serotonin pathway as one possible mechanism in the etiology of TD.

Until the recent discovery of a dominant negative non-sense mutation in the *HDC* gene co-segregating with TD in a large family, histaminergic (HA) neurotransmission was not considered a top candidate for TD etiology (25). However, other findings provide additional support for the involvement of HA neurotransmission in TD. For example, single nucleotide polymorphisms (SNPs) within the *HDC* gene region showed association with TD (26). Also, rare copy number variants (CNVs) found in TD patients were enriched in chromosomal regions harboring HA pathway genes (27). Furthermore, mice lacking the *Hdc* gene exhibited tic-like behaviors (28). Even though no evidence showed direct actions of serotonin and histamine on movements, it is proposed that serotonin and histamine pathways might indirectly regulate movements by modulating the dopamine system in the substantia nigra. In particular, both serotoninergic and HA innervations are observed in the substantia nigra (29, 30). Also, serotonin and histamine receptors are expressed on nigrostriatal dopaminergic neurons (30, 31).

Aside from the neurotransmitter dysregulation hypothesis in TD, developmental and neuroimmunological findings also provide a context for assessing the relevance of potential gene findings. Altered distribution of parvalbumin interneurons (21) and reduced numbers of parvalbumin and cholinergic interneurons in basal ganglia were observed in the post-mortem brain samples of TD patients (9), suggesting another possible, perhaps developmental, mechanism for alterations of CSTS circuits. Additionally, a dysregulated brain-immune system involving microglia cells was suggested to contribute to TD (32). Gene expressions of inflammatory factors were examined using post-mortem basal ganglia samples from TD patients and controls (33). An elevated expression of the *CD45* gene was observed in TD patients even though the elevation was not statistically significant. CD45 is a surface marker of microglia and its expression is increased due to the activation of microglia. In another study, transcriptome analysis of post-mortem striatum of TD patients and controls revealed upregulation of microglia-related genes (34).

GENES DISRUPTED IN PATIENTS WITH TOURETTE'S DISORDER

In this section, we will review 15 genes that have been associated in TD (**Table 1**); to suggest how we might move beyond association to establish a role in TD pathogenesis, we will examine what is known about the biological effects of these genes. We group these genes into several categories: (1) neurite outgrowth: *SLITRK1*; (2) histamine pathway: *HDC*; (3) serotonin pathway: *SERT, HTR1A HTR2B*; (4) glutamate pathway: *SLC1A3*; (5) synaptic signal transduction and cell-adhesion pathway: *NLGN4, CDH2, CNTNAP2/CASPR2, DPP6*; (6) mitochondrial functions: *IMMP2L, MRPL3*; and (7) genes associated with other diseases: *DNAJC13* [Parkinson's disease (PD)], *OFCC1* (orofacial clefts), and *HCRTR2 or OX2R* (excessive daytime sleepiness). The diverse functions of these genes – ranging from neurotransmitter synthesis, neuronal migration, synaptic plasticity, cell adhesion, and protein transportation and synthesis – highlight the complexity of unraveling the pathogenesis of TD. However, in addition to the

TABLE 1 | Genes disrupted in TD.

Biological pathways	Gene name	Disruption(s) found in TD patients and references
Neurite outgrowth	*SLITRK1*	Inversion, frameshift variant, Var321 (38) Synonymous variant: 708C > T (39) 3'-UTR variant: 3383G > A (43) 3225 T > C (41) D397G (44)
Histamine	*HDC*	W317X (25) Intronic transition and synonymous variants: 426C > A, 1743G > A (55)
Serotonin	*SERT*	I425V and 5-HTTLPR (24)
	HTR1A	R219L (78)
	HTR2B	M63R, R449Q (79)
Glutamate	*SLC1A3/EAAT1*	E219D (88)
Synaptic signal transduction and cell adhesion	*NLGN4/NLGN4X*	Deletion across exon 4, 5 and 6 (99)
	CDH2	N706S, N845S (106)
	CNTNAP2	Intronic insertion (121)
	DPP6	Microdeletion at exon 1 (128)
Mitochondrial functions	*IMMP2L*	Translocation (141) *De novo* duplication (142) Translocation and cryptic deletion eliminated the exon 1–3 (143) Intragenic deletions (144)
	MRPL3	S75N (150)
Genes associated with other diseases	*DNAJC13* (Parkinson's disease)	A2057S (150)
	OFCC1 (orofacial clefts)	R129G and a novel variant at 5'-UTR (150)
	HCRTR2/OX2R (excessive daytime sleepiness)	P10S (162)

genetic disruptions discussed here, large structural variations, for example copy number variations (CNVs), have also been investigated in TD patients. Genes disrupted by these structural variants have been discovered and indicated as potential TD associated genes (35–37).

Neurite Outgrowth

SLIT and NTRK-Like Family, Member 1 (*SLITRK1*)

In a TD patient with comorbid ADHD, a *de novo* chromosome 13 inversion was identified (38). The *SLITRK1* gene was mapped close to the breakpoints. Targeted sequencing of the *SLITRK1* gene identified a non-coding variant (var321) and a frameshift mutation (38) in another 174 unrelated TD patients but not in a large control sample. The frameshift mutation led to impaired dendrite growth in neurons and the var321 variant may cause reduced SLITRK1 protein expression (38). While the var321 and additional novel variants within *SLITRK1* were found in other TD patients, these associations were not replicated in subsequent studies (39–49).

Members of the SLITRK protein family are transmembrane proteins. They are structurally homologous to the SLIT and the TRK proteins, which are involved in axon guidance pathway and neurodevelopment (50). The *SLITRK1* gene is highly expressed in developing and mature neuronal tissues and promotes neurite outgrowth in culture (51). The SLITRK1 protein is localized to the post-synaptic densities and has been hypothesized to affect synapse formation at excitatory synapses through interactions with the pre-synaptic cellular adhesion molecule LAR-RPTP (52, 53). In *Slitrk1* knockout mice, although stereotypic behaviors were not observed, the mice exhibited anxiety-like and depression-like behaviors, which were attenuated by chemicals modulating noradrenergic neurotransmission (54). Neurochemical abnormalities were also detected in *Slitrk1* knockout mice: norepinephrine and its metabolites were significantly increased in the prefrontal cortex and the nucleus accumbens while choline and acetylcholine levels were significantly lower in the striatum (54). Taken together, the evidence suggests that the *SLITRK1* gene might play a role in neurochemical modulation.

Histamine Pathway

Histidine Decarboxylase

Histamine neurotransmission was first linked to the etiology of TD when a rare non-sense mutation within the *HDC* gene was discovered in a multiplex family in which the father and all eight children were diagnosed with TD. The mutation resulted from a G to A transition at the ninth exon of the *HDC* gene and led to a premature stop codon (W317X) (25). The heterozygous W317X mutation co-segregated with all affected individuals in this family. The W317X mutation was not found in 3360 unrelated individuals unaffected with TD or another 720 TD patients, suggesting this is a very rare cause for TD. *In vitro* enzymatic assay demonstrated that the truncated protein produced by the mutation lost histidine decarboxylase (HDC) activity and had a dominant negative effect on the activity of wild-type HDC protein. After the initial finding, more TD patients were screened for mutations in the *HDC* gene in different studies. Only an intronic variant and two synonymous variants were identified in a study involving 120 TD patients (55). However, an association of the *HDC* gene and TD phenotypes was reported in a study including 520 TD nuclear families (26). Also, rare, genic CNVs identified in 460 TD patients were enriched for HA pathway genes (27), supporting the potential involvement of the histamine pathway in TD etiology.

In the adult human central nervous system, the *HDC* gene is exclusively expressed in the soma and axon varicosities of HA neurons mostly originating from the tuberomammillary nucleus in the posterior hypothalamic region of the brain (30). The HDC homodimer converts L-histidine into histamine in the soma of HA neurons. Histamine-containing neuronal fibers are seen in many brain areas in rodents and human including cerebral cortex (56, 57). Therefore, loss-of-function mutations at the *HDC* gene will likely cause a lack of histamine in the widespread brain regions receiving HA innervation. In addition to serving as a neurotransmitter, histamine is a neuromodulator, inhibiting dopamine release by striatal dopaminergic neurons through binding to the H3 receptors expressed on these neurons in mice (58). Given the hypothesis that hyperactivity of nigrostriatal dopaminergic neurons is responsible for tic generation (12), it is reasonable that histamine dysregulation may contribute to TD.

Since HDC protein functions as a homodimer (59), individuals harboring the W317X mutation have approximately 25% residual HDC activity remaining compared to the healthy controls. Therefore, the *Hdc* knockout mice may recapitulate the behavioral outcomes caused by the W317X mutation in humans. As expected, the *Hdc* knockout mice show tic-like stereotypic behaviors after psychostimulant administration and reduced prepulse inhibition (28). Interestingly, the striatal dopamine level was increased in the *Hdc* knockout mice during the dark cycle, which could be decreased by administration of histamine in the knockout mice. Also, higher levels of dopamine D2 receptor occupancy were found in the basal ganglia of TD patients carrying the W317X mutations, the *Hdc* knockout mice and the *Hdc* heterozygous mice, indicating that the dopamine release in the basal ganglia of the brain might be disinhibited due to histamine depletion (28). Taken together, parallel studies in TD subjects and mice demonstrated that lack of histamine results in dopamine dysregulation, providing a potential mechanism for the proposed role of dopamine disruption in TD (12).

Serotonin Pathway

Serotonin Transporter (*SLC6A4* or *SERT*)

Given the effectiveness of the SSRIs in reducing OCD symptoms, the *SERT* gene has been studied as candidate gene for OCD (60–64). Serotonin-transporter-linked polymorphic region (5-HTTLPR) polymorphisms and a gain-of-function missense mutation I425V have been associated with OCD (65–69). Sequence variants of the *SERT* gene were first associated with TD in a two-generation pedigree (24). In this family, the heterozygous "long" 5-HTTLPR variant and the I425V mutation perfectly segregated with TD individuals in a dominant pattern. The "long" 5-HTTLPR produces higher *SERT* mRNA level compared to the "short" 5-HTTLPR (70). The I425V mutation results in constitutive activation of the SERT protein whose activity is regulated by cGMP-dependent protein kinase (71). Therefore, carrying both "long" 5-HTTLPR and the I425V mutation is expected to have a synergistic effect that increases the expression of *SERT* mRNA and increases the amount of activated SERT protein.

In the mammalian central nervous system, the *SERT* gene is primarily expressed in the serotonergic neurons that originate from the raphe nucleus in the hindbrain and project widely to other parts of the nervous system, descending to the spinal cord and ascending to the forebrain (72). The human SERT protein is a transmembrane protein (73, 74). Cell surface expression of SERT protein can be regulated by SERT antagonists and substrates (75). The serotonergic axons can innervate and regulate other neurotransmission systems. For example, serotonin can facilitate or inhibit dopamine release in the striatum in a direct or indirect manner (76). Therefore, dysregulation of SERT expression on the plasma membrane may affect dopamine transmission (77). So far, no other sequence variants in the *SERT* gene have been associated with TD and no corresponding transgenic mice are available for *in vivo* studies.

Serotonin Receptor 1A (*HTR1A*) and Serotonin Receptor 2B (*HTR2B*)

In addition to the SERT gene, other serotonin pathway genes have been examined in TD patients. A missense mutation causing an amino acid change from arginine to leucine was identified in the serotonin receptor 1A gene (*HTR1A*) in one TD patient. However, the mutation was not predicted to change the receptor activity (78). Two novel non-synonymous missense variants and three known SNPs in the serotonin receptor 2B (*HTR2B*) gene were also found in 132 Caucasian and 128 Chinese Han TD individuals, though the associations were not statistically significant (79).

There are currently 14 known serotonin receptors and these are categorized into seven classes (80, 81). The *HTR1A* and *HTR2B*, both of which are G protein-coupled receptors, belong to class I and class II, respectively (81). The HTR1A receptor is highly expressed in the brain. Lower brain expression of the HTR1A receptor has been associated with mood disorders in humans. *Htr1a* knockout mice exhibit depression- and anxiety-like behaviors and have been used for antidepressant drug screening (82, 83). The HTR1A receptors are located at both pre-synaptic and post-synaptic neurons in the CNS. Activation of the pre-synaptic HTR1A receptors on the serotonergic neurons leads to inhibition of serotonergic neuron firing and reduced serotonin release whereas activation of the post-synaptic HTR1A can modulate the release of other neurotransmitters (84). Compared to the HTR1A receptor, the role that HTR2B plays in the CNS is not well understood. However, there is evidence suggesting that HTR2B may regulate SERT activity by phosphorylating SERT protein (85). In mice, the HTR2B receptor may be involved in modulating serotonin release from the serotonergic neurons. (86). Taken together, dysfunction of the HTR1A or the HTR2B receptor might lead to abnormal serotonin release in the CNS.

Glutamate Pathway

Excitatory Amino Acid Transporter 1 (*SLC1A3* or *EAAT1*)

Altered cortico-striatal-thalamo-cortical (CSTC) circuitry is believed to provide the neurobiological basis for TD (7, 87). Glutamate is the major excitatory neurotransmitter in CSTS circuitry. A missense mutation (E219D) in the glutamate transporter gene (*SLC1A3*) was associated with TD in a case-control study (88). In the same study, cells transfected with the E219D mutant glutamate transporter gene exhibited increased glutamate uptake activity compared to cells transfected with the wild-type gene. The proposed mechanism for the increased glutamate uptake activity was elevated glutamate transporter expression at the plasma membrane due to the E219D mutation. However, whether TD might be associated with hypo- or hyper-glutamate activity is still controversial.

One of the five subtypes of glutamate transporters, EAAT1, is responsible for the reuptake of the excitatory neurotransmitter, L-Glutamate, from the synapses back into cells. Dysfunction of glutamate transporters may lead to imbalanced extracellular glutamate levels, further affecting downstream glutamate neurotransmission or causing glutamate excitotoxicity to neurons (89, 90). EAAT1 is primarily expressed in glial cells. Regionally, EAAT1 proteins are found in neocortex, striatum, cerebellum, and spinal cord (91). *Eaat1* knockout mice showed hyperactivity and reduced acoustic startle response compared with the wild-type mice (92) but did not exhibit the altered prepulse inhibition behavior, which has been found in TD patients (93). No *Eaat1* gain-of-function mutant mice are available to test the "hypo-glutamate activity" hypothesis in TD.

Synaptic Signal Transduction and Cell-Adhesion Pathways

Neuroligin 4, X Linked (*NLGN4* or *NLGN4X*)

Mutations in the neuroligin (NLGN) family members have been identified in patients with neuropsychiatric disorders such as ASD (94–97) and schizophrenia (98). A small deletion in the *NLGN4* gene was detected in a mother and her two sons (99), one of whom was diagnosed with autism while the other was diagnosed with TD and ADHD. Their mother, who also carried the deletion, had a learning disability, depression, and anxiety. The deletion spanned exon 4, 5, and 6 of the *NLGN4* gene, resulting in a truncated protein. No other known genes were affected by the deletion.

Neuroligins are cell adhesion molecules located on the plasma membrane of the pre-synaptic and post-synaptic neurons. By interacting with neurexins, another family of cell adhesion proteins, NLGNs modulate proper signal transmission between pre-synaptic and post-synaptic neurons (100).Reduced expression of NLGNs in cultured neurons or mice cause deficits in synaptic maturation and plasticity (101, 102). *Nlgn4* knockout mice have been studied at both the behavioral and cellular levels. Because *Nlgn4* gene disruptions had been associated with ASD, the *Nlgn4* knockout mice were tested for ASD-like behaviors. As expected, *Nlgn4* knockout mice exhibited deficits in social interactions and reduced ultrasonic vocalizations compared to the wild-type mice (103). In another study, the *Nlgn4* knockout mice displayed reduced neural network response upon stimulation in both excitatory and inhibitory circuits (104). More interestingly, the *Nlgn4* knockout mice also showed stereotypic repetitive behaviors and increased obsessive compulsive like behaviors (105), supporting the possibility that disruption of the *NLGN4* gene might play a role in TD or related disorders.

Cadherin 2, Type1, N-Cadherin (*CDH2*)

Cadherin 2 (CDH2), also known as N-Cadherin, is another cell adhesion protein that has been associated with TD. CDH2 participates in neuron–neuron communication and in synaptogenesis. In a recent study, exons of the *CDH2* gene were sequenced in 160 OCD probands and 160 controls (106). Four variants in the *CDH2* gene were identified in subjects with OCD or TD. Two mutations were of particular interest: the N706S and the N845S variants. N706S is a rare and novel mutation close to the predicted proteolytic cleavage site of the CDH2 protein while the N845S variant is located at the β-catenin interacting region. Both mutations reduced the CDH2 protein level by more than 50% in transfected HEK293 cells (106), suggesting possible adhesion deficits in cells.

Cadherin 2 is a calcium-dependent cell–cell adhesion glycoprotein. CDH2 primarily mediates neurite outgrowth and axon guidance of neurons on myotubes (107) and on the surface of astrocytes (108, 109). The cytosolic domain of the CDH2 protein forms complexes with catenin proteins (110), and these complexes regulate synaptogenesis in both pre- and post-synaptic neurons (111, 112). Additionally, the cleaved C-terminal domain of the CDH2 is a repressor of CBP/CREB-mediated transcription whose target genes are critical in neural development and plasticity (113). The complete knockout of the *Cdh2* gene is an embryonic lethal in mice whereas *Cdh2* heterozygous null mice do not exhibit obvious morphological defects during development (114). Conditional knockout of the *Cdh2* gene in the cerebral cortex of mice caused disrupted cortical structure (115). Thus far, behavioral analyses in the *Cdh2+/−* mice or *Cdh2* conditional knockout mice have not been conducted.

Contactin-Associated Protein-Like 2 (*CNTNAP2/CASPR2*)

Variants in the *CNTNAP2* gene have been associated with ASD in several family based studies (116–119). Also, putative deleterious mutations were found in the *CNTNAP2* gene in ASD patients (120). In one family, an insertion on chromosome 7p35–p36, disrupting intron 8 of the *CNTNAP2* gene, was shared by a father and his two children, all three of whom were diagnosed with TD (121). However, a translocation disrupting intron 11 of *CNTNAP2* did not cause TD phenotypes in another three generation family (122).

CNTNAP2, a transmembrane protein, belongs to the neurexin superfamily and is highly expressed in neurons and localized to the axonal membrane of the juxtaparanodal region. The CNTNAP2 protein interacts with clustered Shaker-type potassium channels and plays an important role in the axon-glia septate-like junction (123). It is required for normal action potential propagation along myelinated axons of the neurons (124), and it has been hypothesized that malfunctions of the CNTNAP2 protein leads to deficits of electric signal transduction between neurons (121, 125, 126).

Behavioral assessments of *Cntnap2* knockout mice led to stereotypic motor movements (127). Interestingly, a reduced number of GABAergic interneurons were reported in the striatum of the *Cntnap2* knockout mice, which is consistent with previous post-mortem studies showing a reduction in the number of striatal GABAergic interneurons in TD patients (9, 21). Therefore, understanding the molecular mechanism of neuronal loss caused by disruption of CNTNAP2 may help to pinpoint biological pathways altered in TD.

Dipeptidyl-Peptidase 6

A heterozygous microdeletion at the first exon of the *DPP6* gene was identified in a boy with TD as well as the boy's father and paternal uncle both of whom were diagnosed with tic disorder and ADHD (128). The microdeletion led to decreased *DPP6* mRNA level in the boy's blood cells. *DPP6* has also been associated with other neuropsychiatric disorders such as ASD (95, 129) and schizophrenia (130).

Dipeptidyl-peptidase 6 (DPP6) is a transmembrane protein belonging to a family of serine proteases. However, DPP6 does not have protease activity (131). DPP6's expression is enriched in the brain and different isoforms have different distributions in the brain. (132). DPP6 proteins interact with A-type voltage-gated potassium channels, specifically the Kv4 subunit (133, 134). The A-type potassium channels participate in the modulation of dendritic signal transmission (135, 136). Moreover, the A-type potassium channel was reported to control the tonic dopamine release by substantia nigra dopaminergic neurons (137). Even though DPP6 has no peptidase activity, it may have novel functions and play essential roles in Kv4 intracellular trafficking, membrane expression, and proper function of the A-type potassium channels (138). *Dpp6* knockout mice show abnormal synaptogenesis (139), and knocking down the *Dpp6* gene specifically in the mouse brain caused impaired learning and memory abilities (140).

Mitochondria Functions

Inner Mitochondrial Membrane Peptidase 2 Like

A familial translocation segregating with TD or tics (141) and a *de novo* duplication in a TD patient with other developmental and mental phenotypes implicated *IMMP2L* as a possible TD candidate gene (142). This was the first mitochondria-related gene in TD. Subsequently, a cryptic deletion eliminating exons 1–3 of the *IMMP2L* gene and 21 other genes was identified in a TD patient with learning and speech difficulties (143). Also, a case-control study of copy number variations reported intragenic deletions at the *IMMP2L* gene in seven TD patients (144). Among the seven, three deletions at intron 3 led to production of a shorter *IMMP2L* mRNA transcript due to alternative splicing. In the same study, the expression of both the short and the long transcripts was examined by reverse transcription PCR in 19 regions of the human brain. While the long transcript was ubiquitously expressed in all 19 brain regions, the short transcript was selectively expressed at a lower level in only 10 brain regions, suggesting that the short transcript might have a more specific role in the human central nervous system (144).

The human inner mitochondrial membrane peptidase 2 like (IMMP2L) protein is one of the catalytic subunits of the inner mitochondrial membrane peptidase (IMP) complex (145, 146). The IMP complex participates in the cleavage of the inner mitochondrial membrane targeting signal sequence from its protein substrates, allowing maturation of the substrates. Loss of any subunit will cause the decomposition of the whole complex (147). Expression and function of the mammalian IMMP2L protein have been studied in animal models and human tissues. *Immp2l* knockout mice exhibit mitochondrial dysfunction, increased ischemic brain damage, and infertility (148, 149).The human *IMMP2L* mRNAs are ubiquitously expressed in various tissues except for adult liver and lungs. Unlike other TD associated genes, there is no enriched *IMMP2L* mRNA expression in the brain compared to other tissues (142). However, linking mitochondrial dysfunction to TD might lead to further speculation about the varied etiology of TD.

Mitochondrial Ribosomal Protein L3

Whole exome sequencing of a multiplex TD family showed three rare novel non-synonymous mutations in the *MRPL3*, *DNAJC13*, and the *OFCC1* genes (150). The three variants were not found in controls or dbSNPs/1000 Genomes databases. However, a targeted-sequencing study of the same three variants in Han Chinese TD patients did not replicate these findings (151).

Mitochondrial ribosomal protein L3 (MRPL3) is a mitochondrial ribosome protein involved in mitochondrial protein translation (152). Compound heterozygous mutations in the *MRPL3* gene were associated with mitochondrial respiratory chain deficiency in a pedigree of French origin (153), but no psychiatric diseases were reported.

Genes Associated with Other Diseases

DnaJ (Hsp40) Homolog, Subfamily C, Member 13 (*DNAJC13*)

A missense variant (A2057S) in the *DNAJC13* gene was found to segregate with TD or chronic tic disorder (CTD) in a multiplex pedigree (150). Subsequently, a novel missense mutation Asn855Ser in the *DNAJC13* gene was found in a multi-generation family with PD and in an additional four other PD patients (154). Human DNAJC13 is a membrane-associated protein involved in endocytosis, specifically in the process of early endosome-mediated membrane trafficking (155, 156). Knocking down the *DNAJC13* gene in mammalian cells did not cause obvious dysfunction of endocytosis. However, introducing a C-terminus truncated mutant DNAJC13 protein into the cells did affect the normal distribution and formation of early endosomes (156). No *DNAJC13* knockout animal model is available.

Orofacial Cleft 1 Candidate 1

After an initial study suggesting that the *OFCC1* gene led to orofacial clefts (157), it was later linked to schizophrenia (158). Recently, a genome-wide association study (GWAS) of OCD found a significant association with *OFCC1* (159). Sequence variants in *OFCC1* have been found in patients with neurodevelopmental or neuropsychiatric disorders: a missense mutation (R129G) segregating with TD and CTD in a multiplex family (150) and a non-sense and a missense mutation were found in a single autism family (160).

The function of the orofacial cleft 1 candidate 1 (OFCC1) protein is unclear but one study suggested that the OFCC1 protein was an interacting partner and methylation substrate of protein arginine methyltransferase 1 (161). However, *Ofcc1* knockout mice did not show any behavioral abnormalities (158).

Hypocretin (Orexin) Receptor 2 (*HCRTR2/OX2R*)

The coding regions of the orexin-1/hypocretin-1 (*OX1R*) receptor gene, the orexin-2/hypocretin-2 (*OX2R*) gene, and the prepro-orexin gene were examined in patients with Excessive Daytime Sleepiness, TD, or ADHD and healthy controls (162). A C29T nucleotide change in the *OX2R* gene producing a Pro10Ser amino acid substitution was detected in only one TD patient with comorbid ADHD. The Pro10Ser variant reduces responsiveness of the Orexin2 receptor to its ligands, Orexin-A, and Orexin-B. The Orexin receptor 2 is a G protein-coupled receptor that participates the regulation of feeding and sleep-wakefulness in mammalian brains (163). *Ox2r* knockout mice do not show any tic-like behaviors (164).

FUNCTIONAL ANALYSES OF GENES DISRUPTED IN TD

As indicated in the previous section, evidence for TD susceptibility genes exists. The mutations discussed were found in only a small number of individuals with TD, and replication remains elusive. This lack of replication may be due to the extreme locus heterogeneity, similar to what has been found in ASD (165). What evidence beyond stronger statistical association might help establish their potential role in TD pathogenesis? Some of these genes are found within neurobiological pathways that are presumed to be disrupted in TD (e.g., neural signal transmission/modulation) while others are found in novel pathways. Hence, the evidence that these genes are true susceptibility genes remains insufficient. Consequently, more convincing functional studies are needed to determine how variants in these genes could contribute to TD. In this next section, we review the *in vitro* and *in vivo* functional studies and techniques (beyond the knock out experiments referred to above) that will likely be useful to evaluate the consequences of mutations found in these presumptive TD susceptibility genes and for discovery of cellular and molecular phenotypes in disease.

Transgenic Mammalian Cell Lines

Functional studies using neuronal cells from individuals with TD can provide insights into the molecular basis of TD and potentially help to clarify the biological pathways altered in TD. However, one of the difficulties is the inability to obtain relevant biomaterials (e.g., neurons or neural stem cells) from affected individuals. Since TD is not a lethal disorder, there is very limited access to neural tissue from individuals with TD, particularly from individuals with a known causal variant.

Transgenic human non-neuronal cell lines have been used to characterize the cellular and molecular phenotypes resulting from specific mutations. Typically, plasmids carrying a wild type or a mutant gene of interest are delivered into the cell lines. Once the protein products of the transgene are expressed in the cells, assays are developed to evaluate the functional consequences of the mutant proteins. For example, in the *CDH2* gene, both the wild type and mutant *CDH2* genes were cloned into expression plasmids and subsequently delivered into human embryonic kidney (HEK293) cells and reduced expression of mutant CDH2 proteins was reported (106). While easily done, functional studies in non-neuronal cell lines are suboptimal for a variety of reasons. During transgenesis, the gene of interest is often transiently overexpressed or is controlled by a conditional and/or inducible gene expression system (166). Therefore, the level of transgene expression might not faithfully represent the endogenous gene expression level. Also, the expression levels of many genes are tissue-specific (167). This is particularly relevant for genes with multiple transcript isoforms where the isoform expression pattern in transgenic cell lines may not be comparable to patterns in neurons. Furthermore, because transgenic cells would not be expected to have the same gene expression profile as neurons, they may not provide relevant cellular environment for the transgene to execute its genuine neuronal function(s). Neuronal samples from TD patients are therefore preferred for *in vitro* functional studies but these are very difficult if not impossible to obtain. A recent technological advance, induced pluripotent stem cells (iPSCs), now makes functional studies of neuronal samples with a known causal variant possible.

Induced Pluripotent Stem Cells

Use of iPSC-Derived Neuronal Cells to Model Neuropsychiatric and Neurodevelopmental Disorders

The relatively new reprograming technique that converts human somatic cells into iPSCs allows researchers to model diseases *in vitro* using patient-derived cells. Since the first generation of iPSCs from mouse fibroblasts (168), the ability to produce differentiated cells from iPSCs has been intensively studied and improved. Recently, iPSC neuronal differentiation has become routine (169). Generating patient-specific neurons carrying mutations in disease candidate genes is invaluable for researchers who wish to study the cell-autonomous effects of mutations and to understand the cellular basis of neurological and neuropsychiatric disorders. To date, no study using iPSC-derived neurons to model TD has been published. However, mutations associated with other neuropsychiatric disorders have been studied in iPSC-derived neurons, and cellular abnormalities have been demonstrated (170–174). For example, Rett syndrome is a neurodevelopmental disorder occurring mainly in females characterized by mental retardation. Loss-of-function mutations in the methyl-CpG binding protein 2 (*MeCP2*) gene were reported in the majority of Rett Syndrome cases (170). Therefore, neurons with functional null mutation in the *MeCP2* gene were generated from the iPSCs of an individual with Rett Syndrome. In culture, the neurons showed smaller soma size (171). Similarly, iPSC-derived neurons have been used to understand ASD. In an individual with ASD, a balanced translocation spanning the transient receptor potential 6 channel (*TRPC6*) gene was identified. Neurons derived from the iPSCs exhibited decreased *TRPC6* expression, altered morphology and reduced Ca^{2+} influx (172). In schizophrenia, the *DISC1* gene has been considered an important risk factor (175) and in iPSC-derived *DISC1* mutant neurons, pre-synaptic vesicle release was impaired (173).

Unfortunately, *in vitro* neural differentiation from iPSCs yields mixed populations of neurons rather than a homogenous population. For diseases with clear neuropathology, pure cultures of the specific neuron types involved in the disorder are preferred in order to recapitulate disease-related cellular phenotypes. For instance, PD is characterized by loss of substantia nigra dopamine neurons (176). Cultures containing a high percentage of dopaminergic neurons were generated from PD patients who carry monogenic mutations (177–180), and defects in cellular functions such as autophagy, mitophagy, oxidative stress response, and dopamine release were found in these neurons. In patients with amyotrophic lateral sclerosis (ALS), motor neurons degenerate. Therefore, motor neurons were derived from iPSCs of ALS patients carrying known casual mutations (174, 181). As hypothesized, the mutant motor neurons exhibited neurite degeneration (181).

Use of Single-Cell Analysis to Overcome Culture Heterogeneity

One method to overcome cell culture heterogeneity is to analyze single cells, all of the same type. Looking at the transcriptome of single cells using microarray or RNA-seq analysis holds promise of detecting gene dysregulation in particular populations of neurons, which might not be identified by analyzing heterogeneous mixtures of cells. For instance, single-cell gene expression analysis of iPSC-derived dopamine neurons from PD patients with a LRKK2 mutation unveiled dysregulation of oxidative stress genes in mutant dopamine neurons (182). In another study, neurons were generated from the iPSCs of Timothy Syndrome patients with a mutation in the *CACNA1C* gene. Single cells were taken from the culture containing mixed neuron populations, and gene expression was analyzed by microarray. As a result, the distribution of neuron subtypes was altered in the Timothy Syndrome neuronal culture compared to the control cells (183). Compared to microarray, RNA-seq is gaining greater popularity for analyzing the transcriptome of single cells due to its ability to unbiasedly detect any transcript in cells within a broader dynamic range of expression. Generally, there are four important steps to achieve single-cell RNA-seq: (1) single-cell isolation, (2) RNA capture, (3) cDNA synthesis and, (4) next generation sequencing. The microfluidic system is becoming popular for single-cell RNA-seq because it can isolate single cells, lyse the cells, purify RNA, synthesize cDNA or even conduct gene expression analysis all in one run (184, 185).

Use of iPSC-Derived Cerebral Organoids to Model Neuropsychiatric and Neurodevelopmental Disorders

In contrast to PD or ALS, the neuropathology of many neurodevelopmental and neuropsychiatric disorders, such as TD or ASD, is unclear or is heterogeneous (18). As described above, mutations associated with TD indicate dysregulations of various neurotransmitter pathways or of neural circuits involving multiple brain regions. Hence, studying specific type of neurons may not help to explain the pathogenesis of TD. The recently developed "cerebral organoid" cellular system enables the differentiation of iPSCs into a three-dimensional miniature organ in a bioreactor, with minimum external interferences (186). Such self-organized spherical structures resemble the human brain at very early stages of development. In comparison to monolayer neuronal cultures, the cerebral organoids contain more diverse neuronal populations that define distinct brain regions. Also, within the cerebral organoid, neuronal migration and human-specific brain structures (e.g., the outer subventricular zone) were observed (187). Therefore, the cerebral organoid has been used to model neurodevelopmental diseases. For microcephaly, premature neural differentiation was recapitulated in organoids derived from microcephaly patients' iPSCs (187). In cases of idiopathic ASD, overproduction of GABAergic inhibitory neurons in patient-derived cerebral organoids was reported (188). At the molecular level, the cellular phenotype was explained by overexpression of the transcription factor FOXG1. However, use of cerebral organoids to model neurodevelopmental diseases has limitations. The various "brain regions" in the organoids are fairly disorganized. Therefore, the cerebral organoid would not be suitable to study neural circuits. Furthermore, neuronal cells within the organoids are mostly neural progenitor cells, and their differentiation is restricted by limited growth of the organoids, which in turn is probably due to the lack of internal nutrient and oxygen supply. More importantly, each organoid is "unique" because the self-organization process is random and is not controlled by external factors. This "uniqueness" will generate variation among organoids, which may mask phenotypic differences between normal and patient-derived cells.

Use of Genome Editing to Generate Isogenic Control iPSC Lines

One challenge in identifying the phenotypic effects of a given mutation in iPSC-derived neurons is finding an appropriate control sample. While age, gender, and ethnicity-matched control samples with the wild-type allele are typically available, they are not matched for all of the other common genomic variants. Failure to control for such variability in genetic background can lead to spurious results. The recent technological advance of highly specific genome editing now allows the production of more comparable isogenic controls for functional studies. Several genome editing systems, such as zinc finger nuclease (189, 190), TALEN, and CRISPR-Cas9 (191, 192), are able to reverse the mutation to wild type at one genomic locus at a time in iPSCs. Comparing neuronal cells generated from mutant iPSCs and their edited, isogenic control neuronal cells with the mutation removed allows identification of molecular and cellular changes that are due only to the mutation (180). However, "off target" mutations at unrelated loci inadvertently introduced by editing remain a potentially important technological hurdle (193).

Gene Expression and Gene Network Analyses

The major goal of genomic sequencing of patients with neurodevelopmental and neuropsychiatric disorders is to identify disease-associated mutations. Once such genes are found, systematic approaches including genome-wide gene expression analysis and gene network analyses can be used to implicate common biological pathways altered in patients with different mutant genes.

Gene Expression Analysis

Gene expression analysis, primarily through the RNA-seq approach, aims to quantify transcript level of target genes or of the whole transcriptome in biological samples from patients and healthy controls to identify genes dysregulated in human diseases (194). For neurodevelopmental disorders, post-mortem brain samples are often used for the transcriptomic analyses. The first transcriptomic analysis of TD patients' post-mortem striatum samples revealed that interneuron disruption might be involved in the pathophysiology of TD (34). However, to evaluate particular mutations, post-mortem samples meeting specific research criteria are usually difficult or virtually impossible to obtain. With the emergence of somatic cell reprograming techniques, iPSC-derived neurons with and without a putative disease-causing mutation can be produced *in vitro* (195). The transcriptomes of these iPSC-derived neurons can be compared by microarray or RNA sequencing (RNA-seq) (172, 173). To further dissect the cellular phenotype at single neuron level and to detect abnormalities only shown in particular populations of neurons, single-cell transcriptome analysis can also be performed (182, 183). Multiple bioinformatic tools have been developed for RNA-seq data to detect differentially expressed genes (DEGs) from distinct cell types or under different experimental conditions (196–198). Among these RNA-seq analysis methods, none outperforms the others in all aspects. Selecting an optimal method for a study requires an understanding of the benefits and limitations of each method as well as the parameters of the study (196). Once the DEGs between experimental conditions are determined, gene and pathway annotation tools, gene and protein expression and interaction databases can help to explore the gene pathways underlying the disorder. Gene and pathway annotations tools such as IPA[1], KEGG (199, 200), DAVID (201, 202), ConsensusPathDB (203) report biological pathways in which DEGs are enriched or reduced and take these into account to predict how these pathways might be affected. However, the data from which these tools were constructed come from non-neuronal samples which could lead to associations not found in neuronal tissues or failure to detect neuronal associations (204). In order to annotate neuronal gene expression in a temporal and spatial manner, human brain gene expression databases, for example, the Allen Human Brain Atlas (205), BrainSpan (206), GTEx (207) were built using microarray and RNA-seq data from post-mortem brain samples. Mapping DEGs identified in neuronal samples of patients with neurodevelopmental disorders to human brain gene expression databases revealed specific brain regions and neural developmental stages that were affected (34, 208). A more detailed human brain gene expression atlas that annotates gene expression at single cell level has been initiated by a group in Stanford University (209). Single-cell RNA-seq was used to analyze neurons from human adult and fetal cerebral cortex and it identified more diverse populations of neurons within the cortical region (209). Constructing a comprehensive human brain gene expression database at single neuron resolution is quite challenging due to limited access to healthy human brain samples and the high cost of single-cell RNA-seq. Therefore, collaborative work with standardized experimental protocols is required.

Gene Network Analysis

Differential gene expression from transcriptome analysis is sample-dependent and tissue-specific. In order to explore the etiology of complex neurodevelopmental disorders such as TD, disease-associated genes can be mapped to gene networks to visualize relationships between disease candidate genes and, further, to pinpoint annotated or novel pathways. The gene networks can be gene co-expression networks (205, 206), gene regulatory networks[2], protein–protein interaction networks (210) or networks constructed with combined criteria (203, 211). For example, in ASD, disease-associated genes have been evaluated using spatiotemporal gene co-expression networks constructed from BrainSpan (206) and were found to be enriched in sub-networks that represent specific brain regions and time periods during human brain development (212). Furthermore, ASD-associated mutations identified by previous genetic studies were mapped to a "background network" which scores each pair of human genes based on very comprehensive information about every known human gene (211). Cell types and brain areas affected in ASD were implicated (213). With a growing number of mutations associated with TD, the same approaches could be utilized in TD.

Animal Models

Another approach to the study of the functional effects of a specific mutation in a gene is to use animal models. Most often, a putative disease gene is knocked out or modified in the animal model. Then, the mutant and wild type animals from the same genetic background are compared. (Some such animal knock-out studies of putative TD genes have been described above). Conventional animal models are designed to study a small number of genes, usually one or two genes at a time. If, however, TD is caused by the combined effect of multiple variant genes, multi-transgenic animals, whose genomes are modified at multiple loci, would be required. Although more challenging, generation of such multi-transgenic animals can be achieved by genome editing as well. (214, 215).

In order to model TD in animals, the following criteria should be met: (1) the gene to be studied is strongly associated with the disease; (2) the gene and the neurological component phenotypes involved in TD are relatively well conserved between humans and the animal; (3) the gene is thought to have similar functions in both humans and the model animals; and (4) the disease phenotype can be experimentally characterized in the model animals by biochemical and/or behavioral approaches (216). One mouse model in TD that meets these criteria is *HDC*. As indicated previously, a rare dominant non-sense mutation W317X in *HDC* cosegregated with all TD individuals in a two generation pedigree. (25). Subsequently, a study using *HDC* knockout mice demonstrated behavioral and molecular abnormalities caused by the loss of the HDC activity in the brain (28). The knockout and heterozygous mice showed tic-like stereotypic movements after psychostimulant administration. Also, the striatal dopaminergic pathway was dysregulated due to the HDC deficiency. Specifically, the dysregulation of dopamine receptors in the basal ganglia region of the *HDC* knockout and heterozygous mice recapitulated the dysregulation of the same types of dopamine receptors in TD patients carrying the W317X mutation.

SUMMARY AND FUTURE DIRECTIONS

Tourette's disorder is likely caused by a complex multigenic inheritance pattern that includes locus and allelic heterogeneity of both common and rare variants that interact with environmental factors (14, 217, 218). Despite long-standing interest in the genetic contribution to TD, the overall genetic architecture of TD remains elusive. Some of the genes identified as causal of TD are involved in neurotransmitter pathways presumed to be altered in TD, while others are novel. In this respect, the genetics of TD may resemble that of other complex neuropsychiatric disorders. Indeed, there is evidence of some overlap with subsets of similar genes involved in multiple disorders. Furthermore, there also appears to be an increased rate of comorbidity between some such

[1] www.qiagen.com/ingenuity
[2] http://www.braineac.org/

disorders, such as TD and ASD (27, 219). It may also be that current DSM-based psychiatric nosology does not sufficiently "carve nature at its joints," and that other classification schemes, such as Research Domain Criteria (RDoC)(220–224), might reveal etiologically more coherent groupings of disorders or patients.

International consortiums including the Tourette International Collaborative Genetics (TIC Genetics), the Tourette Syndrome Association International Consortium for Genetics (TSAICG), the European Multicenter Tics in Children Studies (EMTICS), the European Society for the Study of Tourette Syndrome (ESSTS), the Tourette Syndrome Genetics The Southern and Eastern Europe initiative (TSGeneSEE), and sharing repositories (New Jersey Center for Tourette Syndrome Repository) (225, 226) have initiated large collaborations to collect many patient and family samples in an effort to understand the genetics of TD. Continued efforts in gene discovery from large open-access repositories are needed to find additional risk variants.

AUTHOR CONTRIBUTIONS

All authors wrote, reviewed, and critiqued the manuscript.

ACKNOWLEDGMENTS

This study was supported by a Grant from the National Institute of Mental Health (R01MH092293) and the New Jersey Center for Tourette Syndrome and Associated Disorders (NJCTS).

FUNDING

National Institute of Mental Health (R01MH092293); New Jersey Center for Tourette Syndrome and Associated Disorders (NJCTS) (Center of Excellence for Tourette Syndrome & Associated Disorders Genetics Repository).

REFERENCES

1. Robertson MM. Diagnosing Tourette syndrome: is it a common disorder? *J Psychosom Res* (2003) **55**(1):3–6. doi:10.1016/S0022-3999(02)00580-9
2. Scharf JM, Miller LL, Gauvin CA, Alabiso J, Mathews CA, Ben-Shlomo Y. Population prevalence of Tourette syndrome: a systematic review and meta-analysis. *Mov Disord* (2015) **30**(2):221–8. doi:10.1002/mds.26089
3. Robertson MM. The Gilles de la Tourette syndrome: the current status. *Arch Dis Child Educ Pract Ed* (2012) **97**(5):166–75. doi:10.1136/archdischild-2011-300585
4. Shaw ZA, Coffey BJ. Tics and tourette syndrome. *Psychiatr Clin North Am* (2014) **37**(3):269–86. doi:10.1016/j.psc.2014.05.001
5. Freeman RD, Fast DK, Burd L, Kerbeshian J, Robertson MM, Sandor P. An international perspective on Tourette syndrome: selected findings from 3,500 individuals in 22 countries. *Dev Med Child Neurol* (2000) **42**(7):436–47. doi:10.1017/S0012162200000839
6. Paschou P, Fernandez TV, Sharp F, Heiman GA, Hoekstra PJ. Genetic susceptibility and neurotransmitters in Tourette syndrome. *Int Rev Neurobiol* (2013) **112**:155–77. doi:10.1016/B978-0-12-411546-0.00006-8
7. Leckman JF, Bloch MH, Smith ME, Larabi D, Hampson M. Neurobiological substrates of Tourette's disorder. *J Child Adolesc Psychopharmacol* (2010) **20**(4):237–47. doi:10.1089/cap.2009.0118
8. Wang ZS, Maia TV, Marsh R, Colibazzi T, Gerber A, Peterson BS. The neural circuits that generate tics in Tourette's syndrome. *Am J Psychiatry* (2011) **168**(12):1326–37. doi:10.1176/appi.ajp.2011.09111692
9. Kataoka Y, Kalanithi PSA, Grantz H, Schwartz ML, Saper C, Leckman JF, et al. Decreased number of parvalbumin and cholinergic interneurons in the striatum of individuals with Tourette syndrome. *J Comp Neurol* (2010) **518**(3):277–91. doi:10.1002/cne.22206
10. Priori A, Giannicola G, Rosa M, Marceglia S, Servello D, Sassi M, et al. Deep brain electrophysiological recordings provide clues to the pathophysiology of Tourette syndrome. *Neurosci Biobehav Rev* (2013) **37**(6):1063–8. doi:10.1016/j.neubiorev.2013.01.011
11. Pogorelov V, Xu MY, Smith HR, Buchanan GF, Pittenger C. Corticostriatal interactions in the generation of tic-like behaviors after local striatal disinhibition. *Exp Neurol* (2015) **265**:122–8. doi:10.1016/j.expneurol.2015.01.001
12. Buse J, Schoenefeld K, Munchau A, Roessner V. Neuromodulation in Tourette syndrome: dopamine and beyond. *Neurosci Biobehav Rev* (2013) **37**(6):1069–84. doi:10.1016/j.neubiorev.2012.10.004
13. Surmeier DJ, Ding J, Day M, Wang Z, Shen W. D1 and D2 dopamine-receptor modulation of striatal glutamatergic signaling in striatal medium spiny neurons. *Trends Neurosci* (2007) **30**(5):228–35. doi:10.1016/j.tins.2007.03.008
14. Bloch M, State M, Pittenger C. Recent advances in Tourette syndrome. *Curr Opin Neurol* (2011) **24**(2):119–25. doi:10.1097/WCO.0b013e328344648c
15. Roessner V, Plessen KJ, Rothenberger A, Ludolph AG, Rizzo R, Skov L, et al. European clinical guidelines for Tourette syndrome and other tic disorders. Part II: pharmacological treatment. *Eur Child Adolesc Psychiatry* (2011) **20**(4):173–96. doi:10.1007/s00787-011-0163-7
16. Minzer K, Lee O, Hong JJ, Singer HS. Increased prefrontal D2 protein in Tourette syndrome: a postmortem analysis of frontal cortex and striatum. *J Neurol Sci* (2004) **219**(1–2):55–61. doi:10.1016/j.jns.2003.12.006
17. Yoon DY, Gause CD, Leckman JF, Singer HS. Frontal dopaminergic abnormality in Tourette syndrome: a postmortem analysis. *J Neurol Sci* (2007) **255**(1–2):50–6. doi:10.1016/j.jns.2007.01.069
18. Felling RJ, Singer HS. Neurobiology of tourette syndrome: current status and need for further investigation. *J Neurosci* (2011) **31**(35):12387–95. doi:10.1523/JNEUROSCI.0150-11.2011
19. Anderson GM, Pollak ES, Chatterjee D, Leckman JF, Riddle MA, Cohen DJ. Brain monoamines and amino acids in Gilles de la Tourette's syndrome: a preliminary study of subcortical regions. *Arch Gen Psychiatry* (1992) **49**(7):584–6. doi:10.1001/archpsyc.1992.01820070078016
20. Singer HS, Morris C, Grados M. Glutamatergic modulatory therapy for Tourette syndrome. *Med Hypotheses* (2010) **74**(5):862–7. doi:10.1016/j.mehy.2009.11.028
21. Kalanithi PS, Zheng W, Kataoka Y, DiFiglia M, Grantz H, Saper CB, et al. Altered parvalbumin-positive neuron distribution in basal ganglia of individuals with Tourette syndrome. *Proc Natl Acad Sci U S A* (2005) **102**(37):13307–12. doi:10.1073/pnas.0502624102
22. Pittenger C, Bloch MH. Pharmacological treatment of obsessive-compulsive disorder. *Psychiatr Clin North Am* (2014) **37**(3):375–91. doi:10.1016/j.psc.2014.05.006
23. Roessner V, Schoenefeld K, Buse J, Bender S, Ehrlich S, Munchau A. Pharmacological treatment of tic disorders and Tourette syndrome. *Neuropharmacology* (2013) **68**:143–9. doi:10.1016/j.neuropharm.2012.05.043
24. Moya PR, Wendland JR, Rubenstein LM, Timpano KR, Heiman GA, Tischfield JA, et al. Common and rare alleles of the serotonin transporter gene, SLC6A4, associated with Tourette's disorder. *Mov Disord* (2013) **28**(9):1263–70. doi:10.1002/mds.25460
25. Ercan-Sencicek AG, Stillman AA, Ghosh AK, Bilguvar K, O'Roak BJ, Mason CE, et al. L-histidine decarboxylase and Tourette's syndrome. *N Engl J Med* (2010) **362**(20):1901–8. doi:10.1056/NEJMoa0907006
26. Karagiannidis I, Dehning S, Sandor P, Tarnok Z, Rizzo R, Wolanczyk T, et al. Support of the histaminergic hypothesis in Tourette syndrome: association of the histamine decarboxylase gene in a large sample of families. *J Med Genet* (2013) **50**(11):760–4. doi:10.1136/jmedgenet-2013-101637
27. Fernandez TV, Sanders SJ, Yurkiewicz IR, Ercan-Sencicek AG, Kim YS, Fishman DO, et al. Rare copy number variants in tourette syndrome disrupt genes in histaminergic pathways and overlap with autism. *Biol Psychiatry* (2012) **71**(5):392–402. doi:10.1016/j.biopsych.2011.09.034
28. Castellan Baldan L, Williams KA, Gallezot JD, Pogorelov V, Rapanelli M, Crowley M, et al. Histidine decarboxylase deficiency causes tourette

syndrome: parallel findings in humans and mice. *Neuron* (2014) **81**(1):77–90. doi:10.1016/j.neuron.2013.10.052
29. Parent M, Wallman MJ, Gagnon D, Parent A. Serotonin innervation of basal ganglia in monkeys and humans. *J Chem Neuroanat* (2011) **41**(4):256–65. doi:10.1016/j.jchemneu.2011.04.005
30. Haas HL, Sergeeva OA, Selbach O. Histamine in the nervous system. *Physiol Rev* (2008) **88**(3):1183–241. doi:10.1152/physrev.00043.2007
31. Di Giovanni G, Di Matteo V, Esposito E. Serotonin-dopamine interaction: experimental evidence and therapeutic relevance. Preface. *Prog Brain Res* (2008) **172**:ix. doi:10.1016/S0079-6123(08)00931-X
32. Frick LR, Williams K, Pittenger C. Microglial dysregulation in psychiatric disease. *Clin Dev Immunol* (2013) **2013**:608654. doi:10.1155/2013/608654
33. Morer A, Chae W, Henegariu O, Bothwell AL, Leckman JF, Kawikova I. Elevated expression of MCP-1, IL-2 and PTPR-N in basal ganglia of Tourette syndrome cases. *Brain Behav Immun* (2010) **24**(7):1069–73. doi:10.1016/j.bbi.2010.02.007
34. Lennington JB, Coppola G, Kataoka-Sasaki Y, Fernandez TV, Palejev D, Li Y, et al. Transcriptome analysis of the human striatum in Tourette syndrome. *Biol Psychiatry* (2014). doi:10.1016/j.biopsych.2014.07.018
35. Sundaram SK, Huq AM, Wilson BJ, Chugani HT. Tourette syndrome is associated with recurrent exonic copy number variants. *Neurology* (2010) **74**(20):1583–90. doi:10.1212/WNL.0b013e3181e0f147
36. Nag A, Bochukova EG, Kremeyer B, Campbell DD, Muller H, Valencia-Duarte AV, et al. CNV analysis in Tourette syndrome implicates large genomic rearrangements in COL8A1 and NRXN1. *PLoS One* (2013) **8**(3):e59061. doi:10.1371/journal.pone.0059061
37. Bertelsen B, Stefansson H, Riff Jensen L, Melchior L, Mol Debes N, Groth C, et al. Association of AADAC deletion and Gilles de la Tourette syndrome in a large European cohort. *Biol Psychiatry* (2015). doi:10.1016/j.biopsych.2015.08.027
38. Abelson JF, Kwan KY, O'Roak BJ, Baek DY, Stillman AA, Morgan TM, et al. Sequence variants in SLITRK1 are associated with Tourette's syndrome. *Science* (2005) **310**(5746):317–20. doi:10.1126/science.1116502
39. Deng H, Le WD, Xie WJ, Jankovic J. Examination of the SLITRK1 gene in Caucasian patients with Tourette syndrome. *Acta Neurol Scand* (2006) **114**(6):400–2. doi:10.1111/j.1600-0404.2006.00706.x
40. Verkerk AJ, Cath DC, van der Linde HC, Both J, Heutink P, Breedveld G, et al. Genetic and clinical analysis of a large Dutch Gilles de la Tourette family. *Mol Psychiatry* (2006) **11**(10):954–64. doi:10.1038/sj.mp.4001877
41. Chou IC, Wan L, Liu SC, Tsai CH, Tsai FJ. Association of the slit and Trk-like 1 gene in Taiwanese patients with Tourette syndrome. *Pediatr Neurol* (2007) **37**(6):404–6. doi:10.1016/j.pediatrneurol.2007.06.017
42. Scharf JM, Moorjani P, Fagerness J, Platko JV, Illmann C, Galloway B, et al. Lack of association between SLITRK1var321 and Tourette syndrome in a large family-based sample. *Neurology* (2008) **70**(16 Pt 2):1495–6. doi:10.1212/01.wnl.0000296833.25484.bb
43. Zimprich A, Hatala K, Riederer F, Stogmann E, Aschauer HN, Stamenkovic M. Sequence analysis of the complete SLITRK1 gene in Austrian patients with Tourette's disorder. *Psychiatr Genet* (2008) **18**(6):308–9. doi:10.1097/YPG.0b013e3283060f6f
44. Miranda DM, Wigg K, Kabia EM, Feng Y, Sandor P, Barr CL. Association of SLITRK1 to Gilles de la Tourette syndrome. *Am J Med Genet B Neuropsychiatr Genet* (2009) **150B**(4):483–6. doi:10.1002/ajmg.b.30840
45. O'Roak BJ, Morgan TM, Fishman DO, Saus E, Alonso P, Gratacos M, et al. Additional support for the association of SLITRK1 var321 and Tourette syndrome. *Mol Psychiatry* (2010) **15**(5):447–50. doi:10.1038/mp.2009.105
46. Yasmeen S, Melchior L, Bertelsen B, Skov L, Mol Debes N, Tumer Z. Sequence analysis of SLITRK1 for var321 in Danish patients with Tourette syndrome and review of the literature. *Psychiatr Genet* (2013) **23**(3):130–3. doi:10.1097/YPG.0b013e328360c880
47. Inai A, Tochigi M, Kuwabara H, Nishimura F, Kato K, Eriguchi Y, et al. Analysis of SLITRK1 in Japanese patients with Tourette syndrome using a next-generation sequencer. *Psychiatr Genet* (2015) **25**(6):256–8. doi:10.1097/YPG.0000000000000104
48. Keen-Kim D, Mathews CA, Reus VI, Lowe TL, Herrera LD, Budman CL, et al. Overrepresentation of rare variants in a specific ethnic group may confuse interpretation of association analyses. *Hum Mol Genet* (2006) **15**(22):3324–8. doi:10.1093/hmg/ddl408
49. Karagiannidis I, Rizzo R, Tarnok Z, Wolanczyk T, Hebebrand J, Nothen MM, et al. Replication of association between a SLITRK1 haplotype and Tourette syndrome in a large sample of families. *Mol Psychiatry* (2012) **17**(7):665–8. doi:10.1038/mp.2011.151
50. Proenca CC, Gao KP, Shmelkov SV, Rafii S, Lee FS. Slitrks as emerging candidate genes involved in neuropsychiatric disorders. *Trends Neurosci* (2011) **34**(3):143–53. doi:10.1016/j.tins.2011.01.001
51. Aruga J, Mikoshiba K. Identification and characterization of Slitrk, a novel neuronal transmembrane protein family controlling neurite outgrowth. *Mol Cell Neurosci* (2003) **24**(1):117–29. doi:10.1016/S1044-7431(03)00129-5
52. Yim YS, Kwon Y, Nam J, Yoon HI, Lee K, Kim DG, et al. Slitrks control excitatory and inhibitory synapse formation with LAR receptor protein tyrosine phosphatases. *Proc Natl Acad Sci U S A* (2013) **110**(10):4057–62. doi:10.1073/pnas.1209881110
53. Um JW, Kim KH, Park BS, Choi Y, Kim D, Kim CY, et al. Structural basis for LAR-RPTP/Slitrk complex-mediated synaptic adhesion. *Nat Commun* (2014) **5**:5423. doi:10.1038/ncomms6423
54. Katayama K, Yamada K, Ornthanalai VG, Inoue T, Ota M, Murphy NP, et al. Slitrk1-deficient mice display elevated anxiety-like behavior and noradrenergic abnormalities. *Mol Psychiatry* (2010) **15**(2):177–84. doi:10.1038/mp.2008.97
55. Lei J, Deng X, Zhang J, Su L, Xu H, Liang H, et al. Mutation screening of the HDC gene in Chinese Han patients with Tourette syndrome. *Am J Med Genet B Neuropsychiatr Genet* (2012) **159B**(1):72–6. doi:10.1002/ajmg.b.32003
56. Panula P, Airaksinen MS, Pirvola U, Kotilainen E. A histamine-containing neuronal system in human brain. *Neuroscience* (1990) **34**(1):127–32. doi:10.1016/0306-4522(90)90307-P
57. Watanabe T, Taguchi Y, Shiosaka S, Tanaka J, Kubota H, Terano Y, et al. Distribution of the histaminergic neuron system in the central nervous system of rats; a fluorescent immunohistochemical analysis with histidine decarboxylase as a marker. *Brain Res* (1984) **295**(1):13–25. doi:10.1016/0006-8993(84)90811-4
58. Schlicker E, Fink K, Detzner M, Gothert M. Histamine inhibits dopamine release in the mouse striatum via presynaptic H3 receptors. *J Neural Transm Gen Sect* (1993) **93**(1):1–10. doi:10.1007/BF01244933
59. Komori H, Nitta Y, Ueno H, Higuchi Y. Structural study reveals that Ser-354 determines substrate specificity on human histidine decarboxylase. *J Biol Chem* (2012) **287**(34):29175–83. doi:10.1074/jbc.M112.381897
60. Zohar J, Insel TR. Drug treatment of obsessive-compulsive disorder. *J Affect Disord* (1987) **13**(2):193–202. doi:10.1016/0165-0327(87)90023-1
61. Lieberman J. Evidence for a biological hypothesis of obsessive-compulsive disorder. *Neuropsychobiology* (1984) **11**(1):14–21. doi:10.1159/000118043
62. Zohar J, Insel TR, Zohar-Kadouch RC, Hill JL, Murphy DL. Serotonergic responsivity in obsessive-compulsive disorder. Effects of chronic clomipramine treatment. *Arch Gen Psychiatry* (1988) **45**(2):167–72. doi:10.1001/archpsyc.1988.01800260081011
63. Billett EA, Richter MA, King N, Heils A, Lesch KP, Kennedy JL. Obsessive compulsive disorder, response to serotonin reuptake inhibitors and the serotonin transporter gene. *Mol Psychiatry* (1997) **2**(5):403–6. doi:10.1038/sj.mp.4000257
64. McDougle CJ, Epperson CN, Price LH, Gelernter J. Evidence for linkage disequilibrium between serotonin transporter protein gene (SLC6A4) and obsessive compulsive disorder. *Mol Psychiatry* (1998) **3**(3):270–3. doi:10.1038/sj.mp.4000391
65. Bengel D, Greenberg BD, Cora-Locatelli G, Altemus M, Heils A, Li Q, et al. Association of the serotonin transporter promoter regulatory region polymorphism and obsessive-compulsive disorder. *Mol Psychiatry* (1999) **4**(5):463–6. doi:10.1038/sj.mp.4000550
66. Di Bella D, Erzegovesi S, Cavallini MC, Bellodi L. Obsessive-compulsive disorder, 5-HTTLPR polymorphism and treatment response. *Pharmacogenomics J* (2002) **2**(3):176–81. doi:10.1038/sj.tpj.6500090
67. Ozaki N, Goldman D, Kaye WH, Plotnicov K, Greenberg BD, Lappalainen J, et al. Serotonin transporter missense mutation associated with a complex neuropsychiatric phenotype. *Mol Psychiatry* (2003) **8**(11):933–6. doi:10.1038/sj.mp.4001415
68. Wendland JR, Moya PR, Kruse MR, Ren-Patterson RF, Jensen CL, Timpano KR, et al. A novel, putative gain-of-function haplotype at SLC6A4 associates with obsessive-compulsive disorder. *Hum Mol Genet* (2008) **17**(5):717–23. doi:10.1093/hmg/ddm343

69. Voyiaziakis E, Evgrafov O, Li D, Yoon HJ, Tabares P, Samuels J, et al. Association of SLC6A4 variants with obsessive-compulsive disorder in a large multicenter US family study. *Mol Psychiatry* (2011) **16**(1):108–20. doi:10.1038/mp.2009.100
70. Hu XZ, Lipsky RH, Zhu G, Akhtar LA, Taubman J, Greenberg BD, et al. Serotonin transporter promoter gain-of-function genotypes are linked to obsessive-compulsive disorder. *Am J Hum Genet* (2006) **78**(5):815–26. doi:10.1086/503850
71. Kilic F, Murphy DL, Rudnick G. A human serotonin transporter mutation causes constitutive activation of transport activity. *Mol Pharmacol* (2003) **64**(2):440–6. doi:10.1124/mol.64.2.440
72. Jacobs BL, Azmitia EC. Structure and function of the brain serotonin system. *Physiol Rev* (1992) **72**(1):165–229.
73. Blakely RD, De Felice LJ, Hartzell HC. Molecular physiology of norepinephrine and serotonin transporters. *J Exp Biol* (1994) **196**:263–81.
74. Lesch KP, Wolozin BL, Estler HC, Murphy DL, Riederer P. Isolation of a cDNA encoding the human brain serotonin transporter. *J Neural Transm Gen Sect* (1993) **91**(1):67–72. doi:10.1007/BF01244919
75. Kittler K, Lau T, Schloss P. Antagonists and substrates differentially regulate serotonin transporter cell surface expression in serotonergic neurons. *Eur J Pharmacol* (2010) **629**(1–3):63–7. doi:10.1016/j.ejphar.2009.12.010
76. Esposito E, Di Matteo V, Di Giovanni G. Serotonin-dopamine interaction: an overview. *Prog Brain Res* (2008) **172**:3–6. doi:10.1016/S0079-6123(08)00901-1
77. Daw ND, Kakade S, Dayan P. Opponent interactions between serotonin and dopamine. *Neural Netw* (2002) **15**(4–6):603–16. doi:10.1016/S0893-6080(02)00052-7
78. Lam S, Shen Y, Nguyen T, Messier TL, Brann M, Comings D, et al. A serotonin receptor gene (5HT1A) variant found in a Tourette's syndrome patient. *Biochem Biophys Res Commun* (1996) **219**(3):853–8. doi:10.1006/bbrc.1996.0322
79. Guo Y, Deng X, Jankovic J, Su L, Zhang J, Le W, et al. Mutation screening of the HTR2B gene in patients with Tourette syndrome. *Neurosci Lett* (2012) **526**(2):150–3. doi:10.1016/j.neulet.2012.08.013
80. Hannon J, Hoyer D. Molecular biology of 5-HT receptors. *Behav Brain Res* (2008) **195**(1):198–213. doi:10.1016/j.bbr.2008.03.020
81. McCorvy JD, Roth BL. Structure and function of serotonin G protein-coupled receptors. *Pharmacol Ther* (2015) **150**:129–42. doi:10.1016/j.pharmthera.2015.01.009
82. Ramboz S, Oosting R, Amara DA, Kung HF, Blier P, Mendelsohn M, et al. Serotonin receptor 1A knockout: an animal model of anxiety-related disorder. *Proc Natl Acad Sci U S A* (1998) **95**(24):14476–81. doi:10.1073/pnas.95.24.14476
83. Toth M. 5-HT1A receptor knockout mouse as a genetic model of anxiety. *Eur J Pharmacol* (2003) **463**(1–3):177–84. doi:10.1016/S0014-2999(03)01280-9
84. Popova NK, Naumenko VS. 5-HT1A receptor as a key player in the brain 5-HT system. *Rev Neurosci* (2013) **24**(2):191–204. doi:10.1515/revneuro-2012-0082
85. Launay JM, Schneider B, Loric S, Da Prada M, Kellermann O. Serotonin transport and serotonin transporter-mediated antidepressant recognition are controlled by 5-HT2B receptor signaling in serotonergic neuronal cells. *FASEB J* (2006) **20**(11):1843–54. doi:10.1096/fj.06-5724com
86. Doly S, Valjent E, Setola V, Callebert J, Herve D, Launay JM, et al. Serotonin 5-HT2B receptors are required for 3,4-methylenedioxymethamphetamine-induced hyperlocomotion and 5-HT release in vivo and in vitro. *J Neurosci* (2008) **28**(11):2933–40. doi:10.1523/JNEUROSCI.5723-07.2008
87. Singer HS, Minzer K. Neurobiology of Tourette's syndrome: concepts of neuroanatomic localization and neurochemical abnormalities. *Brain Dev* (2003) **25**(Suppl 1):S70–84. doi:10.1016/S0387-7604(03)90012-X
88. Adamczyk A, Gause CD, Sattler R, Vidensky S, Rothstein JD, Singer H, et al. Genetic and functional studies of a missense variant in a glutamate transporter, SLC1A3, in Tourette syndrome. *Psychiatr Genet* (2011) **21**(2):90–7. doi:10.1097/YPG.0b013e328341a307
89. Manev H, Favaron M, Guidotti A, Costa E. Delayed increase of Ca2+ influx elicited by glutamate: role in neuronal death. *Mol Pharmacol* (1989) **36**(1):106–12.
90. O'Shea RD. Roles and regulation of glutamate transporters in the central nervous system. *Clin Exp Pharmacol Physiol* (2002) **29**(11):1018–23. doi:10.1046/j.1440-1681.2002.03770.x
91. Furuta A, Rothstein JD, Martin LJ. Glutamate transporter protein subtypes are expressed differentially during rat CNS development. *J Neurosci* (1997) **17**(21):8363–75.
92. Karlsson RM, Tanaka K, Saksida LM, Bussey TJ, Heilig M, Holmes A. Assessment of glutamate transporter GLAST (EAAT1)-deficient mice for phenotypes relevant to the negative and executive/cognitive symptoms of schizophrenia. *Neuropsychopharmacology* (2009) **34**(6):1578–89. doi:10.1038/npp.2008.215
93. Zebardast N, Crowley MJ, Bloch MH, Mayes LC, Wyk BV, Leckman JF, et al. Brain mechanisms for prepulse inhibition in adults with Tourette syndrome: initial findings. *Psychiatry Res* (2013) **214**(1):33–41. doi:10.1016/j.pscychresns.2013.05.009
94. Zhang C, Milunsky JM, Newton S, Ko J, Zhao G, Maher TA, et al. A neuroligin-4 missense mutation associated with autism impairs neuroligin-4 folding and endoplasmic reticulum export. *J Neurosci* (2009) **29**(35):10843–54. doi:10.1523/JNEUROSCI.1248-09.2009
95. Marshall CR, Noor A, Vincent JB, Lionel AC, Feuk L, Skaug J, et al. Structural variation of chromosomes in autism spectrum disorder. *Am J Hum Genet* (2008) **82**(2):477–88. doi:10.1016/j.ajhg.2007.12.009
96. Laumonnier F, Bonnet-Brilhault F, Gomot M, Blanc R, David A, Moizard MP, et al. X-linked mental retardation and autism are associated with a mutation in the NLGN4 gene, a member of the neuroligin family. *Am J Hum Genet* (2004) **74**(3):552–7. doi:10.1086/382137
97. Jamain S, Quach H, Betancur C, Rastam M, Colineaux C, Gillberg IC, et al. Mutations of the X-linked genes encoding neuroligins NLGN3 and NLGN4 are associated with autism. *Nat Genet* (2003) **34**(1):27–9. doi:10.1038/ng1136
98. Kim JE, O'Sullivan ML, Sanchez CA, Hwang M, Israel MA, Brennand K, et al. Investigating synapse formation and function using human pluripotent stem cell-derived neurons. *Proc Natl Acad Sci U S A* (2011) **108**(7):3005–10. doi:10.1073/pnas.1007753108
99. Lawson-Yuen A, Saldivar JS, Sommer S, Picker J. Familial deletion within NLGN4 associated with autism and Tourette syndrome. *Eur J Hum Genet* (2008) **16**(5):614–8. doi:10.1038/sj.ejhg.5202006
100. Sudhof TC. Neuroligins and neurexins link synaptic function to cognitive disease. *Nature* (2008) **455**(7215):903–11. doi:10.1038/nature07456
101. Varoqueaux F, Aramuni G, Rawson RL, Mohrmann R, Missler M, Gottmann K, et al. Neuroligins determine synapse maturation and function. *Neuron* (2006) **51**(6):741–54. doi:10.1016/j.neuron.2006.09.003
102. Chih B, Engelman H, Scheiffele P. Control of excitatory and inhibitory synapse formation by neuroligins. *Science* (2005) **307**(5713):1324–8. doi:10.1126/science.1107470
103. Jamain S, Radyushkin K, Hammerschmidt K, Granon S, Boretius S, Varoqueaux F, et al. Reduced social interaction and ultrasonic communication in a mouse model of monogenic heritable autism. *Proc Natl Acad Sci U S A* (2008) **105**(5):1710–5. doi:10.1073/pnas.0711555105
104. Delattre V, La Mendola D, Meystre J, Markram H, Markram K. Nlgn4 knockout induces network hypo-excitability in juvenile mouse somatosensory cortex in vitro. *Sci Rep* (2013) **3**:2897. doi:10.1038/srep02897
105. El-Kordi A, Winkler D, Hammerschmidt K, Kastner A, Krueger D, Ronnenberg A, et al. Development of an autism severity score for mice using Nlgn4 null mutants as a construct-valid model of heritable monogenic autism. *Behav Brain Res* (2013) **251**:41–9. doi:10.1016/j.bbr.2012.11.016
106. Moya PR, Dodman NH, Timpano KR, Rubenstein LM, Rana Z, Fried RL, et al. Rare missense neuronal cadherin gene (CDH2) variants in specific obsessive-compulsive disorder and Tourette disorder phenotypes. *Eur J Hum Genet* (2013) **21**(8):850–4. doi:10.1038/ejhg.2012.245
107. Hatta K, Okada TS, Takeichi M. A monoclonal antibody disrupting calcium-dependent cell-cell adhesion of brain tissues: possible role of its target antigen in animal pattern formation. *Proc Natl Acad Sci U S A* (1985) **82**(9):2789–93. doi:10.1073/pnas.82.9.2789
108. Reichardt LFN-. Cadherin and integrins: two receptor systems that mediate neuronal process outgrowth on astrocyte surfaces. *Neuron* (2008) **60**(3):398–9. doi:10.1016/j.neuron.2008.10.030
109. Tomaselli KJ, Neugebauer KM, Bixby JL, Lilien J, Reichardt LF. N-cadherin and integrins: two receptor systems that mediate neuronal process outgrowth on astrocyte surfaces. *Neuron* (1988) **1**(1):33–43. doi:10.1016/0896-6273(88)90207-3

110. Arikkath J, Reichardt LF. Cadherins and catenins at synapses: roles in synaptogenesis and synaptic plasticity. *Trends Neurosci* (2008) **31**(9):487–94. doi:10.1016/j.tins.2008.07.001
111. Bamji SX, Shimazu K, Kimes N, Huelsken J, Birchmeier W, Lu B, et al. Role of beta-catenin in synaptic vesicle localization and presynaptic assembly. *Neuron* (2003) **40**(4):719–31. doi:10.1016/S0896-6273(03)00718-9
112. Okuda T, Yu LM, Cingolani LA, Kemler R, Goda Y. beta-Catenin regulates excitatory postsynaptic strength at hippocampal synapses. *Proc Natl Acad Sci U S A* (2007) **104**(33):13479–84. doi:10.1073/pnas.0702334104
113. Marambaud P, Wen PH, Dutt A, Shioi J, Takashima A, Siman R, et al. A CBP binding transcriptional repressor produced by the PS1/epsilon-cleavage of N-cadherin is inhibited by PS1 FAD mutations. *Cell* (2003) **114**(5):635–45. doi:10.1016/j.cell.2003.08.008
114. Radice GL, Rayburn H, Matsunami H, Knudsen KA, Takeichi M, Hynes RO. Developmental defects in mouse embryos lacking N-cadherin. *Dev Biol* (1997) **181**(1):64–78. doi:10.1006/dbio.1996.8443
115. Kadowaki M, Nakamura S, Machon O, Krauss S, Radice GL, Takeichi M. N-cadherin mediates cortical organization in the mouse brain. *Dev Biol* (2007) **304**(1):22–33. doi:10.1016/j.ydbio.2006.12.014
116. Arking DE, Cutler DJ, Brune CW, Teslovich TM, West K, Ikeda M, et al. A common genetic variant in the neurexin superfamily member CNTNAP2 increases familial risk of autism. *Am J Hum Genet* (2008) **82**(1):160–4. doi:10.1016/j.ajhg.2007.09.015
117. Alarcon M, Abrahams BS, Stone JL, Duvall JA, Perederiy JV, Bomar JM, et al. Linkage, association, and gene-expression analyses identify CNTNAP2 as an autism-susceptibility gene. *Am J Hum Genet* (2008) **82**(1):150–9. doi:10.1016/j.ajhg.2007.09.005
118. Strauss KA, Puffenberger EG, Huentelman MJ, Gottlieb S, Dobrin SE, Parod JM, et al. Recessive symptomatic focal epilepsy and mutant contactin-associated protein-like 2. *N Engl J Med* (2006) **354**(13):1370–7. doi:10.1056/NEJMoa052773
119. Penagarikano O, Geschwind DH. What does CNTNAP2 reveal about autism spectrum disorder? *Trends Mol Med* (2012) **18**(3):156–63. doi:10.1016/j.molmed.2012.01.003
120. Bakkaloglu B, O'Roak BJ, Louvi A, Gupta AR, Abelson JF, Morgan TM, et al. Molecular cytogenetic analysis and resequencing of contactin associated protein-like 2 in autism spectrum disorders. *Am J Hum Genet* (2008) **82**(1):165–73. doi:10.1016/j.ajhg.2007.09.017
121. Verkerk AJ, Mathews CA, Joosse M, Eussen BH, Heutink P, Oostra BA. CNTNAP2 is disrupted in a family with Gilles de la Tourette syndrome and obsessive compulsive disorder. *Genomics* (2003) **82**(1):1–9. doi:10.1016/S0888-7543(03)00097-1
122. Belloso JM, Bache I, Guitart M, Caballin MR, Halgren C, Kirchhoff M, et al. Disruption of the CNTNAP2 gene in a t(7;15) translocation family without symptoms of Gilles de la Tourette syndrome. *Eur J Hum Genet* (2007) **15**(6):711–3. doi:10.1038/sj.ejhg.5201824
123. Poliak S, Gollan L, Martinez R, Custer A, Einheber S, Salzer JL, et al. Caspr2, a new member of the neurexin superfamily, is localized at the juxtaparanodes of myelinated axons and associates with K+ channels. *Neuron* (1999) **24**(4):1037–47. doi:10.1016/S0896-6273(00)81049-1
124. Bhat MA, Rios JC, Lu Y, Garcia-Fresco GP, Ching W, St Martin M, et al. Axon-glia interactions and the domain organization of myelinated axons requires neurexin IV/Caspr/Paranodin. *Neuron* (2001) **30**(2):369–83. doi:10.1016/S0896-6273(01)00294-X
125. Mink JW. Basal ganglia dysfunction in Tourette's syndrome: a new hypothesis. *Pediatr Neurol* (2001) **25**(3):190–8. doi:10.1016/S0887-8994(01)00262-4
126. Mink JW. Neurobiology of basal ganglia circuits in Tourette syndrome: faulty inhibition of unwanted motor patterns? *Adv Neurol* (2001) **85**:113–22.
127. Penagarikano O, Abrahams BS, Herman EI, Winden KD, Gdalyahu A, Dong H, et al. Absence of CNTNAP2 leads to epilepsy, neuronal migration abnormalities, and core autism-related deficits. *Cell* (2011) **147**(1):235–46. doi:10.1016/j.cell.2011.08.040
128. Prontera P, Napolioni V, Ottaviani V, Rogaia D, Fusco C, Augello B, et al. DPP6 gene disruption in a family with Gilles de la Tourette syndrome. *Neurogenetics* (2014) **15**(4):237–42. doi:10.1007/s10048-014-0418-9
129. Egger G, Roetzer KM, Noor A, Lionel AC, Mahmood H, Schwarzbraun T, et al. Identification of risk genes for autism spectrum disorder through copy number variation analysis in Austrian families. *Neurogenetics* (2014) **15**(2):117–27. doi:10.1007/s10048-014-0394-0
130. Tanaka S, Syu A, Ishiguro H, Inada T, Horiuchi Y, Ishikawa M, et al. DPP6 as a candidate gene for neuroleptic-induced tardive dyskinesia. *Pharmacogenomics J* (2013) **13**(1):27–34. doi:10.1038/tpj.2011.36
131. Kin Y, Misumi Y, Ikehara Y. Biosynthesis and characterization of the brain-specific membrane protein DPPX, a dipeptidyl peptidase IV-related protein. *J Biochem* (2001) **129**(2):289–95. doi:10.1093/oxfordjournals.jbchem.a002856
132. Nadal MS, Amarillo Y, Vega-Saenz de Miera E, Rudy B. Differential characterization of three alternative spliced isoforms of DPPX. *Brain Res* (2006) **1094**(1):1–12. doi:10.1016/j.brainres.2006.03.106
133. Strop P, Bankovich AJ, Hansen KC, Garcia KC, Brunger AT. Structure of a human A-type potassium channel interacting protein DPPX, a member of the dipeptidyl aminopeptidase family. *J Mol Biol* (2004) **343**(4):1055–65. doi:10.1016/j.jmb.2004.09.003
134. Clark BD, Kwon E, Maffie J, Jeong HY, Nadal M, Strop P, et al. DPP6 localization in brain supports function as a Kv4 channel associated protein. *Front Mol Neurosci* (2008) **1**:8. doi:10.3389/neuro.02.008.2008
135. Schoppa NE, Westbrook GL. Regulation of synaptic timing in the olfactory bulb by an A-type potassium current. *Nat Neurosci* (1999) **2**(12):1106–13. doi:10.1038/16033
136. Johnston D, Hoffman DA, Magee JC, Poolos NP, Watanabe S, Colbert CM, et al. Dendritic potassium channels in hippocampal pyramidal neurons. *J Physiol* (2000) **525**(Pt 1):75–81. doi:10.1111/j.1469-7793.2000.00075.x
137. Liss B, Franz O, Sewing S, Bruns R, Neuhoff H, Roeper J. Tuning pacemaker frequency of individual dopaminergic neurons by Kv4.3L and KChip3.1 transcription. *EMBO J* (2001) **20**(20):5715–24. doi:10.1093/emboj/20.20.5715
138. Nadal MS, Ozaita A, Amarillo Y, Vega-Saenz de Miera E, Ma Y, Mo W, et al. The CD26-related dipeptidyl aminopeptidase-like protein DPPX is a critical component of neuronal A-type K+ channels. *Neuron* (2003) **37**(3):449–61. doi:10.1016/S0896-6273(02)01185-6
139. Lin L, Sun W, Throesch B, Kung F, Decoster JT, Berner CJ, et al. DPP6 regulation of dendritic morphogenesis impacts hippocampal synaptic development. *Nat Commun* (2013) **4**:2270. doi:10.1038/ncomms3270
140. Liao C, Fu F, Li R, Yang WQ, Liao HY, Yan JR, et al. Loss-of-function variation in the DPP6 gene is associated with autosomal dominant microcephaly and mental retardation. *Eur J Med Genet* (2013) **56**(9):484–9. doi:10.1016/j.ejmg.2013.06.008
141. Boghosian-Sell L, Comings DE, Overhauser J. Tourette syndrome in a pedigree with a 7;18 translocation: identification of a YAC spanning the translocation breakpoint at 18q22.3. *Am J Hum Genet* (1996) **59**(5):999–1005.
142. Petek E, Windpassinger C, Vincent JB, Cheung J, Boright AP, Scherer SW, et al. Disruption of a novel gene (IMMP2L) by a breakpoint in 7q31 associated with Tourette syndrome. *Am J Hum Genet* (2001) **68**(4):848–58. doi:10.1086/319523
143. Patel C, Cooper-Charles L, McMullan DJ, Walker JM, Davison V, Morton J. Translocation breakpoint at 7q31 associated with tics: further evidence for IMMP2L as a candidate gene for Tourette syndrome. *Eur J Hum Genet* (2011) **19**(6):634–9. doi:10.1038/ejhg.2010.238
144. Bertelsen B, Melchior L, Jensen LR, Groth C, Glenthoj B, Rizzo R, et al. Intragenic deletions affecting two alternative transcripts of the IMMP2L gene in patients with Tourette syndrome. *Eur J Hum Genet* (2014) **22**(11):1283–9. doi:10.1038/ejhg.2014.24
145. Gakh O, Cavadini P, Isaya G. Mitochondrial processing peptidases. *Biochim Biophys Acta* (2002) **1592**(1):63–77. doi:10.1016/S0167-4889(02)00265-3
146. Burri L, Strahm Y, Hawkins CJ, Gentle IE, Puryer MA, Verhagen A, et al. Mature DIABLO/Smac is produced by the IMP protease complex on the mitochondrial inner membrane. *Mol Biol Cell* (2005) **16**(6):2926–33. doi:10.1091/mbc.E04-12-1086
147. Nunnari J, Fox TD, Walter P. A mitochondrial protease with two catalytic subunits of nonoverlapping specificities. *Science* (1993) **262**(5142):1997–2004. doi:10.1126/science.8266095
148. Lu B, Poirier C, Gaspar T, Gratzke C, Harrison W, Busija D, et al. A mutation in the inner mitochondrial membrane peptidase 2-like gene (Immp2l) affects mitochondrial function and impairs fertility in mice. *Biol Reprod* (2008) **78**(4):601–10. doi:10.1095/biolreprod.107.065987
149. Ma Y, Mehta SL, Lu B, Li PA. Deficiency in the inner mitochondrial membrane peptidase 2-like (Immp21) gene increases ischemic brain damage and impairs mitochondrial function. *Neurobiol Dis* (2011) **44**(3):270–6. doi:10.1016/j.nbd.2011.06.019

150. Sundaram SK, Huq AM, Sun Z, Yu W, Bennett L, Wilson BJ, et al. Exome sequencing of a pedigree with Tourette syndrome or chronic tic disorder. *Ann Neurol* (2011) **69**(5):901–4. doi:10.1002/ana.22398
151. Guo Y, Deng X, Zhang J, Su L, Xu H, Luo Z, et al. Analysis of the MRPL3, DNAJC13 and OFCC1 variants in Chinese Han patients with TS-CTD. *Neurosci Lett* (2012) **517**(1):18–20. doi:10.1016/j.neulet.2012.03.097
152. Gruschke S, Grone K, Heublein M, Holz S, Israel L, Imhof A, et al. Proteins at the polypeptide tunnel exit of the yeast mitochondrial ribosome. *J Biol Chem* (2010) **285**(25):19022–8. doi:10.1074/jbc.M110.113837
153. Galmiche L, Serre V, Beinat M, Assouline Z, Lebre AS, Chretien D, et al. Exome sequencing identifies MRPL3 mutation in mitochondrial cardiomyopathy. *Hum Mutat* (2011) **32**(11):1225–31. doi:10.1002/humu.21562
154. Vilarino-Guell C, Rajput A, Milnerwood AJ, Shah B, Szu-Tu C, Trinh J, et al. DNAJC13 mutations in Parkinson disease. *Hum Mol Genet* (2014) **23**(7):1794–801. doi:10.1093/hmg/ddt570
155. Girard M, Poupon V, Blondeau F, McPherson PS. The DnaJ-domain protein RME-8 functions in endosomal trafficking. *J Biol Chem* (2005) **280**(48):40135–43. doi:10.1074/jbc.M505036200
156. Fujibayashi A, Taguchi T, Misaki R, Ohtani M, Dohmae N, Takio K, et al. Human RME-8 is involved in membrane trafficking through early endosomes. *Cell Struct Funct* (2008) **33**(1):35–50. doi:10.1247/csf.07045
157. Davies SJ, Wise C, Venkatesh B, Mirza G, Jefferson A, Volpi EV, et al. Mapping of three translocation breakpoints associated with orofacial clefting within 6p24 and identification of new transcripts within the region. *Cytogenet Genome Res* (2004) **105**(1):47–53. doi:10.1159/000078008
158. Ohnishi T, Yamada K, Watanabe A, Ohba H, Sakaguchi T, Honma Y, et al. Ablation of Mrds1/Ofcc1 induces hyper-gamma-glutamyl transpeptidasemia without abnormal head development and schizophrenia-relevant behaviors in mice. *PLoS One* (2011) **6**(12):e29499. doi:10.1371/journal.pone.0029499
159. Mattheisen M, Samuels JF, Wang Y, Greenberg BD, Fyer AJ, McCracken JT, et al. Genome-wide association study in obsessive-compulsive disorder: results from the OCGAS. *Mol Psychiatry* (2015) **20**:337–44. doi:10.1038/mp.2014.43
160. Cukier HN, Dueker ND, Slifer SH, Lee JM, Whitehead PL, Lalanne E, et al. Exome sequencing of extended families with autism reveals genes shared across neurodevelopmental and neuropsychiatric disorders. *Mol Autism* (2014) **5**(1):1. doi:10.1186/2040-2392-5-1
161. Weimann M, Grossmann A, Woodsmith J, Ozkan Z, Birth P, Meierhofer D, et al. A Y2H-seq approach defines the human protein methyltransferase interactome. *Nat Methods* (2013) **10**(4):339–42. doi:10.1038/nmeth.2397
162. Thompson MD, Comings DE, Abu-Ghazalah R, Jereseh Y, Lin L, Wade J, et al. Variants of the orexin2/hcrt2 receptor gene identified in patients with excessive daytime sleepiness and patients with Tourette's syndrome comorbidity. *Am J Med Genet B Neuropsychiatr Genet* (2004) **129B**(1):69–75. doi:10.1002/ajmg.b.30047
163. Willie JT, Chemelli RM, Sinton CM, Yanagisawa M. To eat or to sleep? Orexin in the regulation of feeding and wakefulness. *Annu Rev Neurosci* (2001) **24**:429–58. doi:10.1146/annurev.neuro.24.1.429
164. Tsujino N, Sakurai T. Role of orexin in modulating arousal, feeding, and motivation. *Front Behav Neurosci* (2013) **7**:28. doi:10.3389/fnbeh.2013.00028
165. Geschwind DH. Autism: many genes, common pathways? *Cell* (2008) **135**(3):391–5. doi:10.1016/j.cell.2008.10.016
166. Gossen M, Bujard H. Tight control of gene expression in mammalian cells by tetracycline-responsive promoters. *Proc Natl Acad Sci U S A* (1992) **89**(12):5547–51. doi:10.1073/pnas.89.12.5547
167. Mele M, Ferreira PG, Reverter F, DeLuca DS, Monlong J, Sammeth M, et al. Human genomics. The human transcriptome across tissues and individuals. *Science* (2015) **348**(6235):660–5. doi:10.1126/science.aaa0355
168. Takahashi K, Yamanaka S. Induction of pluripotent stem cells from mouse embryonic and adult fibroblast cultures by defined factors. *Cell* (2006) **126**(4):663–76. doi:10.1016/j.cell.2006.07.024
169. Young-Pearse TL, Morrow EM. Modeling developmental neuropsychiatric disorders with iPSC technology: challenges and opportunities. *Curr Opin Neurobiol* (2015) **36**:66–73. doi:10.1016/j.conb.2015.10.006
170. Amir RE, Van den Veyver IB, Wan M, Tran CQ, Francke U, Zoghbi HY. Rett syndrome is caused by mutations in X-linked MECP2, encoding methyl-CpG-binding protein 2. *Nat Genet* (1999) **23**(2):185–8. doi:10.1038/13810
171. Cheung AY, Horvath LM, Grafodatskaya D, Pasceri P, Weksberg R, Hotta A, et al. Isolation of MECP2-null Rett syndrome patient hiPS cells and isogenic controls through X-chromosome inactivation. *Hum Mol Genet* (2011) **20**(11):2103–15. doi:10.1093/hmg/ddr093
172. Griesi-Oliveira K, Acab A, Gupta AR, Sunaga DY, Chailangkarn T, Nicol X, et al. Modeling non-syndromic autism and the impact of TRPC6 disruption in human neurons. *Mol Psychiatry* (2015) **20**(11):1350–65. doi:10.1038/mp.2014.141
173. Wen Z, Nguyen HN, Guo Z, Lalli MA, Wang X, Su Y, et al. Synaptic dysregulation in a human iPS cell model of mental disorders. *Nature* (2014) **515**(7527):414–8. doi:10.1038/nature13716
174. Egawa N, Kitaoka S, Tsukita K, Naitoh M, Takahashi K, Yamamoto T, et al. Drug screening for ALS using patient-specific induced pluripotent stem cells. *Sci Transl Med* (2012) **4**(145):145ra04. doi:10.1126/scitranslmed.3004052
175. Thomson PA, Malavasi EL, Grunewald E, Soares DC, Borkowska M, Millar JK. DISC1 genetics, biology and psychiatric illness. *Front Biol* (2013) **8**(1):1–31. doi:10.1007/s11515-012-1254-7
176. Hornykiewicz O. Brain monoamines and Parkinsonism. *Psychopharmacol Bull* (1975) **11**(3):34–5.
177. Jiang H, Ren Y, Yuen EY, Zhong P, Ghaedi M, Hu Z, et al. Parkin controls dopamine utilization in human midbrain dopaminergic neurons derived from induced pluripotent stem cells. *Nat Commun* (2012) **3**:668. doi:10.1038/ncomms1669
178. Beevers JE, Caffrey TM, Wade-Martins R. Induced pluripotent stem cell (iPSC)-derived dopaminergic models of Parkinson's disease. *Biochem Soc Trans* (2013) **41**(6):1503–8. doi:10.1042/BST20130194
179. Su YC, Qi X. Inhibition of excessive mitochondrial fission reduced aberrant autophagy and neuronal damage caused by LRRK2 G2019S mutation. *Hum Mol Genet* (2013) **22**(22):4545–61. doi:10.1093/hmg/ddt301
180. Reinhardt P, Schmid B, Burbulla LF, Schondorf DC, Wagner L, Glatza M, et al. Genetic correction of a LRRK2 mutation in human iPSCs links parkinsonian neurodegeneration to ERK-dependent changes in gene expression. *Cell Stem Cell* (2013) **12**(3):354–67. doi:10.1016/j.stem.2013.01.008
181. Chen H, Qian K, Du Z, Cao J, Petersen A, Liu H, et al. Modeling ALS with iPSCs reveals that mutant SOD1 misregulates neurofilament balance in motor neurons. *Cell Stem Cell* (2014) **14**(6):796–809. doi:10.1016/j.stem.2014.02.004
182. Nguyen HN, Byers B, Cord B, Shcheglovitov A, Byrne J, Gujar P, et al. LRRK2 mutant iPSC-derived DA neurons demonstrate increased susceptibility to oxidative stress. *Cell Stem Cell* (2011) **8**(3):267–80. doi:10.1016/j.stem.2011.01.013
183. Pasca SP, Portmann T, Voineagu I, Yazawa M, Shcheglovitov A, Pasca AM, et al. Using iPSC-derived neurons to uncover cellular phenotypes associated with Timothy syndrome. *Nat Med* (2011) **17**(12):1657–62. doi:10.1038/nm.2576
184. White AK, VanInsberghe M, Petriv OI, Hamidi M, Sikorski D, Marra MA, et al. High-throughput microfluidic single-cell RT-qPCR. *Proc Natl Acad Sci U S A* (2011) **108**(34):13999–4004. doi:10.1073/pnas.1019446108
185. White AK, Heyries KA, Doolin C, Vaninsberghe M, Hansen CL. High-throughput microfluidic single-cell digital polymerase chain reaction. *Anal Chem* (2013) **85**(15):7182–90. doi:10.1021/ac400896j
186. Lancaster MA, Knoblich JA. Generation of cerebral organoids from human pluripotent stem cells. *Nat Protoc* (2014) **9**(10):2329–40. doi:10.1038/nprot.2014.158
187. Lancaster MA, Renner M, Martin CA, Wenzel D, Bicknell LS, Hurles ME, et al. Cerebral organoids model human brain development and microcephaly. *Nature* (2013) **501**(7467):373–9. doi:10.1038/nature12517
188. Mariani J, Coppola G, Zhang P, Abyzov A, Provini L, Tomasini L, et al. FOXG1-dependent dysregulation of GABA/glutamate neuron differentiation in autism spectrum disorders. *Cell* (2015) **162**(2):375–90. doi:10.1016/j.cell.2015.06.034
189. Bobis-Wozowicz S, Osiak A, Rahman SH, Cathomen T. Targeted genome editing in pluripotent stem cells using zinc-finger nucleases. *Methods* (2011) **53**(4):339–46. doi:10.1016/j.ymeth.2010.12.019
190. Soldner F, Laganiere J, Cheng AW, Hockemeyer D, Gao Q, Alagappan R, et al. Generation of isogenic pluripotent stem cells differing exclusively at two early onset Parkinson point mutations. *Cell* (2011) **146**(2):318–31. doi:10.1016/j.cell.2011.06.019

191. Smith C, Abalde-Atristain L, He C, Brodsky BR, Braunstein EM, Chaudhari P, et al. Efficient and allele-specific genome editing of disease loci in human iPSCs. *Mol Ther* (2015) **23**(3):570–7. doi:10.1038/mt.2014.226
192. Byrne SM, Mali P, Church GM. Genome editing in human stem cells. *Methods Enzymol* (2014) **546**:119–38. doi:10.1016/B978-0-12-801185-0.00006-4
193. Fu Y, Foden JA, Khayter C, Maeder ML, Reyon D, Joung JK, et al. High-frequency off-target mutagenesis induced by CRISPR-Cas nucleases in human cells. *Nat Biotechnol* (2013) **31**(9):822–6. doi:10.1038/nbt.2623
194. Costa V, Aprile M, Esposito R, Ciccodicola A. RNA-Seq and human complex diseases: recent accomplishments and future perspectives. *Eur J Hum Genet* (2013) **21**(2):134–42. doi:10.1038/ejhg.2012.129
195. Marchetto MC, Brennand KJ, Boyer LF, Gage FH. Induced pluripotent stem cells (iPSCs) and neurological disease modeling: progress and promises. *Hum Mol Genet* (2011) **20**(R2):R109–15. doi:10.1093/hmg/ddr336
196. Soneson C, Delorenzi M. A comparison of methods for differential expression analysis of RNA-seq data. *BMC Bioinformatics* (2013) **14**:91. doi:10.1186/1471-2105-14-91
197. Trapnell C, Hendrickson DG, Sauvageau M, Goff L, Rinn JL, Pachter L. Differential analysis of gene regulation at transcript resolution with RNA-seq. *Nat Biotechnol* (2013) **31**(1):46–53. doi:10.1038/nbt.2450
198. Trapnell C, Williams BA, Pertea G, Mortazavi A, Kwan G, van Baren MJ, et al. Transcript assembly and quantification by RNA-Seq reveals unannotated transcripts and isoform switching during cell differentiation. *Nat Biotechnol* (2010) **28**(5):511–5. doi:10.1038/nbt.1621
199. Kanehisa M, Goto S, Sato Y, Kawashima M, Furumichi M, Tanabe M. Data, information, knowledge and principle: back to metabolism in KEGG. *Nucleic Acids Res* (2014) **42**(Database issue):D199–205. doi:10.1093/nar/gkt1076
200. Kanehisa M, Goto S. KEGG: kyoto encyclopedia of genes and genomes. *Nucleic Acids Res* (2000) **28**(1):27–30. doi:10.1093/nar/28.1.27
201. Huang da W, Sherman BT, Lempicki RA. Systematic and integrative analysis of large gene lists using DAVID bioinformatics resources. *Nat Protoc* (2009) **4**(1):44–57. doi:10.1038/nprot.2008.211
202. Huang da W, Sherman BT, Lempicki RA. Bioinformatics enrichment tools: paths toward the comprehensive functional analysis of large gene lists. *Nucleic Acids Res* (2009) **37**(1):1–13. doi:10.1093/nar/gkn923
203. Kamburov A, Wierling C, Lehrach H, Herwig R. ConsensusPathDB – a database for integrating human functional interaction networks. *Nucleic Acids Res* (2009) **37**(Database issue):D623–8. doi:10.1093/nar/gkn698
204. Parikshak NN, Gandal MJ, Geschwind DH. Systems biology and gene networks in neurodevelopmental and neurodegenerative disorders. *Nat Rev Genet* (2015) **16**(8):441–58. doi:10.1038/nrg3934
205. Hawrylycz MJ, Lein ES, Guillozet-Bongaarts AL, Shen EH, Ng L, Miller JA, et al. An anatomically comprehensive atlas of the adult human brain transcriptome. *Nature* (2012) **489**(7416):391–9. doi:10.1038/nature11405
206. Kang HJ, Kawasawa YI, Cheng F, Zhu Y, Xu X, Li M, et al. Spatio-temporal transcriptome of the human brain. *Nature* (2011) **478**(7370):483–9. doi:10.1038/nature10523
207. Keen JC, Moore HM. The genotype-tissue expression (GTEx) project: linking clinical data with molecular analysis to advance personalized medicine. *J Pers Med* (2015) **5**(1):22–9. doi:10.3390/jpm5010022
208. Cotney J, Muhle RA, Sanders SJ, Liu L, Willsey AJ, Niu W, et al. The autism-associated chromatin modifier CHD8 regulates other autism risk genes during human neurodevelopment. *Nat Commun* (2015) **6**:6404. doi:10.1038/ncomms7404
209. Darmanis S, Sloan SA, Zhang Y, Enge M, Caneda C, Shuer LM, et al. A survey of human brain transcriptome diversity at the single cell level. *Proc Natl Acad Sci U S A* (2015) **112**(23):7285–90. doi:10.1073/pnas.1507125112
210. Stark C, Breitkreutz BJ, Reguly T, Boucher L, Breitkreutz A, Tyers M. BioGRID: a general repository for interaction datasets. *Nucleic Acids Res* (2006) **34**(Database issue):D535–9. doi:10.1093/nar/gkj109
211. Gilman SR, Iossifov I, Levy D, Ronemus M, Wigler M, Vitkup D. Rare de novo variants associated with autism implicate a large functional network of genes involved in formation and function of synapses. *Neuron* (2011) **70**(5):898–907. doi:10.1016/j.neuron.2011.05.021
212. Willsey AJ, Sanders SJ, Li M, Dong S, Tebbenkamp AT, Muhle RA, et al. Coexpression networks implicate human midfetal deep cortical projection neurons in the pathogenesis of autism. *Cell* (2013) **155**(5):997–1007. doi:10.1016/j.cell.2013.10.020
213. Chang J, Gilman SR, Chiang AH, Sanders SJ, Vitkup D. Genotype to phenotype relationships in autism spectrum disorders. *Nat Neurosci* (2015) **18**(2):191–8. doi:10.1038/nn.3907
214. Platt RJ, Chen S, Zhou Y, Yim MJ, Swiech L, Kempton HR, et al. CRISPR-Cas9 knockin mice for genome editing and cancer modeling. *Cell* (2014) **159**(2):440–55. doi:10.1016/j.cell.2014.09.014
215. Yang H, Wang H, Shivalila CS, Cheng AW, Shi L, Jaenisch R. One-step generation of mice carrying reporter and conditional alleles by CRISPR/Cas-mediated genome engineering. *Cell* (2013) **154**(6):1370–9. doi:10.1016/j.cell.2013.08.022
216. Godar SC, Mosher LJ, Di Giovanni G, Bortolato M. Animal models of tic disorders: a translational perspective. *J Neurosci Methods* (2014) **238**:54–69. doi:10.1016/j.jneumeth.2014.09.008
217. Comings DE, Wu S, Chiu C, Ring RH, Gade R, Ahn C, et al. Polygenic inheritance of Tourette syndrome, stuttering, attention deficit hyperactivity, conduct, and oppositional defiant disorder: the additive and subtractive effect of the three dopaminergic genes – DRD2, D beta H, and DAT1. *Am J Med Genet* (1996) **67**(3):264–88. doi:10.1002/(SICI)1096-8628(19960531)67:3<264::AID-AJMG4>3.0.CO;2-N
218. Paschou P. The genetic basis of Gilles de la Tourette syndrome. *Neurosci Biobehav Rev* (2013) **37**(6):1026–39. doi:10.1016/j.neubiorev.2013.01.016
219. Clarke RA, Lee S, Eapen V. Pathogenetic model for Tourette syndrome delineates overlap with related neurodevelopmental disorders including autism. *Transl Psychiatry* (2012) **2**:e158. doi:10.1038/tp.2012.75
220. Yee CM, Javitt DC, Miller GA. Replacing DSM categorical analyses with dimensional analyses in psychiatry research: the research domain criteria initiative. *JAMA Psychiatry* (2015) **72**(12):1159–60. doi:10.1001/jamapsychiatry.2015.1900
221. Kraemer HC. Research domain criteria (RDoC) and the DSM-two methodological approaches to mental health diagnosis. *JAMA Psychiatry* (2015) **72**(12):1163–4. doi:10.1001/jamapsychiatry.2015.2134
222. Insel T, Cuthbert B, Garvey M, Heinssen R, Pine DS, Quinn K, et al. Research domain criteria (RDoC): toward a new classification framework for research on mental disorders. *Am J Psychiatry* (2010) **167**(7):748–51. doi:10.1176/appi.ajp.2010.09091379
223. Casey BJ, Oliveri ME, Insel T. A neurodevelopmental perspective on the research domain criteria (RDoC) framework. *Biol Psychiatry* (2014) **76**(5):350–3. doi:10.1016/j.biopsych.2014.01.006
224. Cuthbert BN. Research domain criteria: toward future psychiatric nosologies. *Dialogues Clin Neurosci* (2015) **17**(1):89–97.
225. Heiman GA, King RA, Tischfield JA. New Jersey center for Tourette syndrome sharing repository: methods and sample description. *BMC Med Genomics* (2008) **1**:58. doi:10.1186/1755-8794-1-58
226. Dietrich A, Fernandez TV, King RA, State MW, Tischfield JA, Hoekstra PJ, et al. The Tourette International Collaborative Genetics (TIC Genetics) study, finding the genes causing Tourette syndrome: objectives and methods. *Eur Child Adolesc Psychiatry* (2015) **24**(2):141–51. doi:10.1007/s00787-014-0543-x

14

Cross-Disorder Genetic Analysis of Tic Disorders, Obsessive–Compulsive and Hoarding Symptoms

Nuno R. Zilhão[1,2], Dirk J. Smit[2,3], Dorret I. Boomsma[2] and Danielle C. Cath[1,4]*

[1] Department of Clinical and Health Psychology, Utrecht University, Utrecht, Netherlands, [2] Department of Biological Psychology, Vrije Universiteit, Amsterdam, Netherlands, [3] Neuroscience Campus Amsterdam, Vrije Universiteit, Amsterdam, Netherlands, [4] Altrecht Academic Anxiety Center, Utrecht, Netherlands

Edited by:
Peristera Paschou,
Democritus University
of Thrace, Greece

Reviewed by:
Biju Viswanath,
National Institute of Mental Health
and Neuro Sciences, India
Suhash Chakraborty,
Hindustan Aeronautics
Limited Hospital, India

***Correspondence:**
Nuno R. Zilhão
n.rodrigueszilhaonogueira@vu.nl

Hoarding, obsessive–compulsive disorder (OCD), and Tourette's disorder (TD) are psychiatric disorders that share symptom overlap, which might partly be the result of shared genetic variation. Population-based twin studies have found significant genetic correlations between hoarding and OCD symptoms, with genetic correlations varying between 0.1 and 0.45. For tic disorders, studies examining these correlations are lacking. Other lines of research, including clinical samples and GWAS or CNV data to explore genetic relationships between tic disorders and OCD, have only found very modest if any shared genetic variation. Our aim was to extend current knowledge on the genetic structure underlying hoarding, OC symptoms (OCS), and lifetime tic symptoms and, in a trivariate analysis, assess the degree of common and unique genetic factors contributing to the etiology of these disorders. Data have been gathered from participants in the Netherlands Twin Register comprising a total of 5293 individuals from a sample of adult monozygotic ($n = 2460$) and dizygotic ($n = 2833$) twin pairs (mean age 33.61 years). The data on Hoarding, OCS, and tic symptoms were simultaneously analyzed in Mplus. A liability threshold model was fitted to the twin data, analyzing heritability of phenotypes and of their comorbidity. Following the criteria for a probable clinical diagnosis in all phenotypes, 6.8% of participants had a diagnosis of probable hoarding disorder (HD), 6.3% of OCS, and 12.8% of any probable lifetime tic disorder. Genetic factors explained 50.4, 70.1, and 61.1% of the phenotypic covariance between hoarding-OCS, hoarding-tics, and OCS-tics, respectively. Substantial genetic correlations were observed between hoarding and OCS (0.41), hoarding and tics (0.35), and between OCS and tics (0.37). These results support the contribution of genetic factors in the development of these disorders and their comorbidity. Furthermore, tics were mostly influenced by specific environmental factors unshared with OCS and HD.

Keywords: tic, hoarding, obsessive–compulsive symptoms, heritability, trivariate, twin

INTRODUCTION

Current classification systems of psychiatric disorders are primarily based on consensus statements with respect to clinical symptom diagnostics by physicians. These classification systems, i.e., the International Classification of Diseases (ICD) (1) and the Diagnostic and Statistical Manual of Mental Disorders (DSM) (2), have rendered the separate and categorical entities we know as disorders – including obsessive–compulsive disorder (OCD), Tourette's disorder (TD), and (starting from DSM-5) hoarding disorder (HD).

More specifically, OCD, HD, and tic disorders/TD are complex neuropsychiatric disorders; all characterized by repetitive behaviors that show substantial comorbidity, i.e., co-occurring more often than expected by chance (3–6). OCD is a neurodevelopmental disorder characterized by recurrent intrusive thoughts (obsessions) and repetitive behaviors (compulsions) designed to relieve either tension or anxiety stemming from the obsessions (7, 8). HD has since long been classified as a symptom dimension of OCD, and – to a lesser extent – as a characteristic of obsessive–compulsive personality disorder (7). However, it was later suggested that (1) HD presents mostly (in up to 80% of cases) without concurrent OCD (9) and (2) the neurological mechanisms underlying hoarding might be distinct from OCD (9, 10). Therefore, it was included in DSM-5 as a distinct disorder in the category of OCD spectrum disorders and characterized by the inability to discard an excessive amount of items of no significant value, combined with excessive acquisition and clutter to such an extent that living spaces of an individual are occupied (2). Tic disorders are characterized by recurrent motor and/or vocal tics that occur in a stereotypical fashion against a background of normal motor/phonic activity, with onset in childhood and tendency to decrease in intensity and frequency during adolescence (11).

Prevalence rates for these disorders range between 0.1 and 0.8% for TD (12–19), 2 and 6% for compulsive hoarding (20, 21), and 0.5 and 2.0% for OCD (7, 22).

With respect to comorbidity rates between HD and OCD, in clinical and epidemiological studies of OCD, between 18 and 42% of patients report hoarding behaviors, depending on phenotypic definition (23–26), and reversely, in 12–20% of HD patients, OCD is reported (27–29). In TD/chronic tic disorders, OCD is very common, with estimates ranging from 28 to 49% of OCD/OC symptoms (OCS) in TD, and reversely, of 10–20% of tics in OCD (30, 31). In sum, these comorbidity estimates are well above expected comorbidity rates if the three disorders would be etiologically distinct. Finally, in tic disorders, no studies on hoarding comorbidity have been performed nor have studies been performed on tic comorbidity in HD.

Family studies and genetic epidemiological twin studies on each separate disorder have shown substantial genetic contribution to each separate phenotype, with heritability estimates from twin studies ranging between 0.30 and 0.58 (OCD) (31–35), 0.35 and 0.50 (HD) (20, 28, 33), and.25 and 0.58 (tic disorders) (36–40). A next question is whether the high proportions of co-occurrence between the three phenotypes reflect overlap in genetic or environmental contributions between OCD, HD, and tics. Multivariate twin/family studies are particularly suitable for this, making use of correlations between MZ and DZ twins on the various traits to partition the relative contribution of shared vs. unique genetic and environmental factors that influence multiple traits (41).

Despite recent advances in psychiatric genetics, twin studies specifically investigating shared genetic and environmental influences between OCS, hoarding behavior, and tics are scarce. Two studies by Iervolino et al. in a sample consisting predominantly of female twins from the TwinsUk twin registry (4459 female twins, mean age of 55.0 years) have specifically examined the genetic and environmental overlap between OCS and HD behavior (20, 33). It was found that 45% of the genetic variance was shared between HD and OCS dimensions. Furthermore, hoarding had the lowest loading on the common factor with only 55% of the total variance in OC symptom dimensions being hoarding-specific. A recent twin study of our group within the Netherlands twin Register (NTR), which overlaps with our sample, assessed the unique and shared genetic contributions for HD and OCS in a sample of 7567 twins (2270 males, 5297 females, mean age of 33.2 years) (29). The authors found significant genetic contributions to the comorbidity across both traits, although a low genetic correlation (0.10) was found. Finally, a recent population-based twin family study with data from the Swedish Twin Register (n = 20.821) specifically addressed the proportion of shared genetic and environmental factors underlying the liability to chronic tics, ADHD, and OCS (42). Tics were broadly defined based on the number of *total* tics ("no tic score," "tic score = 1," and "tic score > 1"). A substantial correlation of 0.45 between tics and OCS was found.

From another line of research, Genome-wide association study (GWAS) data from samples of TD and OCD patients were analyzed to find a genetic correlation between OCS and TD of 0.41 (43), which was relatively high in light of what has been described for other complex disorders (44). However, this correlation might have been an overestimation, as the SE of this estimate was large (SE = 0.15) and, in addition, the co-occurence between tics and OCD appeared relatively high (13% of OCD had co-occurring tics/TD, and reversely, 43% of TD had OCD) Furthermore, in this same sample, Yu et al. sought to characterize common genetic variants shared among TD and OCD. Although no specific variants were identified, the combined GWAS signals were significantly enriched for functional alleles, suggesting that there is some proportion of TD–OCD-shared genetic risk variants (45).

So far, genetic epidemiological twin family studies to estimate the shared respective unique contributions of genetic and environmental factors between tic-HD symptoms and between tic-HD–OCS are lacking, as are molecular genetic studies to estimate shared genetic contributions from SNPs across TD, OCS, and HD phenotypes.

Therefore, the main aim of this study was to extend the available data so far with respect to shared etiology between OCS and hoarding behavior (29) by expanding with the tic phenotype, in a large population-based twin sample that includes male, female, and opposite sex twin pairs using diagnostic methods that assess the full range of the symptomatology of these disorders to better address their shared underlying etiology. Specifically, we aimed at (1) replicating previous quantifications of shared and independent genetic contributions to OCS-hoarding behavior; (2) quantifying shared and independent genetic contributions to hoarding behavior and tics; (3) quantifying shared and independent genetic contributions to OCS and tics; and (4) quantifying shared and independent genetic contribution to OCS-hoarding behavior and tics.

MATERIALS AND METHODS

Subjects

Participants included in this study are registered with the NTR. Since 1991, twins and their family members receive surveys by mail and are assessed with questionnaires about health, personality, and lifestyle (46, 47). For these analyses, we used data collected in 2008, corresponding to the survey 8 wave of collection, on obsessive–compulsive symptoms, hoarding, and tic symptoms (henceforth named as "tics"). A total of 16,930 participants from 7400 different families completed the questionnaires. Twins encompassed 8047 individuals (2511 males and 5536 females). This study has been approved by the Medical Ethical Committee of the VU Medical Center Amsterdam.

Measurements

The assessment instruments used were the Hoarding Rating Scale-Self-Report (HRS-SR) for hoarding, the Padua Inventory Abbreviated Revised (PI-ABBR) for OCS, and an abbreviated self-report questionnaire (the Schedule for Tourette and Other Behavioral Syndromes – STOBS-ABBR) based on the Schedule for Tourette and Other Behavioral Syndromes (STOBS) for tics. The HRS-SR questionnaire consists of five items, each scoring on a 0–8 scale, that assess cluttering, difficulty in discarding items, excessive acquisition or collecting, distress derived from hoarding symptoms, and functional impairment (48). The distress item was discarded due to approval restriction on the items to be included in the larger questionnaire. The PI-ABBR questionnaire has been derived from the Padua Inventory-Revised, a 41-item self-report instrument that measures OCS on a scale from 0 to 4, and 5 subsequent subscales (washing, checking, rumination, precision, and impulses). The PI-ABBR has been abbreviated to 12 items that include 2–3 items from each of the five OCS dimensions mentioned above (49). These subscales refer to four main factors of obsessions and compulsions – "impaired control," "fear of contamination," "checking behavior," and "urge/worry of losing control" (50).

The STOBS consists of a semi-structured assessment on tics and has been widely used in data collections by the Tourette Syndrome Association International Consortium for Genetics (TSAICG). It consists of 36 tic items (rated as current/lifetime, not present), generating lifetime tic information (51). For the NTR 2008 survey, the STOBS was abbreviated to a 12-item tic questionnaire on the 9 most frequent tics occurring in clinical samples (11, 52). Additionally, three items were added on age at onset of symptoms, tic severity, and whether the tic persisted for more than a year. Using the STOBS-ABBR, a diagnosis of probable chronic tic disorder was established if the person had (1) one or more chronic motor or one or more vocal tic that (2) occurred before age 21, and (3) had been present for >1 year. Probable TD diagnosis was established when two or more motor and one or more vocal tics were reported that occurred before age 21 and had lasted for >1 year, and probable transient tic disorder was established when motor and/or vocal tics had occurred before age 21 for <1 year. Participants who reported at least one tic, but without an age at onset ≤21, and/or with a tic duration of <1 year were categorized as a probable tic disorder NOS. We use the term "probable" since tic diagnoses were not confirmed by a face-to-face interview by an experienced clinician.

We fitted a liability threshold model, using, for each phenotype, a categorical variable derived from several cut points applied to the full distribution of sum scores (for OCS and HD) and defining the presence/absence of a tic disorder (for tics). The liability threshold model assumes an unobserved (and not measured) liability (or risk) to disease, normally distributed in the population (53, 54). The categories function as a (indirect) measure of this liability, representing the susceptibility to the true underlying distribution of the disease. Four categories were used for both the HRS-SR and PI-ABBR. The HRS-SR was divided into categories that more closely resemble the clinical patterns of symptomatology (no hoarding symptoms, mild symptoms, subclinical hoarding, and clinically significant hoarding or probable HD) having unequal distributions in each category (scores of 0, 1–5, 6–16, and ≥17) (20). For a probable HD diagnosis, we used the cutoff proposed by Tolin to define caseness (48). In this work, a receiver operating characteristic (ROC) analysis determined that the best threshold separating HD from non-HD cases was a sum-score over the cutoff of 17 with a sensitivity and a specificity of 0.95. The scores for PI-ABBR (0, 1–6, 7–15, and ≥16) have been previously described in the literature (49). In brief, ROC determined that the best threshold separating OCD from non-OCD cases was a sum-score over the cutoff of 16 with a sensitivity of 0.74 and a specificity of 0.72. For tics, we derived a dichotomous variable defining the presence or absence of any of the tic disorders described here above, according to a definition of "probable tic disorder," as defined by the STOBS-ABBR. For further details on the phenotype definition for tics, please refer to (Zilhao et al., submitted[1]). Briefly, the probable tic disorder dichotomous variable consists of the most lenient definition defined for caseness, in which lifetime probable chronic tic disorder, probable TD, and probable transient tic disorder are included.

Statistical Analysis

Univariate Twin Analysis

Prevalences, means, and distributions for the three phenotypes were calculated in the entire sample of 16,930 individuals. Performing these analyses on clinically defined significant symptoms has the advantage of increasing the generalizability of the results. Polychoric correlations (correlations on the liability scale) were calculated in Mplus (55) for the PI-ABBR, HRS-SR, and STOBS-ABBR, both in MZ and DZ twin pairs by sex, and in all twins for both sexes. Data from both complete and incomplete twin pairs were included in the analysis. Univariate analyses for each phenotype were performed separately using the software OpenMx (56) to estimate the relative contributions from additive genetic (A), shared environment (C), and non-shared environment (E) to each phenotype. Maximum-likelihood model fitting procedures were carried out, as is standard in structural equation modeling, in which the phenotype was a function of the A, C, and E factors and polychoric correlations, according to the liability threshold

[1] Zilhao NR, Olthof MC, Smit DJA, Cath DC, Mathews CA, Delucchi K, et al. Heritability of Tic Disorders: a Twin-Family Study (submitted).

model described above. We investigated the potential influence of twin-specific and gender-specific (sex differences) environment by constraining correlations across zygosity groups to be equal, for all three phenotypes. The effect of covariates (age and sex) on the thresholds was univariately assessed for each phenotype.

Multivariate Twin Analyses

Using the Mplus software, we then fitted a trivariate genetic model to the data with the weighted least square mean and variance adjusted estimation option (WLSMV) (55), using the described liability threshold models. Covariances between the three phenotypes were partitioned into the relative contributions of shared additive genetic (A), common environmental (C), and non-shared environmental (E) influences to the etiology of the three phenotypes. The influence of common environmental factors and of genetic dominance were tested by comparing a nested AE model with either the ACE or the ADE model using the Chi-square difference test.

Lastly, we performed a single factor analysis on the covariance matrices partitioned between the phenotypes. This analysis gives a representation in terms of the components shared by the three phenotypes.

RESULTS

Descriptives

Means and Distributions

The mean age of the entire sample was 33.61 years (SD = 14.56); for males the mean age was 33.11 years (SD = 14.66) and for females 33.84 years (SD = 14.51). The mean average score for HRS-SF was 5.74 (SD = 5.6) and for the PI-ABBR was 6.89 (SD = 5.2). Males had on average higher scores than females on both the HRS-SF and the PI-ABBR. Also for tics, the prevalence rates were higher in males (13.0%) than in females (12.6%). **Table 1** summarizes the demographics in males and females for the PI-ABBR, HRS-SF, and STOBS-ABBR.

Prevalence and Phenotype "Overlap"

Table 2 shows prevalence rates for the three phenotypes for MZ and DZ twins, as estimated according to the diagnostic criteria. Of the entire sample, 5.0% had clinically significant HD, 6.0% had clinically significant OCS, and 13.5% had any probable tic disorder according to the STOBS-ABBR. The threshold used to determine caseness in a probable HD disorder diagnosis rendered population prevalence rates that closely resemble previous estimates for clinical HD (20, 21). Furthermore, among individuals with OCS, 18.0% had co-occurring HD and 12.1% had tics; among individuals with HD, 15.0% had OCS and 8.72% had tics; among individuals with tics, 27.1% had OCS and 23.3% had HD. Lastly, in the entire sample, 0.31% ($n = 25$) of individuals had the co-occurrence of all three disorders.

TABLE 1 | Sample demographics for the data included in the analysis.

	MZ twins		DZ twins	
	Male	**Female**	**Male**	**Female**
Mean age	35.09 (15.27)	35.63 (15.20)	31.57 (13.98)	31.88 (13.45)
Mean HRS	5.85	5.5	6.08	5.79
Mean PADUA	6.99	6.7	7.04	6.99
Tics (prevalence)	192	188	175	162

Univariate Results

Twin Correlations

Table 3 shows the polychoric correlations as calculated on the observed data for the five zygosity groups, on the HRS-SR, PI-ABBR, and the STOBS-ABBR. Overall, when comparing MZ and DZ pairs on the three phenotypes, an average twofold increase for MZ twins when compared to DZ twins is observed. The greater similarity for MZ twins is an indication of a genetic basis influencing the phenotypes. Also, the moderate MZ correlations suggest the influence of non-shared environmental factors for all three phenotypes.

Specific gender/twin environments were tested univariately for each phenotype. As expected from the twin correlations across all zygosities, the fit statistics results show that correlations could be equated across twins and sex, with no twin-specific or sex-specific environments observed (**Table 4**).

Heritabilities and Fit Statistics

The total heritability estimates were 0.33 (SE = 0.05, $p < 0.001$) for clinically significant HD, 0.38 (SE = 0.05, $p < 0.001$) for OCS, and 0.37 for any tic disorder (SE = 0.05, $p < 0.001$) (off-diagonal in **Table 5**). For non-shared environment, the estimates were 0.67 (SE = 0.05, $p < 0.001$) for clinically significant HD, 0.62 for OCS (SE = 0.05, $p < 0.001$), and 0.63 (SE = 0.05,

TABLE 2 | Prevalence rates for HD (HRS-SR), OCS (PI-R-ABBR), and tics (YGTSS) for the total sample included in the analysis.

	Category	MZ ($n = 3990$) *N* (%)	DZ ($n = 4057$) *N* (%)
HD ($n = 5221$) symptom scores	0	673 (22.8)	435 (19.1)
	1–5	1059 (36)	826 (36.2)
	6–16	1079 (36.6)	880 (38.6)
	>16	137 (4.6)	132 (5.7)
OCS ($n = 5167$) symptom scores	0	190 (6.5)	140 (6.3)
	1–4	1447 (49.6)	1077 (48.0)
	5–15	1107 (37.9)	898 (39.9)
	>15	175 (6.0)	133 (5.9)
Probable tic disorder ($n = 5297$) affected/non-affected	TD	15 (0.5)	14 (0.6)
	Chr motor tic	39 (1.3)	35 (1.5)
	Chr vocal tic	17 (0.6)	16 (0.7)
	Transient tic disorder	159 (5.4)	138 (5.9)
	Tic disorder NOS	150 (5.0)	134 (5.7)

TABLE 3 | Polychoric twin correlations for observed data for HD, OCS, and tics.

	MZ	MZM	MZF	DZ	DZM	DZF	DOS
HD (HRS-SR)	0.336	0.379	0.325	0.177	0.247	0.151	0.048
OCS (PI-R-ABBR)	0.384	0.379	0.386	0.177	0.197	0.139	0.214
Tics (STOBS)	0.37	0.242	0.414	0.19	0.238	0.172	0.114

$p < 0.001$) for tics. No evidence was found for an effect of common environment.

Cross-Disorder Correlations

Examining the cross-disorder correlations (cross-twin cross-trait) again suggests that the genetic factors are involved in the correlations between traits (**Table 5**). The MZ cross-twin cross-trait correlations were 0.14 (HD vs. OCS), 0.12 (HD vs. tics), and 0.16 (OCS vs. tics), while the DZ correlations were 0.07 (HD vs. OCS), 0.05 (HD vs. tics), and 0.02 (OCS vs. tics). The within-person cross-trait correlations (phenotypic correlation) were 0.30 (HD vs. OCS), 0.15 (HD vs. tics), and 0.25 (OCS vs. tics) (**Table 5**).

A trivariate ACE model was fitted to the data in order to examine the relative contributions from shared genetic and environmental contributions to the covariance among the traits. Again, as suggested by patterns of twin correlations, no evidence for common environment was found, and the C parameter could be dropped when compared to the more parsimonious AE model [AE vs. ACE model: χ^2 (6) = 0.876, p = 0.99 and AE vs. ADE model: χ^2 (6) = 2.994, p = 0.81]. Hence, the best-fitting model to the data was one in which the covariation between the three phenotypes can be explained by a set of common A and E factors. **Table 5** and **Figure 1** show the estimates of the relative contributions of genes and non-shared environment factors, calculated from the best-fitting model. The total variance for each variable was constrained to 1, in order to estimate the proportion of individual liability due to shared vs. common genetic/environmental factors. Bivariate heritability results (**Table 5**) show that 50% of the covariance between HD and OCS, 70% of the covariance between HD and tics, and 61% of the covariance between OCS and tics are due to genetic factors. The remaining variance is accounted for by non-shared environmental factors. Furthermore, the genetic correlations were 0.41 (HD vs. OCS), 0.35 (HD vs. tics), and 0.37 (OCS vs. tics). **Figure 1** depicts the path diagram in terms of correlated A and E factors.

Lastly, single factor analysis for the A and E component revealed the degree of genetic and environmental overlap shared by the three phenotypes (**Figure 2**). As shown, between 31.5 and 43% of the total genetic variance of each phenotype is due to genetic factors shared among all three phenotypes. Specific genetic variance unshared with other phenotypes was 60.7% (HD), 57.0% (OCS), and 68.5% (tics). Furthermore, 43.2 and 41.8% of the total environmental variance is due to unique environmental factors shared between HD and OCS, respectively, whereas for tics, this amounts only to 4.4% of the total environmental variance – in other words, tics had the lowest loading on the common factor and were mostly influenced by tic-specific environmental effects (**Figure 2**).

TABLE 4 | Model fit indices for the univariate models, examining the role of sex and zygosity, of each phenotype separately.

Model	NP	−2LL	Versus model	χ^2	df	p
1. Hoarding, saturated	10	–	–	–	–	–
2. Hoarding, equal sex, and zygosities	7	3250.51	Hoarding, saturated	3.83	3	0.28
3. OCS, saturated	10	–	–	–	–	–
4. OCS, equal sex, and zygosities	7	840.18	OCS, saturated	1.07	3	0.78
5. Tics, saturated	10	–	–	–	–	–
6. Tics, equal sex, and zygosities	7	16,091.12	Tics, saturated	5.45	3	0.14

NP, number of parameters; −2LL, −2 × log-likelihood; df, degrees of freedom for χ^2 test.

DISCUSSION

In this study, we sought to examine the extent to which shared genetic and environmental factors contribute to clinically significant OCS, HD, and tic symptomatology. We had at our disposal the largest twin pair sample available to date in which these three phenotypes were measured at the same wave of data collection. The present results extend previous work in the same NTR sample on shared genetic contributions to OCS and HD (29).

Our univariate prevalence rates for clinical significant HD symptoms and OCS are in the expected range when compared to the literature (49, 57). For tics, we note that our somewhat higher prevalence rates than described in the literature might be due to the fact that they reflect lifetime tic disorders, and therefore a somewhat lenient definition for caseness, reflecting our approach to generate optimal results with respect to phenotypic validity, in light of the self-report measures used in the NTR.

Our comorbidity prevalence rates (8.0% of OCS patients reported co-occurring HD, and reversely, 15.0% of HD patients reported co-occurring OCS; 12.1% of OCS patients reported co-occurring tics, and reversely, 27.1% of TD/chronic tic disorders reported co-occurring OCS) are within the expected range when compared with the epidemiological literature (23–31). For HD/tics, to the best of our knowledge, we report here the first comorbidity prevalence rate estimate – 8.72% of HD individuals having co-occurring tics and 23.3% of tic individuals having HD.

The Univariate Model Fitting Results

Previous results with data from the NTR, using by and large the same sample, have yielded heritabilities of 0.40–0.50 for OCS

TABLE 5 | Relative contributions of additive genetic and non-shared environmental influences on the trait variance (diagonal) and covariance cross-trait (off-diagonal) for HD (HRS-SR), OCS (PI-R-ABBR), and tics (YGTSS).

	Phenotypic correlation		CTCT (MZ below, DZ above diagonal)			Additive genetic effects (A)			Non-shared environmental effects (E)		
	HD	OCS	HD	OCS	Tics	HD	OCS	Tics	HD	OCS	Tics
HD	–		–	0.07	0.05	0.326	–	–	0.674	–	–
OCS	0.3	–	0.14	–	0.02	0.504	0.375	–	0.496	0.625	–
Tics	0.15	0.25	0.12	0.16	–	0.701	0.611	0.367	0.299	0.389	0.633

CTCT, cross-twin-cross-trait correlations.

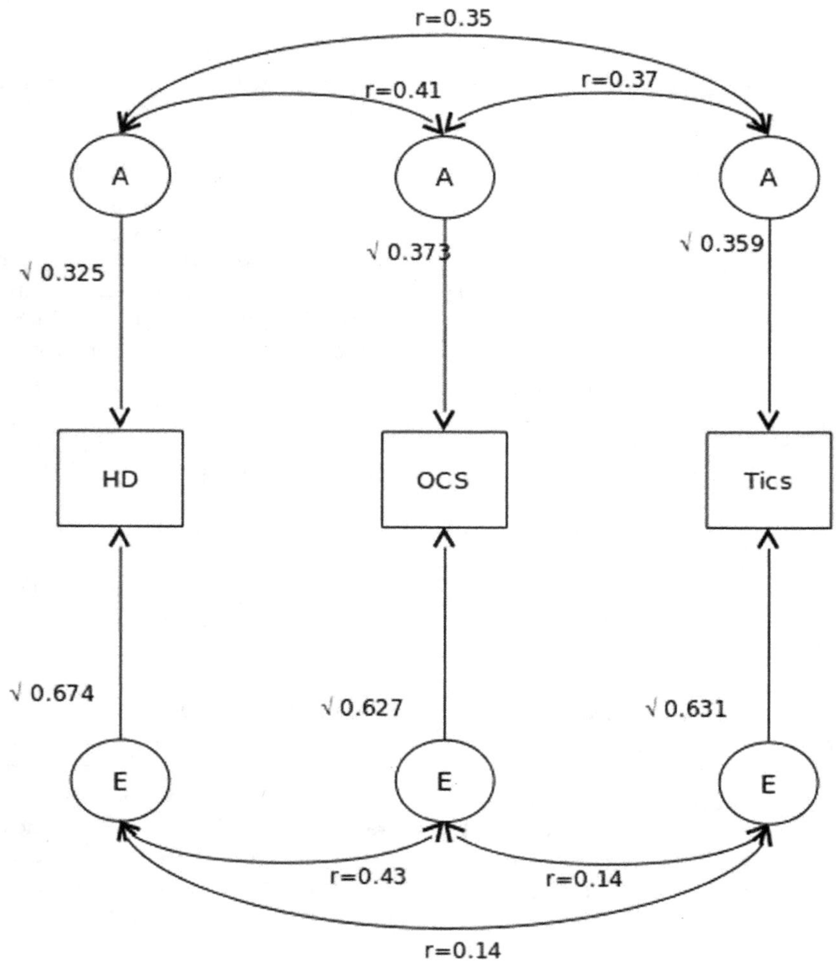

FIGURE 1 | Path diagram for the best-fitting model. Squaring these paths gives the proportion of variance accounted by each of the A and E components. Also indicated are the correlations among each A and E component for each of the three phenotypes. A indicates additive genetic factors and E indicates non-shared environmental factors.

(49, 58), 0.36 for HD (29), and 0.30 for tics (see footnote text 1). Other previous twin/family studies have rendered comparable estimates (0.26–0.55 for OCS, 0.35–0.50 for hoarding, and 0.28–0.56 for tics) (42, 59, 60). We found no evidence for sex differences in twin correlations for any of the phenotypes. Similar findings have been reported for OCS (32, 33, 61), whereas for HD results have been mixed (20, 28); for tics, to the best of our knowledge, the issue of sex differences in twin correlations has not yet been addressed. Our results here show that the genetic contributions to these phenotypes are consistent across both sexes.

Bivariate Analyses

Second, our results provide evidence for shared genetic variation between the phenotypes. The phenotypic correlation between OCS and HD was of 0.30. As expected, we observed a higher phenotypic correlation between OCS and tics (0.25) than between HD and tics (0.15). The genotypic correlations also mirrored this – there was higher shared genetic variance between OCS and HD (0.41) than both OCS and HD with tics (0.37 and 0.35, respectively). Interestingly, a relatively high proportion of the phenotypic correlations were attributable to genetic factors. In other words, although the genetic overlap (expression of same genes) between tics and both OCS and HD is moderate, a substantial proportion of the phenotypic correlation is mediated by their shared genetic variance (61 and 70%, respectively).

Importantly, Iervolino et al. recently reported a genetic correlation between OCS and HD of 0.45, combined with their data suggesting that HD was mostly influenced by specific genetic effects (54.5% specific) (33). The authors argued that this supports the notion of these disorders constituting two etiologically distinct, although related, entities (20, 33). Furthermore, Mathews et al. reported a substantially lower genetic correlation of 0.10 (29). Our current findings of all cross-twin cross-trait genetic correlations being below 0.2 and the within-person cross-trait correlations being all below 0.35 are mostly in line with those in the study by Iervolino et al. (33). Iervolino et al. argue that the

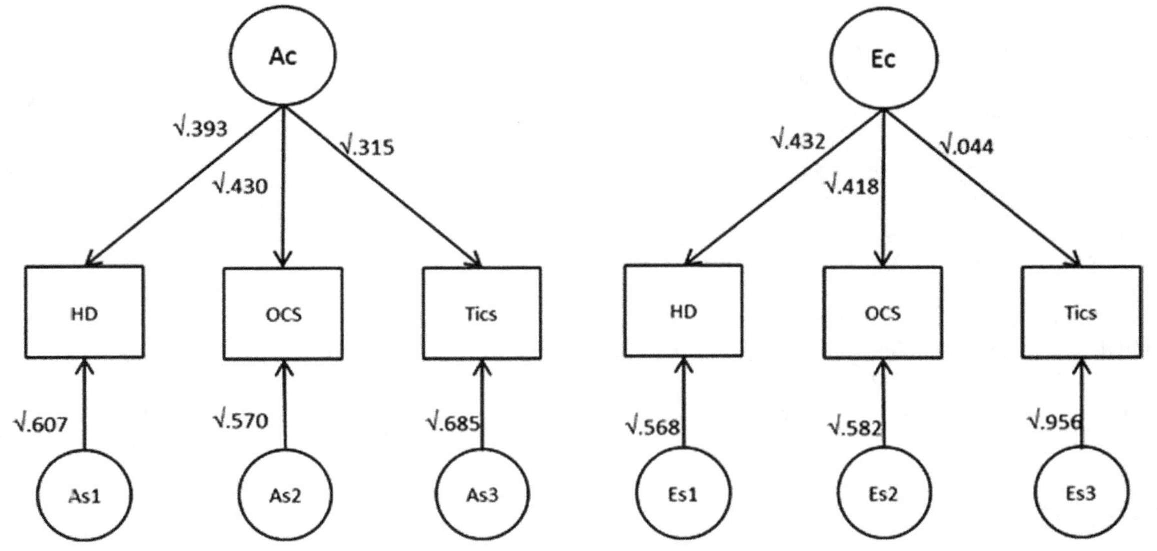

FIGURE 2 | Single factor representation for the each of the A and E component for the best-fitting model. Numbers indicate the proportion (for both A and E components) shared by the three phenotypes. Ac indicates common additive genetic factors and Ec indicates common non-shared environmental factors.

magnitude of these genetic correlations is lower than the shared genetic variance of 0.55 between OCD and other internalizing disorders. i.e., panic disorder, generalized anxiety, phobias, and PTSD (33, 62). They reason that a genetic overlap just under 0.50 argues in favor of HD being a separate, but related entity, as it is currently defined in DSM-5. Our data on the relationship between HD and OCS are in support of this view.

Our estimates of genetic correlations between OCS and tics (0.37) are somewhat lower than the genetic correlations (0.45) as found by Pinto et al. (42). The differences in estimates might be explained by the different phenotypic tic definitions requiring an age of onset before 21 resulting in a prevalence of 13.5%, whereas their multinomial definition of lifetime tics into categories "no tic," "one tic," and "two or more tics" resulted in prevalences of 16% at the first and 6% at the second threshold. Furthermore, our results are not fully in line with tic/OCS-enriched clinical family studies reporting very high genetic correlations between TD and OCS (genetic correlation = 0.92), although the SEs in this study were high (SE = 0.42) (39).

With respect to the shared genetic and environmental contributions to HD and tics, to our knowledge, this is the first twin-family study partitioning the covariance between tics and HD in its relative genetic and environmental components. Our moderate correlation estimate (0.35) supports the argument of viewing TD as distinct from HD.

Third, the common factor model further supports the view of shared genetic etiology between the three phenotypes. Neuroimaging studies have reported structural and functional dysfunctions in the cortico–striato–thalamo–cortical (CSTC) circuitries across all three disorders that have negative implications for motor response inhibition and interference control in these disorders, which might underlie the phenotypic behaviors of all these three disorders (63–65). Our results raise the interesting possibility that a common genetic architecture defines underlying CSTC dysfunctions across the three disorders. Follow-up genome-wide studies may investigate whether specific genetic variants involved in all three disorders are differentially expressed in these brain areas as a result of non-shared environmental influences. In support of this, interestingly, OCS and HD showed low environmental correlations with tics, suggesting that tic disorders have specific environmental contributors invoking tic symptoms. In other words, non-familial (unique) environmental experiences may determine the development of tics, separately from the broader obsessive–compulsive-related disorders, as currently defined in DSM-5 (2).

Finally, our results are relevant for the field of molecular genetics. The lack of power to detect specific genetic risk variants is a recurrent issue in genome-wide studies. One way to overcome this limitation is to combine related phenotypes therefore increasing sample sizes, with consequent power gains. A crucial point here is the balance between power gains from increased sample sizes and power losses from increased heterogeneity (44, 66). Our results suggest that although these disorders share substantial genetic overlap, a substantial proportion of the genetic risk variance contributing to the liability to each disorder is independent from each other, and care should be taken when combining the phenotypes as studied in this paper.

Limitations

These results should be considered in the light of some limitations, mainly considering the phenotypes. Because this is a population-based study, the data collected are based on self-report measures, rather than on clinician-administered structural interviews. The cutoffs have been empirically derived, and are therefore somewhat arbitrary. The cutoffs to determine symptom thresholds (in the case of OCS and HD), by considering the entire range of age available, may have rendered different prevalence estimates, which might have affected estimations of genetic and environmental effects. However, we note that although these threshold cut-offs do not represent definite clinical diagnoses, they do correspond to clinical significant symptoms. Moreover, investigation of dimensions rather than true/false categorical diagnosis is consistent with the ideas forwarded in the NIMH Research Domain Criteria (RDoC) (67).

To conclude, OCS, HD, and tics share etiologic variance that can be explained by substantial genetic correlations. Tics are mostly influenced by specific environmental effects unshared with neither OCS or HD, suggesting that specific environmental stressors might cause the development of tics separate from OCS and HD. Our results are in line with the literature supporting the current definition in DSM-5 of separating these disorders into different, although related, entities.

AUTHOR CONTRIBUTIONS

Acquisition of data, study conception and design, analysis and interpretation of data, drafting of manuscript. All authors listed, have made substantial, direct and intellectual contribution to the work, and approved it for publication.

FUNDING

We are grateful to the twins and siblings for their participation. Furthermore, we thank Dr. Conor Dolan for his critical support of the statistical analyses and overall shaping of the paper. This project has been financed by FP7-People-2012-ITN, project: TS-Eurotrain, grant number 316978; BBR Foundation (NARSAD) 21668; ZonMW (Addiction) 31160008; and European Research Council (ERC-230374).

REFERENCES

1. World Health Organization. *The ICD-10 Classification of Mental and Behavioural Disorders: Clinical Descriptions and Diagnostic Guidelines*. Geneva: World Health Organization (1992).
2. American Psychiatric Association. *DSM 5*. (2013). Available from: http://doi.org/10.1176/appi.books.9780890425596.744053
3. Frost RO, Msw GS, Ab LW, Frost RO. Hoarding: a community health problem. *Health Soc Care Community* (1999) 8(4):229–34. doi:10.1046/j.1365-2524.2000.00245.x
4. Horwath E, Weissman MM. The epidemiology and cross-national presentation of obsessive-compulsive disorder. *Psychiatr Clin North Am* (2000) 23:493–507. doi:10.1016/S0193-953X(05)70176-3
5. Scahill L, Sukhodolsky DG, Williams SK, Leckman JF. Public health significance of tic disorders in children and adolescents. *Adv Neurol* (2005) 96:240–8.
6. Tolin DF, Frost RO, Steketee G, Fitch KE. Family burden of compulsive hoarding: results of an internet survey. *Behav Res Ther* (2008) 46:334–44. doi:10.1016/j.brat.2007.12.008
7. APA. *Diagnostic and Statistical Manual of Mental Disorders*. 4th ed. Washington, DC: American Psychiatric Association (1994). p. 69–81.
8. World Health Organization. *World Health Statistics 2007*. Geneva: World Health Organization (2007).
9. Pertusa A, Fullana MA, Singh S, Alonso P, Menchón JM, Mataix-Cols D. Compulsive hoarding: OCD symptom, distinct clinical syndrome, or both? *Am J Psychiatry* (2008) 165:1289–98. doi:10.1176/appi.ajp.2008.07111730
10. Mataix-Cols D, Frost RO, Pertusa A, Clark LA, Saxena S, Leckman JF, et al. Hoarding disorder: a new diagnosis for DSM-V? *Depress Anxiety* (2010) 27:556–72. doi:10.1002/da.20693
11. Cath DC, Hedderly T, Ludolph AG, Stern JS, Murphy T, Hartmann A, et al. European clinical guidelines for Tourette syndrome and other tic disorders. Part I: assessment. *Eur Child Adolesc Psychiatry* (2011) 20:155–71. doi:10.1007/s00787-011-0164-6
12. Apter A, Pauls DL, Bleich A, Zohar AH, Kron S, Ratzoni G, et al. An epidemiologic study of Gilles de la Tourette's syndrome in Israel. *Arch Gen Psychiatry* (1993) 50:734–8. doi:10.1001/archpsyc.1993.01820210068008
13. Bar-Dayan Y, Arnson Y, Elishkevits K. Screening for common neurologic diseases among Israeli adolescents. *J Child Neurol* (2010) 25:348–51. doi:10.1177/0883073809339878
14. Eapen V, Laker M, Anfield A, Dobbs J, Robertson MM. Prevalence of tics and Tourette syndrome in an inpatient adult psychiatry setting. *J Psychiatry Neurosci* (2001) 26:417–20.
15. Robertson MM, Verril M, Mercer M, James B, Pauls DL. Tourette's syndrome in New Zealand. A postal survey. *Br J Psychiatry* (1994) 164:263–6. doi:10.1192/bjp.164.2.263
16. Scahill L, Dalsgaard S, Bradbury K. The prevalence of Tourette syndrome and its relationship to clinical features. In: Martino D, Leckman JF, editors. *Tourette Syndrome*. Oxford: Oxford University Press (2013). p. 121–33.
17. Schlander M, Schwarz O, Rothenberger A, Roessner V. Tic disorders: administrative prevalence and co-occurrence with attention-deficit/hyperactivity disorder in a German community sample. *Eur Psychiatry* (2011) 26:370–4. doi:10.1016/j.eurpsy.2009.10.003
18. Wenning GK, Kiechl S, Seppi K, Müller J, Högl B, Saletu M, et al. Prevalence of movement disorders in men and women aged 50-89 years (Bruneck study cohort): a population-based study. *Lancet Neurol* (2005) 4:815–20. doi:10.1016/S1474-4422(05)70226-X
19. Zohar AH, Ratzoni G, Pauls DL, Apter A, Bleich A, Kron S, et al. An epidemiological study of obsessive-compulsive disorder and related disorders in Israeli adolescents. *J Am Acad Child Adolesc Psychiatry* (1992) 31(6):1057–61. doi:10.1097/00004583-199211000-00010
20. Iervolino AC, Perroud N, Fullana MA, Guipponi M, Cherkas L, Collier DA, et al. Prevalence and heritability of compulsive hoarding: a twin study. *Am J Psychiatry* (2009) 166:1156–61. doi:10.1176/appi.ajp.2009.08121789
21. Timpano K, Exner C, Glaesmer H, Rief W, Keshaviah A, Brahler E, et al. The epidemiology of the proposed DSM-5 hoarding disorder: exploration of the acquisition specifier, associated features, and distress. *J Clin Psychiatry* (2011) 72(6):780–6. doi:10.4088/JCP.10m06380
22. Ayuso-mateos JL. *Global Burden of Obsessive-Compulsive Disorder in the Year 2000*. Geneva: Global Programme on Evidence for Health Policy (2001). p. 1–10.
23. Frost R, Hartl T. A cognitive-behavioral model of compulsive hoarding. *Behav Res Ther* (1996) 34(4):341–50. doi:10.1016/0005-7967(95)00071-2
24. Lochner C, Kinnear C, Hemmings S, Seller C, Niehaus D, Knowles J, et al. Hoarding in obsessive-compulsive disorder: clinical and genetic correlates. *J Clin Psychiatry* (2005) 66(9):1155–60. doi:10.4088/JCP.v66n0911
25. Rasmussen S, Eisen J. Clinical features and phenomenology of obsessive compulsive disorder. *Psychiatr Ann* (1989) 19(2):67–73. doi:10.3928/0048-5713-19890201-06
26. Samuels J, Bienvenu OJ, Riddle MA, Cullen BAM. Hoarding in obsessive compulsive disorder: results from a case-control study. *Behav Res Ther* (2002) 40:517–28. doi:10.1016/S0005-7967(01)00026-2
27. Frost RO, Steketee G, Tolin DF. Comorbidity in hoarding disorder. *Depress Anxiety* (2011) 28:876–84. doi:10.1002/da.20861
28. Ivanov VZ, Mataix-Cols D, Serlachius E, Lichtenstein P, Anckarsäter H, Chang Z, et al. Prevalence, comorbidity and heritability of hoarding symptoms in adolescence: a population based twin study in 15-year olds. *PLoS One* (2013) 8:e69140. doi:10.1371/journal.pone.0069140
29. Mathews CA, Delucchi K, Cath DC, Willemsen G, Boomsma DI. Partitioning the etiology of hoarding and obsessive-compulsive symptoms. *Psychol Med* (2014) 44(13):2867–76. doi:10.1017/S0033291714000269
30. Como P, LaMarsh J, O'Brien K. Obsessive-compulsive disorder in Tourette's syndrome. *Adv Neurol* (2005) 96:249–61.
31. Do Rosario-Campos MC, Leckman JF, Curi M, Quatrano S, Katsovitch L, Miguel EC, et al. A family study of early-onset obsessive-compulsive disorder. *Am J Med Genet B Neuropsychiatr Genet* (2005) 136B:92–7. doi:10.1002/ajmg.b.30149

32. Hudziak JJ, Van Beijsterveldt CEM, Althoff RR, Stanger C, Rettew DC, Nelson EC, et al. Genetic and environmental contributions to the child behavior checklist obsessive-compulsive scale: a cross-cultural twin study. *Arch Gen Psychiatry* (2004) 61:608–16. doi:10.1001/archpsyc.61.6.608
33. Iervolino AC, Rijsdijk FV, Cherkas L, Fullana MA, Mataix-Cols D. A multivariate twin study of obsessive-compulsive symptom dimensions. *Arch Gen Psychiatry* (2011) 68:637–44. doi:10.1001/archgenpsychiatry.2011.54
34. Pauls DL, Alsobrook JP, Goodman W, Rasmussen S, Leckman JF. A family study of obsessive-compulsive disorder. *Am J Psychiatry* (1995) 152:76–84. doi:10.1176/ajp.152.1.76
35. Zilhao NR, Smit DJA, Den Braber A, Dolan CV, Willemsen G, Boomsma DI, et al. Genetic and environmental contributions to stability in adult obsessive compulsive behavior. *Twin Res Hum Genet* (2014) 18(1):52–60. doi:10.1017/thg.2014.77
36. de Haan MJ, Delucchi KL, Mathews CM, Cath DC. Tic symptom dimensions and their heritabilities in Tourette's syndrome. *Psychiatr Genet* (2015) 25:112–8. doi:10.1097/YPG.0000000000000084
37. Hirschtritt ME, Lee PC, Pauls DL, Dion Y, Grados MA, Illmann C, et al. Lifetime prevalence, age of risk, and genetic relationships of comorbid psychiatric disorders in Tourette syndrome. *JAMA Psychiatry* (2015) 72(4):325–33. doi:10.1001/jamapsychiatry.2014.2650
38. Mataix-Cols D, Isomura K, Pérez-Vigil A, Chang Z, Rück C, Larsson KJ, et al. Familial risks of Tourette syndrome and chronic tic disorders: a population-based cohort study. *JAMA Psychiatry* (2015) 72(8):787–93. doi:10.1001/jamapsychiatry.2015.0627
39. Mathews CA, Grados MA. Familiality of Tourette syndrome, obsessive-compulsive disorder, and attention-deficit/hyperactivity disorder: heritability analysis in a large sib-pair sample. *J Am Acad Child Adolesc Psychiatry* (2011) 50(1):46–54. doi 10.1016/j.jaac.2010.10.004
40. Pauls DL, Raymond CL, Stevenson JM, Leckman JF. A family study of Gilles de la Tourette syndrome. *Am J Hum Genet* (1991) 48:154–63.
41. Van Dongen J, Slagboom PE, Draisma HHM, Martin NG. The continuing value of twin studies in the omics era. *Nat Rev Genet* (2012) 13(9):640–53. doi:10.1038/nrg3243
42. Pinto R, Monzani B, Leckman JF, Christian R, Serlachius E, Lichtenstein P, et al. Understanding the covariation of tics, attention-deficit/hyperactivity, and obsessive-compulsive symptoms: a population-based adult twin study. *Am J Med Genet B Neuropsychiatr Genet* (2016). doi:10.1002/ajmg.b.32436
43. Davis LK, Yu D, Keenan CL, Gamazon ER, Konkashbaev AI, Derks EM, et al. Partitioning the heritability of Tourette syndrome and obsessive compulsive disorder reveals differences in genetic architecture. *PLoS Genet* (2013) 9(10):e1003864. doi:10.1371/journal.pgen.1003864
44. Wray NR, Maier R. Genetic basis of complex genetic disease: the contribution of disease heterogeneity to missing heritability. *Curr Epidemiol Rep* (2014) 1(4):220–7. doi:10.1007/s40471-014-0023-3
45. Yu D, Mathews CA, Neale BM, Ph D, Davis LK, Gamazon ER, et al. Cross-disorder genome-wide analyses suggest a complex genetic relationship between Tourette's syndrome and OCD. *Am J Psychiatry* (2015) 172: 82–93. doi:10.1176/appi.ajp.2014.13101306
46. Boomsma DI, de Geus EJC, Vink JM, Stubbe JH, Distel MA, Hottenga JJ, et al. Netherlands twin register: from twins to twin families. *Twin Res Hum Genet* (2006) 9:849–57. doi:10.1375/twin.9.6.849
47. Willemsen G, Vink JM, Abdellaoui A, den Braber A, van Beek JHDA, Draisma HHM, et al. The adult Netherlands twin register: twenty-five years of survey and biological data collection. *Twin Res Hum Genet* (2013) 16:271–81. doi:10.1017/thg.2012.140
48. Tolin DF, Frost RO, Steketee G. A brief interview for assessing compulsive hoarding: the hoarding rating scale-interview. *Psychiatry Res* (2010) 178(1):147–52. doi:10.1016/j.psychres.2009.05.001
49. Cath DC, van Grootheest DS, Willemsen G, van Oppen P, Boomsma DI. Environmental factors in obsessive-compulsive behavior: evidence from discordant and concordant monozygotic twins. *Behav Genet* (2008) 38(2): 108–20. doi:10.1007/s10519-007-9185-9
50. Sanavio E. Obsessions and compulsions: the Padua inventory. *Behav Res Ther* (1988) 26:169–77. doi:10.1016/0005-7967(88)90116-7
51. Pauls DL, Hurst C. *Schedule for Tourette and Other Behavioral Disorders, Revised.* New Haven, CT: Child Study Center, Yale University (1993).
52. Freeman RD, Fast DK, Burd L, Kerbeshian J, Robertson MM, Sandor P. An international perspective on Tourette syndrome: selected findings from 3,500 individuals in 22 countries. *Dev Med Child Neurol* (2000) 42:436–47. doi:10.1111/j.1469-8749.2000.tb00346.x
53. Falconer DS. The inheritance of liability to certain diseases, estimated from the incidence among relatives. *Ann Hum Genet* (1965) 29:51–76. doi:10.1111/j.1469-1809.1965.tb00500.x
54. Falconer DS. The inheritance of liability to diseases with variable age of onset, with particular reference to diabetes mellitus. *Ann Hum Genet* (1967) 31:1–20. doi:10.1111/j.1469-1809.1967.tb01249.x
55. Prescott CA. Using the Mplus computer program to estimate models for continuous and categorical data from twins. *Behav Genet* (2004) 34(1):17–40. doi:10.1023/B:BEGE.0000009474.97649.2f
56. Boker S, Neale M, Maes H, Wilde M, Spiegel M, Brick T, et al. OpenMx: an open source extended structural equation modeling framework. *Psychometrika* (2011) 76:306–17. doi:10.1007/s11336-010-9200-6
57. Samuels JF, Bienvenu OJ, Grados MA, Cullen B, Riddle MA, Liang K, et al. Prevalence and correlates of hoarding behavior in a community-based sample. *Behav Res Ther* (2008) 46(7):836–44. doi:10.1016/j.brat.2008.04.004
58. van Grootheest DS, Cath D, Hottenga JJ, Beekman AT, Boomsma DI. Genetic factors underlie stability of obsessive-compulsive symptoms. *Twin Res Hum Genet* (2009) 12(5):411–9. doi:10.1375/twin.12.5.411
59. Taylor S, Jang K, Asmundson G. Etiology of obsessions and compulsions: a behavioral-genetic analysis. *J Abnorm Psychol* (2010) 119:672–82. doi:10.1037/a0021132
60. van Grootheest DS, Cath DC, Beekman AT, Boomsma DI. Twin studies on obsessive-compulsive disorder: a review. *Twin Res Hum Genet* (2005) 8(5):450–8. doi:10.1375/183242705774310060
61. Bolton D, Rijsdijk F, O'Connor TG, Perrin S, Eley TC. Obsessive-compulsive disorder, tics and anxiety in 6-year-old twins. *Psychol Med* (2007) 37:39–48. doi:10.1017/S0033291706008816
62. Tambs K, Czajkowsky N, Røysamb E, Neale MC, Reichborn-Kjennerud T, Aggen SH, et al. Structure of genetic and environmental risk factors for dimensional representations of DSM–IV anxiety disorders. *Br J Psychiatry* (2010) 195(4):301–7. doi:10.1192/bjp.bp.108.059485
63. Posner J, Marsh R, Maia TV, Peterson BS, Simpson HB. Reduced functional connectivity within the limbic cortico-striato-thalamo-cortical loop in unmedicated adults with obsessive-compulsive disorder. *Hum Brain Mapp* (2014) 35(6):2852–60. doi:10.1002/hbm.22371.Reduced
64. Van Velzen LS, Vriend C, De Wit SJ, Van Den Heuvel OA. Response inhibition and interference control in obsessive-compulsive spectrum disorders. *Front Hum Neurosci* (2014) 8:419. doi:10.3389/fnhum.2014.00419
65. Wang Z, Ph D, Maia TV, Ph D, Marsh R, Ph D, et al. The neural circuits that generate tics in Tourette's syndrome. *Am J Psychiatry* (2011) 168(12):1326–37. doi:10.1176/appi.ajp.2011.09111692
66. Manchia M, Cullis J, Turecki G, Rouleau GA, Uher R, Alda M. The impact of phenotypic and genetic heterogeneity on results of genome wide association studies of complex diseases. *PLoS One* (2013) 8:e76295. doi:10.1371/journal.pone.0076295
67. Patrick CJ, Hajcak G. Reshaping clinical science: introduction to the special issue on psychophysiology and the NIMH research domain criteria (RDoC) initiative. *Psychophysiology* (2016) 53(3):281–5. doi:10.1111/psyp.12613

15

No Association between Cortical Gyrification or Intrinsic Curvature and Attention-deficit/ Hyperactivity Disorder in Adolescents and Young Adults

Natalie J. Forde[1,2*], Lisa Ronan[3], Marcel P. Zwiers[2], Aaron F. Alexander-Bloch[3,4], Stephen V. Faraone[5,6], Jaap Oosterlaan[7], Dirk J. Heslenfeld[7,8], Catharina A. Hartman[1], Jan K. Buitelaar[2,9†] and Pieter J. Hoekstra[1†]

[1] Department of Psychiatry, University of Groningen, University Medical Center Groningen, Groningen, Netherlands, [2] Department of Cognitive Neuroscience, Donders Institute for Brain, Cognition and Behaviour, Radboud University Medical Center, Nijmegen, Netherlands, [3] Brain Mapping Unit, Department of Psychiatry, University of Cambridge, Cambridge, UK, [4] Child Psychiatry Branch, National Institute of Mental Health, Bethesda, MD, USA, [5] Departments of Psychiatry and of Neuroscience and Physiology, SUNY Upstate Medical University, Syracuse, NY, USA, [6] Department of Biomedicine, K.G. Jebsen Centre for Research on Neuropsychiatric Disorders, University of Bergen, Bergen, Norway, [7] Clinical Neuropsychology Section, Department of Clinical, Neuro and Developmental Psychology, Vrije Universiteit Amsterdam, Amsterdam, Netherlands, [8] Department of Experimental and Applied Psychology, Vrije Universiteit Amsterdam, Amsterdam, Netherlands, [9] Karakter Child and Adolescent Psychiatry University Centre, Nijmegen, Netherlands

Edited by:
Kirsten R. Müller-Vahl, Hannover Medical School, Germany

Reviewed by:
Veit Roessner, TU Dresden, Germany
Kerstin Jessica Plessen, University of Copenhagen, Denmark

***Correspondence:**
Natalie J. Forde
j.n.forde@umcg.nl

[†]Joint last author.

Magnetic resonance imaging (MRI) studies have highlighted subcortical, cortical, and structural connectivity abnormalities associated with attention-deficit/hyperactivity disorder (ADHD). Gyrification investigations of the cortex have been inconsistent and largely negative, potentially due to a lack of sensitivity of the previously used morphological parameters. The innovative approach of applying intrinsic curvature analysis, which is predictive of gyrification pattern, to the cortical surface applied herein allowed us greater sensitivity to determine whether the structural connectivity abnormalities thus far identified at a centimeter scale also occur at a millimeter scale within the cortical surface. This could help identify neurodevelopmental processes that contribute to ADHD. Structural MRI datasets from the NeuroIMAGE project were used [n = 306 ADHD, n = 164 controls, and n = 148 healthy siblings of individuals with ADHD (age in years, mean(sd); 17.2 (3.4), 16.8 (3.2), and 17.7 (3.8), respectively)]. Reconstructions of the cortical surfaces were computed with FreeSurfer. Intrinsic curvature (taken as a marker of millimeter-scale surface connectivity) and local gyrification index were calculated for each point on the surface (vertex) with Caret and FreeSurfer, respectively. Intrinsic curvature skew and mean local gyrification index were extracted per region; frontal, parietal, temporal, occipital, cingulate, and insula. A generalized additive model was used to compare the trajectory of these measures between groups over age, with sex, scanner site, total surface area of hemisphere, and familiality accounted for. After correcting for sex, scanner site, and total surface area no group differences were found in the developmental trajectory of intrinsic curvature or local gyrification index. Despite the increased sensitivity of intrinsic curvature, compared to gyrification measures, to subtle morphological abnormalities of the cortical surface we found no milimeter-scale connectivity abnormalities associated with ADHD.

Keywords: ADHD, intrinsic curvature, biomarker, connectivity, gyrification, development

INTRODUCTION

Attention-deficit/hyperactivity disorder (ADHD) is a common neurodevelopmental disorder affecting~5% of the school age population (Polanczyk et al., 2007) and characterized by pervasive inattention and/or hyperactivity and impulsivity leading to impairments of functioning (American Psychiatric Association, 2013).

ADHD has been proposed to be a dysconnectivity disorder (Konrad and Eickhoff, 2010) where neural circuits are implicated rather than regions, and there has been a move toward investigating ADHD, and other disorders, in terms of connectivity and integration instead of segregation; where specific regional abnormalities are implicated (Friston, 2011). This shift has come in both functional and structural studies, with recent diffusion magnetic resonance imaging (dMRI) analysis concentrating on network connectivity based on white matter tracts as opposed to the traditional voxel-based or region-of-interest analyses (Cao et al., 2013; Hong et al., 2014). A meta-analysis and contemporary review of the available dMRI data revealed that multiple white matter tracts are affected in ADHD, including the anterior corona radiata, forceps minor, and superior and inferior longitudinal fasciculi (Liston et al., 2011; van Ewijk et al., 2012). These white matter tracts consist of bundles of long-range axonal fibers that connect distant gray matter regions (e.g., cortical to sub-cortical structures, inter-hemispheric connections, or frontal to parietal lobes, etc.). However, it is not established whether these long-range white matter connectivity differences are echoed in short-range connections within the cortex. Interestingly, despite the cortex generally being associated with cell bodies rather than connections 95% of connections in the brain are found in the cortex in the form of short-range connections (Braitenberg and Schüz, 1998). Within this study we therefore ask; are these long range abnormalities echoed in the short range connections within the cortex?

Evidence from previous studies does suggest abnormalities of the cortex in those with ADHD. To date many routine markers, such as cortical thickness and volume, have been used to report structural changes in the cortex of individuals with ADHD; however, these results are non-specific in relation to connectivity or the underlying cytoarchitecture of the cortex and sometimes inconsistent (Shaw et al., 2007, 2013; Wolosin et al., 2009; Nakao et al., 2011; Frodl and Skokauskas, 2012; Schweren et al., 2015). Studies into cortical thickness and surface area measures suggest that cortical development has a delayed developmental trajectory in ADHD, with both surface area and cortical thickness reaching their peak later in individuals with ADHD (Shaw et al., 2007, 2012).

It is, however, not clear whether previous cortical findings also relate to connectivity abnormalities within the cortex. To address this we used cortical intrinsic curvature. This is a morphological measure of the intrinsic deformation of the surface and as such may be interpreted in terms of the underlying connectivity of the cortex (Ronan et al., 2011, 2012). This is in contrast to extrinsic measures, such as gyrification, which are related to the embedding of the cortex in three-dimensional space rather than the engrained curvature of the surface (**Figure 1**). These distinct metrics of surface shape are measured at the millimeter-scale (intrinsic curvature) and centimeter-scale respectively (gyrification). The important distinction between these parameters is the nature of the shape they capture. Intrinsic curvature is measure of deformation—i.e., the stretching or compression of the surface, while gyrification (indexed here by the local gyrification index) is a marker of folding. Importantly folding does not deform the surface itself (i.e., distances along the surface remain the same; think of a line drawn on a piece of paper—the length of the line is not changed whether the paper is folded or not). On the other hand deformation (as captured by intrinsic curvature) changes distances along the surface (again, the length of a line on a surface is changed if the surface is stretched or compressed). With the application of intrinsic curvature analysis of the cortical surface we are able to investigate the millimeter-scale connectivity of axonal processes within the gray matter of the cortex. Differential expansion is the process whereby the surface does not expand uniformly but instead has various rates of expansion across the cortex during development resulting in a fluctuating pattern of positive and negative intrinsic curvatures. This differential expansion underlies intrinsic curvature and also results in a greater range of inter-neuronal distances which skews the length distribution toward having a higher proportion of shorter connections, from which more efficient connectivity may be inferred (**Figure 1**, Ronan et al., 2011, 2012). We could therefore make use of the relationship of differential expansion to both intrinsic curvature and connectivity to use one (intrinsic curvature) as a quantifiable measure of the other (connectivity). Describing intrinsic curvature abnormalities associated with ADHD would therefore support the dysconnectivity theory of ADHD by implicating the involvement of short range connections. Intrinsic curvature could then potentially be used clinically as a biological marker of ADHD. Null findings in relation to ADHD would suggest that connectivity abnormalities are constrained to long range connections within the white matter. Either way, this would aid in furthering our understanding of ADHD and its etiology.

Abbreviations: ADHD, attention-deficit/hyperactivity disorder.

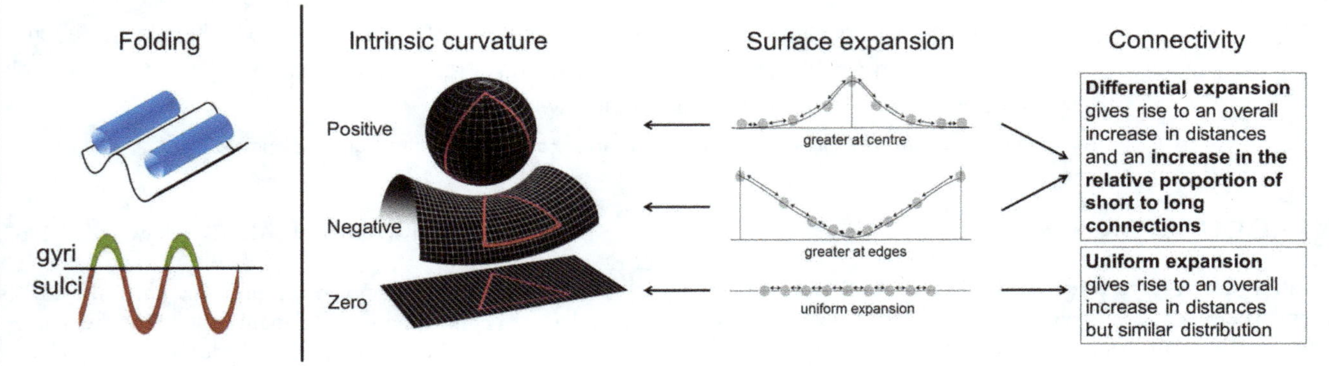

FIGURE 1 | Intrinsic curvature and folding. Folding of the cortical surface, indexed by gyrification measures, relates to extrinsic curvature i.e., how the surface is bent in 3-dimensional space. No intrinsic curvature of the surface is required for folding. Surface expansion is depicted schematically in the above figure with points on a line, equal distribution of points before expansion is assumed. Arrows between points can be interpreted as connections. Differential expansion of the cortex results in either positive or negative intrinsic curvature values depending on whether expansion is faster at the center or edges of the surface. Uniform expansion (zero intrinsic curvature) results in an overall increase in distances between points but no change in the proportion of long to short connections. Differential expansion (positive or negative intrinsic curvature) also results in an increase in the overall distance between points but more importantly it also increases the relative proportion of short to long connections. Figure adapted in part from Ronan et al. (2011, 2012).

Intrinsic curvature has previously been used and shown to be sensitive to cortical differences related to connectivity in patients affected by schizophrenia compared to healthy controls (Ronan et al., 2012) and in a study of healthy participants with various combinations of the *brain derived neurotrophic factor* (*BDNF*) val66met polymorphism (Forde et al., 2014). Furthermore, the related measure of *wiring cost* was found altered in a group of adults with autism spectrum disorder (ASD; Ecker et al., 2013). ASD has also been associated with gyrification and long range connectivity abnormalities (Anagnostou and Taylor, 2011; Schaer et al., 2013). ADHD and ASD share many characteristics as neurodevelopmental disorders and, at least partly, their heritability (Rommelse et al., 2010, 2011), adding weight to our hypothesis that there may be short range connectivity abnormalities in the cortex of individuals with ADHD.

Intrinsic curvature is distinct from, though related to, the overall degree of gyrification (Ronan et al., 2012). While gyrification abnormalities in the left medial temporal region (Mous et al., 2014) and folding abnormalities in the right frontal lobe (Wolosin et al., 2009) have been reported in children with ADHD in two small studies, such abnormalities were not seen in a larger study of gyrification by Shaw et al. (2012). It has been demonstrated that the move in scale-sensitivity using intrinsic curvature, from centimeter to millimeter, increases the power to detect subtle shape differences in the cortex indicative of abnormal neurodevelopment (Ronan et al., 2012). We therefore investigated both local gyrification index and intrinsic curvature in the current study with the assumption that the largely negative previous gyrification studies of ADHD (Shaw et al., 2012) may have been obfuscated by the scale of morphological parameters employed. We thus hypothesized that an investigation of gyrification within the current study would similarly show no group differences while intrinsic curvature would detect subtle morphological alterations indicative of short range dysconnectivity in ADHD.

ADHD is a highly heritable (~80%), genetically complex and heterogeneous disorder (Faraone et al., 2005). Endophenotypes, biologically based phenotypes, hold much promise as less genetically complex markers underlying psychiatric conditions thereby allowing the pathophysiology of conditions to be elucidated (Gottesman and Gould, 2003). As endophenotypes can be thought of as markers of the genetic liability of a disorder they should appear in those with a shared genetic heritage irrespective of diagnosis, for instance the unaffected relatives of an affected individual (Gottesman and Gould, 2003). We therefore took this opportunity to additionally explore the potential of intrinsic curvature as an endophenotypic marker of ADHD by including healthy siblings of those with ADHD, along with the individuals with ADHD and healthy controls in our study design.

METHODOLOGY

Participants

This study was undertaken under the remit of the NeuroIMAGE study, for details see von Rhein et al. (2014) and the study website (www.neuroimage.nl). Briefly the NeuroIMAGE study is the follow up, within the Netherlands, of the International Multicenter ADHD Genetics study (IMAGE; Müller et al., 2011a,b). Initially families who had an individual with ADHD-combined type and healthy control families were recruited to the IMAGE study; all participants were Caucasian, aged 6–18 years and had an IQ $\geq$ 70. Exclusion criteria were a diagnosis of autism, epilepsy and brain, or genetic disorders. Within the ADHD families, individuals with psychiatric diagnoses (other than ADHD) were excluded except for oppositional defiant disorder (ODD), conduct disorder (CD), and pervasive developmental disorder not otherwise specified (PDD-NOS). One or more subjects with ADHD and one or more healthy sibling of those with ADHD from the same family were included. Similarly, multiple healthy subjects were included from healthy control families to balance the familial effect across groups. An extensive battery of diagnostic and neuropsychological tests as well as genetic data were acquired for all participants. From the Dutch sites (Vrije Universiteit [VU] in Amsterdam and Radboud UMC in Nijmegen), all initial participants were invited to participate in the follow up (mean follow up 5.9 years), namely NeuroIMAGE, where neuroimaging data were acquired in addition to behavioral data similar to the initial visit. Note that all ADHD participants were required to still meet criteria for an ADHD diagnosis at time of scanning, therefore those who remitted were omitted from this analysis.

There were 618 full datasets from 374 different families available for the current analysis. Of these there were 306 participants with ADHD (mean [*SD*] age 17.2 [3.4] years), 148 healthy siblings of an individual with ADHD (mean [*SD*] age 17.7 [3.8] years), and 164 healthy controls (mean [*SD*] age 16.8 [3.2] years), see **Table 1** for full demographic details.

At the time of follow-up, all participants in the study were similarly assessed using a combination of a semi-structured diagnostic interview conducted by trained professionals (Dutch translation of the Schedule for Affective Disorders and Schizophrenia for School-Age Children—Present and Lifetime Version K-SADS; Kaufman et al., 1997) and combination of Conners' ADHD questionnaires, these rating were collected of children's functioning off medication. Each child was assessed with a parent-rated questionnaire (Conners' Parent Rating Scale—Revised: Long version CPRS-R:L; Conners et al., 1998a) combined with either a teacher-rating (Conners' Teacher Rating Scale—Revised: Long version CTRS-R:L; Conners et al., 1998b) or a self-report (Conners' Adult ADHD Rating Scales—Self-Report:Long Version CAARS-S:L; Conners et al., 1999).

A diagnostic algorithm was applied to combine symptom counts from the K-SADS and Conners' questionnaires. ADHD diagnosis was given to participants with a combined total symptom count of ≥ 6 (≥ 5 for participants ≥ 18 years) of hyperactive/impulsive and/or inattentive behavior, provided they also: (a) met the DSM-IV criteria for pervasiveness, impact of the disorder and onset-age before 12, and (b) scored $T \geq 63$ on at least one of the Conners' questionnaires (parent, teacher, or self-rating). Healthy control participants were required to score $T < 63$ on both of the Conners' questionnaires, and have ≤ 3 (≤ 2 for participants ≥ 18 years). The K-SADS was additionally used to assess ODD, CD, and presence of tics. Full details can be found in von Rhein et al. (2014).

Structural MRI Acquisition

Two T1-weighted MPRAGE scans were acquired for each participant at one of the two test sites (Amsterdam and Nijmegen). Similar 1.5 Tesla MRI scanners were employed (Siemens SONATA and Siemens AVANTO; Siemens, Erlangen, Germany), using identical head coils (8-channel Phase Array Head Coil). Images were acquired with a sagittal, 3-dimentional GRAPPA parallel imaging sequence with the following parameters: TE = 2.95 ms, TR = 2730 ms, TI = 1000 ms, flip angle = 7°, voxel dimension = 1 × 1 × 1 mm and acquisition time 6.21 min.

Quality Assessment

Image quality was assessed manually by two independent judges. The better quality scan was selected for each participant and those with poor quality scans were omitted ($n = 14$; already excluded from the demographic descriptions).

Surface Reconstruction

The cortical surfaces were reconstructed using FreeSurfer v5.3 (Dale et al., 1999; Fischl et al., 1999a,b; Fischl and Dale, 2000), a programme specifically designed for cortical reconstruction and volumetric segmentation (Dale et al., 1999; Fischl et al., 1999a,b; Fischl and Dale, 2000). The raw images were fed into

TABLE 1 | Group Demographics.

	ADHD		Siblings	Control	Test statistic	*p*-value
n	306		148	164	–	–
Age in years, mean (*SD*)	17.2 (3.4)		17.7 (3.8)	16.8 (3.2)	K-W $\chi^2 = 4.71$	0.095
Sex, m/f	208/98		62/86	87/77	$\chi^2 = 29.85$	<0.001***
IQ, mean (*SD*)	97.0 (15.2)		102.8 (14.3)	105.6 (13.5)	K-W $\chi^2 = 36.71$	<0.001***
Scanner site Ams/Nij	150/156		78/70	105/59	$\chi^2 = 9.78$	0.008*
Handedness r/l/a	269/33/3		124/18/3	146/13/4	$\chi^2 = 3.31$	0.51
ADHD Symptom count, *n (SD)*	13.2 (3.0)		1.2 (1.9)	0.8 (1.7)	K-W $\chi^2 = 484.61$	<0.001***
[a]Stimulant use (never/previous/current)	41/112/147		134/8/1	145/0/0		
Comorbidities	No	Yes	–	–	–	–
	147	159	–	–	–	–
ODD &/or CD only		116	–	–	–	–
[b]Multiple or other		43	–	–	–	–

*SD, standard deviation, m/f–male/female, r/l/a–right/left/ambidextrous, ODD, oppositional defiant disorder, CD, conduct disorder, K–W, Kruskal-Wallis test, χ^2–chi squared test. Scanner site relates to the number of data sets that were acquired at each of the two sites in the study; Ams, VU Amsterdam and Nij, Radboud UMC, Nijmegen. [a]Medication data were not available for all participants (missing for: 6, 5, and 19 participants from the ADHD, sibling and healthy control groups, respectively). [b]This included 22 additional cases of ODD &/or CD along with 10 cases of tic disorders and 33 cases of mood disorders. *p < 0.05, ***p < 0.001.*

the programme where the voxels were subsampled to voxels of 1 mm^3, normalized for intensity, RF-bias field inhomogeneities were removed and the images skull stripped. The gray-white border was then identified followed by the hemispheres being separated, tessellated and deformed resulting in a smooth representation of the pial and white matter surfaces.

Intrinsic Curvature

Intrinsic curvature was calculated per vertex of each participants FreeSurfer reconstruction using Caret software (v5.65, http://brainvis.wustl.edu/wiki/index.php/Caret:About). This process has been detailed previously (Forde et al., 2014; Ronan et al., 2014). The Caret-generated files of intrinsic curvature were imported to MatLab where they underwent filtering to remove outlier curvature values that were not feasible given the resolution of cortical reconstruction (Ronan et al., 2012, 2014). Absolute values of the remaining per vertex intrinsic curvature measures were calculated. Per region the skew of the curvature distribution was then calculated (Ronan et al., 2012, 2014). These regions (frontal, parietal, occipital, temporal, cingulate, and insula) were generated by combining labels from the Desikan-Killiany Atlas (Desikan et al., 2006) which is supplied with the FreeSurfer package. Cortical intrinsic curvature has a distribution highly skewed toward zero intrinsic curvature (Pienaar et al., 2008; Ronan et al., 2011, 2012), therefore the less skewed the distribution, the greater the degree of intrinsic curvature and differential expansion.

Local Gyrification Index

Gyrification index (GI) is the ratio of the amount of cortical surface exposed as opposed to buried within sulcal folds. A large GI indicates a highly folded surface. Local gyrification index (lGI) quantifies GI at each vertex on the surface and is computed in a 3D fashion by using a region of interest around each vertex within the FreeSurfer software (Schaer et al., 2008). Mean local gyrification index was then extracted per region.

Statistical Analysis

R statistics programme was used for all statistical analysis and graph generation. Continuous group demographics; age, IQ, and symptom count were investigated for normality of distribution (Shapiro-Wilks test) and homogeneity of variance (Bartlett's test). Following this, if the assumptions of normality and homogeneity were met, group differences were investigated with an one-way analysis of variance (ANOVA) or, if one or more of the assumptions were violated, with the non-parametric equivalent, the Kruskal-Wallis test.

The non-linear trajectories of intrinsic curvature skew and local gyrification index over age, based on our cross-sectional data, were modeled per group using a generalized additive mixed-effect (GAM) model approach (Wood, 2006) allowing us to compare the developmental trajectories for the different groups. Applying a GAM model allowed the non-linear modeling of the relationship between age and intrinsic curvature skew with greater flexibility than the standard polynomial form of the growth curve. This method has previously been effectively applied in neuroimaging data (Alexander-Bloch et al., 2014). Briefly, penalized spline mixed-effect models were used to fit the developmental trajectories for each group in each region. This was done using the gamm4 (Wood and Scheipl, 2014) and mcgv (Wood, 2011) packages in R statistics with sex, scanner site, and surface area included as possible confounders. Total cortical surface area was included to control for brain size as both intrinsic curvature and gyrification develop as a function of surface expansion. The non-independence of family members was accounted for by including family as a random factor. IQ, stimulant use, comorbidity, and symptom severity were added to the model to investigate their effect. Due to the nature of additive models group-by-age and group-by-sex interactions could not be appropriately modeled within the GAM model and were instead modeled using a linear mixed effect model (LME) with similar settings to the GAM model. As there were no hemisphere-by-group interactions, measures were collapsed from left and right to give an average intrinsic curvature skew or average local gyrification index per region which was used for analyses. To account for multiple comparisons (two measures each tested in six regions) the alpha level was adjusted to 0.004 for all tests.

Sensitivity Analysis

Due to the possible confounds of having groups ill matched for sex and scanner site a sensitivity analysis was undertaken. Individuals were carefully matched on sex, scanner site, and age which resulted in a subset of participants (n = 66 per group, see **Table 2**). Furthermore, all participants with ADHD and a comorbid condition (ODD, CD, tic disorder etc.) were excluded. The above statistical methods were then reapplied to this subset.

RESULTS

Demographics

Groups did not differ significantly with respect to age. Groups did differ with respect to the proportion of males to females, the distribution of subjects across the two scanner sites and IQ. Therefore, these measures were included in further analysis (**Table 1**). Also approximately half of the ADHD group had one or more comorbid conditions. A total of 138 participants

TABLE 2 | Demographics from matched groups.

	ADHD	Siblings	Control	Test stat	p-value
n	66	66	66	–	–
Age in years, mean (SD)	16.97 (2.67)	17.03 (2.73)	17.07 (2.67)	0.02	0.98
Age in years, range	11.3–22.0	11.3–22.2	11.5–22.5	–	–
Sex, m/f	38/28	38/28	38/28	–	–
Scanner site, Ams/Nij	29/37	29/37	29/37	–	–
IQ, mean (SD)	99.45 (14.1)	99.6 (14.1)	103.6 (11.5)	2.06	0.13
Handedness r/l/a	59/7/0	55/7/1	60/4/2		
Symptom count, n (SD)	13.08 (2.94)	1.39 (2.03)	0.79 (1.77)		

SD, standard deviation, m/f, male/female, r/l/a, right/left/ambidextrous.

with ADHD had comorbid ODD and/or CD, including 130 subjects with ODD and 46 subjects with a diagnosis of CD. Ten participants with ADHD also presented with tics. Thirty-three were also diagnosed with a mood disorder. There were 147 participants with ADHD and no comorbidities. Those with comorbidities were excluded from the sensitivity analysis to remove the possibility that these had an effect on findings.

Intrinsic Curvature

There was no main effect of group on intrinsic curvature (**Table 3**, **Figure 2**). Indicating no difference in the degree of differential expansion, and therefore the underlying cytoarchitechture and connectivity of the cortex, between individuals with ADHD, their siblings and controls. There was a very strong main effect of age in all regions (**Table 3**). There was also a main effect of sex in the frontal region (intrinsic curvature skew higher in females; $t = 4.11$, $p = 4.57 \times 10^{-5}$) while in the temporal and cingulate regions total surface area was also significant ($t = -5.78$, $p = 1.19 \times 10^{-8}$ and $t = 3.47$, $p = 0.0006$, respectively).

Local Gyrification Index

Similarly, there was no main effect of group on local gyrification (**Table 3**, **Figure 3**). This implies there is no differences in the degree of cortical folding between participants with ADHD, their siblings and controls. There was a very strong main effect of age (**Table 3**) and total surface area (frontal: $t = 14.12$, $p = 2.37 \times 10^{-39}$, parietal: $t = 17.11$, $p = 8.25 \times 10^{-54}$, temporal: $t = 19.31$, $p = 4.17 \times 10^{-65}$, occipital: $t = 14.50$, $p = 4.41 \times 10^{-41}$, cingulate: $t = 13.13$, $p = 7.90 \times 10^{-35}$, and insula: $t = 14.07$, $p = 4.10 \times 10^{-39}$) in all regions.

Neither IQ, symptom severity, comorbidity nor stimulant status had an effect on the intrinsic curvature or local gyrification models. There were also no significant group-by-age or group-by-sex interactions in either the intrinsic curvature or local gyrification analyses as modeled with a LME model. Finally, the sensitivity analysis to ensure that neither the covariates (sex and scanner site) nor comorbidities were confounding our study revealed no group differences between the carefully matched groups (**Table 4**). Furthermore, data analyzed per test site and per sex showed similar findings in each case (see Supplementary Tables 1–4).

Tics

Only 10 members of the ADHD group were also seen to have tics, this low number (3.3%) may relate to the older age of participants (average 17.22 years) and method of recruiting (specifically recruiting families affected by ADHD) and meant statistical analysis between those with and without tics was deemed futile due to the lack of power.

DISCUSSION

We applied measures of cortical intrinsic curvature and local gyrification to investigate differences in cortical brain development, related to cortical connectivity, between people with ADHD, their healthy siblings and unrelated healthy controls. We found no difference between the groups with respect to either intrinsic curvature or local gyrification index within any of the regions investigated.

These negative findings indicate that developmental abnormalities previously found in the cortex of those with ADHD (Shaw et al., 2007, 2012) are not due to underlying differences in differential expansion. ADHD has been associated with cortical developmental delay of measures such as cortical thickness and surface area (Shaw et al., 2007, 2012) and cross sectional abnormalities of cortical volume and thickness (Filipek et al., 1997; Makris et al., 2007; Wolosin et al., 2009; Almeida et al., 2010; Proal et al., 2011; Almeida Montes et al., 2012; Frodl and Skokauskas, 2012), this includes cortical thickness deficits bilaterally in the medial temporal cortex that have previously been reported in this study cohort (Schweren et al., 2015). This large study of gyrification is in keeping with a previous longitudinal study that showed no maturational differences in gyrification between individuals with ADHD compared to healthy controls (Shaw et al., 2012). However, two smaller studies have previously reported differences between those with ADHD and controls; in gyrification of the left medial temporal region (Mous et al., 2014) and folding index globally and in the right frontal lobe (Wolosin et al., 2009). Inconsistency in findings may relate to various methods having been employed. We proposed that intrinsic curvature analysis may have been more sensitive than gyrification measures to detect cortical differences between groups if present, however, our results concur with

TABLE 3 | Results.

	Intrinsic curvature				Local gyrification index			
Region	**Group F**	**Group *p***	**Age F**	**Age *p***	**Group F**	**Group *p***	**Age F**	**Age *p***
Frontal	0.41	0.66	128.75	9.6×10^{-25}***	0.63	0.53	326.90	1.3×10^{-60}***
Parietal	1.96	0.14	108.31	3.0×10^{-21}***	0.41	0.67	407.01	2.2×10^{-74}***
Temporal	0.74	0.48	63.95	5.6×10^{-15}***	0.26	0.77	192.43	5.0×10^{-36}***
Occipital	2.61	0.07	10.58	0.001*	0.71	0.49	116.53	5.6×10^{-22}***
Cingulate	2.94	0.05	40.31	4.4×10^{-8}***	0.66	0.52	92.26	1.3×10^{-20}***
Insula	0.56	0.57	60.20	3.3×10^{-14}***	1.83	0.16	129.14	3.3×10^{-24}***

*Test statistics and p-values are reported for the main effects of group and age on intrinsic curvature and local gyrification index in each region for the full sample ($n = 618$). Adjusted $p = 0.004$. *$p < 0.004$, ***$p < 8 \times 10^{-5}$.*

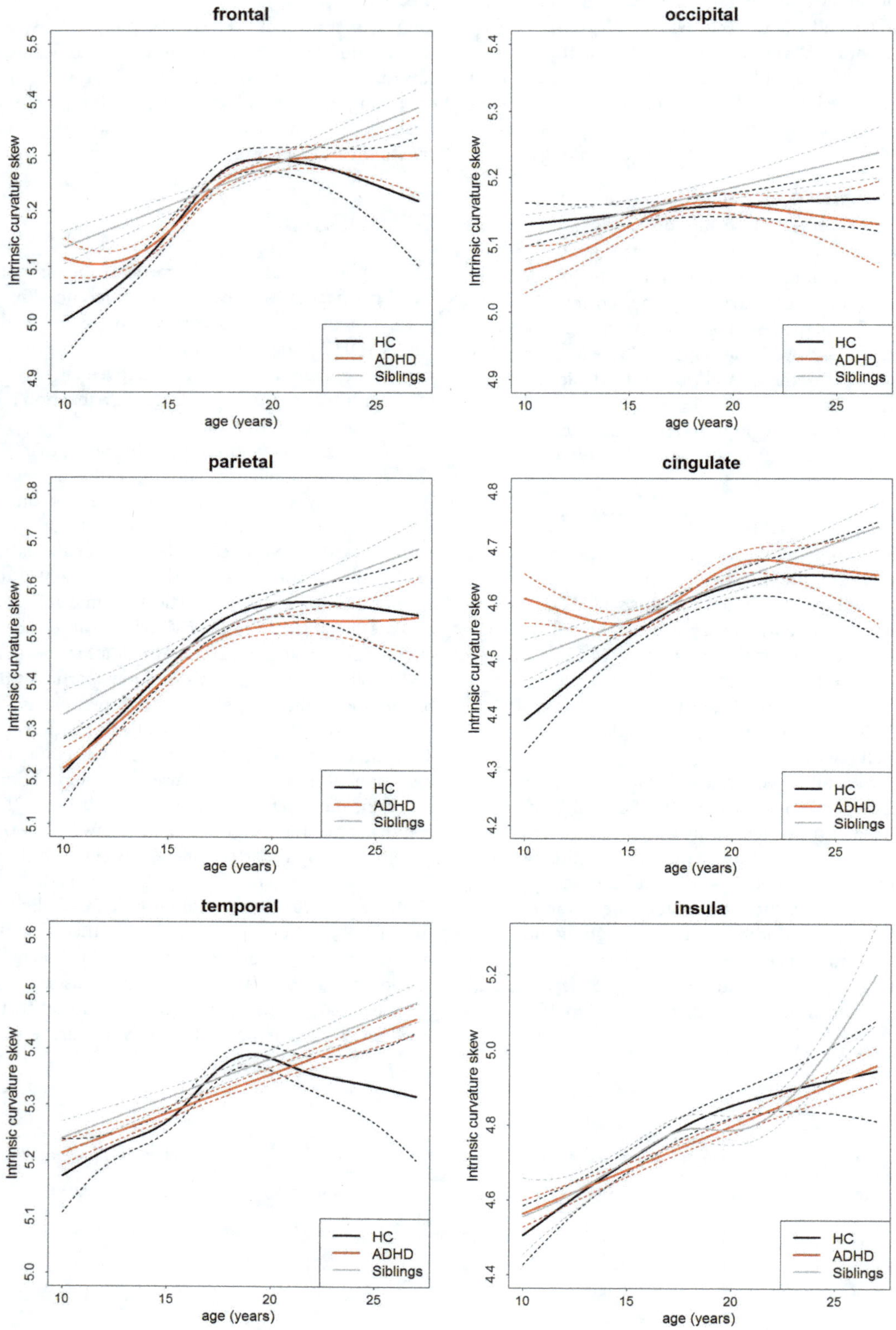

FIGURE 2 | Age-curves of intrinsic curvature skew per group for each region. Differences between groups were not significant. Caution must be taken when viewing these graphs as a very small proportion of the participants were under the age of 12 or over 23 years of age thus the apparent differences at these ages are driven by a few individuals only. Broken lines represent the standard error for each group. HC, healthy control (black lines), ADHD, Attention-deficit/hyperactivity disorder (red lines), Siblings, healthy siblings of ADHD participant (gray lines).

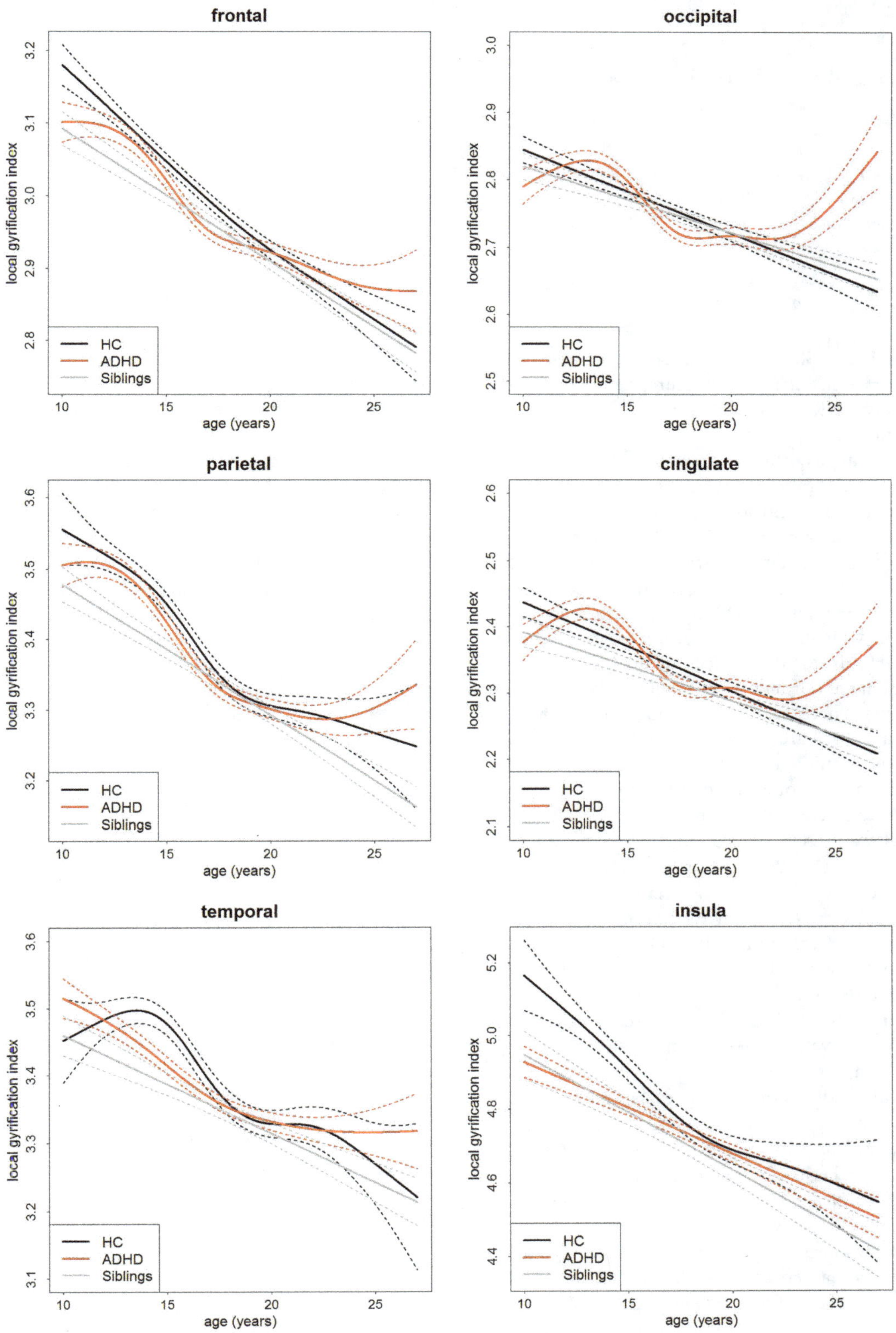

FIGURE 3 | Age-curves of local gyrification index per group for each region. Differences between groups were not significant. Caution must be taken when viewing these graphs as a very small proportion of the participants were under the age of 12 or over 23 years of age thus the apparent differences at these ages are driven by a few individuals only. Broken lines represent the standard error for each group. HC, healthy control (black lines), ADHD, Attention-deficit/hyperactivity disorder (red lines), Siblings, healthy siblings of ADHD participant (gray lines).

TABLE 4 | Matched results.

Region	Intrinsic curvature				Local gyrification index			
	Group F	**Group *p***	**Age F**	**Age *p***	**Group F**	**Group *p***	**Age F**	**Age *p***
Frontal	0.15	0.86	36.55	6.8×10^{-9}***	0.32	0.72	90.98	1.2×10^{-16}***
Parietal	1.04	0.36	37.91	3.8×10^{-9}***	0.29	0.75	103.33	1.5×10^{-18}***
Temporal	1.16	0.32	29.50	1.6×10^{-7}***	0.06	0.94	47.12	7.1×10^{-11}***
Occipital	0.52	0.59	4.28	0.04	0.90	0.41	15.88	9.5×10^{-5}**
Cingulate	2.25	0.11	20.99	8.1×10^{-6}***	1.32	0.27	15.35	1.2×10^{-4}**
Insula	2.23	0.11	6.98	0.009	0.13	0.88	37.70	4.6×10^{-8}***

*Test statistics and p-values are reported for the main effects of group and age on intrinsic curvature and local gyrification index in each region for the matched sample ($n = 198$). Adjusted $p = 0.004$. *$p < 0.004$, **$p < 8 \times 10^{-4}$, ***$p < 8 \times 10^{-5}$.*

the previous finding of Shaw et al. (2012) in that we found no diagnostic difference in intrinsic curvature, which is predictive of gyrification pattern (Ronan et al., 2014).

In contrast to our hypothesis we can infer from this that there are no short range cortico-cortico connectivity differences within the gray matter of the cortex between those with ADHD, their siblings or healthy controls. Previous reports have found evidence of white matter connectivity abnormalities in ADHD when long range connections between distinct gray matter regions were analyzed. Our findings suggest that these changes do not similarly occur at a smaller within gray matter scale but are constrained to the white matter. Furthermore, this finding helps differentiate ADHD from ASD which has been associated with cortical connectivity abnormalities in adults (Ecker et al., 2013) and schizophrenia where the cortical connectivity differences seen (Ronan et al., 2012) are proposed to relate to the abnormal cytoarchitechture present in schizophrenia (Selemon et al., 1995, 1998). As well as cortical connectivity differences, abnormalities in white matter tracts have been shown in schizophrenia (Ellison-Wright and Bullmore, 2009; Ellison-Wright et al., 2014) and ASD (Barnea-Goraly et al., 2004; Alexander et al., 2007). While larger scale connectivity differences also occur in ADHD (Konrad and Eickhoff, 2010) from this study we can infer that, unlike in schizophrenia and ASD, there are no short range connectivity abnormalities in the cortical gray matter of ADHD patients. This implies that despite a shared heritability between ASD and ADHD (Rommelse et al., 2010) there are, at least partially, different abnormal developmental mechanisms at play in the respective conditions.

Given our null findings of differences between groups the use of either IC or LGI alone do not seem to be sensitive endophenotypic markers for ADHD. However, despite this, considering the high heritability of cortical indices (Thompson et al., 2001; Panizzon et al., 2009; Rogers et al., 2010) the inclusion of these measures along with various other biological and cognitive indices in more complex data driven approaches may aid in identifying biomarkers and endophenotypes for ADHD.

Intrinsic curvature holds much potential as a sensitive marker of cortical connectivity and abnormal cortical development. However, it has not yet been widely used and how the measure changes over the lifetime in healthy participants needs further quantification. Although our study had substantial numbers of participants ($n = 618$) we lacked the power to detect differences in the early adolescent and early adulthood stages of development. This is due to our age range being normally distributed about our mean, resulting in robust findings through mid to late adolescents but reduced power in early adolescence and adulthood. Finally, interactions between group and age were modeled using a standard linear mixed-effects model, which showed no significant interactions, instead of the GAM model. This was due to the nature of additive models which by definition do not allow interactions. However, there remains the possibility that there may well be an interaction between group and age but that this is not discernible with a linear model.

In conclusion, we found there are no short range connectivity differences within the cortical gray matter, as inferred from intrinsic curvature measures, between participants with ADHD, their unaffected siblings and healthy controls.

ETHICS STATEMENT

The protocol was approved by the Commissie Mensgebonden Onderzoek (CMO) Regio Arnhem-Nijmegen and the medical ethical committee of the VU University Medical Center. For children between 12 and 18 both parents and children gave written informed consent. For participants below 12 parents gave written informed consent.

AUTHOR CONTRIBUTIONS

NF analyzed these data and wrote the manuscript. LR, MZ, and AA significantly contributed to the processing and/or analysis of data. SF, JO, DH, CH, JB, and PH were all involved with the conception and funding of the NeuroIMAGE project. CH and LR further acted as statistical experts. While JB and PH supervised the study and critically evaluated the manuscript.

ACKNOWLEDGMENTS

The NeuroIMAGE project was supported by NIH Grant R01MH62873 (to SF), NWO Large Investment Grant 1750102007010 and ZonMW Grant 60-60600-97-193, and NWO grants 433-09-242 and 056-13-015 (to JB) and grants from Radboud University Medical Center Nijmegen, University

Medical Center Groningen, Accare and VU University Medical Center Amsterdam. Further funding has been received from the European Union under the Seventh Framework People Programme (TS-EUROTRAIN, GA 316978, and TACTICS, GA 278948).

SUPPLEMENTARY MATERIAL

The Supplementary Material for this article can be found online at: http://journal.frontiersin.org/article/10.3389/fnins.2017.00218/full#supplementary-material

REFERENCES

Alexander, A. L., Lee, J. E., Lazar, M., Boudos, R., DuBray, M. B., Oakes, T. R., et al. (2007). Diffusion tensor imaging of the corpus callosum in Autism. *Neuroimage* 34, 61–73. doi: 10.1016/j.neuroimage.2006.08.032

Alexander-Bloch, A. F., Reiss, P. T., Rapoport, J., McAdams, H., Giedd, J. N., Bullmore, E. T., et al. (2014). Abnormal cortical growth in schizophrenia targets normative modules of synchronized development. *Biol. Psychiatry* 76, 438–446. doi: 10.1016/j.biopsych.2014.02.010

Almeida, L. G., Ricardo-Garcell, J., Prado, H., Barajas, L., Fernández-Bouzas, A., Ávila, D., et al. (2010). Reduced right frontal cortical thickness in children, adolescents and adults with ADHD and its correlation to clinical variables: a cross-sectional study. *J. Psychiatr. Res.* 44, 1214–1223. doi: 10.1016/j.jpsychires.2010.04.026

Almeida Montes, L. G., Prado Alcántara, H., Martínez García, R. B., De La Torre, L. B., Avila Acosta, D., Duarte, M. G., et al. (2012). Brain cortical thickness in ADHD: age, sex, and clinical correlations. *J. Atten. Disord.* 17, 641–654. doi: 10.1177/1087054711434351

American Psychiatric Association (2013). *Diagnostic and Statistical Manual of Mental Disorders. 5th Edn*, Washington, DC.

Anagnostou, E., and Taylor, M. J. (2011). Review of neuroimaging in autism spectrum disorders: what have we learned and where we go from here. *Mol. Autism* 2:4. doi: 10.1186/2040-2392-2-4

Barnea-Goraly, N., Kwon, H., Menon, V., Eliez, S., Lotspeich, L., and Reiss, A. L. (2004). White matter structure in autism: preliminary evidence from diffusion tensor imaging. *Biol. Psychiatry* 55, 323–326. doi: 10.1016/j.biopsych.2003.10.022

Braitenberg, V., and Schüz, A. (1998). *Cortex: Statistics and Geometry of Neuronal Connectivity*. Berlin; Heidelberg: *Springer Berlin Heidelberg*.

Cao, Q., Shu, N., An, L., Wang, P., Sun, L., Xia, M.-R., et al. (2013). Probabilistic diffusion tractography and graph theory analysis reveal abnormal white matter structural connectivity networks in drug-naive boys with attention deficit/hyperactivity disorder. *J. Neurosci.* 33, 10676–10687. doi: 10.1523/JNEUROSCI.4793-12.2013

Conners, C. K., Erhardt, D., and Sparrow, E. (1999). *Conners Adult ADHD Rating Scale - Self Report, Long Version (CAARS-S-L)*. Multi-Health Systems, Inc.

Conners, C. K., Sitarenios, G., Parker, J. D., and Epstein, J. N. (1998a). Revision and restandardization of the conners teacher rating scale (CTRS-R): factor structure, reliability, and criterion validity. *J. Abnorm. Child Psychol.* 26, 279–291. doi: 10.1023/A:1022606501530

Conners, C. K., Sitarenios, G., Parker, J. D., and Epstein, J. N. (1998b). The revised Conners' Parent Rating Scale (CPRS-R): factor structure, reliability, and criterion validity. *J. Abnorm. Child Psychol.* 26, 257–268. doi: 10.1023/A:1022602400621

Dale, A. M., Fischl, B., and Sereno, M. I. (1999). Cortical surface-based analysis. I. Segmentation and surface reconstruction. *Neuroimage* 9, 179–194. doi: 10.1006/nimg.1998.0395

Desikan, R. S., Ségonne, F., Fischl, B., Quinn, B. T., Dickerson, B. C., Blacker, D., et al. (2006). An automated labeling system for subdividing the human cerebral cortex on MRI scans into gyral based regions of interest. *Neuroimage* 31, 968–980. doi: 10.1016/j.neuroimage.2006.01.021

Ecker, C., Ronan, L., Feng, Y., Daly, E., Murphy, C., Ginestet, C. E., et al. (2013). Intrinsic gray-matter connectivity of the brain in adults with autism spectrum disorder. *Proc. Natl. Acad. Sci. U.S.A.* 110, 13222–13227. doi: 10.1073/pnas.1221880110

Ellison-Wright, I., and Bullmore, E. (2009). Meta-analysis of diffusion tensor imaging studies in schizophrenia. *Schizophr. Res.* 108, 3–10. doi: 10.1016/j.schres.2008.11.021

Ellison-Wright, I., Nathan, P. J., Bullmore, E. T., Zaman, R., Dudas, R. B., Agius, M., et al. (2014). Distribution of tract deficits in schizophrenia. *Biomed. Cent. Psychiatry* 14:99. doi: 10.1186/1471-244x-14-99

Faraone, S. V., Perlis, R. H., Doyle, A. E., Smoller, J. W., Goralnick, J. J., Holmgren, M. A., et al. (2005). Molecular genetics of attention-deficit/hyperactivity disorder. *Biol. Psychiatry* 57, 1313–1323. doi: 10.1016/j.biopsych.2004.11.024

Filipek, P. A., Semrud-Clikeman, M., Steingard, R. J., Renshaw, P. F., Kennedy, D. N., and Biederman, J. (1997). Volumetric MRI analysis comparing subjects having attention-deficit hyperactivity disorder with normal controls. *Neurology* 48, 589–601. doi: 10.1212/WNL.48.3.589

Fischl, B., and Dale, A. M. (2000). Measuring the thickness of the human cerebral cortex from magnetic resonance images. *Proc. Natl. Acad. Sci. U.S.A.* 97, 11050–11055. doi: 10.1073/pnas.200033797

Fischl, B., Sereno, M. I., and Dale, A. M. (1999a). Cortical surface-based analysis. II: *inflation, flattening, and a surface-based coordinate system.* Neuroimage 9, 195–207. doi: 10.1006/nimg.1998.0396

Fischl, B., Sereno, M. I., Tootell, R. B., and Dale, A. M. (1999b). High-resolution intersubject averaging and a coordinate system for the cortical surface. *Hum. Brain Mapp.* 8, 272–284. doi: 10.1002/(SICI)1097-0193(1999)8:4<272::AID-HBM10>3.0.CO;2-4

Forde, N. J., Ronan, L., Suckling, J., Scanlon, C., Neary, S., Holleran, L., et al. (2014). Structural neuroimaging correlates of allelic variation of the BDNF val66met polymorphism. *Neuroimage* 90, 280–289. doi: 10.1016/j.neuroimage.2013.12.050

Friston, K. J. (2011). Functional and effective connectivity: a review. *Brain Connect.* 1, 13–36. doi: 10.1089/brain.2011.0008

Frodl, T., and Skokauskas, N. (2012). Meta-analysis of structural MRI studies in children and adults with attention deficit hyperactivity disorder indicates treatment effects. *Acta Psychiatr. Scand.* 125, 114–126. doi: 10.1111/j.1600-0447.2011.01786.x

Gottesman, I. I., and Gould, T. D. (2003). Reviews and overviews the endophenotype concept in psychiatry : etymology and strategic intentions. *Am. J. Psychiatry* 160, 636–645. doi: 10.1176/appi.ajp.160.4.636

Hong, S.-B., Zalesky, A., Fornito, A., Park, S., Yang, Y.-H., Park, M.-H., et al. (2014). Connectomic disturbances in attention-deficit/hyperactivity disorder: a whole-brain tractography analysis. *Biol. Psychiatry* 76, 656–663. doi: 10.1016/j.biopsych.2013.12.013

Kaufman, J., Birmaher, B., Brent, D., Rao, U., Flynn, C., Moreci, P., et al. (1997). Schedule for affective disorders and schizophrenia for school-age children-present and lifetime version (K-SADS-PL): initial reliability and validity data. *J. Am. Acad. Child Adolesc. Psychiatry* 36, 980–988. doi: 10.1097/00004583-199707000-00021

Konrad, K., and Eickhoff, S. B. (2010). Is the ADHD brain wired differently? A review on structural and functional connectivity in attention deficit hyperactivity disorder. *Hum. Brain Mapp.* 31, 904–916. doi: 10.1002/hbm.21058

Liston, C., Malter Cohen, M., Teslovich, T., Levenson, D., and Casey, B. J. (2011). Atypical prefrontal connectivity in attention-deficit/hyperactivity disorder: pathway to disease or pathological end point? *Biol. Psychiatry* 69, 1168–1177. doi: 10.1016/j.biopsych.2011.03.022

Makris, N., Biederman, J., Valera, E. M., Bush, G., Kaiser, J., Kennedy, D. N., et al. (2007). Cortical thinning of the attention and executive function networks in adults with attention-deficit/hyperactivity disorder. *Cereb. Cortex* 17, 1364–1375. doi: 10.1093/cercor/bhl047

Mous, S. E., Karatekin, C., Kao, C.-Y., Gottesman, I. I., Posthuma, D., and White, T. (2014). Gyrification differences in children and adolescents with velocardiofacial syndrome and attention-deficit/hyperactivity disorder: a pilot study. *Psychiatry Res.* 221, 169–171. doi: 10.1016/j.pscychresns.2013.12.002

Müller, U. C., Asherson, P., Banaschewski, T., Buitelaar, J. K., Ebstein, R. P., Eisenberg, J., et al. (2011a). The impact of study design and diagnostic approach in a large multi-centre ADHD study. Part 1: ADHD symptom patterns. *BMC Psychiatry* 11:54. doi: 10.1186/1471-244X-11-54

Müller, U. C., Asherson, P., Banaschewski, T., Buitelaar, J. K., Ebstein, R. P., Eisenberg, J., et al. (2011b). The impact of study design and diagnostic approach in a large multi-centre ADHD study: part 2: DImensional measures of psychopathology and intelligence. *BMC Psychiatry* 11:55. doi: 10.1186/1471-244X-11-55

Nakao, T., Radua, J., Rubia, K., and Mataix-Cols, D. (2011). Gray matter volume abnormalities in ADHD: voxel-based meta-analysis exploring the effects of age and stimulant medication. *Am. J. Psychiatry* 168, 1154–1163. doi: 10.1176/appi.ajp.2011.11020281

Panizzon, M. S., Fennema-Notestine, C., Eyler, L. T., Jernigan, T. L., Prom-Wormley, E., Neale, M., et al. (2009). Distinct genetic influences on cortical surface area and cortical thickness. *Cereb. Cortex* 19, 2728–2735. doi: 10.1093/cercor/bhp026

Pienaar, R., Fischl, B., Caviness, V., Makris, N., and Grant, P. E. (2008). A methodology for analyzing curvature in the developing brain from preterm to adult. *Int. J. Imaging Syst. Technol.* 18, 42–68. doi: 10.1002/ima.20138

Polanczyk, G., de Lima, M. S., Horta, B. L., Biederman, J., and Rohde, L. A. (2007). The worldwide prevalence of ADHD: a systematic review and metaregression analysis. *Am. J. Psychiatry* 164, 942–948. doi: 10.1176/ajp.2007.164.6.942

Proal, E., Reiss, P. T., Klein, R. G., Mannuzza, S., Gotimer, K., Ramos-Olazagasti, M. A., et al. (2011). Brain gray matter deficits at 33-year follow-up in adults with attention-deficit/hyperactivity disorder established in childhood. *Arch. Gen. Psychiatry* 68, 1122–1134. doi: 10.1001/archgenpsychiatry.2011.117

Rogers, J., Kochunov, P., Zilles, K., Shelledy, W., Lancaster, J., Thompson, P., et al. (2010). On the genetic architecture of cortical folding and brain volume in primates. *Neuroimage* 53, 1103–1108. doi: 10.1016/j.neuroimage.2010.02.020

Rommelse, N. N. J., Franke, B., Geurts, H. M., Hartman, C. A, and Buitelaar, J. K. (2010). Shared heritability of attention-deficit/hyperactivity disorder and autism spectrum disorder. *Eur. Child Adolesc. Psychiatry* 19, 281–295. doi: 10.1007/s00787-010-0092-x

Rommelse, N. N. J., Geurts, H. M., Franke, B., Buitelaar, J. K., and Hartman, C. A. (2011). A review on cognitive and brain endophenotypes that may be common in autism spectrum disorder and attention-deficit/hyperactivity disorder and facilitate the search for pleiotropic genes. *Neurosci. Biobehav. Rev.* 35, 1363–1396. doi: 10.1016/j.neubiorev.2011.02.015

Ronan, L., Pienaar, R., Williams, G., Bullmore, E., Crow, T. J., Roberts, N., et al. (2011). Intrinsic curvature: a marker of millimeter-scale tangential cortico-cortical connectivity? *Int. J. Neural Syst.* 21, 351–366. doi: 10.1142/S0129065711002948

Ronan, L., Voets, N. L., Hough, M., Mackay, C., Roberts, N., Suckling, J., et al. (2012). Consistency and interpretation of changes in millimeter-scale cortical intrinsic curvature across three independent datasets in schizophrenia. *Neuroimage* 63, 611–621. doi: 10.1016/j.neuroimage.2012.06.034

Ronan, L., Voets, N., Rua, C., Alexander-Bloch, A., Hough, M., Mackay, C., et al. (2014). Differential tangential expansion as a mechanism for cortical gyrification. *Cereb. Cortex* 24, 2219–2228. doi: 10.1093/cercor/bht082

Schaer, M., Bach Cuadra, M., Tamarit, L., Lazeyras, F., Eliez, S., and Thiran, J. P. (2008). A surface-based approach to quantify local cortical gyrification. *IEEE Trans. Med. Imaging* 27, 161–170. doi: 10.1109/TMI.2007.903576

Schaer, M., Ottet, M.-C., Scariati, E., Dukes, D., Franchini, M., Eliez, S., et al. (2013). Decreased frontal gyrification correlates with altered connectivity in children with autism. *Front. Hum. Neurosci.* 7:750. doi: 10.3389/fnhum.2013.00750

Schweren, L. J. S., Hartman, C. A., Heslenfeld, D. J., van der Meer, D., Franke, B., Oosterlaan, J., et al. (2015). Thinner medial temporal cortex in adolescents with attention-deficit/hyperactivity disorder and the effects of stimulants. *J. Am. Acad. Child Adolesc. Psychiatry* 54, 1–8. doi: 10.1016/j.jaac.2015.05.014

Selemon, L. D., Rajkowska, G., and Goldman-Rakic, P. S. (1995). Abnormally high neuronal density in the schizophrenic cortex. *Arch. Gen. Psychiatry* 52, 805. doi: 10.1001/archpsyc.1995.03950220015005

Selemon, L. D., Rajkowska, G., and Goldman-Rakic, P. S. (1998). Elevated neuronal density in prefrontal area 46 in brains from schizophrenic patients: application of a three-dimensional, stereologic counting method. *J. Comp. Neurol.* 392, 402–412. doi: 10.1002/(SICI)1096-9861(19980316)392:3<402::AID-CNE9>3.0.CO;2-5

Shaw, P., Eckstrand, K., Sharp, W., Blumenthal, J., Lerch, J. P., Greenstein, D., et al. (2007). Attention-deficit/hyperactivity disorder is characterized by a delay in cortical maturation. *Proc. Natl. Acad. Sci. U.S.A.* 104, 19649–19654. doi: 10.1073/pnas.0707741104

Shaw, P., Malek, M., Watson, B., Greenstein, D., de Rossi, P., and Sharp, W. (2013). Trajectories of cerebral cortical development in childhood and adolescence and adult attention-deficit/hyperactivity disorder. *Biol. Psychiatry* 74, 599–606. doi: 10.1016/j.biopsych.2013.04.007

Shaw, P., Malek, M., Watson, B., Sharp, W., Evans, A., and Greenstein, D. (2012). Development of cortical surface area and gyrification in attention-deficit/hyperactivity disorder. *Biol. Psychiatry* 72, 191–197. doi: 10.1016/j.biopsych.2012.01.031

Thompson, P. M., Cannon, T. D., Narr, K. L., van Erp, T., Poutanen, V. P., Huttunen, M., et al. (2001). Genetic influences on brain structure. *Nat. Neurosci.* 4, 1253–1258. doi: 10.1038/nn758

van Ewijk, H., Heslenfeld, D. J., Zwiers, M. P., Buitelaar, J. K., and Oosterlaan, J. (2012). Diffusion tensor imaging in attention deficit/hyperactivity disorder: a systematic review and meta-analysis. *Neurosci. Biobehav. Rev.* 36, 1093–1106. doi: 10.1016/j.neubiorev.2012.01.003

von Rhein, D., Mennes, M., van Ewijk, H., Groenman, A. P., Zwiers, M. P., Oosterlaan, J., et al. (2014). The NeuroIMAGE study: a prospective phenotypic, cognitive, genetic and MRI study in children with attention-deficit/hyperactivity disorder. Design and descriptives. *Eur. Child Adolesc. Psychiatry* 24, 265–281. doi: 10.1007/s00787-014-0573-4

Wolosin, S. M., Richardson, M. E., Hennessey, J. G., Denckla, M. B., and Mostofsky, S. H. (2009). Abnormal cerebral cortex structure in children with ADHD. *Hum. Brain Mapp.* 30, 175–184. doi: 10.1002/hbm.20496

Wood, S. N. (2006). *Generalized Additive Models: An Introduction with R.* Boca Raton; London; New York, NY: Chapman & Hall/CRC.

Wood, S. N. (2011). Fast stable restricted maximum likelihood and marginal likelihood estimation of semiparametric generalized linear models. *J. R. Stat. Soc. Ser. B Stat. Methodol.* 73, 3–36. doi: 10.1111/j.1467-9868.2010.00749.x

Wood, S. N., and Scheipl, F. (2014). *gamm4: Generalized Additiove Mixed Models using mgcv and lme4.* Available online at: https://cran.r-project.org/web/packages/gamm4/index.html (Accessed October 21, 2015).

16

Toward a Symptom-Guided Neurostimulation for Gilles de la Tourette Syndrome

*Nicole Pedroarena-Leal and Diane Ruge**

Department of Psychology and Neurosciences, Leibniz Research Centre for Working Environment and Human Factors, Technical University Dortmund, Dortmund, Germany

Edited by:
Kirsten R. Müller-Vahl, Hannover Medical School, Germany

Reviewed by:
Joachim K. Krauss, Hannover Medical School, Germany
Michael Okun, University of Florida Health, USA

***Correspondence:**
Diane Ruge
ruge@ifado.de

Therapy resistance of approximately one-third of patients with Gilles de la Tourette syndrome (GTS) requires consideration of alternative therapeutic interventions. This article provides a condensed review of the invasive and non-invasive stimulation techniques that have been applied, to date, for treatment and investigation of GTS. Through this perspective and short review, the article discusses potential novel applications for neurostimulation techniques based on a symptom-guided approach. The concept of considering the physiological basis of specific symptoms when using stimulation techniques will provide a platform for more effective non-pharmacological neuromodulation of symptoms in GTS.

Keywords: neuropsychiatry, physiology, symptom, cerebellum, therapy, Gilles de la Tourette syndrome

INTRODUCTION

The use of non-invasive and invasive brain stimulation techniques for relief of specific symptomatology in neuropsychiatric disorders should be considered as a young therapeutic intervention. The motivation for such a proposal stems from the need for alternatives to current pharmaceutical neuromodulation for Gilles de la Tourette syndrome (GTS), as approximately one-third of patients with GTS demonstrate therapy resistance or side effects to conventional neuropharmaceuticals, with limited current alternatives for symptom management. When considering the role of circuit components in learning and plasticity processes, brain stimulation becomes a strategic and valuable technique for investigating potential treatment options for neuropsychiatric disorders, since particular neural circuits have demonstrated abnormal excitability related to symptom manifestation and have been linked to aberrations in plasticity-induced learning (1). Such results offer a physiological approach to understanding and analyzing circuit aberrancies that are observed clinically as symptoms of specific neuropsychiatric disorders. The relationship between specific symptom manifestation and the underlying nodal or network participation that accounts for alterations in neural firing is a question worth posing, as such differences in analysis would personalize and thereby improve the current approach to the application and use of neurostimulation.

Of particular interest is the potential to use neurostimulation in a more discrete and motivated manner. Specifically, regions that are analyzed to participate in specific motor and cognitive functions are targeted as regions of interest, an approach guided by the concept of "personalized intervention" in neuropsychiatric disorders. This deviates from the current dominating avenues where a particular structure is chosen for stimulation. Analysis of resulting behavior and physiology, usually at a group level, follows. This paper provides an overview of the application, to date, of both invasive and non-invasive neurostimulation to GTS patients and reflects on the potential benefits and challenges of considering nodal and network participation in aberrant behavior as a potential guide for individualized patient stimulation.

FUNCTION, STRUCTURE, AND SYMPTOMATOLOGY FOR MOTIVATED APPLICATION

The consideration of structures' functions in the underling neural circuit producing symptomatology is not trivial: stimulation *via* electric currents to a complex electrochemical, dynamic structure that the brain represents prevents simple prediction of potential neurostimulation effects on behavior and symptoms. In essence, this process involves at least three steps: (i) the analysis of the effect of neurostimulation on physiology and (ii) the effect of changes in neurophysiology on behavior or symptoms. These last two steps are preceded by one challenging, cardinal step (A), which in the era of computational neuroscience is often discounted or overlooked: the analysis of the behavioral problem by an experienced pattern recognizer, a clinician. However, some approaches are currently on the way in an attempt to replace or improve human pattern recognition.

So far, in therapeutic neurostimulation for GTS, solid mechanistic rationale for its use is often spared, one reason being that applicators are rarely trained in the previously mentioned aspects, which include (a) clinical pattern recognition, (b) neurophysiology read-outs, and (c) sophisticated stimulation strategies. This delays the development of more effective stimulation protocols. Thus, the need for unconventional options to available treatment can perhaps be best understood by reorienting the manner in which GTS symptomatology is analyzed and framed.

The cardinal behavioral symptoms in GTS are tics. Tics can be sudden and meaningless movements, simple movements (such as blinking, eye rolling, and head nodding) or complex (touching, jumping, squatting, etc.). Often motor tics, including eye blinking and neck turning, are only abnormal and different from regular movements due to the intensity of reoccurrence and frequency (2). Many can develop over time into more purposeful, longer duration movements (complex motor tics). Consequently, *a tic is not a tic is not a tic* and, hence, requires initial analysis in step (A). To add to the complexity, a scenario like this would inadequately reduce the abnormal motor behavior to a one-dimensional behavioral problem (tic), which in GTS, with its frequent comorbidities (obsessions, compulsions, etc.), is often a mixture of faulty motor patterns.

For example, in children, throat clearing and other cold-related behavior is often reported by parents as persisting after the cold recedes and observed to adopt a recurrent and frequent inclusion in motor tic repertoire. Such repeated activation of potentially learned motor memories seems to occur with various motor actions that, if not for their frequent repetition or misplaced execution, would otherwise be considered as regular movements (2). It could be hypothesized that these represent "invasive motor memories," i.e., learned and stored patterns. Clinical observations such as these frame GTS symptomatology in such a way that allows for a more inclusive approach to analyzing underlying causes of symptoms, as it aims to bridge the underlying physiology with the clinical manifestation reflecting neural aberrancies.

Traditionally, neural nodes that have been attributed to GTS symptoms are elements forming part of the cortico-basal ganglia (BG) network. Such models suggest that involuntary movements are related to decreased inhibitory output from the BG. This reduction in output is thought to underlie excessive frontal cortical activity (2–5). More recently, contributing models have been extended to include cerebellar circuits using functional magnetic resonance imaging (6) and animal models (7). The specific timing with a tic-preceding time interval in the cerebellum and primary motor cortex suggests that both structures function as origins of tic movement release. Furthermore, the match in latency of cerebellar and primary motor cortex discharges proposes that tic expression can be considered to represent a "global network dysrhythmia." By contrast, local field potential discharges have been recorded in the BG outside tic expression (7). Such difference of involvement in tic production suggests that different nodes function in distinct ways and at varying time points, implying tic-generating networks encompass multiple and distributed areas in neural circuits.

Can both, clinical observation with potential underlying contribution of these various, mentioned nodes to circuit involvement exemplifies be considered in combination? The apparent and observable lack of movement extinction (i.e., in the case of tics: the erasure or inhibition of the undesired movement patterns) could be a faulty pattern in negative reinforcement mediated by aberrant BG processes. Yet, it could be speculated that the early manifestation of tics is mediated *via* cerebellar learning abnormalities, such as the deficient, early correction of error signals and cerebellar eye blink, conditioning type of learning. By contrast, the BG are crucial for the persistence or retention of these same aberrant movements that are impeded from full erasure due to deviant punishment and reinforcement learning. Moreover, the role of the cerebellum and its interaction with anterior nodes, including the amygdala, hippocampus, and prefrontal cortex for extinction of learned movements, but also emotion, fear, and cognitive patterns, has to be taken into consideration. The involvement of different nodes in distinct characteristics of the manifesting symptoms points to the importance and need of considering inter-individual differences in patient tic repertoire or behavioral problems, as such dissimilarities in manifestations among patients could point to variations in nodal participation. Looking at the individual development of tics over time and based on the knowledge we have on learning mechanisms, it becomes plausible that the source of such varied and diverse symptomatology as that present in GTS patients can not be solely attributed to one structure, rather, should be tied to the involvement of wider neural circuit involvement.

How do these patterns, however, persist long enough to be integrated into motor tic repertoire? The nature of certain tics hints at a more diffuse and interconnected network involved in more complex repertoires of tics. These inquiries point to the multidimensional system that is contributing to symptom manifestation. A multidimensional view allows for the consideration that early manifestation of tics is mediated *via* other nodes, for example, the cerebellum, with cerebellar learning abnormalities manifesting as deficient, early correction of error signals and classical conditioning type of learning, while the BG are crucial for the persistence or retention of aberrant movements that cannot be extinguished because of deviant punishment and reinforcement learning.

Parsing out of specific symptom characteristics and their corresponding possible origin allows for a more precisely guided contribution to analyzing nodal participation and circuit level involvement. Such dissection is crucial when considering the application of stimulation, especially in the often comorbid nature of GTS and associated symptoms. This reflection raises two questions: (i) How would stimulating one component of the circuit imply network level effects in remote areas? and (ii) In what way can effects on aberrant motor behavior be extrapolated? One approach to answering such questions could be to shift the focus of stimulation from specific brain targets to stimulation of particular brain networks.

INVASIVE AND NON-INVASIVE NEUROSTIMULATION FOR GTS TREATMENT

Neurostimulation for GTS has thus far been applied without much mechanistic rationale with regard to the underlying neurophysiology mentioned, the specific contribution of nodes and time points in a neural network, nor has the knowledge gap between neurophysiological effects and behavioral effect—if present—been bridged. The following gives a short overview of the approaches that have been used to ameliorate symptoms. This overview provides insight into the fact that stimulation thus far has been target driven stimulation not fully rooted in clear physiological rationale. This serves as a basis for understanding the perspective of symptom-guided targeted neurostimulation explained in previous sections.

Discrete stimulation of anatomical structures to improve aberrant movements has been examined in a wide array of disorders yet, a personalized consideration of the role these areas play as participating nodes in wider neural circuits, and how these circuits come to manifest certain symptoms over others, has not been explicitly attempted nor analyzed in GTS. If clinical benefits outweigh the possible lack of response to stimulation or side effects, this could be considered acceptable, but not having a deeper understanding of underlying mechanism delays progress in development of efficient treatment and leads to dead ends. A tighter analysis of the connection between specific symptom manifestation and nodal structures that could be stimulated for symptom improvement, therefore, could be more fully explored to ground results in physiology and not just in potential epiphenomena.

Relevance of a discussion of DBS or other neurostimulation for movement disorders other than GTS becomes clearer when considering parallels in regards to certain symptomatology. For example, dystonic muscle contractions cause abnormal posturing of limbs, as can occur in certain GTS motor tics. Additionally, dystonic symptoms can resemble GTS tics in their repetitive and involuntary nature. Certain GTS patients also manifest dystonic tics, with movements that are relatively slow and temporarily persistent actions, such as twisting, pulling, or squeezing movements, resembling movements in dystonia patients. Patients exhibiting typical (i.e., clonic) tics have been found to manifest dystonic tics, a common motor manifestation present in 57% of the cohort studied (8). Potentially, this points to similarities in their contributing physiological cause and motivates approaches to studying the application of respective neurostimulation techniques to GTS patients.

In the case of invasive stimulation specifically for GTS, treatment has been applied for severe cases of the disorder. DBS of various thalamic nuclei, the centromedian–parafascicular (CM–pf) and the internal portion of the ventralis oralis anterior, has been used to treat refractory GTS patients (9). Additionally, there have been further tic reduction surgeries for refractory GTS patients following DBS to the anteromedial and postero-ventrolateral portions of the internal globus pallidus, the anterior limb of the internal capsule, subthalamic nucleus, and nucleus accumbens [for an overview, see also Ref. (10) and more recently (11)].

Although such stimulation results indicate the presence of participating anatomical centers in the manifestation of aberrant movement, there appears to be a lacking amount of analysis in terms of the role these various structures have on the production of such erroneous movement, one of the missing factors previously mentioned as necessary for providing neurophysiological backing for stimulating one anatomical component over the other. This lack of bridging between symptomatology and physiological activity indicates that there should be a growing consideration for the stimulation of different, discrete structures for various movement disorders depending on (a) the symptom being targeted and (b) the known, or hypothesized, physiology of nodes of participation in wider neurocircuits underlying such aberrations.

The aforementioned consideration of DBS application in disorders other than GTS sustains relevance when considering similarities. DBS applied to the ventral intermediate nucleus (Vim) of the thalamus has more or less replaced the use of thalamotomy to treat essential tremor (12). In dystonia, the application of DBS to subcortical structures has been used (13). DBS has also been applied to the ventral anterior internal capsule and subgenual cingulate white matter to treat medically intractable forms of certain neuropsychiatric disorders, such as obsessive–compulsive disorder and depression (14). The amygdala has also been proposed as a participating mediator of various neuropsychiatric disorders including anxiety and depression (15). In terms of its role in GTS symptomatology, projections from the superficial nuclei of the amygdala have been considered as important for tic suppression due to the nuclei's interactions with the frontal cortex (16). Such a neuromodulatory role in tic suppression would implicate the amygdala as another node in the participating circuitry for GTS.

Apart from invasive techniques such as DBS, other physiologically grounded and non-invasive approaches have permitted a relation between symptom manifestation and underlying neural circuits. Abnormal excitability related to symptom manifestation has been linked to aberrations in plasticity-induced learning using transcranial magnetic stimulation (TMS) (1). The electromagnetic stimulation techniques offer both measurement and potential for modulation of neurophysiology using minimal risk and high tolerability methodology. The use of such non-invasive stimulation techniques has been used to activate Purkinje cell circuits of the cerebellar cortex, potentially inducing inhibition of the disynaptic, dentate–thalamocortical facilitatory connection and production of inhibition of the primary motor cortex (M1) (17–19).

Additionally, other stimulation studies have quantified activity of specific structures, such as the cerebellum, involved in aberrant neural circuits and correlated this activity with the severity of specific symptoms, such as motor tics. Such assessment permits relevant circuit activity to be monitored, facilitating targeted application for potential neuromodulation. Specific paradigms have been developed to monitor and quantify structural activity non-invasively. For example, the use of TMS for cerebellar conditioning in healthy subjects, when implemented 5–7 ms prior to the test stimulus, results in inhibition of motor-evoked potentials (20, 21), a decrease in amplitude referred to as cerebellar brain inhibition (CBI). This type of inhibition is mediated through pathways between the cerebellum and M1.

The CBI protocol is an example of a non-invasive neurostimulation paradigm that allows quantification of structural (cerebellar) activity. The amount of activity assessed by the CBI paradigm might be correlated with tic severity, potentially demonstrating that more selective modulation of certain aberrant pathways can be achieved.

Studies have shown that the application of 1-Hz, low-frequency repetitive TMS (rTMS) over the supplementary motor area (SMA) of the cortex in children with GTS led to amelioration of motor tics, with tic symptoms improving over the 12 weeks of the study duration (22). Such improvement is attributed to normalization of bihemispheric hyperexcitability (23). Clinical applications are supported by TMS studies demonstrating that decreased motor inhibition is present in GTS patients, who show physiological differences from non-GTS patients, with a shorter cortical silent period when using cortical inhibition TMS paradigms (24). Additionally, the use of short interval short intracortical inhibition TMS paradigms on children with GTS shows that cortical inhibition is inversely associated with severity of motor tics (25).

Additionally, low-frequency (1 Hz) rTMS has also been applied to normalize overactive motor cortical regions (specifically, the SMA) (26) and improve GTS symptoms. This is based on imaging studies showing that metabolism is increased in premotor, prefrontal, and motor cortex during tic suppression and tics, indicating increased activity in these regions which implicates that hyperexcitability is tied to tic manifestation (27–29). Yet, it has been shown that higher intensities of stimulation (100% of resting motor threshold) administered over more than 2 days has a more significant, long-lasting, and beneficial effect on tics (30) than that of lower frequencies (31). Subjects with GTS who were treated with this TMS paradigm showed clinical improvement during the first week of rTMS and continued to improve during the second week of treatment. This improvement in symptoms was correlated with a significant increase in resting motor threshold, which remained stable 3 months following the study. Clinical improvement is attributed to normalization of the right hemisphere hyperexcitability present in these patients, potentially indicating a restoration of hemispheric symmetry (30).

However, the use of TMS for clinical application remains limited, in part due to the rather narrow interpretation of how these techniques can be best applied. Current problems with stimulation can perhaps be considered to be rooted in the bottom-up approach to its application rather than the top-down proposal previously mentioned: that is, observing clinical manifestation of behavior in order to propose underlying circuits that have structures accessible for specific neurostimulation paradigms designed to modulate particular aberrant firing. The benefit of such a proposal is that it allows consideration of individual symptoms as guides to the physiology involved in their production.

The application of non-invasive neurostimulation techniques for premeditated, symptom-guided application correlated with known or proposed circuit level participation in aberrant physiology has not been clearly described as the prime motivation behind structure targeting or specific clinical improvements. As a result, although there are improvements in certain symptoms resulting from the application of neurostimulation to various anatomical components participating in the underlying circuits of aberrant movements, it must be noted that without a clearer, symptom-guided application of neurostimulation to participating circuit nodes, such modulation of symptoms to specific paradigms or parameters applied cannot decisively be attributed to the resulting changes.

Gilles de la Tourette syndrome patients have been treated with DBS since 1999, and approximately 48 published studies report some degree of motor tic reduction (32). While initial trials have been promising, the mechanisms subserving the effectiveness of DBS in reducing GTS signs and symptoms have yet to be identified. A condensed list of invasive stimulation is provided in **Table 1**.

Current models of GTS hypothesize that thalamocortical–BG dysfunction is a key network underlying many of its symptoms. A recent study provided evidence that different types of tics, for example, are paralleled by different types of electrophysiological signatures (47): studied patients with GTS implanted with bilateral DBS electrodes with depth leads in the CM–pF as well as subdural strips over the precentral gyrus. Low-frequency (1–10 Hz) CM–pf activity was observed during tics, as well as modulations in beta rhythms over the motor cortex. The division of tics in the study (three categories: long complex, complex, and simple) showed that long complex tics, tics involving multiple body regions and lasting longer than 5 s were synchronized with detectable thalamocortical signatures. Such symptom-categorized monitoring of neural activity in circuitry implicated in GTS physiology highlights the need for more discrete and motivated application of neuromodulation and monitoring, so as to provide firmly guided evidence for prioritizing stimulation and ideally predicting potential outcomes. Acute trials of closed loop stimulation using the human tic detector are currently underway. Such results further indicate that there is neurophysiological evidence for divergent symptom signatures rooted in particular network-firing aberrancies.

TABLE 1 | Examples of Invasive Stimulation in GTS. The table provides a condensed overview of invasive stimulation approaches presented in this article, as well as additional studies of interest, that have been used thus far to ameliorate or investigate symptoms in GTS.

Reference	*n*	Target	Outcome
Visser-Vandewalle et al. (33)	3	Thalamus: centromedian nucleus, substantia periventricularis, and nucleus ventro-oralis internus	Tic reduction ranging from 72.2 to 90.1% reduction at long-term follow-up, although specific tic persistence was reported for the 3 patients
Maciunas et al. (34)	5	Thalamus: centromedian–parafascicular (CM–Pf) and ventralis oral complex (Voi)	3 out of 5 patients' improvement in [Yale Global Tic Severity Scale (YGTSS) and TS Symptom List scores]. 2 patients did not improve after 3-month follow-up
Servello et al. (35)	18	Thalamus: bilateral CM–Pf and Voi	6 patients showed progressive improvement in tic severity, and 12 showed recurrent motor and phonic tics after stimulation, with 3 showing waxing and waning of symptoms
Welter et al. (36)	3	Thalamus: bilateral CM–Pf GPi: ventromedial locations	YGTSS showed that GPi stimulation reduced tic severity to 65, 96, and 74%, respectively. Bilateral stimulation of the CM–Pf produced a 64, 30, and 40%, respectively, reduction in tic severity. In patient 2, the improvement decreased after 2 months
Porta et al. (37)	15	Thalamus: bilateral CM–Pf and Voi	15 out of 18 patients improved in tic severity and behavioral ratings (including anxiety and depression) Data not available for 3 patients
Kwon et al. (23)		Transcranial magnetic stimulation (TMS). Supplementary motor area (SMA) of the cortex	Normalization of the right hemisphere hyperexcitability leading to clinical improvement
Martínez-Fernández et al. (38)	5	GPi: 2 patients in the bilateral posterolateral location, 2 patients in the bilateral anteromedial location, 1 initially in the posterolateral was switched to the anteromedial location after 18 months	2 patients with stimulation the bilateral posterolateral location: 1 patient showed a 54.7% reduction in motor tics and the second patient only showed a plateau in motor and phonic tics but still interfered with lifestyle according to YGTSS 2 patients in stimulation in bilateral anteromedial location: 1 patient showed a 60% reduction in motor tics. Motor and phonic tics resolved for the second patient 1 patient with anteromedial location switch after 18 months: only a 19% reduction for motor tics in the YGTSS
Cannon et al. (39)	11	GPi: bilateral anteromedial globus pallidus internus	10 patients (91%) showed improvement in tic severity, with a 48% reduction in motor tics and a 56.5% reduction in phonic tics. 6 patients (54.5%) had more than 50% reduction; sustained for at least 3 months in YGSS. 2 patients required pharmacotherapy for tics after surgery. 1 patient was a non-responder
Maling et al. (40)	5	Thalamus: bilateral CM–Pf and Voi	3 out of 5 patients showed significant YGTSS decrease. The remaining 2 showed only a small clinical improvement corresponding to small changes in gamma power
Porta et al. (41)	18	Thalamus: bilateral CM–Pf and Voi	Reduction in tic severity, as well as improvements in the comorbid obsessive–compulsive behaviors (OCB), and co-existing psychopathologies (anxiety and depressive symptomatology). However, only 7 out of 15 patients did the overall global assessment of improvement indicate improvement
Huys et al. (42)	8	Thalamus: bilateral for 6 patients; ventral anterior and ventrolateral motor areas	YGTSS showed a 51% reduction in motor tics and a 53% in vocal tics, with a total of 58% reduction score compared to baseline
Dehning et al. (43)	6	GPi: bilateral postero-ventrolateral location	2 patients did not respond to stimulation, and the mean YGTSS score for the remaining 4 patients was 29.5 at the last follow-up, with a mean Tourette Syndrome Quality-of-Life Scale (TSQOL) of 7.75
Zhang et al. (44)	13	GPi: bilateral posterolateral location	YGTSS scores at the last visit compared with baseline were reduced in all 13 patients by a mean of 52.1%. 12 of the 13 showed a mean TSQOL of 45.7%, with 1 patient denying improvement. Only 6 patients reported a significantly high response with overall marked reduction in all tic types
Bloch and Levkovitz (45)	12	TMS. Bilateral SMA inhibition	Improvement in clinical symptoms in children with GTS for at least 6 months
Kefalopoulou et al. (46)	15	GPi: bilateral anteromedial location	Mild improvement in YGTSS, with 80.7 for the off-stimulation period, and 68.3 for the on-stimulation period form a baseline of 87.9. No significant improvement in mean quality-of-life scores (GTS-QOL)

The table provides a condensed overview of invasive stimulation approaches presented in this article, as well as additional studies of interest, that have been used thus far to ameliorate or investigate symptoms in GTS. Beyond the demonstration of DBS as a therapeutic option, the number of insufficient responders is shown.

A recent study by the same group also modified the stimulation patterns to intermittent stimulation of the thalamus and despite reached responder status in the majority of the small patient group (48). A recent review discusses the relevance of different anatomical structures and modes of stimulation, closed loop, open loop, etc. (49).

THERAPEUTIC APPLICATION OF NEUROSTIMULATION TECHNIQUES BASED ON PLASTICITY-INDUCED LEARNING

The relevance of such physiological considerations versus epiphenomena of therapeutic neurostimulation can be illustrated by reflecting on the possible symptom improvement outcomes of such a circuit-based model of application, i.e., demonstration of causality relationships of stimulation, effects on physiology (perhaps using non-invasive stimulation), and ultimately effects on behavior.

Considering differences in learning specialization, one can propose that targeting particular nodes based on their involvement in specific tic repertoire might be a more efficient manner of using currently available neurostimulation techniques. The cerebellum is important during early phases of abnormal motor learning based on faulty encoding of errors. BG might point to a more context dependent role in the reinforcement of tics, such as reward-based reinforcement (50). As a result, abnormal reinforcement may facilitate repetitive behaviors and may be involved in higher cognitive symptoms of GTS.

Additionally, it is also crucial to consider neural mechanisms that occur offline, more specifically, a consideration of the process of forgetting such retained movements (tics). When contemplating the effects on symptomatology related to such potential decrease in "forgetting mechanisms" (51), aberrancies in this type of synaptic modulation could be proposed to manifest, or at least retain, the erroneous reinforcement of aberrant movements (tics) in these patients.

Therefore, when contemplating the therapeutic application of neurostimulation for GTS symptomology, it is worth considering that plasticity-induced learning is faulty in GTS in more than one way and might originate symptoms that require stimulation of particular nodes over others. There is no simple extrapolation possible to predict an outcome on behavior with current strategies. The analysis to the use and application of neurostimulation requires an interdisciplinary approach to patient symptoms, one in which there is a bridging between clinical eye and investigative complex methods of studying effects on neurophysiology and behavior.

CONCLUSION

The parameters for therapeutic use of neurostimulation in neuropsychiatric disorders, as well as the reliability of stimulating certain nodes over other regions for specific symptoms, have yet to be established. Regardless of these present uncertainties of the benefits of neurostimulation techniques for neuropsychiatric disorders and the exact role of certain structures in GTS symptomatology, it is apparent that promising therapeutic alternatives for patients can be developed by considering the application of brain stimulation to neural circuits. However, such application is dependent on finding its use on the modulation of plasticity mechanisms and alteration of learning at a circuit level. Although the benefits of applying neurostimulation techniques as therapy remain to be precisely defined, it is evident that utilizing non-pharmacological neuromodulation techniques is a consideration worth making.

AUTHOR CONTRIBUTIONS

All authors were involved in the study concept and design, analysis and interpretation of manuscript, critical revision of manuscript for intellectual content, literature review, acquisition of data, and drafting of the manuscript.

ACKNOWLEDGMENTS

The authors would like to express their gratitude to The Dorothy Feiss Scientific Research Grant. The authors would like to thank the Editor-in-Chief of Frontiers (*Frontiers in Psychiatry*) for the opportunity to submit this paper to the journal.

FUNDING

The publication of this article was funded by the Open Access Fund of the Leibniz Association and by the Open Access Fund of the Technical University of Dortmund.

REFERENCES

1. Pedroarena-Leal N, Ruge D. Cerebellar neurophysiology in Gilles de la Tourette syndrome and its role as a target for therapeutic intervention. *J Neuropsychol* (2015). doi:10.1111/jnp.12091
2. Leckman JF, Cohen DJ, editors. *Tourette's Syndrome – Tics, Obsessions, Compulsions: Developmental Psychopathology and Clinical Care*. New York: John Wiley & Sons (1999).
3. Albin RL, Mink JW. Recent advances in Tourette syndrome research. *Trends Neurosci* (2006) 29(3):175–82. doi:10.1016/j.tins.2006.01.001
4. DeLong MR. Primate models of movement disorders of basal ganglia origin. *Trends Neurosci* (1990) 13(7):281–5. doi:10.1016/0166-2236(90)90110-V
5. Mink JW. Basal ganglia dysfunction in Tourette's syndrome: a new hypothesis. *Pediatr Neurol* (2001) 25(3):190–8. doi:10.1016/S0887-8994(01)00262-4
6. Bohlhalter S, Goldfine A, Matteson S, Garraux G, Hanakawa T, Kansaku K, et al. Neural correlates of tic generation in Tourette syndrome: an event-related functional MRI study. *Brain* (2006) 129(Pt 8):2029–37. doi:10.1093/brain/awl050
7. McCairn KW, Iriki A, Isoda M. Global dysrhythmia of cerebro-basal ganglia-cerebellar networks underlies motor tics following striatal disinhibition. *J Neurosci* (2013) 33(2):697–708. doi:10.1523/JNEUROSCI.4018-12.2013
8. Jankovic J, Stone L. Dystonic tics in patients with Tourette's syndrome. *Mov Disord* (1991) 6(3):248–52. doi:10.1002/mds.870060309
9. Vandewalle V, van der Linden C, Groenewegen H, Caemaert J. Stereotactic treatment of Gilles de la Tourette syndrome by high frequency stimulation of thalamus. *Lancet* (1999) 353(9154):724. doi:10.1016/S0140-6736(98)05964-9
10. Cavanna AE, Eddy CM, Mitchell R, Pall H, Mitchell I, Zrinzo L, et al. An approach to deep brain stimulation for severe treatment-refractory Tourette syndrome: the UK perspective. *Br J Neurosurg* (2011) 25(1):38–44. doi:10.3109/02688697.2010.534200
11. Deeb W, Rossi RJ, Porta M, Visser-Vandewalle V, Servello D, Silburn P, et al. The international deep brain stimulation registry and database for Gilles de la Tourette syndrome: how does it work? *Front Neurosci* (2016) 10:170. doi:10.3389/fnins.2016.00170

12. Zhang K, Bhatia S, Oh MY, Cohen D, Angle C, Whiting D. Long-term results of thalamic deep brain stimulation for essential tremor. *J Neurosurg* (2010) 112(6):1271–6. doi:10.3171/2009.10.JNS09371
13. Gross RE, Lozano AM. Advances in neurostimulation for movement disorders. *Neurol Res* (2000) 22(3):247–58.
14. Lujan JL, Chaturvedi A, McIntyre CC. Tracking the mechanisms of deep brain stimulation for neuropsychiatric disorders. *Front Biosci* (2008) 13:5892–904.
15. Ball T, Rahm B, Eickhoff SB, Schulze-Bonhage A, Speck O, Mutschler I. Response properties of human amygdala subregions: evidence based on functional MRI combined with probabilistic anatomical maps. *PLoS One* (2007) 2(3):e307. doi:10.1371/journal.pone.0000307
16. Werner CJ, Stöcker T, Kellermann T, Wegener HP, Schneider F, Shah NJ, et al. Altered amygdala functional connectivity in adult Tourette's syndrome. *Eur Arch Psychiatry Clin Neurosci* (2010) 260(S2):95–9. doi:10.1007/s00406-010-0161-7
17. Groiss SJ, Ugawa Y. Cerebellar stimulation in ataxia. *Cerebellum* (2012) 11(2):440–2. doi:10.1007/s12311-011-0329-3
18. Iwata NK, Ugawa Y. The effects of cerebellar stimulation on the motor cortical excitability in neurological disorders: a review. *Cerebellum* (2005) 4(4):218–23. doi:10.1080/14734220500277007
19. Ugawa Y, Terao Y, Hanajima R, Sakai K, Furubayashi T, Machii K, et al. Magnetic stimulation over the cerebellum in patients with ataxia. *Electroencephalogr Clin Neurophysiol* (1997) 104(5):453–8. doi:10.1016/S0168-5597(97)00051-8
20. Ugawa Y, Day BL, Rothwell JC, Thompson PD, Merton PA, Marsden CD. Modulation of motor cortical excitability by electrical stimulation over the cerebellum in man. *J Physiol* (1991) 441(1):57–72.
21. Ugawa Y, Uesaka Y, Terao Y, Hanajima R, Kanazawa I. Magnetic stimulation over the cerebellum in humans. *Ann Neurol* (1995) 37(6):703–13. doi:10.1002/ana.410370603
22. Le K, Liu L, Sun M, Hu L, Xiao N. Transcranial magnetic stimulation at 1 Hertz improves clinical symptoms in children with Tourette syndrome for at least 6 months. *J Clin Neurosci* (2013) 20(2):257–62. doi:10.1016/j.jocn.2012.01.049
23. Kwon HJ, Lim WS, Lim MH, Lee SJ, Hyun JK, Chae J-H, et al. 1-Hz low frequency repetitive transcranial magnetic stimulation in children with Tourette's syndrome. *Neurosci Lett* (2011) 492(1):1–4. doi:10.1016/j.neulet.2011.01.007
24. Moll GH, Wischer S, Heinrich H, Tergau F, Paulus W, Rothenberger A. Deficient motor control in children with tic disorder: evidence from transcranial magnetic stimulation. *Neurosci Lett* (1999) 272(1):37–40.
25. Gilbert DL, Bansal AS, Sethuraman G, Sallee FR, Zhang J, Lipps T, et al. Association of cortical disinhibition with tic, ADHD, and OCD severity in Tourette syndrome. *Mov Disord* (2004) 19(4):416–25. doi:10.1002/mds.20044
26. Chen R, Classen J, Gerloff C, Celnik P, Wassermann EM, Hallett M, et al. Depression of motor cortex excitability by low-frequency transcranial magnetic stimulation. *Neurology* (1997) 48(5):1398–403. doi:10.1212/WNL.48.5.1398
27. Peterson BS, Skudlarski P, Anderson AW, Zhang H, Gatenby JC, Lacadie CM, et al. A functional magnetic resonance imaging study of tic suppression in Tourette syndrome. *Arch Gen Psychiatry* (1998) 55(4):326–33.
28. Pourfar M, Feigin A, Tang CC, Carbon-Correll M, Bussa M, Budman C, et al. Abnormal metabolic brain networks in Tourette syndrome. *Neurology* (2011) 76(11):944–52. doi:10.1212/WNL.0b013e3182104106
29. Stern E, Silbersweig DA, Chee KY, Holmes A, Robertson MM, Trimble M, et al. A functional neuroanatomy of tics in Tourette syndrome. *Arch Gen Psychiatry* (2000) 57(8):741–8.
30. Mantovani A, Lisanby SH, Pieraccini F, Ulivelli M, Castrogiovanni P, Rossi S. Repetitive transcranial magnetic stimulation (rTMS) in the treatment of obsessive-compulsive disorder (OCD) and Tourette's syndrome (TS). *Int J Neuropsychopharmacol* (2006) 9(1):95–100. doi:10.1017/S1461145705005729
31. Munchau A, Bloem BR, Thilo KV, Trimble MR, Rothwell JC, Robertson MM. Repetitive transcranial magnetic stimulation for Tourette syndrome. *Neurology* (2002) 59(11):1789–91. doi:10.1212/01.WNL.0000036615.25044.50
32. Schrock LE, Mink JW, Woods DW, Porta M, Servello D, Visser-Vandewalle V, et al. Tourette syndrome deep brain stimulation: a review and updated recommendations. *Mov Disord* (2015) 30(4):448–71. doi:10.1002/mds.26094
33. Visser-Vandewalle V, Temel Y, Boon P, Vreeling F, Colle H, Hoogland G, et al. Chronic bilateral thalamic stimulation: a new therapeutic approach in intractable Tourette syndrome. Report of three cases. *J Neurosurg* (2003) 99(6):1094–100. doi:10.3171/jns.2003.99.6.1094
34. Maciunas RJ, Maddux BN, Riley DE, Whitney CM, Schoenberg MR, Ogrocki PJ, et al. Prospective randomized double-blind trial of bilateral thalamic deep brain stimulation in adults with Tourette syndrome. *J Neurosurg* (2007) 107(5):1004–14. doi:10.3171/JNS-07/11/1004
35. Servello D, Porta M, Sassi M, Brambilla A, Robertson MM. Deep brain stimulation in 18 patients with severe Gilles de la Tourette syndrome refractory to treatment: the surgery and stimulation. *J Neurol Neurosurg Psychiatry* (2008) 79(2):136–42. doi:10.1136/jnnp.2006.104067
36. Welter ML, Mallet L, Houeto JL, Karachi C, Czernecki V, Cornu P, et al. Internal pallidal and thalamic stimulation in patients with Tourette syndrome. *Arch Neurol* (2008) 65(7):952–7. doi:10.1001/archneur.65.7.952
37. Porta M, Brambilla A, Cavanna AE, Servello D, Sassi M, Rickards H, et al. Thalamic deep brain stimulation for treatment-refractory Tourette syndrome: two-year outcome. *Neurology* (2009) 73(17):1375–80. doi:10.1212/WNL.0b013e3181bd809b
38. Martínez-Fernández R, Zrinzo L, Aviles-Olmos I, Hariz M, Martinez-Torres I, Joyce E, et al. Deep brain stimulation for Gilles de la Tourette syndrome: a case series targeting subregions of the globus pallidus internus. *Mov Disord* (2011) 26(10):1922–30. doi:10.1002/mds.23734
39. Cannon E, Silburn P, Coyne T, O'Maley K, Crawford JD, Sachdev PS. Deep brain stimulation of anteromedial globus pallidus interna for severe Tourette's syndrome. *Am J Psychiatry* (2012) 169(8):860–6. doi:10.1176/appi.ajp.2012.11101583
40. Maling N, Hashemiyoon R, Foote KD, Okun MS, Sanchez JC. Increased thalamic gamma band activity correlates with symptom relief following deep brain stimulation in humans with Tourette's syndrome. *PLoS One* (2012) 7(9):e44215. doi:10.1371/journal.pone.0044215
41. Porta M, Servello D, Zanaboni C, Anasetti F, Menghetti C, Sassi M, et al. Deep brain stimulation for treatment of refractory Tourette syndrome: long-term follow-up. *Acta Neurochir* (2012) 154(11):2029–41. doi:10.1007/s00701-012-1497-8
42. Huys D, Bartsch C, Koester P, Lenartz D, Maarouf M, Daumann J, et al. Motor improvement and emotional stabilization in patients with Tourette syndrome after deep brain stimulation of the ventral anterior and ventrolateral motor part of the thalamus. *Biol Psychiatry* (2016) 79(5):392–401. doi:10.1016/j.biopsych.2014.05.014
43. Dehning S, Leitner B, Schennach R, Müller N, Bötzel K, Obermeier M, et al. Functional outcome and quality of life in Tourette's syndrome after deep brain stimulation of the posteroventrolateral globus pallidus internus: long-term follow-up. *World J Biol Psychiatry* (2014) 15(1):66–75. doi:10.3109/15622975.2013.849004
44. Zhang JG, Ge Y, Stead M, Zhang K, Yan S, Hu W, et al. Long-term outcome of globus pallidus internus deep brain stimulation in patients with Tourette syndrome. *Mayo Clin Proc* (2014) 89(11):1506–14. doi:10.1016/j.mayocp.2014.05.019
45. Bloch Y, Levkovitz Y. Deep-TMS add-on treatment for intractable Tourette syndrome: a feasibility study. *Brain Stimulat* (2015) 8(2):324. doi:10.1016/j.brs.2015.01.052
46. Kefalopoulou Z, Zrinzo L, Jahanshahi M, Candelario J, Milabo C, Beigi M, et al. Bilateral globus pallidus stimulation for severe Tourette's syndrome: a double-blind, randomised crossover trial. *Lancet* (2015) 14(6):595–605. doi:10.1016/S1474-4422(15)00008-3
47. Shute JB, Okun MS, Opri E, Molina R, Rossi PJ, Martinez-Ramirez D, et al. Thalamocortical network activity enables chronic tic detection in humans with Tourette syndrome. *Neuroimage Clin* (2016) 12:165–72. doi:10.1016/j.nicl.2016.06.015
48. Rossi JP, Opri E, Shute JB, Molina R, Bowers D, Ward H, et al. Scheduled, intermittent stimulation of thalamus reduces tics in Tourette syndrome. *Parkinsonism Relat Disord* (2016) 29(2016):35–41. doi:10.1016/j.parkreldis.2016.05.033
49. Almeida L, Martinez-Ramirez D, Rossi PJ, Peng Z, Gunduz A, Okun MS. Chasing tics in the human brain: development of open, scheduled and closed loop responsive approaches to deep brain stimulation for Tourette syndrome. *J Clin Neurol* (2015) 11(2):122–31. doi:10.3988/jcn.2015.11.2.122

50. Doya K. Complementary roles of basal ganglia and cerebellum in learning and motor control. *Curr Opin Neurobiol* (2000) 10(6):732–9. doi:10.1016/S0959-4388(00)00153-7
51. Tsumoto T. Long-term depression in cerebral cortex: a possible substrate of "forgetting" that should not be forgotten. *Neurosci Res* (1993) 16(4):263–70. doi:10.1016/0168-0102(93)90036-P

17

GPi Oscillatory Activity Differentiates Tics from the Resting State, Voluntary Movements, and the Unmedicated Parkinsonian State

Joohi Jimenez-Shahed[1], Ilknur Telkes[2], Ashwin Viswanathan[3] and Nuri F. Ince[2]**

[1] Parkinson's Disease Center and Movement Disorders Clinic, Department of Neurology, Baylor College of Medicine, Houston, TX, USA, [2] Department of Biomedical Engineering, University of Houston, Houston, TX, USA, [3] Department of Neurosurgery, Baylor College of Medicine, Houston, TX, USA

Edited by:
Kirsten R. Müller-Vahl,
Hannover Medical School, Germany

Reviewed by:
Andrea A. Kühn,
Charité, Germany
Judith Walters,
National Institute of Neurological Disorders and Stroke, USA

***Correspondence:**
Joohi Jimenez-Shahed
jshahed@bcm.edu
Nuri F. Ince
nfince@uh.edu

Background: Deep brain stimulation (DBS) is an emerging treatment strategy for severe, medication-refractory Tourette syndrome (TS). Thalamic (Cm-Pf) and pallidal (including globus pallidus interna, GPi) targets have been the most investigated. While the neurophysiological correlates of Parkinson's disease (PD) in the GPi and subthalamic nucleus (STN) are increasingly recognized, these patterns are not well characterized in other disease states. Recent findings indicate that the cross-frequency coupling (CFC) between beta band and high frequency oscillations (HFOs) within the STN in PD patients is pathologic.

Methods: We recorded intraoperative local field potentials (LFPs) from the postero-ventrolateral GPi in three adult patients with TS at rest, during voluntary movements, and during tic activity and compared them to the intraoperative GPi-LFP activity recorded from four unmedicated PD patients at rest.

Results: In all PD patients, we noted excessive beta band activity (13–30 Hz) at rest which consistently modulated the amplitude of the co-existent HFOs observed between 200 and 400 Hz, indicating the presence of beta-HFO CFC. In all 3TS patients at rest, we observed theta band activity (4–7 Hz) and HFOs. Two patients had beta band activity, though at lower power than theta oscillations. Tic activity was associated with increased high frequency (200–400 Hz) and gamma band (35–200 Hz) activity. There was no beta-HFO CFC in TS patients at rest. However, CFC between the phase of 5–10 Hz band activity and the amplitude of HFOs was found in two TS patients. During tics, this shifted to CFC between the phase of beta band activity and the amplitude of HFOs in all subjects.

Conclusions: To our knowledge this is the first study that shows that beta-HFO CFC exists in the GPi of TS patients during tics and at rest in PD patients, and suggests that this pattern might be specific to pathologic/involuntary movements. Furthermore, our findings suggest that during tics, resting state 5–10 Hz-HFO CFC shifts to beta-HFO CFC which can be used to trigger stimulation in a closed loop system when tics are present.

Keywords: Tourette syndrome, Parkinson's disease, voluntary movements, tics, globus pallidus interna, local field potentials, deep brain stimulation

INTRODUCTION

Tourette syndrome (TS) is a neuropsychiatric disorder defined by the presence of vocal and motor tics, but characterized by frequent co-morbidities such as attention deficit disorder and obsessive compulsive disorder (Jankovic, 2001). Onset is typically in childhood with a waxing and waning course that is likely to resolve or significantly improve by the late teenage years (Freeman and Tourette Syndrome International Database, 2007). While the worst-ever time period for tics is often 10–12 years of age (Bloch et al., 2006a; Shprecher et al., 2014), 5–10% of patients will continue to experience significant or worsening symptoms into adulthood (Freeman and Tourette Syndrome International Database, 2007).

Predictors of severity or the course of TS are not well understood, though contributing factors may include presence of fine motor skills deficits (Bloch et al., 2006b), reduced caudate volumes (Bloch et al., 2005) or greater tic severity at a younger age (Bloch et al., 2006a). Approximately 5% of individuals with TS in a tertiary referral setting may meet criteria for "malignant" TS in which symptoms are self-injurious or may lead to emergency room visits or hospitalizations (Cheung et al., 2007). Pharmacologic and non-pharmacologic therapies exist for management of TS symptoms, and several new treatments are currently being investigated (Kious et al., 2016).

Deep brain stimulation (DBS) is an emerging therapy for advanced, medication-refractory TS, and consensus criteria for DBS candidacy have recently been revised (Schrock et al., 2015). Considerations include such factors as age, tic severity, tics as the primary source of disability, failure of typical medications and behavioral therapy, psychiatric co-morbidities, and psychosocial factors. While the exact mechanism of action of DBS is unclear, small series have suggested that marked improvement can be achieved (Schrock et al., 2015). Randomized clinical trials (Maciunas et al., 2007; Ackermans et al., 2011; Kefalopoulou et al., 2015) have shown less robust improvements following DBS, but this could be related to difficulties in designing clinical trials to adequately study this complex condition (Jimenez-Shahed, 2015). As a consequence, no consensus exists regarding the optimal site of stimulation in TS. The most studied targets include the globus pallidus interna (GPi) and the centromedian-parafascicular complex of the thalamus (Cm-Pf).

During DBS, an electrical stimulus is applied to a deep nucleus relevant to movement generation and the pathogenesis of tic activity. As with DBS in other movement disorders, a recording microelectrode is advanced into the target while electrical recordings (microelectrode recordings, or MER) are obtained, which are used to identify the optimal location for final electrode placement. MER allows for analysis of single unit neuronal activity (SUA), and different nuclei can be identified by their signature firing rate and pattern, which may also differ by disease state (Gross et al., 2006). Concurrent to the recording and analysis of SUA (Telkes et al., 2015), and also following placement of the DBS macroelectrode (Telkes et al., 2014), local field potential (LFP) recordings can be obtained. LFPs represent the aggregate activity of a group of neurons within the target structure. LFP recordings can also be obtained from the implanted DBS electrode(s) during surgery for replacement of a depleted implantable pulse generator (IPG; Abosch et al., 2012).

LFP analysis in Parkinson's disease (PD) has provided substantial insight into the pathophysiology and treatment of this movement disorder, including identification of the beta band of oscillations as a potential biomarker for the untreated disease state, which is abolished after administration of levodopa (Thompson et al., 2014). Similarly, analysis of intraoperative LFP recordings obtained during DBS electrode placement offers a unique opportunity to study the *in vivo* neurophysiology of tics in TS.

The purpose of this study was to obtain LFP recordings during the resting state, during tic activity, and during voluntary movements in patients with TS, and to compare these recordings to those obtained in the unmedicated resting state of patients with PD undergoing the same surgical procedure in the same brain target. The chosen site of stimulation for TS at our center is the bilateral postero-ventrolateral portion of the globus pallidus interna (pvGPi), based upon our prior experiences (Shahed et al., 2007) and anatomic considerations relating this nucleus to basal ganglia circuitry and TS phenomenology (Viswanathan et al., 2012), including "dystonic" tics. For a number of years, pvGPi DBS has also been a well-established treatment for patients with advanced PD (Deep-Brain Stimulation for Parkinson's Disease Study Group, 2001; Weaver et al., 2009). We hypothesized that LFP spectral characteristics and non-linear interactions between different frequency bands can distinguish tic activity from the resting and parkinsonian states, as well as from voluntary movements.

METHODS

Patients with medication refractory TS are considered for surgery at our center during consensus review by a team of Movement Disorders Neurologists, Neurosurgeons, and Neuropsychologists, and according to accepted criteria. In both TS and PD patients, comprehensive pre-operative neurologic and neuropsychological assessments are performed and reviewed by the consensus team in order to determine the appropriateness of DBS for each candidate. Experimental procedures related to the recording and analyses of LFPs are approved by the Institutional Review Board of Baylor College of Medicine. Candidates for DBS confirmed by consensus review were approached for participation in the study and written informed consent was obtained.

For both TS and PD patients undergoing an electrode placement procedure, the stereotactic coordinates for the pvGPi are chosen based on direct targeting (Machado et al., 2006). The microelectrode is advanced to the intended target using standard MER techniques. After the optimal location for implantation of the electrode is decided, the DBS macroelectrode (model 3387, Medtronic, Minneapolis, MN) is inserted to the appropriate depth. In PD patients, the electrode placement procedure is performed while "off" medications.

LFP recordings are obtained during the DBS electrode placement procedure in the hemisphere contralateral to the more severe tic activity in TS subjects, and in the left hemisphere of all PD subjects. The DBS macroelectrode is connected to sterile recording cables [a twist-lock cable (Medtronic) and a custom design matching cable (BioCables)] and the LFP recordings are obtained from its four contacts by using a gHIAmp (gTec, Graz, Austria) biosignal amplifier at a sampling rate of 1200 Hz, with 24-bit A/D resolution. Electromyography and electrocardiography is also performed in order to monitor the patient's behavioral state and to identify and remove artifacts from recordings. These signals are entered into the multipurpose neural data acquisition system in order to synchronize behavior with the neural data. For TS patients, video recordings are also made to characterize the phenomenology of any involuntary movements and synchronize LFP activity to the presence, absence, onset and offset of movements. During an IPG replacement procedure, the depleted IPG is first disconnected from the DBS lead extension cables. The distal ends of the extension cables are then connected to sterile recording cables (multiplex adapter cable model 74001 [2x4] and a twist-lock cable (model 3550-03; Medtronic). LFP recordings are obtained thereafter using the same biosignal amplifier, accompanied by electromyography, electrocardiography, and video recordings.

LFPs are recorded before intraoperative test stimulation during a resting period lasting for a minimum of 1 min in both TS and PD patients, and for TS patients, during provocation of spontaneous tics and during voluntary movements. Tic provocation is accomplished by suggestion (discussing tic characteristics or other triggers to provoke spontaneous tic activity). At least 3 repetitions of this sequence are performed. The recordings and motor assessments are conducted over a 10–15 min period. A representative video demonstrating the data and video acquisition system is included in the Supplementary Material (**Video 1**). Once LFP recordings are complete, the recording cable is disconnected and usual surgical procedures continue, including intraoperative testing of stimulation (Machado et al., 2006), to verify the presence of motor benefits and absence of stimulation side effects.

In this investigation, we report LFP analysis from three adult patients with TS and four with PD. LFP recordings from one TS subject (Subject III) were made during an IPG replacement procedure, 3.0 years after initial DBS electrode placement surgery. All other recordings were made during the initial DBS electrode placement surgery.

SIGNAL PROCESSING

All recorded signals were visualized with custom software that was developed in-house, and annotated to distinguish artifact and/or epochs of resting, active movements, and tic activity. Based on these annotations, resting state data from all subjects and tic periods from TS subjects were extracted into MATLAB (Mathworks, Natick, Massachusetts). LFP data from all four contacts were band-pass filtered using an FIR filter with 3 and 500 Hz cutoff frequencies. For elimination of power line artifacts, a 60 Hz notch filter and notch filters at harmonics of 60 Hz were used. During preprocessing of LFP data, raw signals were converted into a bipolar derivation (contacts 0–1, 1–2, 2–3).

The frequency content of the oscillatory LFP activity from the GPi was explored by power spectral analysis. The power spectrum of each bipolar LFP derivation was estimated using the modified Welch periodogram method (Telkes et al., 2014). Specifically, a fast Fourier transform (FFT) was computed with a 2048-sample long Hanning window and the window was shifted with 50% overlap. Since there were multiple segments of tic movements, the power spectra related to each state were averaged. In order to compare the power changes in specific LFP sub-bands between different events, the power in the beta, gamma and high frequency oscillation (HFO) ranges were computed over averaged tic and averaged voluntary hand movement periods separately, and were normalized according to the power of the baseline. The power changes with respect to baseline were represented in decibel (dB) scale,

$$P_{i,j,k}(dB) = 10\,log_{10}\left(\frac{A_k}{R_k}\right) \quad (1)$$

where A_k and R_k represent the active and resting state power of sub-band indexed with k respectively.

In order to quantify the non-linear interactions between different LFP frequency bands, the coupling between the amplitude of HFOs and the phase of low frequency oscillations were investigated by using a phase locking value (PLV) approach (Lachaux et al., 1999). For this particular purpose, LFP signals were filtered with a 2nd order Butterworth filter from 4 to 40 Hz with a 2 Hz band width and 1 Hz shift that constituted 37 bandpass filtered components for the low frequencies. Similarly, the same LFP signal was bandpass filtered from 150 to 500 Hz with another 2nd order Butterworth filter with 80 Hz band width and 25 Hz shift. Thus, 15 bandpass filtered components were obtained for high frequencies. The envelope of these high frequency components was extracted by using the Hilbert transform and the PLV method was used to estimate cross-frequency coupling (CFC) between the phase of low frequency activity and the amplitude of high frequency activity.

An analysis for statistical significance was performed over every single CFC calculated in order to check if the observed value differed from what would be expected due to chance alone. To achieve this, a surrogate analysis was performed by calculating the coupling between randomly selected blocks of both amplitude and phase envelopes. The chance occurrence of coupling between phase and amplitude was estimated by using 100 surrogates, and a z-score was computed for each individual CFC. In order to account for multiple comparisons, Bonferroni's correction was applied (the significance level of the test $\alpha = 0.05/555$, where the number of tests $= 37 \times 15$, or 555).

RESULTS

The clinical characteristics of enrolled subjects are included in **Table 1**. Based upon the tic characteristics and the LFP recording environment (electrode placement surgery vs. IPG replacement), handgrip movements were performed in two subjects and lateral neck movements were used in the other, in order to investigate voluntary movements. The type of voluntary movements and observed tic epochs and their duration are provided in **Table 2**. In all subjects where recordings were made during DBS surgery, the position of the electrode at the time of LFP recording remained unchanged after intraoperative testing of stimulation verified improvement in symptoms and absence of side effects. Test stimulation was performed after LFP recordings were made. Additionally, a contralateral DBS electrode was also successfully placed, and post-operative programming of the device led to reduction in motor symptoms (**Table 1**).

Figure 1 shows representative raw LFP signal characteristics in all three TS patients (Subjects I–III) in the resting state (left-hand side) when no tics or other movements were present, and during tic activity (right-hand side) as characterized by video and surface EMG. The beta, gamma, and high frequency bands are associated with event related desynchronization (ERD) and synchronization (ERS) during tic events. The LFP data filtered between 13 and 30 Hz in Subject I and Subject III indicate the presence of ERD, with lower amplitude beta band oscillations during tic periods compared to the resting state. During tic periods, there is also amplitude enhancement (ERD) in the gamma range (40–150 Hz) and higher frequencies (150–500 Hz) in all subjects. LFP raw data from Subject II filtered in the same frequency bands do not show an ERD-ERS pattern. A clear difference in theta range (4–7 Hz) oscillations between resting and tic periods are also not apparent in Subject II, whereas EMG signals show a clear difference between resting and tic states in all subjects.

We first investigated the LFP power spectra from each bipolar electrode combination (0–1, 1–2, and 2–3) in Subjects I–III, at rest and during tic activity. The greatest power of LFP spectral dynamics was most commonly found in 0–1 and 1–2 bipolar contact derivations. **Figure 2** compares the power spectra in the resting state to that during tic activity and active movement, obtained from the bipolar contact combination with the highest LFP power and across frequency ranges. In Subject I (**Figures 2A,B**), 4 Hz (theta band) and 13 Hz activity (beta band) during rest switches to 5 and 15 Hz activity during tics, and shifts further during voluntary hand movements to a clear peak at 10 Hz with enhancement in the beta band between 20 and 30 Hz. LFP power is broadly decreased in the 13–30 Hz range during voluntary hand movements, correlating with the ERD pattern demonstrated in **Figure 1**. In the HFO range, voluntary hand movements have the highest power (fast HFO) compared to the resting state and tic events. LFP power during tics is broadly higher than baseline between 150 to 450 Hz.

In Subject II, a 3.5 Hz activity peak is consistently seen during all events (**Figures 2C,D**). Even though gamma-ERS occurs during voluntary hand movements, no clear peak is observed. The power of gamma LFPs during averaged tic periods is higher than during the resting state. There is also clear enhancement of slow HFO activity during tic events compared to both baseline and voluntary hand movements. There are no event-related differences in the fast HFO range. In Subject III, compared to the resting state, the power of the theta peak is the highest during active movements, and is only slightly higher during averaged tic periods (**Figures 2E,F**). A clear beta peak is observed during rest, which attenuates during averaged tic periods and active movement. Once again, the power in the HFO range is higher during tics and active movement compared to the resting state.

Figure 3 summarizes the LFP power changes during tics and voluntary hand movements across frequency sub-bands relative to the resting state in each of three TS subjects. Theta band changes relative to the resting state are inconsistent across subjects. Beta band activity was lower during tics and lowest

TABLE 1 | Clinical Characteristics of Subjects receiving pvGPi stimulation.

	Diagnosis	Age at time of surgery, gender	Pre-op motor exam	Motor exam 1-year post-implant (% change)	Hemisphere
Subject I	TS	36 yo M	YGTSS total: 84	YGTSS total: 67 (20.2%)	Left
Subject II	TS	27 yo M	YGTSS total: 88	YGTSS total: 58 (34.1%)	Left
Subject III	TS	22 yo F	YGTSS total: 81	YGTSS total: 45 (44.4%)	Left
Subject IV	PD	51 yo M	MDS-UPDRS3: Off = 72; on = 18	–	Left
Subject V	PD	49 yo F	MDS-UPDRS3: Off = 47; on = 28	–	Left
Subject VI	PD	62 yo M	UPDRS3: Off = not done; on = 40	–	Left
Subject VII	PD	62 yo M	MDS-UPDRS3: Off = 40; on = 19	–	Left

TS, Tourette syndrome; PD, Parkinson's disease; YGTSS, Yale Global Tic Severity Scale; MDS-UPDRS3, Movement Disorders Society Unified Parkinson's Disease Rating Scale Part 3 Motor exam; UPDRS, Unified Parkinson's Disease Rating Scale.

TABLE 2 | Data segments used for the estimation of power spectra and CFC results in TS subjects.

	Tic activity		Voluntary hand movements	
	No. of epochs	Total duration (s)	No. and type of movements	Total duration (s)
Subject I	3	35-17-10	3 sets of handgrips (5 times each)	11-9-8
Subject II	5	25-36-17-27-18	3 sets of handgrips (10, 5, 5 times)	18-11-15
Subject III	2	193-122	2 sets of lateral neck movements (4 and 6 times)	16-15

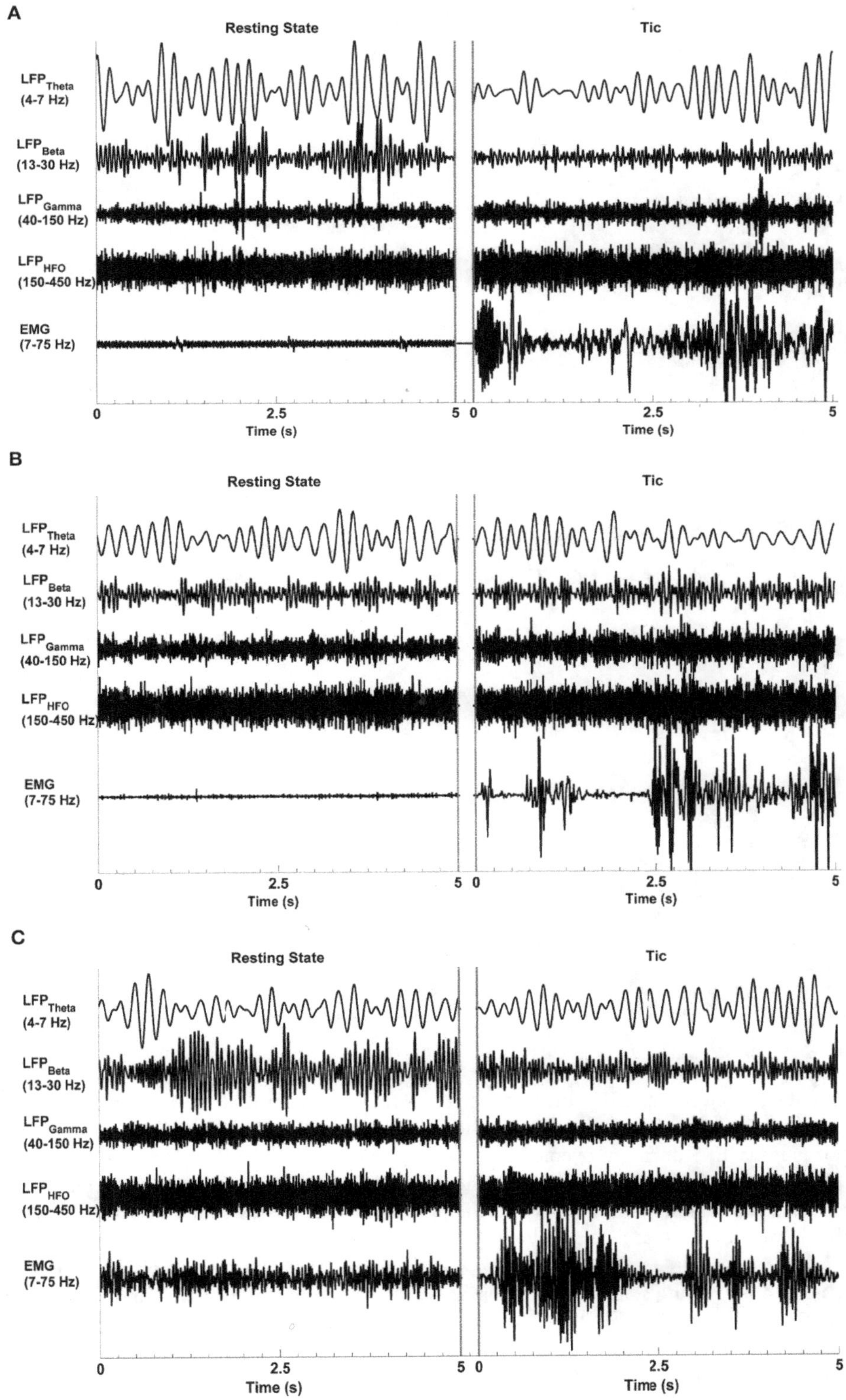

FIGURE 1 | Representative LFP signal characteristics during the resting state and tics. Epochs of each state lasting 5 s are presented, separated by red lines. The raw LFP data was bandpass filtered at the theta (4–7 Hz), beta (13–30 Hz), gamma (40–150 Hz), and high frequency oscillation (HFO, 150–500 Hz) ranges. The EMG signals were filtered between 7 and 75 Hz. Event-related desynchronization and synchronization are evident in Subjects I **(A)** and III **(C)** but not in Subject II **(B)**. All subjects demonstrate a clear increase in EMG activity during tics compared to the resting state. The red lines indicate the end of one epoch and the beginning of another.

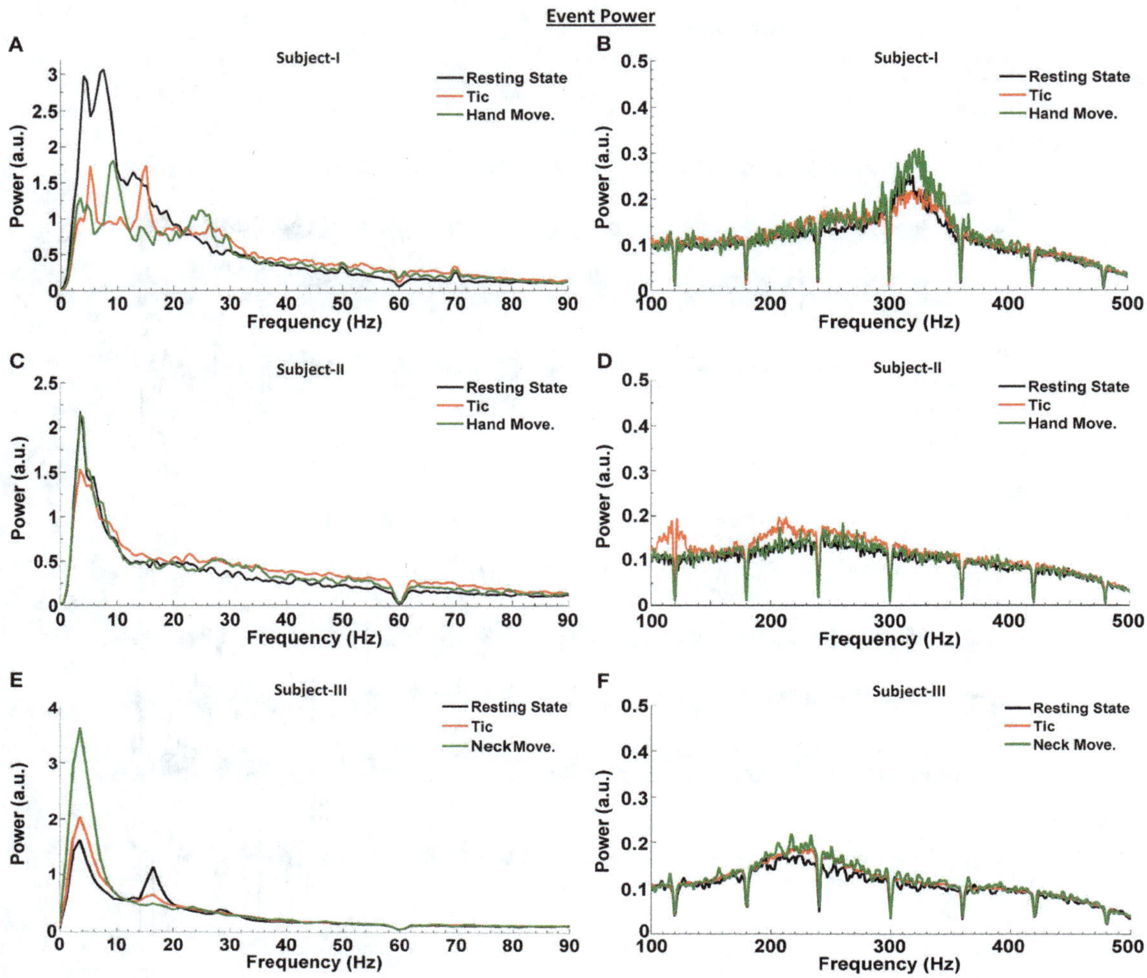

FIGURE 2 | LFP power spectra at rest, during tic activity and during voluntary movements in TS subjects. Spectra are shown in the bipolar contact derivation with the highest power [0–1 (Subjects I and II) and 1–2 (Subject III)]. LFP activity related to the resting state is shown in black, related to tic activity is shown in red, and related to voluntary movements is shown in green, for Subject I **(A,B)**, Subject II **(C,D)**, and Subject III **(E,F)**. The number and the duration of individual tic epochs and active movements which were averaged for spectral analysis are provided in **Table 2**.

during voluntary movements in Subjects I and III, corresponding to the ERD demonstrated in **Figure 1**. By contrast, neither reduced beta activity nor gamma-ERS during movement events were seen in Subject II. HFO activity was consistently higher during tics in all subjects. In Subjects I and III, there is a further increase in power of this frequency sub-band during voluntary movements.

The GPi power spectrum in the resting state for four subjects with PD is shown in **Figure 4**. Two PD Subjects (V and VI) show increased activity around 5 Hz, and one (Subject VII) has a low power peak at 7 Hz. In the beta band, Subjects IV and VI have increased activity between 20 and 30 Hz, while Subject V demonstrates a relatively large and wide range of beta band activity across the 12–30 Hz spectrum. Subject VII shows weak beta band activity. In the HFO range, all PD subjects show broad increases, with two (IV and VII) in the slower HFO spectrum (200–250 Hz) and two (V and VI) in the faster spectrum (250–350 Hz).

Next, in order to characterize the temporal relationships between low frequency (4–40 Hz) and wide HFO (150–500 Hz) bands, we assessed for the presence of CFC. **Figure 5** depicts the GPi CFC comodulograms for each TS subject, and **Figure 6** for each PD subject. In subjects with TS, CFC was investigated at rest (**Figures 5A,C,E**) and during tics (**Figures 5B,D,F**). The strongest CFC was seen in Subject I during the resting state, at a phase frequency between 5 and 10 Hz, coupled to the HFO amplitude at 250–400 Hz ($p < 0.05$) (**Figure 5A**). Interestingly, this range overlaps substantially with the theta range LFP frequency peaks seen during the resting state in this individual (**Figure 2A**). Significant CFC was also seen during tics, but at a higher beta frequency phase (13–33 Hz, $p < 0.05$) and remaining coupled to the amplitude in the

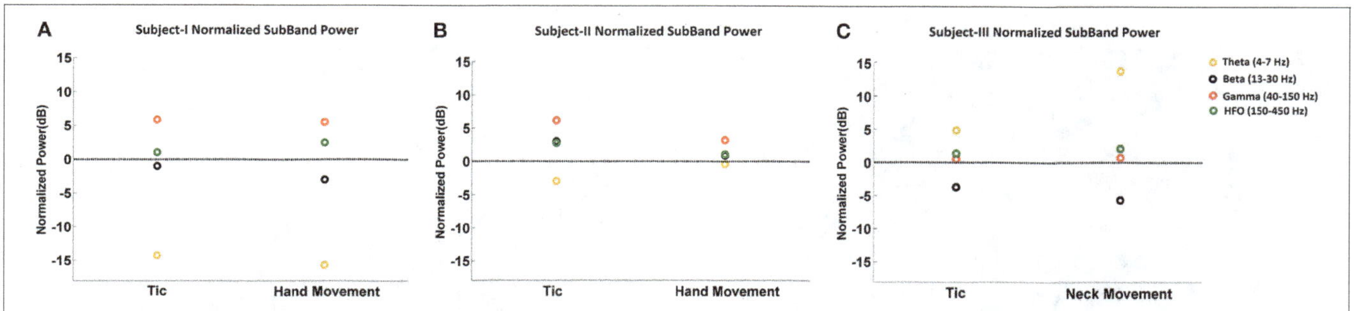

FIGURE 3 | Normalized sub-band power of LFPs during tic and voluntary hand movements relative to the resting state. The sub-band power changes at theta (4–7 Hz), beta (13–30 Hz), gamma (40–150 Hz), and HFO (150–450 Hz) bands are shown for Subject I **(A)**, Subject II **(B)**, and Subject III **(C)**.

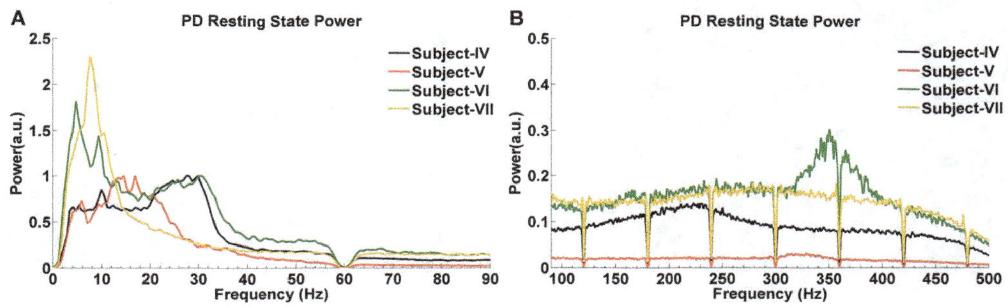

FIGURE 4 | LFP power spectra of PD subjects in the resting state at low (A) and high (B) frequencies.

same range of HFOs (**Figure 5B**). This phase coupling was maximal at 24–26 Hz.

By contrast, no CFC was found in Subject II during the resting state (**Figure 5C**). CFC during tic periods was weak, but still statistically significant ($p < 0.05$) (**Figure 5D**), and still demonstrated coupling between the phase of beta activity (localized at 25 Hz) and the amplitude of HFOs (localized at 325 Hz). In Subject III, the resting state (**Figure 5E**) is characterized by CFC between the phase frequencies localized at 8–10 Hz, and coupled to the amplitude of HFOs at 275–325 Hz ($p <$ 350 Hz), whereas tic periods (**Figure 5F**) are characterized by a shift to beta-HFO CFC to the phase of beta activity localized at 23–24 Hz, and coupled to the amplitude of HFOs at 275–300 Hz ($p < 0.05$). The presence of CFC was also assessed during voluntary movements in all subjects, and none was found across any frequency range (data not shown).

Analysis of CFC in PD patients during the resting state indicates a very strong phase-to-amplitude modulation between the phase of wide beta band activity and the amplitude of HFOs (**Figures 6A–D**). CFC phase frequencies are consistent with the increased LFP power shown in **Figure 6**, as are the amplitude frequencies for HFOs. For example, Subject V (**Figure 6B**) shows stronger and more widespread activity from 10 to 25 Hz than the other PD subjects, which corresponds to the widest phase frequency of CFC. This is coupled to the amplitude of HFOs ranging from 250 to 400 Hz, a range where the LFP power spectra is also greatest (**Figure 4**). On the other hand, Subject VII had the lowest LFP spectral power without a clear beta frequency band peak. This corresponds to the smallest coupling amongst PD subjects, though it was still significant ($p < 0.05$). HFOs were also amongst the lowest frequency range (**Figure 4**).

CONCLUSIONS

In this study we explored the LFP characteristics in the pvGPi of three patients with TS and four patients with PD. Although theta frequency peaks, lesser beta peaks, and HFO activity characterized the resting state in TS subjects, changes in LFP sub-bands did not consistently differentiate tics from active movements or the resting state. However, we did find a substantial difference in CFC between tic periods compared to the resting state, which was not seen during voluntary movements. Specifically, in TS subjects at rest, we found coupling between the phase of theta-low alpha oscillations to the amplitude of HFOs in 2 subjects, and during tic activity we found coupling between the phase of beta oscillations to the amplitude of HFOs in all 3 subjects. Amongst unmedicated PD patients at rest, we demonstrated increased beta band and broad HFO activity, as well as CFC between the phase of these beta oscillations and the amplitude of HFOs.

It is well-recognized that beta frequency oscillations are characteristic of the "off" medication state in PD in both the STN and GPi, and are abolished in the "on" state after administration of levodopa (Brown et al., 2001). The degree of improvement in motor symptoms (bradykinesia and rigidity)

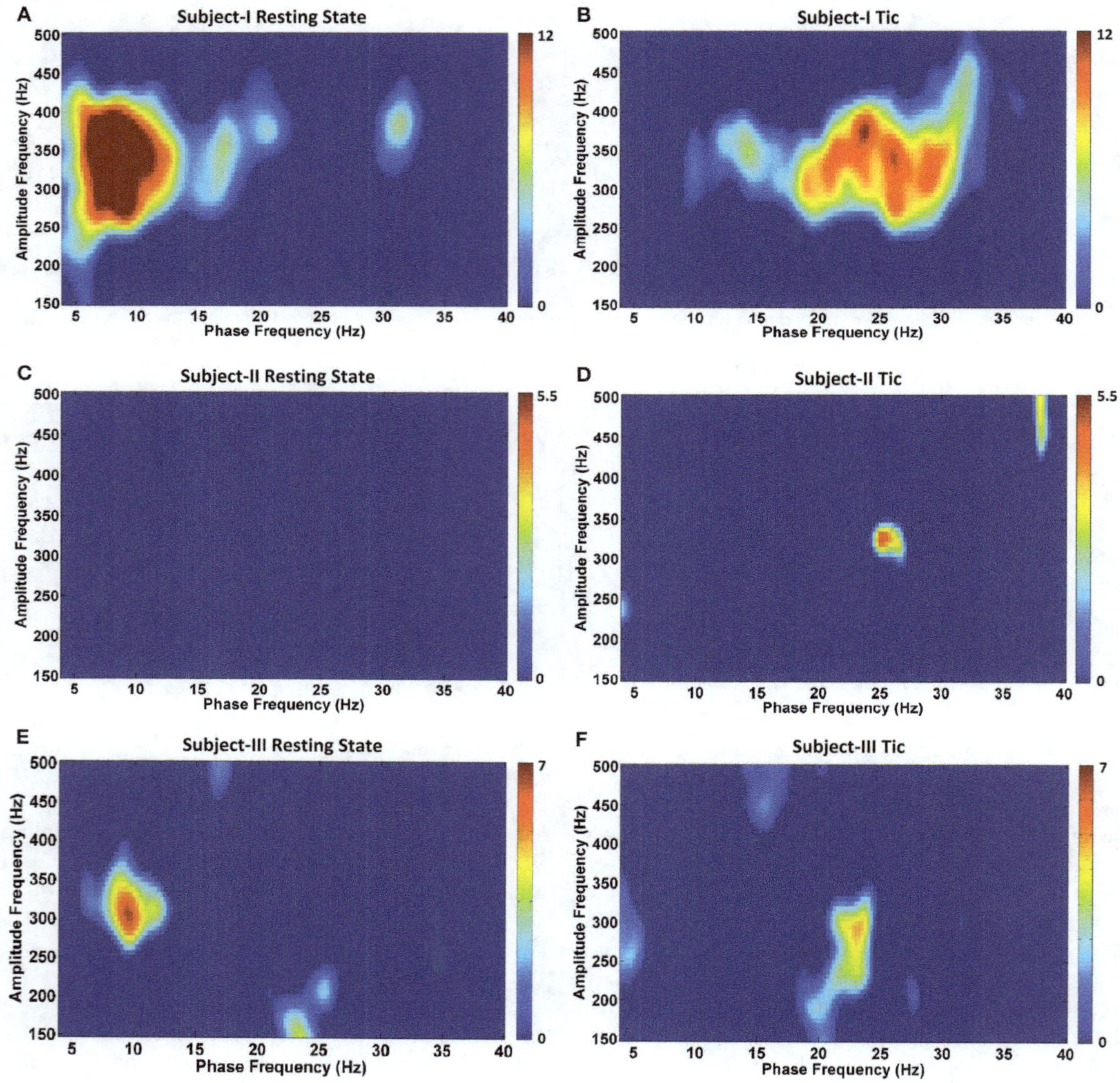

FIGURE 5 | Phase-amplitude coupling comodulograms for three TS subjects during the resting state and tic activity. Panels **(A–F)** demonstrate comodulograms for Subjects I–III respectively.

correlates with the degree of beta band suppression (Weinberger et al., 2006; Ray et al., 2008; Kuhn et al., 2009). Lastly, in the STN, beta ERD occurs upon movement initiation and heightened synchronization occurs upon termination of movements (Alegre et al., 2005; Hsu et al., 2012). As expected, we found excessive beta band activity at rest in our PD subjects with lower power HFOs across a broad range. By contrast, TS is a hyperkinetic movement disorder without features of bradykinesia or rigidity, with abnormal movements occurring in bouts. When the LFP spectra of TS subjects were compared to those of PD subjects, the resting state was found to be characterized by predominant excessive theta activity (3.5 or 4 Hz) in all three subjects, and also with HFOs (200–400 Hz) at lower power. In PD subjects, the main energy of LFPs was in the higher frequencies, except for Subject VI, who also shows high activity ranging from 5 to 13 Hz. Two TS subjects demonstrated beta frequency oscillations but at a lower power than the theta peak. Our findings therefore support the idea that beta band activity relates to relative akinesia.

Previous investigations into the LFP characteristics of TS patients undergoing DBS have focused on the thalamus. Neumann et al. (2013) identified LFP patterns in 5 subjects undergoing GPi and CM-Pf DBS, and found a peak in the 6–10 Hz frequency band. Others have also demonstrated alpha (8–13 Hz) or lower frequency (2–7 Hz) activity in the VO nucleus of the thalamus (Marceglia et al., 2010) and CM-Pf (Maling et al., 2012; Bour et al., 2015), but the clinical correlates of these frequency sub-bands remain unclear.

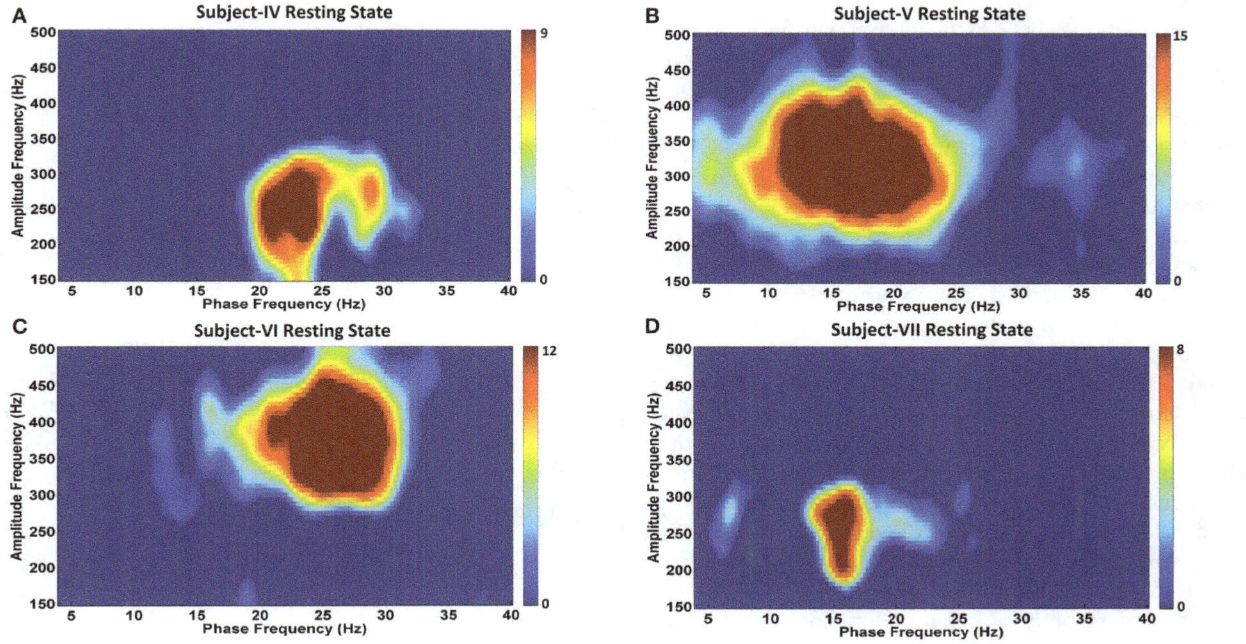

FIGURE 6 | Phase-amplitude coupling comodulgrams for four PD subjects in the resting state. Panels **(A–D)** demonstrate the resting state comodulograms in Subjects IV–VII, respectively, who all have Parkinson's disease, and are "off" medications.

In PD, however, the power of the gamma and HFO spectra increases after levodopa administration, and gamma activity increases in the "off" state during voluntary movement (Brown et al., 2001; Foffani et al., 2003; Kane et al., 2009). Moreover, a cross-frequency coupling (CFC) between the phase of beta oscillations and the amplitude of HFOs has been identified in the STN, which also attenuates following administration of levodopa and is less prominent in patients with milder PD symptoms (Lopez-Azcarate et al., 2010; Ozkurt et al., 2011; Van Wijk et al., 2016). Coupling between phase of beta band oscillations and amplitude of broad band gamma activity (50–200 Hz) has also been demonstrated in the motor cortex of PD patients, but found to be absent in dystonia and epilepsy (De Hemptinne et al., 2013), and is abolished after DBS (De Hemptinne et al., 2015). Gamma band and HFOs therefore were suggested to represent a prokinetic state, while beta-HFO phase amplitude coupling were thought to characterize relative akinesia in patients with PD.

Our investigation identifies the presence of beta-HFO CFC in the pvGPi of four PD subjects during the unmedicated resting state. To our knowledge, this finding has not been previously reported. We were further able to demonstrate, for the first time, that the pattern of CFC in TS subjects at rest differs from that of unmedicated PD, and that this in turn differs from the CFC during tics. In two of three TS subjects, CFC between the phase of 5–10 Hz band activity and the amplitude of HFOs was found during the resting state. The 5–10 Hz range highly overlaps with the excessive theta band activity we observed at rest (**Figure 2**). We further found that this resting state CFC in the same subjects shifts to beta-HFO CFC during tics. Despite the obvious change in the phase index of CFC between the resting state and tic periods, we were unable to identify a consistent or corresponding change in theta band power during voluntary movements or tic periods, compared to the resting state (**Figure 3**). It is possible that the methodologic differences in LFP capture in Subject III (recorded during IPG exchange) may have contributed to this inconsistency. Nonetheless, the consistent beta-HFO CFC seen during tic periods in all three subjects is notable, though found to a lesser extent in Subject II. LFP analysis in Subject II did not show either beta-ERD or gamma-ERS relative to the resting state during movements or any CFC while at rest. Since LFPs recorded from motor territories of the basal ganglia during voluntary movements are associated with beta-ERD (Kuhn et al., 2004), the absence of beta-ERD and gamma-ERS in Subject II suggests that the electrode might not be optimally placed within the pvGPi motor territory, thereby explaining the lack of CFC at rest or strong CFC during tics.

Dystonia is another movement disorder amenable to pvGPi DBS that is characterized by diminished power in the beta band and higher power in the 8–20 Hz range (Silberstein et al., 2003; Weinberger et al., 2012). Liu et al. (2008) showed an increased power of synchronization in the 3–18 Hz range during dystonic spasms compared to the resting state. Neumann et al. (2016) demonstrated that theta (but not beta) frequency peaks in patients with cervical dystonia at rest correlated with symptom severity. CFC in dystonia patients within the GPi has been identified between the phase of theta and the amplitude of gamma oscillations (Moll et al., 2014), though it is unclear if this was found at rest or during dystonic spasms. Barow et al. (2014)

further demonstrated that high frequency stimulation of the pvGPi can suppress theta oscillatory activity in subjects with mobile, phasic dystonia. Excessive theta activity in the pvGPi at rest in both dystonia and TS patients may therefore represent an underlying pathophysiologic similarity that supports the notion that a "dystonic" phenomenology of tics may indeed be treated with pvGPi DBS, similar to idiopathic dystonia, and as demonstrated by our three cases.

Another recent investigation into the LFP dynamics of the subthalamic nucleus (STN) in both PD and dystonia patients (Wang et al., 2016) found similar power spectral densities across multiple frequency ranges, including beta and theta, between the two groups, as well as resting state beta-HFO phase-amplitude coupling. Rather than representing a PD biomarker, this coupling may therefore represent pathologic network activity in patients with movement disorders (such as PD, dystonia and TS), though studies in patients without movement disorders are lacking.

Although the present study is limited to three patients with TS, and lack of information about the response of these LFP and CFC patterns to medications or DBS, our findings have particular relevance to the design of a closed loop, on-demand DBS system based on sensing of *in vivo* neurophysiologic biomarkers of involuntary movements such as tics. Further investigation to distinguish the LFP characteristics between tic and voluntary movement sequences is warranted in order to make the sensing paradigms as precise as possible. However, our findings do suggest the possibility that the shift in phase to amplitude CFC from the resting state (5–10 Hz activity coupled to HFO) to tic activity (beta-HFO) can be used to trigger stimulation in a closed loop system when tics are present. Furthermore, our work provides support for the continued investigation pvGPi DBS in cases of refractory TS as an overall modulator of tics.

AUTHOR CONTRIBUTIONS

JJS, IT, AV, NI: Substantial contributions to the conception or design of the work; substantial contribution to the acquisition, analysis, or interpretation of data for the work; Drafting the work and revising it critically for important intellectual content; Final approval of the version to be published; Agrees to be accountable for all aspects of the work in ensuring that questions related to the accuracy or integrity of any part of the work are appropriately investigated and resolved.

SUPPLEMENTARY MATERIAL

The Supplementary Material for this article can be found online at: http://journal.frontiersin.org/article/10.3389/fnins.2016.00436

Video 1 | This video segment demonstrates a representative example of a tic flurry recording during DBS electrode placement into the pvGPi of Subject II. An initial resting period is followed by the onset of a series of repetitive right hand tics. The real-time neural acquisition system captures raw LFP signals in each bipolar electrode derivation, EMG activity, and an electrocardiogram.

REFERENCES

Abosch, A., Lanctin, D., Onaran, I., Eberly, L., Spaniol, M., and Ince, N. F. (2012). Long-term recordings of local field potentials from implanted deep brain stimulation electrodes. *Neurosurgery* 71, 804–814. doi: 10.1227/NEU.0b013e3182676b91

Ackermans, L., Duits, A., Van Der Linden, C., Tijssen, M., Schruers, K., Temel, Y., et al. (2011). Double-blind clinical trial of thalamic stimulation in patients with Tourette syndrome. *Brain* 134, 832–844. doi: 10.1093/brain/awq380

Alegre, M., Alonso-Frech, F., Rodriguez-Oroz, M. C., Guridi, J., Zamarbide, I., Valencia, M., et al. (2005). Movement-related changes in oscillatory activity in the human subthalamic nucleus: ipsilateral vs. contralateral movements. *Eur. J. Neurosci.* 22, 2315–2324. doi: 10.1111/j.1460-9568.2005.04409.x

Barow, E., Neumann, W. J., Brucke, C., Huebl, J., Horn, A., Brown, P., et al. (2014). Deep brain stimulation suppresses pallidal low frequency activity in patients with phasic dystonic movements. *Brain* 137, 3012–3024. doi: 10.1093/brain/awu258

Bloch, M. H., Leckman, J. F., Zhu, H., and Peterson, B. S. (2005). Caudate volumes in childhood predict symptom severity in adults with Tourette syndrome. *Neurology* 65, 1253–1258. doi: 10.1212/01.wnl.0000180957.98702.69

Bloch, M. H., Peterson, B. S., Scahill, L., Otka, J., Katsovich, L., Zhang, H., et al. (2006a). Adulthood outcome of tic and obsessive-compulsive symptom severity in children with Tourette syndrome. *Arch. Pediatr. Adolesc. Med.* 160, 65–69. doi: 10.1001/archpedi.160.1.65

Bloch, M. H., Sukhodolsky, D. G., Leckman, J. F., and Schultz, R. T. (2006b). Fine-motor skill deficits in childhood predict adulthood tic severity and global psychosocial functioning in Tourette's syndrome. *J. Child Psychol. Psychiatry* 47, 551–559. doi: 10.1111/j.1469-7610.2005.01561.x

Bour, L. J., Ackermans, L., Foncke, E. M., Cath, D., Van Der Linden, C., Visser Vandewalle, V., et al. (2015). Tic related local field potentials in the thalamus and the effect of deep brain stimulation in Tourette syndrome: report of three cases. *Clin. Neurophysiol.* 126, 1578–1588. doi: 10.1016/j.clinph.2014.10.217

Brown, P., Oliviero, A., Mazzone, P., Insola, A., Tonali, P., and Di Lazzaro, V. (2001). Dopamine dependency of oscillations between subthalamic nucleus and pallidum in Parkinson's disease. *J. Neurosci.* 21, 1033–1038.

Cheung, M. Y., Shahed, J., and Jankovic, J. (2007). Malignant Tourette syndrome. *Mov. Disord.* 22, 1743–1750. doi: 10.1002/mds.21599

Deep-Brain Stimulation for Parkinson's Disease Study Group (2001). Deep-brain stimulation of the subthalamic nucleus or the pars interna of the globus pallidus in Parkinson's disease. *N. Engl. J. Med.* 345, 956–963. doi: 10.1056/NEJMoa000827

De Hemptinne, C., Ryapolova-Webb, E. S., Air, E. L., Garcia, P. A., Miller, K. J., Ojemann, J. G., et al. (2013). Exaggerated phase-amplitude coupling in the primary motor cortex in Parkinson disease. *Proc. Natl. Acad. Sci. U.S.A.* 110, 4780–4785. doi: 10.1073/pnas.1214546110

De Hemptinne, C., Swann, N. C., Ostrem, J. L., Ryapolova-Webb, E. S., San Luciano, M., Galifianakis, N. B., et al. (2015). Therapeutic deep brain stimulation reduces cortical phase-amplitude coupling in Parkinson's disease. *Nat. Neurosci.* 18, 779–786. doi: 10.1038/nn.3997

Foffani, G., Priori, A., Egidi, M., Rampini, P., Tamma, F., Caputo, E., et al. (2003). 300-Hz subthalamic oscillations in Parkinson's disease. *Brain* 126, 2153–2163. doi: 10.1093/brain/awg229

Freeman, R. D., and Tourette Syndrome International Database, C. (2007). Tic disorders and ADHD: answers from a world-wide clinical dataset on Tourette syndrome. *Eur. Child Adolesc Psychiatry* 16(Suppl. 1), 15–23. doi: 10.1007/s00787-007-1003-7

Gross, R. E., Krack, P., Rodriguez-Oroz, M. C., Rezai, A. R., and Benabid, A. L. (2006). Electrophysiological mapping for the implantation of deep brain stimulators for Parkinson's disease and tremor. *Mov. Disord.* 21(Suppl. 14), S259–S283. doi: 10.1002/mds.20960

Hsu, Y. T., Lai, H. Y., Chang, Y. C., Chiou, S. M., Lu, M. K., Lin, Y. C., et al. (2012). The role of the sub-thalamic nucleus in the preparation of volitional movement termination in Parkinson's disease. *Exp. Neurol.* 233, 253–263. doi: 10.1016/j.expneurol.2011.10.013

Jankovic, J. (2001). Tourette's syndrome. *N. Engl. J. Med.* 345, 1184–1192. doi: 10.1056/NEJMra010032

Jimenez-Shahed, J. (2015). Design challenges for stimulation trials of Tourette's syndrome. *Lancet Neurol.* 14, 563–565. doi: 10.1016/S1474-4422(15)00043-5

Kane, A., Hutchison, W. D., Hodaie, M., Lozano, A. M., and Dostrovsky, J. O. (2009). Dopamine-dependent high-frequency oscillatory activity in thalamus and subthalamic nucleus of patients with Parkinson's disease. *Neuroreport* 20, 1549–1553. doi: 10.1097/WNR.0b013e32833282c8

Kefalopoulou, Z., Zrinzo, L., Jahanshahi, M., Candelario, J., Milabo, C., Beigi, M., et al. (2015). Bilateral globus pallidus stimulation for severe Tourette's syndrome: a double-blind, randomised crossover trial. *Lancet Neurol.* 14, 595–605. doi: 10.1016/S1474-4422(15)00008-3

Kious, B. M., Jimenez-Shahed, J., Shprecher, D. R. (2016). Treatment-refractory tourette syndrome. *Prog. Neuropsychopharmacol. Biol. Psychiatry* 70, 227–236. doi: 10.1016/j.pnpbp.2016.02.003

Kuhn, A. A., Tsui, A., Aziz, T., Ray, N., Brucke, C., Kupsch, A., et al. (2009). Pathological synchronisation in the subthalamic nucleus of patients with Parkinson's disease relates to both bradykinesia and rigidity. *Exp. Neurol.* 215, 380–387. doi: 10.1016/j.expneurol.2008.11.008

Kuhn, A. A., Williams, D., Kupsch, A., Limousin, P., Hariz, M., Schneider, G. H., et al. (2004). Event-related beta desynchronization in human subthalamic nucleus correlates with motor performance. *Brain* 127, 735–746. doi: 10.1093/brain/awh106

Lachaux, J. P., Rodriguez, E., Martinerie, J., and Varela, F. J. (1999). Measuring phase synchrony in brain signals. *Hum. Brain Mapp.* 8, 194–208.

Liu, X., Wang, S., Yianni, J., Nandi, D., Bain, P. G., Gregory, R., et al. (2008). The sensory and motor representation of synchronized oscillations in the globus pallidus in patients with primary dystonia. *Brain* 131, 1562–1573. doi: 10.1093/brain/awn083

Lopez-Azcarate, J., Tainta, M., Rodriguez-Oroz, M. C., Valencia, M., Gonzalez, R., Guridi, J., et al. (2010). Coupling between beta and high-frequency activity in the human subthalamic nucleus may be a pathophysiological mechanism in Parkinson's disease. *J. Neurosci.* 30, 6667–6677. doi: 10.1523/JNEUROSCI.5459-09.2010

Machado, A., Rezai, A. R., Kopell, B. H., Gross, R. E., Sharan, A. D., and Benabid, A. L. (2006). Deep brain stimulation for Parkinson's disease: surgical technique and perioperative management. *Mov. Disord.* 21(Suppl. 14), S247–S258. doi: 10.1002/mds.20959

Maciunas, R. J., Maddux, B. N., Riley, D. E., Whitney, C. M., Schoenberg, M. R., Ogrocki, P. J., et al. (2007). Prospective randomized double-blind trial of bilateral thalamic deep brain stimulation in adults with Tourette syndrome. *J. Neurosurg.* 107, 1004–1014. doi: 10.3171/JNS-07/11/1004

Maling, N., Hashemiyoon, R., Foote, K. D., Okun, M. S., and Sanchez, J. C. (2012). Increased thalamic gamma band activity correlates with symptom relief following deep brain stimulation in humans with Tourette's syndrome. *PLoS ONE* 7:e44215. doi: 10.1371/journal.pone.0044215

Marceglia, S., Servello, D., Foffani, G., Porta, M., Sassi, M., Mrakic-Sposta, S., et al. (2010). Thalamic single-unit and local field potential activity in Tourette syndrome. *Mov. Disord.* 25, 300–308. doi: 10.1002/mds.22982

Moll, C. K., Galindo-Leon, E., Sharott, A., Gulberti, A., Buhmann, C., Koeppen, J. A., et al. (2014). Asymmetric pallidal neuronal activity in patients with cervical dystonia. *Front. Syst. Neurosci.* 8:15. doi: 10.3389/fnsys.2014.00015

Neumann, W. J., Huebl, J., Brücke, C., Slentz, C., Schneider, G. H., and Kühn, A. A. (2016). Pallidal low frequency activity correlates with dystonic symptoms in patients with cervical dystonia [abstract]. *Mov. Disord.* 31, S1-S697. doi: 10.1002/mds.26688

Neumann, W. J., Hueble, J., Brücke, C., Lutjens, G., Capelle, H. H., Krauss, J. K., et al. (2013). Local field potentials show increased 6–10 Hz activity recorded from the globus pallidus inernus and the thalamus in patients with tourette-syndrome. *Stereotact. Funct. Neurosurg.* 91(Suppl 1), 155–312. doi: 10.1159/000351990

Ozkurt, T. E., Butz, M., Homburger, M., Elben, S., Vesper, J., Wojtecki, L., et al. (2011). High frequency oscillations in the subthalamic nucleus: a neurophysiological marker of the motor state in Parkinson's disease. *Exp. Neurol.* 229, 324–331. doi: 10.1016/j.expneurol.2011.02.015

Ray, N. J., Jenkinson, N., Wang, S., Holland, P., Brittain, J. S., Joint, C., et al. (2008). Local field potential beta activity in the subthalamic nucleus of patients with Parkinson's disease is associated with improvements in bradykinesia after dopamine and deep brain stimulation. *Exp. Neurol.* 213, 108–113. doi: 10.1016/j.expneurol.2008.05.008

Schrock, L. E., Mink, J. W., Woods, D. W., Porta, M., Servello, D., Visser-Vandewalle, V., et al. (2015). Tourette syndrome deep brain stimulation: a review and updated recommendations. *Mov. Disord.* 30, 448–471. doi: 10.1002/mds.26094

Shahed, J., Poysky, J., Kenney, C., Simpson, R., and Jankovic, J. (2007). GPi deep brain stimulation for Tourette syndrome improves tics and psychiatric comorbidities. *Neurology* 68, 159–160. doi: 10.1212/01.wnl.0000250354.81556.90

Shprecher, D. R., Rubenstein, L. A., Gannon, K., Frank, S. A., Kurlan, R. (2014). Temporal course of the tourette syndrome clinical triad. *Tremor Other Hyperkinet. Mov. (N Y).* 4:243. doi: 10.7916/D8HD7SV6

Silberstein, P., Kuhn, A. A., Kupsch, A., Trottenberg, T., Krauss, J. K., Wohrle, J. C., et al. (2003). Patterning of globus pallidus local field potentials differs between Parkinson's disease and dystonia. *Brain* 126, 2597–2608. doi: 10.1093/brain/awg267

Telkes, I., Ince, N. F., Onaran, I., and Abosch, A. (2014). Localization of subthalamic nucleus borders using macroelectrode local field potential recordings. *Conf. Proc. IEEE Eng. Med. Biol. Soc.* 2014, 2621–2624. doi: 10.1109/embc.2014.6944160

Telkes, I., Ince, N. F., Onaran, I., and Abosch, A. (2015). Spatio-spectral characterization of local field potentials in the subthalamic nucleus via multitrack microelectrode recordings. *Conf. Proc. IEEE Eng. Med. Biol. Soc.* 2015, 5561–5564. doi: 10.1109/embc.2015.7319652

Thompson, J. A., Lanctin, D., Ince, N. F., and Abosch, A. (2014). Clinical implications of local field potentials for understanding and treating movement disorders. *Stereotact. Funct. Neurosurg.* 92, 251–263. doi: 10.1159/000364913

Van Wijk, B. C., Beudel, M., Jha, A., Oswal, A., Foltynie, T., Hariz, M. I., et al. (2016). Subthalamic nucleus phase-amplitude coupling correlates with motor impairment in Parkinson's disease. *Clin. Neurophysiol.* 127, 2010–2019. doi: 10.1016/j.clinph.2016.01.015

Viswanathan, A., Jimenez-Shahed, J., Baizabal Carvallo, J. F., and Jankovic, J. (2012). Deep brain stimulation for Tourette syndrome: target selection. *Stereotact. Funct. Neurosurg.* 90, 213–224. doi: 10.1159/000337776

Wang, D. D., De Hemptinne, C., Miocinovic, S., Qasim, S. E., Miller, A. M., Ostrem, J. L., et al. (2016). Subthalamic local field potentials in Parkinson's disease and isolated dystonia: an evaluation of potential biomarkers. *Neurobiol. Dis.* 89, 213–222. doi: 10.1016/j.nbd.2016.02.015

Weaver, F. M., Follett, K., Stern, M., Hur, K., Harris, C., Marks, W. J. Jr., et al. (2009). Bilateral deep brain stimulation vs best medical therapy for patients with advanced Parkinson disease: a randomized controlled trial. *JAMA* 301, 63–73. doi: 10.1001/jama.2008.929

Weinberger, M., Hutchison, W. D., Alavi, M., Hodaie, M., Lozano, A. M., Moro, E., et al. (2012). Oscillatory activity in the globus pallidus internus: comparison between Parkinson's disease and dystonia. *Clin. Neurophysiol.* 123, 358–368. doi: 10.1016/j.clinph.2011.07.029

Weinberger, M., Mahant, N., Hutchison, W. D., Lozano, A. M., Moro, E., Hodaie, M., et al. (2006). Beta oscillatory activity in the subthalamic nucleus and its relation to dopaminergic response in Parkinson's disease. *J. Neurophysiol.* 96, 3248–3256. doi: 10.1152/jn.00697.2006

18

Meta-Analysis of Tourette Syndrome and Attention Deficit Hyperactivity Disorder Provides Support for a Shared Genetic Basis

Fotis Tsetsos[1], *Shanmukha S. Padmanabhuni*[1], *John Alexander*[1], *Iordanis Karagiannidis*[1], *Margaritis Tsifintaris*[1], *Apostolia Topaloudi*[1], *Dimitrios Mantzaris*[1], *Marianthi Georgitsi*[1,2], *Petros Drineas*[3] *and Peristera Paschou*[1]*

[1] Department of Molecular Biology and Genetics, Democritus University of Thrace, Alexandroupolis, Greece, [2] Laboratory of General Biology, Department of Medicine, Aristotle University of Thessaloniki, Thessaloniki, Greece, [3] Computer Science Department, Rensselaer Polytechnic Institute, Troy, NY, USA

Edited by:
Kirsten R. Müller-Vahl, Hannover Medical School, Germany

Reviewed by:
Thomas V. Fernandez, Yale School of Medicine, USA
Suhash Chakraborty, Hindustan Aeronautics Limited Hospital, India

***Correspondence:**
Peristera Paschou
ppaschou@mbg.duth.gr

Gilles de la Tourette Sydrome (TS) is a childhood onset neurodevelopmental disorder, characterized phenotypically by the presence of multiple motor and vocal tics. It is often accompanied by multiple psychiatric comorbidities, with Attention Deficit/Hyperactivity Disorder (ADHD) among the most common. The extensive co-occurrence of the two disorders suggests a shared genetic background. A major step toward the elucidation of the genetic architecture of TS was undertaken by the first TS Genome-wide Association Study (GWAS) reporting 552 SNPs that were moderately associated with TS (p < 1E-3). Similarly, initial ADHD GWAS attempts and meta-analysis were not able to produce genome-wide significant findings, but have provided insight to the genetic basis of the disorder. Here, we examine the common genetic background of the two neuropsychiatric phenotypes, by meta-analyzing the 552 top hits in the TS GWAS with the results of ADHD first GWASs. We identify 19 significant SNPs, with the top four implicated genes being TBC1D7, GUCY1A3, RAP1GDS1, and CHST11. TBCD17 harbors the top scoring SNP, rs1866863 (p:3.23E-07), located in a regulatory region downstream of the gene, and the third best-scoring SNP, rs2458304 (p:2.54E-06), located within an intron of the gene. Both variants were in linkage disequilibrium with eQTL rs499818, indicating a role in the expression levels of the gene. TBC1D7 is the third subunit of the TSC1/TSC2 complex, an inhibitor of the mTOR signaling pathway, with a central role in cell growth and autophagy. The top genes implicated by our study indicate a complex and intricate interplay between them, warranting further investigation into a possibly shared etiological mechanism for TS and ADHD.

Keywords: Tourette Syndrome, ADHD, meta-analysis, cross-disorder, TBC1D7, GUCY1A3, RAP1GDS1, CHST11

1. INTRODUCTION

Gilles de la Tourette Syndrome (TS) is a childhood onset neuropsychiatric disorder characterized by a multitude of motor and vocal tics that last longer than a year. Its international prevalence has been estimated to be approximately 1% (Robertson et al., 2009). A recent systematic review and meta-analysis on the population prevalence of TS, refined its prevalence estimate in children to 0.3–1%

(Scharf et al., 2015). It presents a significant gender bias, with 73% of its patients being male, and the male patients being more likely to develop comorbid disorders (Robertson et al., 2015). TS is often associated with other neuropsychiatric disorders, including Attention Deficit/Hyperactivity Disorder (ADHD), Obsessive Compulsive Disorder (OCD), depression and anxiety (Robertson, 2006).

The first genome-wide association study (GWAS) on TS was undertaken by the Tourette Syndrome Association International Consortium for Genetics (TSAICG) (Scharf et al., 2013). In their primary analysis, no SNPs achieved an association p-value of genome-wide significance, however this study provided the basis for subsequent studies, as the top signals that attained a $p < 10^{-3}$ were found to be significantly enriched for functional variants. The Gilles de la Tourette Syndrome GWAS Replication Initiative (GGRI) undertook a replication (Paschou et al., 2014) of the first GWAS study, by selecting the top LD-independent SNPs and additional SNPs singificantly enriched in eQTL or mQTLs for genotyping in 609 European TS patients and 610 ancestry-matched controls, recruited from different European countries and Canada. This replication study enriched the significance of the selected SNPs and provided more evidence toward the genetic aetiology of TS.

On the other hand, initial GWAS attempts on ADHD also did not yield genome-wide significant results (Neale et al., 2008; Mick et al., 2010; Neale et al., 2010a; Lesch et al., 2008). To that end, a meta-analysis was conducted by Neale et al. (2010b), aggregating the results of the previous GWAS projects and meta-analyzing them. This meta-analysis could not produce any significant results either, but, similar to the TS GWAS, it set the groundwork for the elucidation of the genetic background of ADHD.

The relationship of TS with ADHD is well established (Karagiannidis et al., 2016). Individuals with ADHD commonly present tics, and in individuals with TS and tics, ADHD is a significant commorbidity. ADHD occurs in a significant proportion of TS patients, ranging from 21 to 90% in studied cohorts (Robertson, 2006). This phenotypic association is a major indication of a common genetic background between the two disorders. Furthermore, a recent study investigating the genetic correlation among neuropsychiatric and neurological disease based on GWAS results for each disorder, also recovered a genetic correlation between TS and ADHD (Anttila et al., 2016).

This is the first study to attempt to identify a shared genetic component between TS and ADHD. We used summary statistics from the latest large-scale genomic efforts to unravel the genetic background of TS and ADHD and derived the combined effects of shared polymorphisms between the two datasets, highlighting genes and pathways that may play a role in the shared etiology between the two disorders.

2. MATERIALS AND METHODS

2.1. Data Sources

For our study we focused on the combination of the known effects of SNPs on the phenotypes of TS and ADHD.

Scharf et al in their study (Scharf et al., 2013) performed a GWAS and meta-analysis on a total of 1285 cases and 4964 ancestry-matched controls of European ancestry, genotyped on 484,295 SNPs. The dataset was analyzed in three split cohorts and was subsequently meta-analyzed. The study reported 552 SNPs associated with TS that acquired a $p < 10^{-3}$.

We acquired the ADHD meta-GWAS whole-genome summary statistics from the study conducted by the ADHD subgroup of the Psychiatric GWAS consortium (Neale et al., 2010b; Cross-Disorder Group of the Psychiatric Genomics Consortium, 2013). The total sample size consisted of 896 cases, 2455 controls and 2064 trios genotyped and then imputed to 1,230,536 SNPs.

We used the publically available top SNPs with a $p < 10^{-3}$ associated with TS (Scharf et al., 2013) and meta-analyzed them with the results of the ADHD meta-analysis (Neale et al., 2010b; Cross-Disorder Group of the Psychiatric Genomics Consortium, 2013). We identified 489 SNPs that were overlapping between the two sources to proceed with the meta-analysis.

2.2. Meta-Analytical Procedure

We combined the effects of the SNPs in each phenotype, following a meta-analytic approach, assuming a fixed-effects model, using the Z-Scores as the effect and the number of cases in each study as the weight. The heterogeneity of each analyzed SNP was assessed using Cochran's Q-test and I^2 statistic. The analysis was performed using the METAL (Willer et al., 2010) software. The significance threshold was set using the Bonferroni correction for multiple testing.

2.3. Annotation and Functional Significance

We proceeded to analyze the significant SNPs using the ENSEMBL Variant Effect Predictor (McLaren et al., 2010) to annotate and explore the possible functional characteristics of the associated variants. The genomic positions of the variants were converted to the GRCh38 assembly coordinates. For the investigation of the allelic frequencies, and the linkage disequilibrium (LD) patterns we used data from the 1000Genomes project (1000 Genomes Project Consortium et al., 2015) and the LDlink software (Machiela and Chanock, 2014). To investigate the association of the variants and their respective genes with tissue expression levels we used the GTEx portal (The GTEx Consortium, 2013) and the Expression Atlas database (Petryszak et al., 2014). The annotation and exploration of the genomic structure of the identified loci was further assisted by the use of LdOOKUP, developed by Shaun Purcell (https://purces04.u.hpc.mssm.edu/ldookup/ldookup.cgi).

We have uploaded all codes necessary to confirm our conclusions and they can be found at https://github.com/ftsetsos/tsadhdmeta2016.

3. RESULTS

The meta-analysis produced 19 significant SNPs, out of the total 489 tested. The significance threshold was set using the Bonferroni correction for multiple testing, setting the significance level at a p-value of 0.0001022.

Of these 19 SNPs, five attained the lowest p-values, coupled with no evidence of confounding heterogeneity ($I^2 = 0$). The tested SNPs that present the most significant heterogeneity (Het $p < 0.05$) were the ones that had achieved a $p < 0.05$ in the original ADHD meta-analysis. The annotation showed that the majority of the significant variants are located in introns, two are in regulatory regions, while three are intergenic.

The first and third top hits (rs1866863, *p*:3.23E-07 and rs2458304, *p*:2.54E-06) reside on a LD-block of 54.19 kb on the 6p24.1 region. They show significant linkage disequilibrium between them (*D*′: 0.909, R^2: 0.725). The former is a variant located in the regulatory region downstream of the TBC1D7 gene, and the latter is an intron variant in the same gene. Both are in LD with the rs499818 eQTL (R^2: 0.59 and 0.48 respectively), suggesting an interplay with the expression levels of the gene.

Chromosome 4 hosts the second (rs2705462, *p*:1.44E-06), the fourth (rs17561798, *p*:9.89E-06), and two lower-ranked variants(rs477897, *p*:8.65E-05 and rs2285084, *p*:1.00E-04), each residing in four distinct, LD-independent loci. The most significant variant, rs2705462, is located in the intergenic region upstream of the GUCY1A3 gene in the 4q32.1 region on a LD-block of 46.63 kb. The next variant, rs17561798, resides in the 4q23 region and is an intron variant inside the RAP1GDS1 gene. The variant rs477897 is located within an intron of ADD1 in the region 4p16.3 captures an area of 125.59 kb, implicating the genes H3BP2, ADD1, MFSD10, NOP14. The intron variant rs2285084 is located in the gene ANXA10. The gene is included in the locus 4q32.3 in a high LD region of 330.00 kb that contains also the genes ANXA10, DDX60, DDX60L.

The fifth most significant SNP, rs1650137 (*p*:1.76E-05), is located on 12q23.3 in an intron of the gene CHST11. This region is inside a LD-block that extends for 39.68 kb. The variant rs2246417 came up as the sixth most significant (*p*:1.95E-05), residing in the locus 21q22.3 in a LD-block of 16.29 kb, within an intron of the LINC00316 gene.

The variant rs11716445 (*p*: 8.01E-05) resides in the 3p21.31 region. This region is characterized by a very large area with an extended high-LD block of 1941.64 kb and it contains 70 genes, with the first genes being PLXNB1, CCDC51, TMA7, ATRIP, TREX1, and ending with HYAL2, TUSC2, RASSF1, ZMYND10, NPRL2. The variant itself is located in the intron of the RHOA gene. It is one of the lower-ranked variants that achieved minimal confounding by heterogeneity.

The locus 7p21.3 hosts the intergenic variants rs13244651 (*p*:4.11E-05) and rs17531553 (*p*:7.08E-05) that are part of a LD-block sized at 103.93 kb, albeit with no known genes close to them, and no strong suggestive results for any direct functional implication.

Two genomic regions on chromosome 9 are implicated by our results. A region of 58.16 kb in the 9p24.2 locus contains the variants rs1007021 (*p*: 4.38E-05) and rs1007022 (*p*:7.68E-05) in the introns of KCNV2, showing strong LD between them (*D*′: 1.000 R^2:0.803). The region 9q31.1 contains the intergenic variant rs7858600 (*p*:5.30E-05) inside a region of 27.35 kb.

In the locus 10q21.1, the intergenic variant rs1896373 (*p*:7.46E-05) captures a region of 47.58 kb, in strong LD with the rs1919459 eQTL (R^2: 0.97) that is associated with the regulation of DKK1. The variant rs4789936 (*p*:8.92E-05) is located in the 17q25.3 locsus, in a LD-region 34.19 kb, and is an intron variant of the gene TIMP2 while on it is non-coding exon variant in the gene CEP295NL. In the locus 16q12.1, the variant rs7203818 (*p*:1.01E-04) resides in a LD-block of 21.12 kb within an intron of ZNF423.

On chromosome 13, the LD-associated variants rs7336083 and rs9319159 (*D*′: 0.974 R^2: 0.897) represent an LD-block of 292.34 kb and reside in the introns of the LINC00351 gene. The result is mostly driven by the *p*-value attained in the TS meta-analysis and there is evidence of significant confounding caused by heterogeneity.

We summarize the results of the meta-analysis on **Table 1**. In **Table 2**, we provide the annotation we generated for each significant variant, and in **Table 3** we provide the LD regions associated with the variants. The full results of the meta-analysis on the 489 tested SNPs are described in more detail in the Supplementary Material.

4. DISCUSSION

This is the first study to identify shared genetic factors underlying TS and ADHD, two closely related and often co-occurring neuropsychiatric disorders (Karagiannidis et al., 2016). We meta-analyzed 489 of the top hit SNPs in the first TS GWAS, that had also been tested in ADHD published GWASs and meta-analysis. Our own meta-analysis highlights genes that may play a role in the shared etiology between TS and ADHD. 19 SNPs attained in the meta-analysis a *p*-value lower than the significance threshold, as denoted by the Bonferroni correction approach for multiple testing. All significant SNPs had the same direction of effect, which is indicative of a shared mechanism of disease development. A minority of those had not presented any association with ADHD in the original ADHD meta-analysis, with the resulting combined *p*-value being driven mostly by the *p*-value acquired from the TS study.

The five most significant SNPs had achieved moderate association *p*-values in the original ADHD study, and thus attained high *p*-values with no heterogeneity-based confounding in our meta-analysis, becoming strong candidates for the shared genomic background of the disorders.

TBC1D7 (TBC1 Domain Family, Member 7) is a prominent gene in our results, with two variants achieving the top and the third best *p*-values in our study. The top scoring SNP is located in a regulatory region downstream of the gene, while the third top is located within an intron of the gene. The associated variants have demonstrated linkage disequilibrium with a known eQTL for the expression of the gene, further substantiating their implication into the regulation of the expression profile of the gene. Expression profiling in Expression Atlas and GTEx show significant overexpression in the brain, the heart, the testis and in blood cells. The product of the gene is the third subunit of the TSC1-TSC2 complex with a Rheb-GAP activity, and is ubiquitously present in the complex (Dibble et al., 2012). An eQTL for TBC1D7 has been significantly associated with migraine and migraine without aura in a study of 23,285 individuals with migraine and 95,425 population-matched

TABLE 1 | Significant results of the meta-analysis.

SNP	Chromosome	Position	Allele	TS	ADHD	Meta	Direction	I^2	Het *P*-value
rs1866863	6	13336583	A	6.09E-04	1.51E-04	3.23E-07	–	0	0.9916
rs2705462	4	155648650	T	8.30E-04	5.09E-04	1.44E-06	–	0	0.875
rs2458304	6	13323663	A	3.74E-04	1.77E-03	2.54E-06	–	0	0.5818
rs17561798	4	98314790	A	3.80E-04	6.01E-03	9.89E-06	–	0	0.4226
rs1650137	12	104586532	A	4.01E-04	9.58E-03	1.76E-05	++	0	0.3702
rs2246417	21	45339588	T	2.54E-04	1.42E-02	1.95E-05	++	13.7	0.2816
rs9319159	13	85445305	T	1.15E-05	1.11E-01	3.77E-05	–	79.2	0.02837
rs13244651	7	10308596	T	5.03E-05	6.18E-02	4.11E-05	++	67.8	0.07797
rs1007021	9	2723657	A	5.36E-05	6.26E-02	4.38E-05	++	67.5	0.07919
rs7858600	9	102764080	A	2.26E-04	3.42E-02	5.30E-05	++	42.8	0.1859
rs7336083	13	85429252	A	9.49E-06	1.71E-01	6.88E-05	–	82.3	0.01756
rs17531553	7	10311703	A	9.40E-05	6.73E-02	7.08E-05	++	64.5	0.09348
rs1896373	10	52334599	T	3.46E-04	3.50E-02	7.46E-05	++	35.8	0.2121
rs1007022	9	2723761	A	8.85E-05	7.33E-02	7.68E-05	++	66	0.08647
rs11716445	3	49368662	A	7.95E-04	2.22E-02	8.01E-05	++	0	0.336
rs477897	4	168177763	A	3.10E-04	4.19E-02	8.65E-05	++	42.5	0.1874
rs4789936	17	78901892	T	7.12E-04	2.61E-02	8.92E-05	–	5.1	0.3047
rs2285084	4	2904558	A	8.07E-04	2.66E-02	1.00E-04	–	1	0.3149
rs7203818	16	49610387	A	4.03E-04	4.09E-02	1.01E-04	++	37.1	0.2075

Here we report the p-values attained in each study, the combined p-value after the meta-analysis and the direction of the effect. Alongside these statistics, we also present Cochran's I^2 value and the heterogeneity p-value for each SNP.

TABLE 2 | Functional annotation of the significant SNPs of the meta-analysis.

SNP	Chromosome	Position	*P*-value	Gene	Impact	Global Freq	EUR Freq
rs1866863	6	13336583	3.23E-07	TBC1D7	Regulatory region	A:0.4583	G:0.3907
rs2705462	4	155648650	1.44E-06	GUCY1A3	Intergenic	T:0.2041	T:0.2893
rs2458304	6	13323663	2.54E-06	TBC1D7	Intron	A:0.4287	G:0.3598
rs17561798	4	98314790	9.89E-06	RAP1GDS1	Intron	G:0.0110	G:0.0398
rs1650137	12	104586532	1.76E-05	CHST11	Intron	A:0.2911	A:0.2038
rs2246417	21	45339588	1.95E-05	LINC00316	Intron	C:0.2428	C:0.1461
rs9319159	13	85445305	3.77E-05	LINC00351	Intron	T:0.3259	T:0.3797
rs13244651	7	10308596	4.11E-05	Intergenic	Intergenic	G:0.3724	G:0.4066
rs1007021	9	2723657	4.38E-05	KCNV2	Intron	A:0.1388	A:0.0696
rs7858600	9	102764080	5.30E-05	Intergenic	Intergenic	G:0.3694	A:0.4861
rs7336083	13	85429252	6.88E-05	LINC00351	Intron	A:0.3311	A:0.3668
rs17531553	7	10311703	7.08E-05	Intergenic	Intergenic	G:0.3746	G:0.4066
rs1896373	10	52334599	7.46E-05	Intergenic	Regulatory region	T:0.4994	T:0.4513
rs1007022	9	2723761	7.68E-05	KCNV2	Intron	A:0.0649	A:0.0567
rs11716445	3	49368662	8.01E-05	RHOA	Intron	A:0.03115	A:0.1024
rs477897	4	168177763	8.65E-05	ANXA10	Intron	G:0.1148	G:0.2256
rs4789936	17	78901892	8.92E-05	CEP295NL	Intron	T:0.4407	T:0.5219
rs2285084	4	2904558	1.00E-04	ADD1	Intron	G:0.2414	G:0.2087
rs7203818	16	49610387	1.01E-04	ZNF423	Intron	A:0.2169	A:0.1581

Here we present the genes in which the SNPs are located, along with the frequency of the alleles in global and european populations, according to 1000 Genomes.

controls (Anttila et al., 2013). Interestingly, Anttila et al (Anttila et al., 2016) also picked up a genetic correlation between TS and migraine.

The presence of TBC1D7 in the TSC1/2 complex creates a suggestive functional link between the proteins. The role of the TSC1/2 complex is indicative of TBC1D7's role in the brain and neuropsychiatric disease, as an important component of the active complex. The TSC1 (Tuberous Sclerosis 1) and TSC2 (Tuberous Sclerosis 2) genes have an important role in the aetiology of Tuberous Sclerosis Complex (TSC).

TABLE 3 | LD-regions that are captured by the top SNPs in our study.

SNP	Chromosome	Region	Length (kb)	Gene(s)	eQTL
rs11716445	3	48446237..50387873	1941.64	PLXNB1;...NPRL2	–
rs2705462	4	156557255..156603882	46.63	GUCY1A3	–
rs477897	4	168980017..169310018	330.00	ANXA10; DDX60; DDX60L	–
rs2285084	4	2836195..2961783	125.59	SH3BP2; ADD1; MFSD10; NOP14	–
rs1866863	6	13298395..13352581	54.19	TBC1D7	1.7e-10 (rs499818)
rs17531553	7	10255806..10359733	103.93	–	–
rs7858600	9	105517266..105544614	27.35	–	–
rs1007021	9	2699874..2758034	58.16	KCNV2	–
rs1896373	10	54068904..54116478	47.58	DKK1	2.18e-05 (rs1919459)
rs1650137	12	104977289..105016971	39.68	CHST11	–
rs7336083	13	85893863..86186202	292.34	–	–
rs7203818	16	49637407..49658524	21.12	ZNF423	–
rs4789936	17	76894415..76928600	34.19	TIMP2; LOC100653515	–
rs2246417	21	46744358..46760648	16.29	–	–

Regions that are in linkage disequilibrium with the top SNPs, along with the range of genes residing in those regions and any linked known eQTLs. Genomic coordinates are in reference to the GRCh37 assembly.

TSC is a neurodevelopmental disorder that typically presents with tumours of the brain, skin, heart, lungs, and kidneys, but also neurological disorders such as epilepsy, cognitive disability and autism. The TSC1/2 complex acts as an inhibitor of the mechanistic target of rapamycin (mTOR) signaling pathway which plays a central role in cell growth, proliferation, autophagy and thus also neurodevelopment (Henske et al., 2016). The TSC pathway regulates neuronal structure and function, and is sensitive to gene-dosage effects, showing degrees of haploinsufficiency (Tavazoie et al., 2005). TSC1 has also been implicated in bipolar disorder, without attaining genome-wide significance (Scott et al., 2009). Furthermore, TSC1 has been shown to have a neuroprotective role in hippocampal regions of the brain, protecting against ischemic events (Papadakis et al., 2013).

RAP1GDS1 (RAP1, GTP-GDP dissociation stimulator 1) is a GDP/GTP exchange protein with GTPase activity (Riess et al., 1993). It is located on chromosome 4 and is the third top locus to be implicated in the shared genetic background, with the associated variant residing in the intron of the gene. It is significantly overexpressed in brain and nervous tissues. RAP1GDS1 has been shown to interact with RHO (Ras homolog gene family, member A), that has also been implicated in this study, in a cascade involving interactions with multiple signaling proteins (Vikis et al., 2002; Berg et al., 2010; Hamel et al., 2011). CHST11 (carbohydrate chondroitin 4 sulfotransferase 11) is involved in the sulfation of chondroitin (Klppel, 2010), which is a key element of the brain matrix (Kwok et al., 2012). It is expressed in areas of the brain, including the hippocampus and the caudate nucleus. GUCY1A3 (Guanylate cyclase soluble subunit alpha-3) functions as the main receptor for nitric oxide, and has been implicated in Moyamoya disease, a disease causing constriction in arteries and brain ischemic events (Wallace et al., 2016).

5. CONCLUSION

We investigate, for the first time, the common genetic background between TS and ADHD on a genomewide scale and provide evidence that specific genes may underlie both disorders. The implicated variants lie on genes that appear to have a complex interplay between them. The main theme of the results is the Ras signaling cascade in the brain, with TBC1D7 and RAP1GDS1 being key elements of the brain signaling pathways. Interestingly, an additional theme emerging from the data, is related to brain ischemic response, with GUCY1A3 and the TSC1/2 complex (which includes TBC1D7) as implicated as factors. Intriguingly, one of our top hits, TBC1D7, implicates the mTOR signaling pathway and autophagy processes (Dibble et al., 2012). Furthermore, our analysis also points to CHST11, which has been shown to regulate the brain extracellular matrix, by affecting the chondroitin sulfation levels. Therefore, further investigation in the role of the respective genes in the shared genetic aetiology of TS and ADHD is warranted. Our results provide an intriguing insight into the shared mechanism of common neuropsychiatric disorders.

AUTHOR CONTRIBUTIONS

FT, SP, JA, IK, MT, AT, DM, MG, PD performed data analysis and interpretation, and participated in manuscript writing. PP designed and supervised the study, performed data analysis and interpretation, and participated in manuscript writing. All authors read and approved the final version to be published and agreed to be accountable for all aspects of the work.

FUNDING

This study was supported by the TS-EUROTRAIN and the EMTICS projects, funded by the European Union under the Seventh Framework People Programme (TS-EUROTRAIN, FP7-PEOPLE-2012-ITN, Grant Agr.No.316978 EMTICS, FP7-HEALTH, Grant Agr.No. 278367).

ACKNOWLEDGMENTS

We would like to thank the Psychiatric Genetics Consortium, the Tourette Syndrome Association International Consortium for Genetics and the TS/OCD working group of the Psychiatric Genetics Consortium.

SUPPLEMENTARY MATERIAL

The Supplementary Material for this article can be found online at: http://journal.frontiersin.org/article/10.3389/fnins.2016.00340

REFERENCES

1000 Genomes Project Consortium, Auton, A., Brooks, L. D., Durbin, R. M., Garrison, E. P., Kang, H. M., et al. (2015). A global reference for human genetic variation. *Nature* 526, 68–74. doi: 10.1038/nature15393

Anttila, V., Bulik-Sullivan, B., Finucane, H. K., Bras, J., Duncan, L., Escott-Price, V., et al. (2016). Analysis of shared heritability in common disorders of the brain. *bioRxiv*. doi: 10.1101/048991. [Epub ahead of print].

Anttila, V., Winsvold, B. S., Gormley, P., Kurth, T., Bettella, F., McMahon, G., et al. (2013). Genome-wide meta-analysis identifies new susceptibility loci for migraine. *Nat. Genet.* 45, 912–917. doi: 10.1038/ng.2676

Berg, T. J., Gastonguay, A. J., Lorimer, E. L., Kuhnmuench, J. R., Li, R., Fields, A. P., et al. (2010). Splice variants of SmgGDS control small gtpase prenylation and membrane localization. *J. Biol. Chem.* 285, 35255–35266. doi: 10.1074/jbc.M110.129916

Cross-Disorder Group of the Psychiatric Genomics Consortium (2013). Identification of risk loci with shared effects on five major psychiatric disorders: a genome-wide analysis. *Lancet* 381, 1371–1379. doi: 10.1016/S0140-6736(12)62129-1

Dibble, C. C., Elis, W., Menon, S., Qin, W., Klekota, J., Asara, J. M., et al. (2012). TBC1D7 is a third subunit of the TSC1-TSC2 complex upstream of mTORC1. *Mol. Cell* 47, 535–546. doi: 10.1016/j.molcel.2012.06.009

Hamel, B., Monaghan-Benson, E., Rojas, R. J., Temple, B. R. S., Marston, D. J., Burridge, K., et al. (2011). SmgGDS is a guanine nucleotide exchange factor that specifically activates RhoA and RhoC. *J. Biol. Chem.* 286, 12141–12148. doi: 10.1074/jbc.M110.191122

Henske, E. P., Jóźwiak, S., Kingswood, J. C., Sampson, J. R., and Thiele, E. A. (2016). Tuberous sclerosis complex. *Nat. Rev. Dis. Primers* 2:16035. doi: 10.1038/nrdp.2016.35

Karagiannidis, I., Tsetsos, F., Padmanabhuni, S. S., Alexander, J., Georgitsi, M., and Paschou, P. (2016). The genetics of Gilles de la Tourette syndrome: a common aetiological basis with comorbid disorders? *Curr. Behav. Neurosci. Rep.* 1–14. doi: 10.1007/s40473-016-0088-z

Klppel, M. (2010). The roles of chondroitin-4-sulfotransferase-1 in development and disease. *Prog. Mol. Biol. Transl. Sci.* 93, 113–132. doi: 10.1016/S1877-1173(10)93006-8

Kwok, J. C. F., Warren, P., and Fawcett, J. W. (2012). Chondroitin sulfate: a key molecule in the brain matrix. *Int. J. Biochem. Cell Biol.* 44, 582–586. doi: 10.1016/j.biocel.2012.01.004

Lesch, K. P., Timmesfeld, N., Renner, T. J., Halperin, R., Röser, C., Nguyen, T. T., et al. (2008). Molecular genetics of adult ADHD: converging evidence from genome-wide association and extended pedigree linkage studies. *J. Neural Transm.* 115, 1573–1585. doi: 10.1007/s00702-008-0119-3

Machiela, M. J., and Chanock, S. J. (2014). LDlink: a web-based application for exploring population-specific haplotype structure and linking correlated alleles of possible functional variants. *Bioinformatics* 31, 3555–3557. doi: 10.1093/bioinformatics/btv402

McLaren, W., Pritchard, B., Rios, D., Chen, Y., Flicek, P., and Cunningham, F. (2010). Deriving the consequences of genomic variants with the Ensembl API and SNP Effect Predictor. *Bioinformatics* 26, 2069–2070. doi: 10.1093/bioinformatics/btq330

Mick, E., Todorov, A., Smalley, S., Hu, X., Loo, S., Todd, R. D., et al. (2010). Family-based genome-wide association scan of attention-deficit/hyperactivity disorder. *J. Am. Acad. Child Adolesc. Psychiatry* 49, 898-905.e3. doi: 10.1016/j.jaac.2010.02.014

Neale, B. M., Lasky-Su, J., Anney, R., Franke, B., Zhou, K., Maller, J. B., et al. (2008). Genome-wide association scan of attention deficit hyperactivity disorder. *Am. J. Med. Genet. B Neuropsychiatr. Genet.* 147B, 1337–1344. doi: 10.1002/ajmg.b.30866

Neale, B. M., Medland, S., Ripke, S., Anney, R. J. L., Asherson, P., Buitelaar, J., et al. (2010a). Case-control genome-wide association study of attention-deficit/hyperactivity disorder. *J. Am. Acad. Child Adolesc. Psychiatry* 49, 906–920. doi: 10.1016/j.jaac.2010.06.007

Neale, B. M., Medland, S. E., Ripke, S., Asherson, P., Franke, B., Lesch, K.-P., et al. (2010b). Meta-analysis of genome-wide association studies of attention-deficit/hyperactivity disorder. *J. Am. Acad. Child Adolesc. Psychiatry* 49, 884–897. doi: 10.1016/j.jaac.2010.06.008

Papadakis, M., Hadley, G., Xilouri, M., Hoyte, L. C., Nagel, S., McMenamin, M. M., et al. (2013). Tsc1 (hamartin) confers neuroprotection against ischemia by inducing autophagy. *Nat. Med.* 19, 351–357. doi: 10.1038/nm.3097

Paschou, P., Yu, D., Gerber, G., Evans, P., Tsetsos, F., Davis, L. K., et al. (2014). Genetic association signal near NTN4 in Tourette syndrome. *Ann. Neurol.* 76, 310–315. doi: 10.1002/ana.24215

Petryszak, R., Burdett, T., Fiorelli, B., Fonseca, N. A., Gonzalez-Porta, M., Hastings, E., et al. (2014). Expression Atlas update - A database of gene and transcript expression from microarray- and sequencing-based functional genomics experiments. *Nucleic Acids Res.* 42, D926–D932. doi: 10.1093/nar/gkt1270

Riess, O., Epplen, C., Siedlaczck, I., and Epplen, J. T. (1993). Chromosomal assignment of the human smg GDP dissociation stimulator gene to human chromosome 4q21-q25. *Hum. Genet.* 92, 629–630. doi: 10.1007/BF00420952

Robertson, M. M. (2006). Attention deficit hyperactivity disorder, tics and Tourette's syndrome: the relationship and treatment implications. A commentary. *Eur. Child Adolesc. Psychiatry* 15, 1–11. doi: 10.1007/s00787-006-0505-z

Robertson, M. M., Cavanna, A. E., and Eapen, V. (2015). Gilles de la Tourette syndrome and disruptive behavior disorders: prevalence, associations, and explanation of the relationships. *J. Neuropsychiatry Clin. Neurosci.* 27, 33–41. doi: 10.1176/appi.neuropsych.13050112

Robertson, M. M., Eapen, V., and Cavanna, A. E. (2009). The international prevalence, epidemiology, and clinical phenomenology of Tourette syndrome: a cross-cultural perspective. *J. Psychosom. Res.* 67, 475–483. doi: 10.1016/j.jpsychores.2009.07.010

Scharf, J. M., Miller, L. L., Gauvin, C. A., Alabiso, J., Mathews, C. A., and Ben-Shlomo, Y. (2015). Population prevalence of Tourette syndrome: a systematic review and meta-analysis. *Mov. Disord.* 30, 221–228. doi: 10.1002/mds.26089

Scharf, J. M., Yu, D., Mathews, C. A., Neale, B. M., Stewart, S. E., Fagerness, J. A., et al. (2013). Genome-wide association study of Tourette's syndrome. *Mol. Psychiatry* 18, 721–728. doi: 10.1038/mp.2012.69

Scott, L. J., Muglia, P., Kong, X. Q., Guan, W., Flickinger, M., Upmanyu, R., et al. (2009). Genome-wide association and meta-analysis of bipolar disorder in individuals of European ancestry. *Proc. Natl. Acad. Sci. U.S.A.* 106, 7501–7506. doi: 10.1073/pnas.0813386106

Tavazoie, S. F., Alvarez, V. A., Ridenour, D. A., Kwiatkowski, D. J., and Sabatini, B. L. (2005). Regulation of neuronal morphology and function by the tumor suppressors Tsc1 and Tsc2. *Nat. Neurosci.* 8, 1727–1734. doi: 10.1038/nn1566

The GTEx Consortium (2013). The Genotype-Tissue Expression (GTEx) project. *Nat. Genet.* 45, 580–585. doi: 10.1038/ng.2653

Vikis, H. G., Stewart, S., and Guan, K.-L. (2002). SmgGDS displays differential binding and exchange activity towards different Ras isoforms. *Oncogene* 21, 2425–2432. doi: 10.1038/sj.onc.1205306

Wallace, S., Guo, D.-C., Regalado, E., Mellor-Crummey, L., Bamshad, M., Nickerson, D. A., et al. (2016). Disrupted nitric oxide signaling due to GUCY1A3 mutations increases risk for moyamoya disease, achalasia and hypertension. *Clin. Genet.* doi: 10.1111/cge.12739. [Epub ahead of print].

Willer, C. J., Li, Y., and Abecasis, G. R. (2010). METAL: fast and efficient meta-analysis of genomewide association scans. *Bioinformatics* 26, 2190–2191. doi: 10.1093/bioinformatics/btq340

19

The Fallacy of Univariate Solutions to Complex Systems Problems

Christina N. Lessov-Schlaggar[1]*, *Joshua B. Rubin*[2,3] *and Bradley L. Schlaggar*[1,2,3,4,5]

[1] Department of Psychiatry, Washington University School of Medicine, St. Louis, MO, USA, [2] Department of Neurology, Washington University School of Medicine, St. Louis, MO, USA, [3] Department of Pediatrics, Washington University School of Medicine, St. Louis, MO, USA, [4] Department of Radiology, Washington University School of Medicine, St. Louis, MO, USA, [5] Department of Neuroscience, Washington University School of Medicine, St. Louis, MO, USA

Edited by:
Peristera Paschou,
Democritus University of Thrace,
Greece

Reviewed by:
Ahmad Seif Kanaan,
Max Planck Institute/Hannover
Medical School, Germany
Siyan Fan,
Vrije Universiteit (VU), Amsterdam,
Netherlands

***Correspondence:**
Christina N. Lessov-Schlaggar
schlaggc@psychiatry.wustl.edu

Complex biological systems, by definition, are composed of multiple components that interact non-linearly. The human brain constitutes, arguably, the most complex biological system known. Yet most investigation of the brain and its function is carried out using assumptions appropriate for simple systems—univariate design and linear statistical approaches. This heuristic must change before we can hope to discover and test interventions to improve the lives of individuals with complex disorders of brain development and function. Indeed, a movement away from simplistic models of biological systems will benefit essentially all domains of biology and medicine. The present brief essay lays the foundation for this argument.

Keywords: Tourette syndrome, neuropsychiatric illness, cancer, fMRI, developmental cognitive neuroscience

INTRODUCTION

Non-invasive neuroimaging has invigorated a deep and abiding interest in understanding the human brain, the most complex biological system, in health and disease. This burgeoning research focus has impelled technological innovation in neuroimaging and application of a growing number of mathematical/computational approaches to analysis, which help visualize the complexity of the brain in greater depth than previously possible. From our current vantage point we are compelled to ask whether our capabilities have outstripped the paradigms we use for scientific research, and whether our conceptual and analytical frameworks have become a barrier to understanding complex systems.

A deep understanding of complex biological systems requires conceptual and analytical strategies that respect that complexity. Yet, there continues to be a dominating focus in experimental design and analysis on univariate, linear, and narrowly defined relationships. These approaches, including multivariate linear regression (which is an elaboration on the univariate linear framework), are gratifying because they are conceptually simple and align neatly with the traditional scientific method, in which emphasis is placed on a single isolatable dependent variable. However, the univariate/linear approach will necessarily fail when tasked with providing the basis for deep explanations for complex biological systems.

This essay highlights the need to recognize the fallacy of the univariate conceptual framework with respect to complex systems and to embrace complexity so as to align the problem to be solved with the approach taken. We contend that there are some effective ways to study complex systems through care in study design and sample ascertainment, deep phenotyping, and statistical approaches. However, the shift to individual-level analysis, the basis for personalized medicine, will require both methodological advances and a readiness for investigators and reviewers to eschew biologically implausible reductionist models of complex biology.

ARGUMENTATION

Study Design and Sample Ascertainment

Standard clinical trial design emphasizes a univariate conceptual framework—as the Consolidated Standards of Reporting Trials approach argues (Moher et al., 2001), if randomization is done correctly, the only difference between a treatment and control group is the treatment itself. Then, results are framed to reflect the central tendency of the two groups and whether that central tendency differs for the defined primary outcome. However, the central tendency of a treated group does not necessarily inform the clinician whether the patient currently in the exam room and seeking help is (or is not) likely to respond to the offered therapy, particularly if the patient would not have met study inclusion criteria.

Why would the patient have not been offered entry into the study? Because the study design, inspired by univariate approaches to complex problems, mandates inclusion/exclusion criteria that reduce variability and remove potentially confounding factors, which necessarily makes the study less generalizable to the broader population. Further, it undermines the ability, using study data, to make predictions about treatment response for individual patients. Such single patient/subject level prediction, it seems to us, should be a fundamental and significant priority of clinical trials. Yet, quantifying and characterizing the central tendency at the group level appear to be the principal objectives.

Similarly, a commonly employed study design in cognitive neuroscience is between-group comparison of cases and controls. For some of the authors, case status might comprise tobacco-dependent cigarette smokers or patients with Tourette syndrome (TS), a neurodevelopmental disorder defined by the chronic presence of motor and vocal tics. Controls, by definition, would include non-smokers or individuals without TS, respectively. Comparing cases and controls on brain outcomes would almost certainly uncover group differences (Azizian et al., 2009; Rickards, 2009; Eichele and Plessen, 2013; Fedota and Stein, 2015). However, group differences cannot be ascribed to case/control status alone: both tobacco dependence and TS are complex disorders that do not exist simply on the background of an otherwise typically developed, neuropsychiatrically healthy individual. Tobacco dependent smokers, relative to non-smokers are more likely to abuse other substances (Madden and Heath, 2002; John et al., 2003; Agrawal et al., 2012), to have history of mood or behavioral problems (Grant et al., 2004; Smith et al., 2014), to experience worse socioeconomic indicators, and to have family history of substance use and psychopathology (Lessov et al., 2004; Lawrence et al., 2007; Buu et al., 2009; Xian et al., 2010; CDC, 2011; Zoloto et al., 2012). TS patients, compared to non-TS patients, are more likely to suffer from anxiety and mood disorders, obsessive compulsive disorder (OCD), attention deficit hyperactivity disorder (ADHD), sleep disorders, learning disability, and to have family history of such problems (Mathews and Grados, 2011; O'Rourke et al., 2011; Martino et al., 2013; Mol Debes, 2013; Ghosh et al., 2014; Eysturoy et al., 2015; Hirschtritt et al., 2015). In addition, case status may be but one manifestation that is overt at the moment of investigation. For example, a tobacco dependent adolescent's mood disorder may be subclinical at the time of investigation but emerge later. Or a 2nd grader with a persistent tic disorder may not manifest OCD clinically until middle school. The later emergence of those clinical manifestations belies an earlier determination that the individual is truly free of those clinical burdens. In monogenic genetic disorders, such as Rett Syndrome and CDKL5 epileptic encephalopathy, some individuals with the classic mutation do not necessarily manifest the phenotype (Amir et al., 2000) or may have distinctly different developmental trajectories (Hagebeuk et al., 2015) despite having identical mutations.

Care in sample ascertainment can minimize group differences. One epidemiologically sound approach is to recruit cases and controls from the same demographic area to match socioeconomic characteristics. An alternative approach is to collect sufficient information during screening of potential study participants to identify cases and controls that are matched/similar on background characteristics and to invite the matched subset of participants into the study. One caveat in matching unrelated cases and controls is that individuals who can be matched may represent the tail end of their respective distribution. For example, dependent smokers who can be matched to non-smokers likely do not have burden from known comorbidities and may not be representative of the average dependent smoker; conversely, non-smokers who can be matched to smokers may have greater psychiatric history than the average non-smoker. Another robust approach is to use control individuals who are related to the cases, such as twin or full siblings, to match more closely on genetics, family environment, and other shared history (Lessov-Schlaggar et al., 2013).

In clinical trials, whether random assignment to treatment or control conditions achieves its intended balance is commonly not tested. The commonly employed stringent inclusion criteria that effectively homogenize the study sample likely contribute to the sense of balance in group differences. For example, suppose treatment and control groups are matched on sex (equal numbers of males and females in each group), and socioeconomic status (SES) (equal numbers from low and high SES in each group). On the surface, it would seem that as a consequence of this matching strategy, sex or SES, individually, could not be driving a treatment effect. However, it remains plausible that a sex by SES interaction is lurking such that for the treatment group, 70% of females come from a high SES environment while for the control group, 30% of females come from a high SES environment. Thus, a treatment effect could be driven by a sex by SES interaction that is misattributed. Vigilance in sample ascertainment shows respect for the complexity of human behavior and the neurobiological mechanisms that generate it.

Deep Phenotyping

The co-occurrence of two or more problems is the rule and not the exception in pediatric neuropsychiatric illness (Arcelus and Vostanis, 2003). Comorbidity can be due to shared genetic or environmental mechanisms (Mathews and Grados, 2011; Vrieze et al., 2012), suggesting shared etiology and shared neurobiological mechanisms. For example, brain mechanisms of cognitive control (itself a complex construct) have been implicated in numerous conditions, including drug addiction and TS (Kalivas and Volkow, 2005; Mueller et al., 2006; Church et al., 2009; Garavan and Weierstall, 2012; Jung et al., 2013). Therefore, when comparing cases and controls care in the kind and amount of phenotypic data collection is also necessary. Having data on risk factors allows not only for better matching algorithms, but also for exploration of phenotypic subgroups that differ in behavioral phenomenology. For example, using multiple measures in a large family study of TS, latent class analysis identified five TS subgroups characterized by TS+OCD+ADHD, TS+OCD, TS plus obsessive compulsive behaviors, chronic tics plus OCD, and a subgroup with minimal symptomatology (Grados and Mathews, 2008). Further, only the TS+OCD+ADHD subgroup was significantly heritable (Grados and Mathews, 2008). The differential clustering of symptoms, diagnoses, and heritability estimates, suggest differences in disease etiology or similar proximate etiological mechanisms but disparate additional modifying factors. Identifying potential differences in etiology and modifying factors is paramount to the task of identifying effective therapy. If there is an assumption that all TS manifests from the same underlying cause, then it would necessarily follow—down a garden path argument—that all patients with TS should respond to the same therapy. Of course, inter-individual differences in response to therapy are obvious; such differences could be the consequence of TS as a phenocopy for different etiologies, or could be the consequence of genetic polymorphisms in drug metabolism pathways, unrelated to the etiology of TS. Approaches to understanding therapy optimization require reorienting our approach to investigation so as to determine the reasons that a given patient responds to treatment B and not treatment A.

It is important to recognize that heterogeneity is not limited to atypical populations. It may be discomforting to realize that the composition of a standard group of "healthy controls" is almost certainly heterogeneous. For example, Fair et al. (2012) applied a large neuropsychological battery to a cohort of typically developing children collected as a control sample in a study of ADHD. They then applied an unsupervised clustering algorithm to the psychometric data of each individual and identified subgroups within the cohort of healthy controls that mirrored the subgrouping identified for the ADHD cohort (Fair et al., 2012). The implications of clustering individuals into subgroups based on rich single subject data are substantial given that the standard case/control statistical analysis assumes (incorrectly, most likely) that the case and control groups are each representative of the population of cases and controls, allowing for the application of standard parametric statistics to test group differences.

In another example, using resting state functional connectivity MRI data, groups of typically developing children and children with ADHD could be separated into subgroups based on the pattern of functional connectivity of the nucleus accumbens with the rest of the brain (Costa Dias et al., 2015). Differences between controls and ADHD patients within each subgroup showed different aspects of atypical connectivity in ADHD (Costa Dias et al., 2015); the ADHD subgroup demonstrating atypical connectivity of the nucleus accumbens with attention networks also had higher impulsivity relative to respective controls and to the other ADHD subgroups (Costa Dias et al., 2015) suggesting distinct mechanism(s) that may underlie impulsivity in ADHD.

Using resting state functional connectivity MRI, Laumann and colleagues showed that collecting data from the same individual over multiple occasions achieves high level of measurement accuracy and uncovers individual-specific functional brain organization (Laumann et al., 2015). The functional organization of the individual brain shares similarity to group-level functional organization, in that functional systems are evident on the individual and group-average brain (Laumann et al., 2015). However, the functional organization of the individual brain shows a more complex landscape where adjacent cortical regions belong to two or more functional systems, and not one system as in the group-average brain, as well as differences in functional system boundaries between right and left hemispheres (Laumann et al., 2015). This level of specificity could only can be achieved using a large amount of data from the same individual (see also Poldrack et al., 2015) showing how such an approach can detect inter-individual differences that might be associated with individual differences in behavior, disease mechanism, treatment response, and so forth.

Analysis that embraces complexity provides a richer, more interesting, and likely more biologically relevant model of causal mechanisms. By liberalizing phenotypic definitions and collecting as much data per individual as possible, we will be able to better understand individual differences and to better identify deviant or rare phenotypes.

Statistical Approaches

Often, we see lack of capitalizing on good study design or deep phenotyping when it comes to statistical analysis, such as longitudinal data being analyzed cross-sectionally or comorbidity being treated as a confounding variable. Treating longitudinal data as cross-sectional does not take advantage of the overall reduction in variability and error estimation with repeat assessment of the same individuals. A small mean difference in task-evoked brain activity, as measured by fMRI, between times 1 and 2 may not be significant when analyzed cross-sectionally; however, if each subject's low amplitude response moved in the same direction, the effect could be highly statistically significant when analyzed longitudinally.

Comorbidity is often treated as nuisance variable(s). Investigations by the Tourette Syndrome Association International Consortium for Genetics demonstrate that the neuropsychiatric comorbidities of TS have very complex genetic relationships (Mathews and Grados, 2011). It is simply erroneous to consider comorbidities to superimpose linearly on the diagnosis of interest. Yet the practice of using linear regression or covariance to remove the confounding contribution of a comorbid diagnosis is predicated on such a linear relationship. Comorbidity shares variation with the phenotype of interest that affects outcome, and treating it as a nuisance variable undermines the results by statistically removing informative variation. Further, a covariate only controls for the linear relationship of that variable with outcome. It is likely the case that comorbidity is not captured by additive effects, but is the result of complex interactions of etiological mechanisms. The notion of pure insertion of a phenotype, such as OCD, onto TS, is problematic. In the neuroimaging literature, Friston et al. (1996) discussed the problem of pure insertion in the setting of cognitive subtraction, refuting the implicit assumption employed in many neuroimaging studies that "there are no interactions among the cognitive components of a task."

In the clinical setting, often the most vexing question asked by the parent of a child diagnosed with a persistent tic disorder is "what does the future hold for my child?" The ability to provide real, evidence-based, predictions for that patient and family—not a summary relevant to the central tendency of the population of individuals with persistent tics, but predictions that are specific to the patient in the office—is of paramount importance. Single patient/subject level prediction requires methodological approaches to study design and data analysis that capitalize on the richness afforded by high dimensional data and inter-individual variance, as shown in Laumann et al. (2015), for example.

Our own first efforts in this regard used resting state functional connectivity MRI and support vector machine based multivariate pattern analysis to predict, on a single subject basis, age-group membership (adult vs. child) as well as the brain maturity of single subjects (Dosenbach et al., 2010; Greene et al., 2014). We have applied similar approaches to predict whether an individual has TS or not (Greene et al., 2016). These approaches (Johnston et al., 2015; Kambeitz-Ilankovic et al., 2015; Stock et al., 2015) are orienting the field toward the importance of single subject/patient level prediction. Fair and colleagues (Miranda-Dominguez et al., 2014) introduced a highly compelling recent exemplar, "connectotyping," using resting state functional connectivity MRI, to reveal a functional "fingerprint" of an individual with substantially less data than needed for the deep characterization described in Laumann's (Laumann et al., 2015) and Poldrack's work (Poldrack et al., 2015).

One important caveat regarding multivariate pattern analysis is that, at least to our knowledge, it is not possible to perform what would be considered a standard power analysis—constructs like effect size and measurement variance do not readily translate into the n-dimensional space within which such analysis operates.

Beyond the Cognitive Neurosciences

Potential advantages of single subject, rather than group-level prediction, are important to consider in other diseases with complex phenotypes, like cancer. Driving forces for clinical trial design and conduct included, ethical considerations, statistical models and simplicity in order to ensure consistency across multiple trial sites (Meier, 1975). Missing from the driving forces for trial design is disease biology. Advances in cancer biology have significantly refined our view of causation, such that histological diagnoses are giving way to molecular subtyping within histological diagnostic groups, and patients are being stratified for therapies that target causative genetic events (Bautista et al., 2014; Robinson et al., 2015). While this approach is touted as the foundation for personalized "precision" medicine, in reality it most frequently perpetuates a monolithic view of cancer biology and therapeutic responses that is inconsistent with the state of scientific evidence in cancer biology.

As we are focused here on central nervous system disease we will limit our comments to malignant brain tumors. The combination of surgery, radiation and chemotherapy for glioblastoma, the most common and malignant of brain tumors, was first applied in the late 1940s and first studied in clinical trials in the 1960s (Gunther, 1949; Levin and Wilson, 1976; Walker and Gehan, 1976). The improvement in survival was measured in months and for the vast majority of patients this remains the benefit of therapy today (Stupp et al., 2005). Over the same period of time, our understanding of the biology of glioblastoma has advanced remarkably. The complexity of the mutational landscape has been repeatedly described (Frattini et al., 2013; van Thuijl et al., 2015). The significance of epigenetic modulation of the cancer genome to cancer biology and therapeutic resistance has been recognized (Sturm et al., 2014). The importance of multi-clonality to tumor evolution in response to treatment has been established (Kim et al., 2015), as has impact of cancer immune editing and immunological checkpoints to cancer development (Pellegatta et al., 2011). We also know that this spectrum of intra-tumoral heterogeneity in each patient must also be overlaid on the distinct biologies of males vs. females (Sun et al., 2014) and genome-wide polymorphisms that determine important phenotypic differences between individuals in such things as metabolism and circadian rhythm, which impact on disease risk, progression, and therapeutic responses.

Among the conclusions of this enormous body of research is that each glioblastoma patient has multiple genetically and epigenetically distinct clonal lineages that must be simultaneously targeted for a reasonable chance of cure. Despite this knowledge, we continue to "match" groups of patients and evaluate novel drugs one at a time, and we continue to dramatically fail to improve outcome (Bastien et al., 2015). We have neglected to recognize that the complexity of this disease demands a revolutionary change in approaches to clinical investigation in which the individual is what is being interrogated, not the group. Success may require abandoning current research paradigms and statistical frameworks in favor of models that can be informative for multiple "n's" of one.

CONCLUDING REMARKS

Classical statistics, developed before computers and technologies that can analyze and deliver millions of data points, may be inadequate for analyzing high-dimensional data sets. Inherent in the idea of personalized medicine is a translational approach, whereby basic science and clinical research data can be used together to predict with high accuracy an individual patient's clinical prognosis and treatment. Achieving personalized medicine will almost certainly require a paradigm shift toward embracing complexity and developing and funding complex systems analytics research.

AUTHOR CONTRIBUTIONS

BS co-conceived the thesis of this essay and co-authored it. CL co-conceived the thesis of this essay and co-authored it. JR co-conceived the thesis of this essay and co-authored it.

REFERENCES

Agrawal, A., Budney, A. J., and Lynskey, M. T. (2012). The co-occurring use and misuse of cannabis and tobacco: a review. *Addiction* 107, 1221–1233. doi: 10.1111/j.1360-0443.2012.03837.x

Amir, R. E., Van den Veyver, I. B., Schultz, R., Malicki, D. M., Tran, C. Q., Dahle, E. J., et al. (2000). Influence of mutation type and X chromosome inactivation on Rett syndrome phenotypes. *Ann. Neurol.* 47, 670–679. doi: 10.1002/1531-8249(200005)47:5<670::AID-ANA20>3.0.CO;2-F

Arcelus, J., and Vostanis, P. (2003). Child psychiatric disorders among primary mental health service attenders. *Br. J. Gen. Pract.* 53, 214–216.

Azizian, A., Monterosso, J., O'Neill, J., and London, E. D. (2009). "Magnetic resonance imaging studies of cigarette smoking," in *Nicotine Psychopharmacology*, eds J. E. Henningfield and E. C. S. Pogun (Berlin: Springer-Verlag), 114–138.

Bastien, J. I., McNeill, K. A., and Fine, H. A. (2015). Molecular characterizations of glioblastoma, targeted therapy, and clinical results to date. *Cancer* 121, 502–516. doi: 10.1002/cncr.28968

Bautista, F., Paci, A., Minard-Colin, V., Dufour, C., Grill, J., Lacroix, L., et al. (2014). Vemurafenib in pediatric patients with BRAFV600E mutated high-grade gliomas. *Pediatr. Blood Cancer* 61, 1101–1103. doi: 10.1002/pbc.24891

Buu, A., Dipiazza, C., Wang, J., Puttler, L. I., Fitzgerald, H. E., and Zucker, R. A. (2009). Parent, family, and neighborhood effects on the development of child substance use and other psychopathology from preschool to the start of adulthood. *J. Stud. Alcohol Drugs* 70, 489–498. doi: 10.15288/jsad.2009.70.489

CDC (2011). Vital signs: current cigarette smoking among adults aged ≥18 years–United States, 2005-2010. *MMWR Morb. Mortal. Wkly. Rep.* 60, 1207–1212.

Church, J. A., Wenger, K. K., Dosenbach, N. U., Miezin, F. M., Petersen, S. E., and Schlaggar, B. L. (2009). Task control signals in pediatric tourette syndrome show evidence of immature and anomalous functional activity. *Front. Hum. Neurosci.* 3:38. doi: 10.3389/neuro.09.038.2009

Costa Dias, T. G., Iyer, S. P., Carpenter, S. D., Cary, R. P., Wilson, V. B., Mitchell, S. H., et al. (2015). Characterizing heterogeneity in children with and without ADHD based on reward system connectivity. *Dev. Cogn. Neurosci.* 11, 155–174. doi: 10.1016/j.dcn.2014.12.005

Dosenbach, N. U., Nardos, B., Cohen, A. L., Fair, D. A., Power, J. D., Church, J. A., et al. (2010). Prediction of individual brain maturity using fMRI. *Science* 329, 1358–1361. doi: 10.1126/science.1194144

Eichele, H., and Plessen K. J. (2013). Neural plasticity in functional and anatomical MRI studies of children with Tourette syndrome. *Behav. Neurol.* 27, 33–45. doi: 10.1155/2013/376590

Eysturoy, A. N., Skov, L., and Debes, N. M. (2015). Genetic predisposition increases the tic severity, rate of comorbidities, and psychosocial and educational difficulties in children with Tourette syndrome. *J. Child Neurol.* 30, 320–325. doi: 10.1177/0883073814538668

Fair, D. A., Bathula, D., Nikolas, M. A., and Nigg, J. T. (2012). Distinct neuropsychological subgroups in typically developing youth inform heterogeneity in children with ADHD. *Proc. Natl. Acad. Sci. U.S.A.* 109, 6769–6774. doi: 10.1073/pnas.1115365109

Fedota, J. R., and Stein, E. A. (2015). Resting-state functional connectivity and nicotine addiction: prospects for biomarker development. *Ann. N. Y. Acad. Sci.* 1349, 64–82. doi: 10.1111/nyas.12882

Frattini, V., Trifonov, V., Chan, J. M., Castano, A., Lia, M., Abate, F., et al. (2013). The integrated landscape of driver genomic alterations in glioblastoma. *Nat. Genet.* 45, 1141–1149. doi: 10.1038/ng.2734

ACKNOWLEDGMENTS

We thank our colleague Nico Dosenbach for thoughtful comments on an earlier version of this manuscript.

Friston, K. J., Price, C. J., Fletcher, P., Moore, C., Frackowiak, R. S., and Dolan, R. J. (1996). The trouble with cognitive subtraction. *NeuroImage* 4, 97–104. doi: 10.1006/nimg.1996.0033

Garavan, H., and Weierstall, K. (2012). The neurobiology of reward and cognitive control systems and their role in incentivizing health behavior. *Prev. Med.* 55(Suppl.), S17–S23. doi: 10.1016/j.ypmed.2012.05.018

Ghosh, D., Rajan, P. V., Das, D., Datta, P., Rothner, A. D., and Erenberg, G. (2014). Sleep disorders in children with Tourette syndrome. *Pediatr. Neurol.* 51, 31–35. doi: 10.1016/j.pediatrneurol.2014.03.017

Grados, M. A., and Mathews, C. A. (2008). Latent class analysis of gilles de la tourette syndrome using comorbidities: clinical and genetic implications. *Biol. Psychiatry* 64, 219–225. doi: 10.1016/j.biopsych.2008.01.019

Grant, B. F., Stinson, F. S., Dawson, D. A., Chou, S. P., Dufour, M. C., Compton, W., et al. (2004). Prevalence and co-occurrence of substance use disorders and independent mood and anxiety disorders: results from the national epidemiologic survey on alcohol and related conditions. *Arch. Gen. Psychiatry* 61, 807–816. doi: 10.1001/archpsyc.61.8.807

Greene, D. J., Church, J. A., Dosenbach, N. U., Nielsen, A. N., Adeyemo, B., Nardos, B., et al. (2016). Multivariate pattern classification of pediatric Tourette syndrome using functional connectivity MRI. *Dev. Sci.* doi: 10.1111/desc.12407. [Epub ahead of print].

Greene, D. J., Laumann, T. O., Dubis, J. W., Ihnen, S. K., Neta, M., Power, J. D., et al. (2014). Developmental changes in the organization of functional connections between the basal ganglia and cerebral cortex. *J. Neurosci.* 34, 5842–5854. doi: 10.1523/JNEUROSCI.3069-13.2014

Gunther, J. (1949). *Death Be Not Proud*. New York, NY: Harper Perennial.

Hagebeuk, E. E., Marcelis, C. L., Alders, M., Kaspers, A., and de Weerd, A. W. (2015). Two siblings with a CDKL5 mutation: genotype and phenotype evaluation. *J. Child Neurol.* 30, 1515–1519. doi: 10.1177/0883073815573317

Hirschtritt, M. E., Lee, P. C., Pauls, D. L., Dion, Y., Grados, M. A., Illmann, C., et al. (2015). Lifetime prevalence, age of risk, and genetic relationships of comorbid psychiatric disorders in Tourette syndrome. *JAMA Psychiatry* 72, 325–333. doi: 10.1001/jamapsychiatry.2014.2650

John, U., Hill, A., Rumpf, H. J., Hapke, U., and Meyer, C. (2003). Alcohol high risk drinking, abuse and dependence among tobacco smoking medical care patients and the general population. *Drug Alcohol Depend.* 69, 189–195. doi: 10.1016/S0376-8716(02)00315-0

Johnston, B. A., Steele, J. D., Tolomeo, S., Christmas, D., and Matthews, K. (2015). Structural MRI-based predictions in patients with treatment-refractory depression (TRD). *PLoS ONE* 10:e0132958. doi: 10.1371/journal.pone.0132958

Jung, J., Jackson, S. R., Parkinson, A., and Jackson, G. M. (2013). Cognitive control over motor output in Tourette syndrome. *Neurosci. Biobehav. Rev.* 37, 1016–1025. doi: 10.1016/j.neubiorev.2012.08.009

Kalivas, P. W., and Volkow, N. D. (2005). The neural basis of addiction: a pathology of motivation and choice. *Am. J. Psychiatry* 162, 1403–1413. doi: 10.1176/appi.ajp.162.8.1403

Kambeitz-Ilankovic, L., Meisenzahl, E. M., Cabral, C., von Saldern, S., Kambeitz, J., Falkai, P., et al. (2015). Prediction of outcome in the psychosis prodrome using neuroanatomical pattern classification. *Schizophr. Res.* 173, 159–165. doi: 10.1016/j.schres.2015.03.005

Kim, H., Zheng, S., Amini, S. S., Virk, S. M., Mikkelsen, T., Brat, D. J., et al. (2015). Whole-genome and multisector exome sequencing of primary and post-treatment glioblastoma reveals patterns of tumor evolution. *Genome Res.* 25, 316–327. doi: 10.1101/gr.180612.114

Laumann, T. O., Gordon, E. M., Adeyemo, B., Snyder, A. Z., Joo, S. J., Chen, M. Y., et al. (2015). Functional system and areal organization of a highly sampled individual human brain. *Neuron* 87, 657–670. doi: 10.1016/j.neuron.2015.06.037

Lawrence, D., Fagan, P., Backinger, C. L., Gibson, J. T., and Hartman, A. (2007). Cigarette smoking patterns among young adults aged 18-24 years in the United States. *Nicotine Tob. Res.* 9, 687–697. doi: 10.1080/14622200701365319

Lessov, C. N., Martin, N. G., Statham, D. J., Todorov, A. A., Slutske, W. S., Bucholz, K. K., et al. (2004). Defining nicotine dependence for genetic research: evidence from Australian twins. *Psychol. Med.* 34, 865–879. doi: 10.1017/S0033291703001582

Lessov-Schlaggar, C. N., Lepore, R. L., Kristjansson, S. D., Schlaggar, B. L., Barnes, K. A., Petersen, S. E., et al. (2013). Functional neuroimaging study in identical twin pairs discordant for regular cigarette smoking. *Addict. Biol.* 18, 98–108. doi: 10.1111/j.1369-1600.2012.00435.x

Levin, V. A., and Wilson, C. B. (1976). Nitrosourea chemotherapy for primary malignant gliomas. *Cancer Treat. Rep.* 60, 719–724.

Madden, P. A., and Heath, A. C. (2002). Shared genetic vulnerability in alcohol and cigarette use and dependence. *Alcohol. Clin. Exp. Res.* 26, 1919–1921. doi: 10.1111/j.1530-0277.2002.tb02503.x

Martino, D., Madhusudan, N., Zis, P., and Cavanna, A. E. (2013). An introduction to the clinical phenomenology of Tourette syndrome. *Int. Rev. Neurobiol.* 112, 1–33. doi: 10.1016/B978-0-12-411546-0.00001-9

Mathews, C. A., and Grados, M. A. (2011). Familiality of Tourette syndrome, obsessive-compulsive disorder, and attention-deficit/hyperactivity disorder: heritability analysis in a large sib-pair sample. *J. Am. Acad. Child Adolesc. Psychiatry* 50, 46–54. doi: 10.1016/j.jaac.2010.10.004

Meier, P. (1975). Statistics and medical experimentation. *Biometrics* 31, 511–529. doi: 10.2307/2529434

Miranda-Dominguez, O., Mills, B. D., Carpenter, S. D., Grant, K. A., Kroenke, C. D., Nigg, J. T., et al. (2014). Connectotyping: model based fingerprinting of the functional connectome. *PLoS ONE* 9:e111048. doi: 10.1371/journal.pone.0111048

Moher, D., Schulz, K. F., and Altman, D. (2001). The CONSORT statement: revised recommendations for improving the quality of reports of parallel-group randomized trials. *JAMA* 285, 1987–1991. doi: 10.1001/jama.285.15.1987

Mol Debes, N. M. (2013). Co-morbid disorders in Tourette syndrome. *Behav. Neurol.* 27, 7–14. doi: 10.1155/2013/237513

Mueller, S. C., Jackson, G. M., Dhalla, R., Datsopoulos, S., and Hollis, C. P. (2006). Enhanced cognitive control in young people with Tourette's syndrome. *Curr. Biol.* 16, 570–573. doi: 10.1016/j.cub.2006.01.064

O'Rourke, J. A., Scharf, J. M., Platko, J., Stewart, S. E., Illmann, C., Geller, D. A., et al. (2011). The familial association of tourette's disorder and ADHD: the impact of OCD symptoms. *Am. J. Med. Genet. B Neuropsychiatr. Genet.* 156B, 553–560. doi: 10.1002/ajmg.b.31195

Pellegatta, S., Cuppini, L., and Finocchiaro, G. (2011). Brain cancer immunoediting: novel examples provided by immunotherapy of malignant gliomas. *Expert Rev. Anticancer Ther.* 11, 1759–1774. doi: 10.1586/era.11.102

Poldrack, R. A., Laumann, T. O., Koyejo, O., Gregory, B., Hover, A., Chen, M. Y., et al. (2015). Long-term neural and physiological phenotyping of a single human. *Nat. Commun.* 6, 8885. doi: 10.1038/ncomms9885

Rickards, H. (2009). Functional neuroimaging in Tourette syndrome. *J. Psychosom. Res.* 67, 575–584. doi: 10.1016/j.jpsychores.2009.07.024

Robinson, G. W., Orr, B. A., Wu, G., Gururangan, S., Lin, T., Qaddoumi, I., et al. (2015). Vismodegib exerts targeted efficacy against recurrent sonic hedgehog-subgroup medulloblastoma: results from Phase II pediatric brain tumor consortium studies PBTC-025B and PBTC-032. *J. Clin. Oncol.* 33, 2646–2654. doi: 10.1200/JCO.2014.60.1591

Smith, P. H., Mazure, C. M., and McKee, S. A. (2014). Smoking and mental illness in the U.S. *Popul. Tob. Control* 23, e147–e153. doi: 10.1136/tobaccocontrol-2013-051466

Stock, A. K., Popescu, F., Neuhaus, A. H., and Beste, C. (2015). Single-subject prediction of response inhibition behavior by event-related potentials. *J. Neurophysiol.* 115, 1252–1262. doi: 10.1152/jn.00969.2015

Stupp, R., Mason, W. P., van den Bent, M. J., Weller, M., Fisher, B., Taphoorn, M. J., et al. (2005). Radiotherapy plus concomitant and adjuvant temozolomide for glioblastoma. *N. Engl. J. Med.* 352, 987–996. doi: 10.1056/NEJMoa043330

Sturm, D., Bender, S., Jones, D. T., Lichter, P., Grill, J., Becher, O., et al. (2014). Paediatric and adult glioblastoma: multiform (epi)genomic culprits emerge. *Nat. Rev. Cancer* 14, 92–107. doi: 10.1038/nrc3655

Sun, T., Warrington, N. M., Luo, J., Brooks, M. D., Dahiya, S., Snyder, S. C., et al. (2014). Sexually dimorphic RB inactivation underlies mesenchymal glioblastoma prevalence in males. *J. Clin. Invest.* 124, 4123–4133. doi: 10.1172/JCI71048

van Thuijl, H. F., Mazor, T., Johnson, B. E., Fouse, S. D., Aihara, K., Hong, C., et al. (2015). Evolution of DNA repair defects during malignant progression of low-grade gliomas after temozolomide treatment. *Acta Neuropathol.* 129, 597–607. doi: 10.1007/s00401-015-1403-6

Vrieze, S. I., Hicks, B. M., Iacono, W. G., and McGue, M. (2012). Decline in genetic influence on the co-occurrence of alcohol, marijuana, and nicotine dependence symptoms from age 14 to 29. *Am. J. Psychiatry* 169, 1073–1081. doi: 10.1176/appi.ajp.2012.11081268

Walker, M. D., and Gehan, E. A. (1976). Clinical studies in malignant gliomas and their treatment with the nitrosoureas. *Cancer Treat. Rep.* 60, 713–716.

Xian, H., Scherrer, J. F., Pergadia, M. L., Madden, P. A., Grant, J. D., Sartor, C. E., et al. (2010). Contribution of parental psychopathology to offspring smoking and nicotine dependence in a genetically informative design. *J. Stud. Alcohol Drugs* 71, 664–673. doi: 10.15288/jsad.2010.71.664

Zoloto, A., Nagoshi, C. T., Presson, C., and Chassin, L. (2012). Attention deficit/hyperactivity disorder symptoms and depression symptoms as mediators in the intergenerational transmission of smoking. *Drug Alcohol Depend.* 126, 147–155. doi: 10.1016/j.drugalcdep.2012.05.003

20

Convergent Validity of the PUTS

Valerie Cathérine Brandt[1,2]*, Christian Beck[3], Valeria Sajin[1,2], Silke Anders[3] and Alexander Münchau[1,2]

[1] Department of Paediatric and Adult Movement Disorders and Neuropsychiatry, Center of Brain, Behavior and Metabolism, University of Lübeck, Lübeck, Germany, [2] Department of Neurology, University of Lübeck, Lübeck, Germany, [3] Department of Neurology, Institute of Social and Affective Neuroscience, University of Lübeck, Lübeck, Germany

Edited by:
Peristera Paschou,
Democritus University of Thrace, Greece

Reviewed by:
Kerstin Jessica Plessen,
University of Copenhagen, Denmark
Alka Anand Subramanyam,
Topiwala National Medical College & BYL Nair Charitable Hospital, India

****Correspondence:***
Valerie Cathérine Brandt
valerie.brandt@neuro.uni-luebeck.de

Premonitory urges are a cardinal feature in Gilles de la Tourette syndrome. Severity of premonitory urges can be assessed with the "Premonitory Urge for Tic Disorders Scale" (PUTS). However, convergent validity of the measure has been difficult to assess due to the lack of other urge measures. We investigated the relationship between average real-time urge intensity assessed by an in-house developed real-time urge monitor (RUM), measuring urge intensity continuously for 5 min on a visual analog scale, and general urge intensity assessed by the PUTS in 22 adult Tourette patients (mean age 29.8 ± 10.3 SD, 19 males). Additionally, underlying factors of premonitory urges assessed by the PUTS were investigated in the adult sample using factor analysis and were replicated in 40 children and adolescents diagnosed with Tourette syndrome (mean age 12.05 ± 2.83 SD, 31 males). Cronbach's α for the PUTS 10 was acceptable ($\alpha = 0.79$) in the adult sample. Convergent validity between average real-time urge intensity scores (as assessed with the RUM) and the 10-item version of the PUTS ($r = 0.64$) and the 9-item version of the PUTS ($r = 0.66$) was good. A factor analysis including the 10 items of the PUTS and average real-time urge intensity scores revealed three factors. One factor included the average real-time urge intensity score and appeared to measure urge intensity, whereas the other two factors can be assumed to reflect the (sensory) quality of urges and subjective control, respectively. The factor structure of the 10 PUTS items alone was replicated in a sample of children and adolescents. The results indicate that convergent validity between the PUTS and the real-time urge assessment monitor is good. Furthermore, the results suggest that the PUTS might assess more than one dimension of urges, and it may be worthwhile developing different subscales of the PUTS assessing premonitory urges in terms of intensity and quality, as well as subjectively experienced control over tics and premonitory urges.

Keywords: Tourette syndrome, tic, premonitory urge, PUTS, real-time urge monitor

INTRODUCTION

Premonitory urges, or simply "urges," are aversive subjective sensations that have been described to precede tics in patients suffering from Gilles de la Tourette syndrome (GTS) (1, 2).

In contrast to entirely involuntary movements in other movement disorders, tics can be suppressed for limited time intervals. However, during tic suppression, unpleasant urges tend to increase until relieved by a tic (3–5). Therefore, tics are frequently experienced as voluntary responses to urges (4). Approximately 80–90% of GTS patients report to experience urges (1, 6, 7); hence, urges may play a key role in understanding GTS. Although the onset of urges appears to be delayed relative to tic onset by approximately 3 years, this finding might be due to difficulties assessing urges in 5- to 7-year olds (1, 7). Premonitory urges typically occur at the location where a tic is about to occur, but can also be experienced as a general inner tension (1). They can be experienced as "warm" or "cold," "pressure-like," or "tickling" sensations (8). In terms of intensity or urgency, premonitory urges have been likened to an itch (9).

A decade ago, Woods and Colleagues developed a short questionnaire to capture urge severity in children with tics (6). This questionnaire has been shown to have good psychometric properties (6, 10) and was later validated in adults (2, 11). The items of the Premonitory Urge for Tic Disorders Scale (PUTS) assess different sensory qualities of the urge, such as tickling, rising inner tension, or a "not just right" feeling. Moreover, questions cover the frequency of urge–tic associations, and the relief patients may experience after a tic has been executed.

Assessing convergent and discriminant validity of a new questionnaire are methods typically applied in psychometrics in order to ensure that the questionnaire measures the theoretical construct it was designed to measure and can discriminate between this construct and closely related constructs. However, investigating the convergent validity of the PUTS has been difficult because research concerning urges is relatively young, and there is a lack of instruments measuring a comparable construct. Furthermore, despite the wide use of the instrument, we are not aware of any study addressing the question of whether the PUTS assesses more than one dimension of urge phenomenology. Factor analyses are commonly applied when evaluating whether a questionnaire measures multiple dimensions of a construct or several constructs, especially when the questionnaire has several subscales (e.g., impulsivity, hyperactivity, and attention). The PUTS was designed as a one-dimensional questionnaire assessing urge severity, but studies showing that urge severity measured by the PUTS correlates positively with tic severity, obsessive-compulsive symptoms and anxiety (6, 10, 12, 13) suggest that the PUTS may reflect a multidimensional construct.

The current study uses a newly developed real-time urge monitor (RUM) to examine convergent validity between the PUTS and average tic-related urge intensity measured in real time. Furthermore, we assessed the discriminant validity between the PUTS and measures of attention-deficit hyperactivity disorder (ADHD) and obsessive–compulsive disorder (OCD). Moreover, the study examines whether the PUTS might measure more than one dimension of the urge phenomenon.

MATERIALS AND METHODS

Participants – Clinical Assessment

Twenty-two patients (mean age 29.82 ± 10.34 SD, range = 17–55; 19 males) with a GTS diagnosis according to DSM-5 criteria (14) were included in this study. All patients gave their written informed consent prior to the study. Additionally, questionnaire data of 40 children and adolescents with a GTS diagnosis (mean age 12.05 ± 2.83 SD, range = 7–17; 31 males) were included in the study. Informed written assent was given by the children and written consent was given by their parents. The study was reviewed and approved by the local ethics committee and conformed to the Declaration of Helsinki.

Gilles de la Tourette syndrome symptom severity was assessed using the clinician-rated Yale Global Tic Severity Scale [YGTSS (15)]. In adults, symptoms of ADHD in childhood were rated on the German short version of the "Wender Utah Rating Scale" [WURS-K (16)], whereas current ADHD symptoms were assessed with the German ADHD self-rating scale [ADHD-SB (17)]. Symptoms of OCD were measured with the "Yale–Brown Obsessive–Compulsive Disorder Scale" [Y-BOCS (18)]. In children, symptoms of ADHD were assessed using the German parent-rated "FBB-ADHD" scale ["Diagnostik-System für Psychische Störungen nach ICD 10 und DSM-IV für Kinder und Jugendliche II," DISYPS-II (19)] or the clinician-rated ADHD DSM-IV checklist [ADHD-DC (20)]. Symptoms of OCD were assessed with the "Yale–Brown Obsessive–Compulsive Disorder Scale for Children" [CY-BOCS (18, 21)].

The PUTS Scale

Premonitory urges in general were measured using the validated German version of the PUTS (11). The PUTS is a 10-item self-rating scale and was originally developed to assess the intensity of urge phenomena on a 1–4 Likert rating scale (6). However, the last item has been removed from the PUTS score, because it was found to show small correlations with the rest of the scale (6, 10).

Experimental Procedure of the Real-Time Urge Monitor

Adult patients ($N = 22$) were seated in front of a Sony Vaio laptop (15″ screen) and were familiarized with the task. They were instructed to perform a continuous rating of their urge to tic over a period of 5 min. The right-hand side of the laptop screen showed a vertical intensity scale from 0 to 100, and patients were asked to indicate the intensity level of their current urge to tic, with 0 being no urge at all and 100 being the strongest urge intensity they typically experienced (see **Figure 1**). During the whole

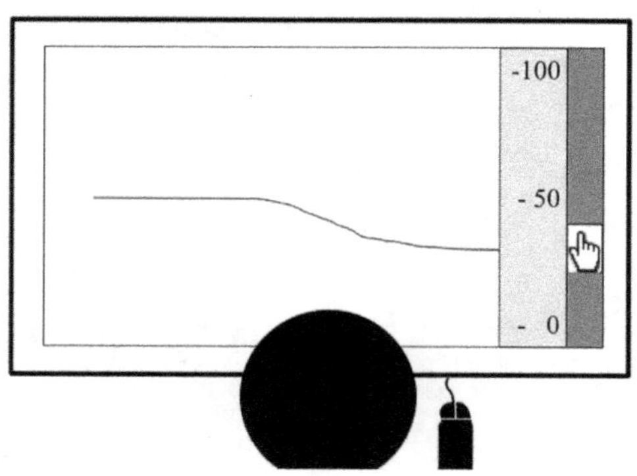

FIGURE 1 | The figure shows an example of the real-time urge monitor. After a countdown, a blue line started moving across the screen continuously. Patients were asked to use the scroll bar on the right to continuously indicate the intensity of their current urge to tic on a scale from 0 to 100, displayed on the right of the screen.

course of the experiment, patients were asked not to suppress any tics and to tic freely.

The task started when patients pressed a button. The button press initiated a countdown (3–2–1–0). At time 0, a blue line moved across the screen (at an intensity level 50), starting on the right-hand side of the screen, crossing the screen within 10 s. Patients were asked to continuously adjust the level of the blue line according to their subjectively experienced urge to tic. Hence, participants could see their urge ratings for the previous 10 s at any time. Data were sampled at 10 Hz. Patients were given the opportunity of a 1-min practice run and were asked to start the task after the experimenter left the room.

Data Analysis

The continuous RUM resulted in 3000 data points per 5 min. The first 10 s (100 urge data points) were excluded in order to allow patients time to adjust the urge level on the screen to the correct level. The remaining 2900 data points were aggregated into a mean real-time urge intensity score.

In order to assess the internal consistency of the PUTS, an indicator of the reliability of a questionnaire, Cronbach's α was calculated. A value of $\alpha > 0.80$ is generally considered good, a value of $\alpha > 0.70$ acceptable. Reliability was assessed in adults and children/adolescents separately.

Convergent validity (the degree to which two measures assessing the same construct are related) between the PUTS and the average real-time urge intensity monitor was assessed by correlating the mean real-time urge intensity scores of the adult sample ($N = 22$) with the PUTS 9 and the PUTS 10 score, respectively, using Pearson's r. Discriminant validity (the degree to which a measure can discriminate between the construct it was designed to measure and the construct it was not designed to measure) between the PUTS and OCD/ADHD measures was assessed using Pearson's r.

In order to assess the discriminatory power of individual PUTS items in the adult GTS sample, i.e., how well individual items of the PUTS capture the construct measured by the questionnaire overall, item-test correlations were performed between items and the PUTS 9 score as well as the PUTS 10 score (part-whole corrected) using Pearson's r. Additionally, the individual PUTS items were correlated with the average real-time urge intensity score in order to investigate which PUTS items best captured urge intensity.

Thereafter, two factor analyses were run. The first included only the 10 items of the PUTS, in order to assess whether the PUTS might reflect more than one dimension of premonitory urges. The second additionally included the real-time urge intensity score as an item, in order to determine which one of the factors might best represent the construct of urge intensity. Finally, a factor analysis including only the 10 items of the PUTS was computed in the young sample ($N = 40$) to assess whether the factor structure was similar in a younger, independent sample.

RESULTS

Clinical Assessment

In the adults sample, mean total tic severity according to the YGTSS (0–50) was 17.05 ± 7.7 SD, and the mean PUTS 9 score (10–36) was 21.05 ± 5.78 SD. Results from the Y-BOCS showed that none of the patients exceeded the overall cut off for clinically relevant OCD symptoms (16), with values ranging from 0 to 14 (3.19 ± 4.85). However, WURS-K values ranged from 0 to 48 (15.98 ± 13.65) indicating that 4 patients scored in the clinical range (cut off = 30); three of these patients also fulfilled DSM-5 criteria for ADHD (14).

In the young sample, mean total tic severity according to the YGTSS50 was 17.77 ± 8.12 SD. The mean PUTS 9 score was 17.83 ± 6.38 SD. Mean ADHD values according to the FBB-ADHD ($N = 25$) scale were 0.96 ± 0.77 SD and according to the ADHD-DC ($N = 13$) scale were 0.15 ± 0.14 SD. Nine out of the 40 children scored in the clinical range and/or had an ADHD diagnosis according to DSM-5 (14). The mean CY-BOCS score ($N = 36$) was 3.03 ± 6.3 SD; five of these patients had a diagnosis in the OCD spectrum.

Internal Consistency of the PUTS

Cronbach's α across the 10 items of the PUTS was acceptable in the adult sample ($\alpha = 0.79$) and good in the young sample ($\alpha = 0.84$).

Item–test correlations between individual PUTS items and the PUTS 9/PUTS 10 score showed that items 1, 6, and 9 consistently did not assess the overall construct of the PUTS as well as the other items (please see **Table 1** for coefficients; for items, see **Table 2**). As previously found, item 10 also showed a very small correlation with the overall test score ($r = -0.02$). Excluding items 1, 6, 9, and 10 increased internal reliability of the PUTS in the adult sample ($\alpha = 0.84$), but not the young sample ($\alpha = 0.84$).

Convergent Validity between the PUTS and Real-Time Urge Intensity

The average real-time urge intensity score was highly correlated with the PUTS 10 ($r = 0.64, p = 0.001$) and the PUTS 9 ($r = 0.66$, $p = 0.001$). PUTS items 1, 9, and 10 showed weak and non-significant correlations with the average real-time urge intensity score ($r < 0.2, p > 0.4$; for a full list of correlations between real-time urge intensity score and single items of the PUTS, please see **Table 1**). Excluding these items increased the overall correlation between the mean real-time urge intensity score and the PUTS 10 ($r = 0.71, p < 0.001$).

The YGTSS motor tic severity score showed medium correlations with the PUTS (PUTS 10: rho = 0.43, $p = 0.048$; PUTS 9: rho = 0.48, $p = 0.025$) and a medium non-significant correlation with real-time urge intensity (rho = 0.37, $p = 0.09$). The number of tics per 5 min (121.36 ± 60.56) correlated significantly with real-time urge intensity ($r = 0.46, p = 0.03$), but not with the PUTS 9 ($r = 0.36, p = 0.103$) or PUTS 10 score ($r = 0.39, p = 0.073$).

Discriminant Validity between Urge Measures and ADHD/OCD Measures

There was a significant correlation between the PUTS 10 and the Y-BOCS (see **Table 1**). Correlations between single items of the PUTS and clinical scores showed that the Y-BOCS was

TABLE 1 | Correlations between PUTS items and RUM/ADHD/OCD measures.

PUTS	RUM	PUTS 9	PUTS 10	Y-BOCS	WURS-K	ADHD-SB	ADHD-A	ADHD-H	ADHD-I
Item 1	**0.13**	0.25	0.28	−0.18	−0.35	−0.01	−0.14	−0.09	0.17
Item 2	**0.55****	0.67**	0.68**	0.25	0.29	0.13	0.002	0.34	−0.01
Item 3	**0.36**	0.58**	0.6**	0.59**	0.56**	0.44*	0.26	0.64**	0.27
Item 4	**0.51***	0.8**	0.79**	0.53*	0.46*	0.27	0.26	0.26	0.15
Item 5	**0.35**	0.72**	0.75**	0.43*	0.27	0.18	0.22	0.22	0.18
Item 6	**0.55****	0.3	0.22	0.08	0.32	0.25	0.24	0.27	0.08
Item 7	**0.6****	0.58**	0.55**	0.09	0.02	0.02	−0.09	0	33
Item 8	**0.67****	0.47*	0.41	−0.11	0.001	0.1	−0.13	0.23	0.35
Item 9	**−0.01**	0.21	0.26	0.5*	0.19	0.09	0.18	−0.11	0.18
Item 10	**−0.17**		−0.02	0.16	−0.23	−0.32	−0.27	−0.25	−0.34
Multitrait-multimethod matrix									
RUM	1								
PUTS 9	0.66**	1							
PUTS 10	0.64**	0.99	1						
Y-BOCS	0.11	0.41	0.43*	1					
WURS-k	0.12	0.35	0.32	0.51*	1				
ADHD-SB	0.2	0.25	0.21	0.34	0.61**	1			
ADHSD-A	−0.01	0.15	0.11	0.38	0.57**	0.89**	1		
ADHD-H	0.26	0.35	0.31	0.28	0.73**	0.83**	0.54*	1	
ADHD-I	0.05	0.3	0.25	0.09	0.58**	0.82**	0.61**	0.67**	1

RUM, real-time urge monitor; PUTS, Premonitory Urge for Tic Disorders Scale; Y-BOCS, Yale–Brown Obsessive–Compulsive Scale; WURS-K, Wender Utah Rating Scale Short Form; ADHD-SB, Attention Deficit Hyperactivity Disorder Self-Rating Scale; ADHD-A, inattention subscale of the ADHD-SB; ADHD-H, hyperactivity subscale of the ADHD-SB; ADHD-I, impulsivity subscale of the ADHD-SB.

**$p < 0.05$.*

***$p < 0.01$.*

TABLE 2 | Rotated factor analysis of the PUTS and the real-time urge measure.

Items	Adult sample			Young sample		
	F1	F2	F3	F1	F2	F3
Item 1: Right before I do a tic I feel like my insides are itchy	0.02	**0.60**	0.59	**0.67**	−0.05	0.09
Item 2: Right before I do a tic I feel pressure inside my brain or body	**0.72**	0.32	0.06	**0.76**	0.4	0.04
Item 3: Right before I do a tic I feel "wound up" or tense inside	**0.85**	0.01	−0.05	0.34	**0.82**	−0.03
Item 4: Right before I do a tic I feel like something is not "just right"	**0.86**	0.27	0.03	0.07	**0.82**	0.28
Item 5: Right before I do a tic I feel like something is not complete	**0.82**	0.18	0.19	0.06	**0.87**	0.17
Item 6: Right before I do a tic I feel like there is energy in my body that needs to get out	0.44	0.18	**−0.76**	0.22	0.09	**0.66**
Item 7: I have these feelings almost all the time before I do a tic	0.27	**0.82**	−0.02	**0.75**	0.22	0.5
Item 8: These feelings happen for every tic I have	0.14	**0.90**	−0.26	**0.83**	0.1	0.16
Item 9: After I do the tic, the itchiness, energy, pressure, tense feelings, or feelings that something is not "just right," or complete go away, at least for a while	0.38	−0.004	**0.62**	0.28	0.07	**0.86**
Item 10: I am able to stop my tics even if only for a short period of time	0.14	−0.22	**0.76**	−0.11	0.39	**0.54**
Real-time urge intensity score	0.46	**0.63**	−0.32			

F, factor; PUTS, Premonitory Urge for Tic Disorders Scale.

significantly correlated with items 3 ($r = 0.59$, $p = 0.004$), 4 ($r = 0.53$, $p = 0.012$), 5 ($r = 0.43$, $p = 0.047$), and 9 ($r = 0.5$, $p = 0.019$; **Table 1**). The WURS-K score correlated significantly with items 3 ($r = 0.56$, $p = 0.006$) and 4 ($r = 0.46$, $p = 0.032$), ADHD-SB also correlated significantly with item 3 ($r = 0.44$, $p = 0.047$), especially with hyperactivity ($r = 0.64$, $p = 0.002$). However, the WURS-K and the Y-BOCS total scores were also significantly correlated ($r = 0.51$, $p = 0.014$; **Table 1**).

There were no significant correlations between the real-time urge intensity score and ADHD/OCD scores (**Table 1**).

Dimensions of the PUTS

A factor analysis with Varimax rotation across the PUTS 10 and the real-time urge intensity score revealed three factors. Items 2, 3, 4, and 5 loaded highest on the first factor, whereas the real-time urge intensity score loaded highest on the second factor together with items 1, 7, and 8. Item 1 did not load clearly on one factor though but was almost equally distributed between factors 2 and 3. Items 6, 9, and 10 loaded highest on the third factor (**Table 2**). The same structure emerged when only the 10 PUTS items were included in the analysis.

A very similar structure of the 10 PUTS items was found in the young sample. The only item that differed was Item 2, loading highest on the intensity factor instead of the quality factor (see **Table 2**).

DISCUSSION

Construct Validity of the PUTS

The current study sought to assess the convergent validity of the PUTS with a measure that assesses urge intensity in real time. Average real-time urge intensity correlated highly with the PUTS 9 and PUTS 10 scores. This shows good convergent validity of the PUTS with a measure that tracks urge intensity over a limited time interval. However, low correlations between urge intensity assessed by the real-time urge intensity monitor and individual items (1, 9, and 10) of the PUTS suggest that not all items of the PUTS tap into the construct of urge intensity. These findings were reflected by the results regarding internal consistency of the PUTS.

Internal consistency of the PUTS 10 was acceptable ($\alpha = 0.79$) in adult GTS patients, replicating previous findings (2, 6). However, consistency could be increased by excluding a number of items that showed small to medium correlations with the overall construct assessed by the PUTS. Item 10, referring to the ability to stop one's tics, was already removed from the PUTS total score in most recent studies (12, 22). Item 1, assessing an "itch-like" urge quality, item 6, characterizing urges as an energy that needs to get out, and item 9, assessing to what degree urges subside after tics, also appeared to assess a different construct than urge intensity. Excluding items 1, 6, 9, and 10 increased internal consistency and convergent validity in the adult sample. However, instead of excluding these items, it might be worthwhile investigating and building on the different underlying dimensions of urges that the PUTS might assess. Factor analyses including all 10 items of the PUTS (with and without real-time urge intensity score) revealed a three-factor solution.

Items loading on the first factor assess whether patients feel "a pressure," "wound up," "like something is not 'just right' or 'incomplete'" and might be interpreted to assess the *quality* of premonitory sensations. The second factor included the average real-time urge intensity score and two items assessing in how far patients had these "feelings almost all the time" before a tic and "for every tic" and might reflect the overall *intensity* of premonitory urges. Item 1 ("*...my insides are itchy*") also loaded highest on the second factor. However, it loaded almost equally high on factor three (0.60 vs. 0.59) and might not clearly reflect any of the underlying dimensions. Surprisingly, it was not included in the first factor, assessing quality of urges.

The third factor comprised item 9, assessing how much tics are associated with a relief in urges and item 10, referring to the patients ability to stop their tics. Additionally, item 6 assesses to what degree patients feel that there is "an energy" in their body that needs to get out before the tic and loaded highly negatively on factor three. The nature of these items suggests that the underlying factor may be related to the perceived *control* over tics and urges.

This pattern was largely replicated in 40 children and adolescents with GTS. In this sample, item 2, referring to urges as a pressure moved from the *quality* factor to the *intensity* factor.

Convergent and Discriminant Validity

The medium correlation between the overall PUTS score and the motor tic severity score of the YGTSS suggests that both questionnaires assess distinct, but related constructs. This cannot strictly be taken as proof of validity of the PUTS because the YGTSS does not aim to assess the same construct as the PUTS. Moreover, previous studies regarding the association between the PUTS and the YGTSS have rendered mixed results (2, 6, 10, 12, 23, 24). This suggests that the relationship between urge severity and tic severity either depends on the sample characteristics (e.g., comorbidities) or that they are not always sufficiently captured by the PUTS and/or the YGTSS to reveal their relationship.

A significant correlation in the medium range between the number of tics assessed in real time and urge intensity assessed in real time supports the notion that tic severity and urge severity are related, but distinct phenomena, independent of the measure used to assess them. The finding that correlations across different measures (real-time urge intensity with YGTSS motor tic severity; real-time number of tics with PUTS scores) were lower and non-significant could be due to the different time windows assessed by questionnaires and real-time instruments. Questionnaires aim to assess phenomena in general, whereas the RUM assesses severity of tics and urges in a small time window. Tics wax and wane and urge severity assessed at a particular point in time can differ from urge severity judged over a longer time period and averaged across all tics that the patient recalls while filling out the questionnaire.

The PUTS 10, but not the PUTS 9 score, correlated significantly with the Y-BOCS, but not with ADHD measures, replicating previous mixed findings on the association between symptoms of OCD or ADHD and urges measured by the PUTS (6, 10, 12, 13, 24, 25). However, we would not classify significant correlations with the Y-BOCS as convergent validity because the questionnaires aim to assess very different constructs. On the contrary, it might be more useful if items assessing urge intensity associated with tics did not tap into related phenomena that might be associated with obsessions or compulsions. Hence, the discriminant validity of the PUTS was not good because it did not clearly measure urge intensity only associated with tics.

The majority of OCD patients with premonitory sensations experience "just-right" sensations (26), whereas the majority of GTS patients describe it as an impulse or urge to move (4). Based on the correlational pattern between single items of the PUTS and measures of OCD and ADHD, it appears likely that specific items, related to the *quality* of urges, tap into phenomena that are typically associated with OCD (i.e., "not just right" feelings or feelings of incompleteness) or ADHD (i.e., feeling "wound up") and not specifically with the urge to tic. Similar associations between PUTS items and OCD symptoms have previously been found (10, 13).

Urge intensity *per se* might not be associated with symptoms of OCD and ADHD. In line with this assumption, items loading on the *intensity* factor of the PUTS and the real-time urge intensity score were not significantly correlated with OCD or ADHD scores, suggesting that urge *intensity* is independent from comorbidities.

Limitations and Future Directions

The main limitation of the study is the sample size. Although this should not be problematic for the results concerning convergent validity between the PUTS and the real-time urge measure, more patients will be required to draw firm conclusions concerning the underlying dimensions assessed by the PUTS. Despite the replication of a very similar three-factor solution in the young sample, it might be useful for researchers to pool their PUTS data and investigate whether these dimensions can be replicated in large samples of at least 50 individuals (27).

If the structure can be replicated, the PUTS might be further developed into several subscales with more items on each scale. The subscale assessing urge intensity should then have high discriminant validity, purely assessing urge intensity regarding tics and not tap into phenomena that might also be associated with comorbidities. The subscales assessing quality of urges and perceived control over urges/tics might be very interesting and useful with regard to comorbidities. For instance, individuals with higher ADHD scores were less likely to say that they could stop their tics in this sample, whereas patients with higher OCD scores were more likely to say that urges subsided after tics. Although correlations with ADHD symptoms were not significant, perceived control might be an interesting question to pursue in the future. Furthermore, intelligence has been shown to be associated with some executive functions (28), and future studies might evaluate the role of intelligence in perceived and actual tic control. Until now, research investigating differences in premonitory urges has mostly focused on the different qualities of the experienced sensation (e.g., just right feeling, impulse, and energy release), and future studies might investigate the underlying dimensions of urges more comprehensively.

AUTHOR CONTRIBUTIONS

VB: conceptualization/design, data acquisition, analysis, interpretation, draft, approval of the manuscript for publication, and agrees to be accountable for all aspects of the work. CB: conceptualization/design, programming of the task, critical revision for important intellectual content, approval of the manuscript for publication, and agrees to be accountable for all aspects of the work. VS: data acquisition, analysis, critical revision for important intellectual content, approval of the manuscript for publication, and agrees to be accountable for all aspects of the work. SA: conceptualization/design, critical revision for important intellectual content, approval of the manuscript for publication, and agrees to be accountable for all aspects of the work. AM: conceptualization/design, critical revision for important intellectual content, approval of the manuscript for publication, and agrees to be accountable for all aspects of the work.

REFERENCES

1. Leckman JF, Walker DE, Cohen DJ. Premonitory urges in Tourette's syndrome. *Am J Psychiatry* (1993) **150**:98–102. doi:10.1176/ajp.150.1.98
2. Crossley E, Seri S, Stern JS, Robertson MM, Cavanna AE. Premonitory urges for tics in adult patients with Tourette syndrome. *Brain Dev* (2014) **36**:45–50. doi:10.1016/j.braindev.2012.12.010
3. Jankovic J. Tourette syndrome. Phenomenology and classification of tics. *Neurol Clin* (1997) **15**:267–75. doi:10.1016/S0733-8619(05)70311-X
4. Kwak C, Dat Vuong K, Jankovic J. Premonitory sensory phenomenon in Tourette's syndrome. *Mov Disord* (2003) **18**:1530–3. doi:10.1002/mds.10618
5. Brandt VC, Beck C, Sajin V, Baaske M, Bäumer T, Beste C, et al. Temporal relationship between premonitory urges and tics in Gilles de la Tourette syndrome. *Cortex* (2016) **77**:24–37. doi:10.1016/j.cortex.2016.01.008
6. Woods DW, Piacentini J, Himle MB, Chang S. Premonitory Urge for Tics Scale (PUTS): initial psychometric results and examination of the premonitory urge phenomenon in youths with tic disorders. *J Dev Behav Pediatr* (2005) **26**:397–403. doi:10.1097/00004703-200512000-00001
7. Robertson MM. Gilles de la Tourette syndrome: the complexities of phenotype and treatment. *Br J Hosp Med (Lond)* (2011) **72**:100–7. doi:10.12968/hmed.2011.72.2.100
8. Banaschewski T, Woerner W, Rothenberger A. Premonitory sensory phenomena and suppressibility of tics in Tourette syndrome: developmental aspects in children and adolescents. *Dev Med Child Neurol* (2003) **45**:700–3. doi:10.1017/S0012162203001294
9. Lang A. Patient perception of tics and other movement disorders. *Neurology* (1991) **41**:223–8. doi:10.1212/WNL.41.2_Part_1.223
10. Reese HE, Scahill L, Peterson AL, Crowe K, Woods DW, Piacentini J, et al. The premonitory urge to tic: measurement, characteristics, and correlates in older adolescents and adults. *Behav Ther* (2014) **45**:177–86. doi:10.1016/j.beth.2013.09.002
11. Rössner V, Müller-Vahl K, Neuner I. PUTS – Premonitory Urge Tics Scale: Fragebogen für Kinder. In: Müller-Vahl K, editor. *Tourette-Syndrom und Andere Tic-Erkrankungen im Kindes- und Erwachsenenalter*. Berlin: MWV Medizinische Wissenschaftliche Verlagsgesellschaft (2010). p. 204.
12. Steinberg T, Shmuel Baruch S, Harush A, Dar R, Woods D, Piacentini J, et al. Tic disorders and the premonitory urge. *J Neural Transm (Vienna)* (2010) **117**:277–84. doi:10.1007/s00702-009-0353-3
13. Rajagopal S, Cavanna AE. Premonitory urges and repetitive behaviours in adult patients with Tourette syndrome. *Neurol Sci* (2014) **35**:969–71. doi:10.1007/s10072-014-1706-8
14. DSM-5. *Diagnostic and Statistical Manual of Mental Disorders*. Arlington, VA: American Psychiatric Publishing (2013).
15. Leckman JF, Riddle MA, Hardin MT, Ort SI, Swartz KL, Stevenson J, et al. The Yale Global Tic Severity Scale: initial testing of a clinician-rated scale of tic severity. *J Am Acad Child Adolesc Psychiatry* (1989) **28**:566–73. doi:10.1097/00004583-198907000-00015
16. Ward MF, Wender PH, Reimherr FW. The Wender Utah Rating Scale: an aid in the retrospective diagnosis of childhood attention deficit hyperactivity disorder. *Am J Psychiatry* (1993) **150**:885–90.
17. Rosler M, Retz W, Retz-Junginger P, Thome J, Supprian T, Nissen T, et al. [Tools for the diagnosis of attention-deficit/hyperactivity disorder in adults. Self-rating behaviour questionnaire and diagnostic checklist]. *Nervenarzt* (2004) **75**:888–95. doi:10.1007/s00115-003-1622-2
18. Goodman WK, Price LH, Rasmussen SA, Mazure C, Fleischmann RL, Hill CL, et al. The Yale-Brown Obsessive Compulsive Scale. I. Development, use, and reliability. *Arch Gen Psychiatry* (1989) **46**:1006–11. doi:10.1001/archpsyc.1989.01810110048007
19. Döpfner M, Görtz-Dorten A, Lehmkuhl G. In: Hogrefe AG, editor. *Diagnostik-System für Psychische Störungen nach ICD-10 und DSM-IV für Kinder und Jugendliche – II*. Bern: Verlag Hans Huber (2008).
20. Rösler M, Retz-Junginger P, Retz W, Stieglitz R-D. *Homburger ADHS-Skalen für Erwachsene (HASE). Manual*. Göttingen: Hogrefe (2008).
21. Scahill L, Riddle MA, McSwiggin-Hardin M, Ort SI, King RA, Goodman WK, et al. Children's Yale-Brown Obsessive Compulsive Scale:

reliability and validity. *J Am Acad Child Adolesc Psychiatry* (1997) **36**:844–52. doi:10.1097/00004583-199706000-00023

22. Capriotti MR, Brandt BC, Turkel JE, Lee HJ, Woods DW. Negative reinforcement and premonitory urges in youth with tourette syndrome: an experimental evaluation. *Behav Modif* (2014) **38**:276–96. doi:10.1177/0145445514531015
23. Ganos C, Kahl U, Schunke O, Kuhn S, Haggard P, Gerloff C, et al. Are premonitory urges a prerequisite of tic inhibition in Gilles de la Tourette syndrome? *J Neurol Neurosurg Psychiatry* (2012) **83**:975–8. doi:10.1136/jnnp-2012-303033
24. Eddy CM, Cavanna AE. Premonitory urges in adults with complicated and uncomplicated tourette syndrome. *Behav Modif* (2014) **38**:264–75. doi:10.1177/0145445513504432
25. Crossley E, Cavanna AE. Sensory phenomena: clinical correlates and impact on quality of life in adult patients with Tourette syndrome. *Psychiatry Res* (2013) **209**:705–10. doi:10.1016/j.psychres.2013.04.019
26. Ferrao YA, Shavitt RG, Prado H, Fontenelle LF, Malavazzi DM, de Mathis MA, et al. Sensory phenomena associated with repetitive behaviors in obsessive-compulsive disorder: an exploratory study of 1001 patients. *Psychiatry Res* (2012) **197**:253–8. doi:10.1016/j.psychres.2011.09.017
27. Bryant FB, Yarnold PR. Principal components analysis and exploratory and confirmatory factor analysis. In: Grimm LG, Yarnold RR, editors. *Reading and Understanding Multivariale Statistics*. Washington, DC: American Psychological Association (1995). p. 99–136.
28. Friedman NP, Miyake A, Corley RP, Young SE, Defries JC, Hewitt JK. Not all executive functions are related to intelligence. *Psychol Sci* (2006) **17**:172–9. doi:10.1111/j.1467-9280.2006.01681.x

21

Targeted Re-Sequencing Approach of Candidate Genes Implicates Rare Potentially Functional Variants in Tourette Syndrome Etiology

John Alexander[1†], Hera Potamianou[1†], Jinchuan Xing[2,3], Li Deng[2,3], Iordanis Karagiannidis[1], Fotis Tsetsos[1], Petros Drineas[4], Zsanett Tarnok[5], Renata Rizzo[6], Tomasz Wolanczyk[7], Luca Farkas[5], Peter Nagy[5], Urszula Szymanska[7], Christos Androutsos[8], Vaia Tsironi[8], Anastasia Koumoula[8], Csaba Barta[9], TSGeneSEE[10], Paul Sandor[11], Cathy L. Barr[12,13], Jay Tischfield[2,3], Peristera Paschou[1], Gary A. Heiman[2,3] and Marianthi Georgitsi[1,14]**

[1] Department of Molecular Biology and Genetics, Democritus University of Thrace, Alexandroupoli, Greece, [2] Department of Genetics, Rutgers, The State University of New Jersey, Piscataway, NJ, USA, [3] Human Genetics Institute of New Jersey, Rutgers, The State University of New Jersey, Piscataway, NJ, USA, [4] Computer Science Department, Purdue University, West Lafayette, USA, [5] Vadaskert Clinic for Child and Adolescent Psychiatry, Budapest, Hungary, [6] Department of Clinical and Experimental Medicine, University of Catania, Catania, Italy, [7] Department of Child Psychiatry, Medical University of Warsaw, Warsaw, Poland, [8] Child and Adolescent Psychiatry Clinic, Sismanoglio General Hospital of Attica, Athens, Greece, [9] Molecular Biology and Pathobiochemistry, Institute of Medical Chemistry, Semmelweis University, Budapest, Hungary, [10] Tourette Syndrome Genetics — Southern and Eastern Europe Initiative (TSGeneSEE Consortium), [11] Department of Psychiatry, University of Toronto, Toronto, ON, Canada, [12] Genetics and Development Division, Krembil Research Institute, University Health Network, Toronto, ON, Canada, [13] Program in Neurosciences and Mental Health, The Hospital for Sick Children, Toronto, ON, Canada, [14] Laboratory of General Biology, Department of Medicine, Aristotle University of Thessaloniki, Thessaloniki, Greece

Edited by:
Ahmet O. Caglayan,
Yale University, USA

Reviewed by:
Munis Dundar,
Erciyes University, Turkey
Romina D'Aurizio,
National Research Council (CNR), Italy

****Correspondence:***
Gary A. Heiman
heiman@dls.rutgers.edu
Marianthi Georgitsi,
margeorgitsi@auth.gr

† These authors have contributed equally to this work.

Although the genetic basis of Tourette Syndrome (TS) remains unclear, several candidate genes have been implicated. Using a set of 382 TS individuals of European ancestry we investigated four candidate genes for TS (*HDC*, *SLITRK1*, *BTBD9*, and *SLC6A4*) in an effort to identify possibly causal variants using a targeted re-sequencing approach by next generation sequencing technology. Identification of possible disease causing variants under different modes of inheritance was performed using the algorithms implemented in VAAST. We prioritized variants using Variant ranker and validated five rare variants via Sanger sequencing in *HDC* and *SLITRK1*, all of which are predicted to be deleterious. Intriguingly, one of the identified variants is in linkage disequilibrium with a variant that is included among the top hits of a genome-wide association study for response to citalopram treatment, an antidepressant drug with off-label use also in obsessive compulsive disorder. Our findings provide additional evidence for the implication of these two genes in TS susceptibility and the possible role of these proteins in the pathobiology of TS should be revisited.

Keywords: next generation sequencing, targeted re-sequencing, genetic susceptibility, rare variants, TS candidate genes, *HDC*, *SLITRK1*

INTRODUCTION

Tourette Syndrome (TS; OMIM #137580) is a complex neurodevelopmental disorder of childhood onset, characterized by motor and vocal tics. It often presents with co-morbidities such as attention deficit hyperactivity disorder (ADHD) and/or obsessive-compulsive disorder (OCD), as well as mood disorders, anxiety and sleep disorders. Apart from various environmental factors that contribute to TS complexity (Hoekstra et al., 2013; Mathews et al., 2014), twin and family studies have long established that TS bears a strong genetic component (Price et al., 1985; Pauls et al., 1991, 2014). However, despite extensive on-going genetic research, concrete evidence supporting specific pathogenetic mechanisms is still largely lacking. Several genes (such as *SLITRK1*, *HDC*, *NLGN4*, *CNTNAP2*, *IMMP2L*, *SLC6A4* also known as *SERT*, and *NTN4*) and chromosomal loci have been implicated to date although, associations between genetic variation and TS are often limited to specific population-based cohorts or may be restricted to extremely rare mutations identified solely in unique multigenerational pedigrees.

A very promising candidate TS susceptibility region was implicated for the first time in 2005 by Abelson et al. (Abelson et al., 2005). The study reported a *de novo* inversion in a TS patient, occurring in the vicinity of the Slit and Trk-like family member 1 (*SLITRK1*) gene. The authors subsequently sequenced *SLITRK1* in 174 unrelated TS probands and identified rare mutations. This spurred intense interest in TS genetics with multiple studies reporting rather mixed results (Abelson et al., 2005; Deng et al., 2006; Keen-Kim et al., 2006; Wendland et al., 2006; Chou et al., 2007; Scharf et al., 2008; Zimprich et al., 2008; O'Roak et al., 2010; Karagiannidis et al., 2012). Recently, our group and others have provided evidence for association of the disorder with common alleles and haplotypes being over-transmitted in TS cases; these findings support the hypothesis of the existence of an as of yet unidentified risk factor in linkage disequilibrium (LD) with the associated markers and possibly lying in gene regulatory regions (Miranda et al., 2009; Karagiannidis et al., 2012).

Abnormalities of cortico-striatal-thalamic-cortical pathways and dysfunction of both dopamine and serotonin neurotransmitter systems have long been considered in association to TS (Peterson et al., 2003; Kalanithi et al., 2005; Muller-Vahl et al., 2005). The recent implication of the *L-histidine decarboxylase* (*HDC*) gene in TS etiology has also raised the intriguing hypothesis of the involvement of histaminergic neural pathways in the onset of the disorder (Ercan-Sencicek et al., 2010; Lei et al., 2012). Moreover, a genome-wide scan for *de novo* or transmitted rare copy number variants in TS had found enrichment of genes within the histamine signaling pathways (Fernandez et al., 2012). Subsequently, our group found evidence for over-transmission of *HDC* alleles and significantly associated haplotypes in trios of European origin (Karagiannidis et al., 2013).

The serotonin transporter gene (*SERT*, 5-HTT), coding for a solute carrier family 6 member 4 protein (*SLC6A4*) was reported to carry both common and rare variants as well as a high-expressing haplotype associated with increased gene expression (5-HTTLPR/rs25531/rs25532) and protein activity (p.I425V), thus potentially contributing to serotonergic abnormalities in TS with or even more so, without OCD (Kilic et al., 2003; Moya et al., 2013). These high-expressing alleles have been previously significantly associated with OCD (Hu et al., 2006; Wendland et al., 2008), which is believed to share a degree of common genetic background with TS (Mathews and Grados, 2011; Yu et al., 2015).

Variants in the BTB/POZ domain-containing protein 9 gene (*BTBD9*) have been previously associated with restless legs syndrome (RLS) (Allen et al., 2005; Winkelmann et al., 2007). High RLS prevalence has also been reported in TS and, similar to TS, it has been linked to frontostriatal circuits dysfunction and is responsive to dopamine neurotransmission modification (Turjanski et al., 1999). *BTBD9* variants were found to be associated with TS in French Canadian and Chinese patient cohorts (Riviere et al., 2009; Guo et al., 2012). Yet, all analysed variants were intronic and thus do not provide direct functional relevance; however, they could be in LD with potentially functional yet unknown variants, such as variants in gene regulatory regions or, tissue and neuroanatomical region-specific, naturally-occurring somatic mutations (Lodato et al., 2015).

The abovementioned TS susceptibility genes have emerged from candidate gene association studies (*SLC6A4*, *BTBD9*), chromosomal aberration studies (*SLITRK1*), and linkage analysis studies (*HDC*). Despite decades of efforts in the field of TS genetics, the overall number of identified variants likely predisposing to TS remains extremely small. With the advent of next-generation sequencing technology, there is a resurging interest toward the identification of rare variants of potentially intermediate-to-high penetrance effects that might aid in explaining part of the missing heritability of the TS phenotype.

In the present study we report results on a targeted re-sequencing approach in a cohort of 382 TS cases of European and Canadian origin, aiming to explore the existence of rare genetic variation across four genes that have attracted considerable interest in the past years, namely *SLITRK1*, *HDC*, *BTBD9*, and *SLC6A4*. Moreover, given the findings from our previous studies on association of *SLITRK1* and *HDC* haplotypes with TS (Karagiannidis et al., 2012, 2013), we wanted to explore whether previously associated risk haplotypes are in linkage with rare coding, and thus directly functional variants in these two genes.

MATERIALS AND METHODS

Study Subjects

A total of 382 individuals with TS were included in the study. The subjects represent affected cases from family trios who had been previously recruited within The Tourette Syndrome Genetics—Southern and Eastern Europe Initiative (TSGeneSEE) and originated from Hungary ($n = 117$), Italy ($n = 95$), Poland ($n = 68$), Greece ($n = 17$), and Albania ($n = 8$). In addition, 77 TS cases originating from Canada were also available. The majority of these individuals have been described previously (Karagiannidis et al., 2013). Assessment was performed by on-site clinicians using the tools provided by the TS Association International Consortium for Genetics (TSAICG, 2007). TS was ascertained according to DSM-IV-TR criteria for Italy, Hungary, Albania, and Greece, and DSM-IV for Poland. For Canadian samples, TS was ascertained using DSM-III-R criteria. Differences between DSM-III-R, DSM-IV, and DSM-IV-TR are minimal; the upper age limit of onset is 18 in DSM-IV (and DSM-IV-TR) and 21 in DSM-III-R, and the "marked distress" criterion, possibly pointing to more severe cases, only appears in DSM-IV (applied only to the Polish cases; Cath et al., 2011). For all samples, collection was approved by local Ethics Boards and written informed consent was taken from all participating individuals or their parents.

Genomic DNA Extraction

Peripheral blood samples were collected in EDTA-containing tubes and genomic DNA was purified using the Qiagen Gentra Puregene kit with minor protocol modifications (Qiagen GmbH, Hilden, Germany).

Exome Capture and Targeted Re-Sequencing

Using the Fluidigm custom panel design pipeline, the four candidate genes (*HDC, SLITRK1, SLC6A4, BTBD9*) were targeted for sequencing and custom primers were designed. For *HDC* and *SLITRK1*, the whole locus including 1 kb upstream and downstream were targeted. For *SLC6A4* and *BTBD9*, exonic regions of the genes were targeted (Table S1).

DNA samples were tagged and amplified using Fluidigm Access Array System (Fluidigm Corporation, South San Francisco, USA). The 48.48 Access Array integrated fluidics circuit (IFC) protocol was followed. The sample mix solution was prepared using 50 ng/uL of genomic DNA. The gDNA was then combined with sample pre-mix and loaded into the 48.48 Access Array IFC. Upon amplification completion, the IFC was placed on the Post-PCR IFC Controller AX and the Harvest (151x) Script was run. After the completion of the script 10 uL of the product was removed and placed into a 96-well PCR plate. Barcoding PCR was then set up using the manufacturer's instructions on a conventional PCR thermal cycler. With the incorporation of a unique identifier or barcode for each sample and the necessary sequencing adaptors, it is possible to process all samples simultaneously on the sequencing platform.

Quality and quantity of the library were evaluated on the Agilent BioAnalyzer (Agilent Technologies, Santa Clara, CA, US) and quantified using KAPA quantification. The sequencing was then completed following the protocol for the Illumina (Illumina, San Diego, CA) MiSeq V3 chemistry 2 × 100-bp paired-end reads. Once the sequencing was completed, de-multiplexing was performed using Illumina's bcl2fastq2 v2.15 to generate sample specific fastq files.

Sequence Alignment and Genotype Calling

Sequence alignment was performed using Burroughs Wheeler alignment (BWA; Li and Durbin, 2009) using the reference human genome build hg19 from UCSC. Samtools (Li et al., 2009) was used to convert BAM alignment files to SAM format and then sort and index them. INDEL realignment was performed using IndelRealigner and base quality score recalibration was performed using BaseRecalibrator from GATK (McKenna et al., 2010). PCR and optical duplicates were removed from samples using Picard (http://picard.sourceforge.net). Variant calling was done on the targeted regions (Table S1) by combining all the samples using the GATK pipeline and following their best practices protocol. Further filtering was applied to keep only the variants that passed the quality control filters and 95% genotype call rate. Sequencing data (BAM files) can be accessed via http://paschou-lab.mbg.duth.gr/share_data.html.

Variant Ranker Analysis

Variants were then annotated using ANNOVAR (Wang et al., 2010) and ranked using Variant Ranker tool (http://paschou-lab.mbg.duth.gr/Software.html). Variant ranker aggregates annotation information based on allelic frequency scores, conservation scores, prediction algorithm scores, and clinical information. Using Variant Ranker, the variants are prioritized on the basis of their effect, novelty, and annotation information. A variant was designated as novel if not present in database of human variation dbSNP build 138 and had a minor allele frequency (MAF) $\leq$0.01 in 1000 Genomes, Exome Aggregation Consortium (ExAC) and National Heart, Lung, and Blood Institute Exome Sequencing Project (NHLBI ESP6500) database.

VAAST Analysis

Scoring and prioritization analysis of deleterious alleles was performed using VAAST 2.0 (Hu et al., 2013). We applied the likelihood ratio test in VAAST using both dominant and recessive disease models of inheritance, with the help of a background file comprising of 189 genomes from 1000 Genomes project (Abecasis et al., 2012), 184 Danish exomes (Li et al., 2010), 10Gen genome dataset (Reese et al., 2010), and 40 whole genomes from the Complete Genomics Diversity Panel.

Identification of Linkage Disequilibrium (LD) SNPs

We used the web-based application LDproxy (Machiela and Chanock, 2015) to identify proxy LD SNPs and LdOOKUP (http://purces04.u.hpc.mssm.edu/ldookup/ldookup.cgi) to browse for variants in LD with other GWAS studies from the Psychiatric Genomics Consortium, brain eQTL data and the NHGRI GWAS catalog (Welter et al., 2014).

Sanger Sequencing

PCR primers were designed using PRIMER3 (http://primer3plus.com) and confirmed to have unique genomic product by UCSC *in-silico* PCR (http://genome.ucsc.edu/cgi-bin/hgPcr), targeting amplicons of sizes between 300 and 400 bp. PCR products were purified using QIAquick PCR purification kit from Qiagen (QIAGEN, CA), followed by Sanger sequencing on an ABI 3730xl sequencer in Genscript (NJ, USA), using the BigDye Terminator v.3.1 chemistry.

RESULTS

Identification of Variants

We explored whether coding variations in four genes, namely, *HDC, SLITRK1, BTBD9* and *SLC6A4* play a role in TS susceptibility. We utilized next-generation sequencing technology to perform targeted sequencing on a total of 60 kilobases, including the entire *HDC* and *SLITRK1* genes, and spanning 15 exons of *SLC6A4* and 11 exons of *BTBD9* genes, across 382 TS cases of Caucasian origin (Table S1). Regarding data quality, more than 95% of bases were sequenced with >99.9% accuracy, covering most amplicons at >100X.

We obtained 336 single nucleotide polymorphisms (SNPs) with 31 exonic SNPs (see summary statistics on **Table 1**). We focused only on functionally important non-synonymous exonic variants and pursued validation via Sanger sequencing. We found a novel rare (MAF = 0.13%) variant in *HDC* residing in exon 12 (*HDC*:NM_002112:exon12:c.A1564C:p.I522L), two rare (MAF = 0.13%) novel *SLITRK1* variants, at positions chr13:g.84454582 (*SLITRK1*:NM_052910:exon1:c.G1061C:p.G354A). and chr13:g.84454485 (*SLITRK1*:NM_052910:exon1:c.G1158T:p.K386N), residing in exon 1 of the gene, and two known rare variants, rs146746846 (MAF = 0.13%) (*SLITRK1*:NM_052910:exon1:c.C892T:p.H298Y) and rs150504822 (MAF = 0.26%; *SLITRK1*:NM_052910:exon1:c.A1252T:p.T418S), also in exon 1 (**Table 2**). The five confirmed variants were ranked within the top six potentially etiologically relevant variants by our Variant Ranker algorithm and were all predicted to be deleterious by MutationTaster functional prediction algorithm (Schwarz et al., 2010; Table S2). One confirmed *SLITRK1* variant (rs146746846) was also identified by VAAST under a recessive model of inheritance (Table S3). Proxy LD SNPs available for rs150504822 on *SLITRK1* were input into LdOOKUP to identify significant variants in other GWAS studies. A variant in LD with rs150504822, namely rs6563353, was identified (Tables S4, S5); rs6563353 has been positively associated (p = 2.06e-6) with increased citalopram-induced general side effect burden, in patients with depression (Adkins et al., 2012). Citalopram is an antidepressant drug of the selective serotonin reuptake inhibitor class, with an off-label use for OCD treatment.

TABLE 1 | Summary of functional annotation of identified variants.

Variant category	Number of variants
Upstream	23
5′UTR	9
Coding (Exonic)	31
Intronic	205
3′UTR	40
Downstream	17
Intergenic	11
Total	336
Nonsynonymous	17
Synonymous	14
Total Coding	31

UTR, Untranslated region.

DISCUSSION

To our knowledge, this is the first study applying next generation sequencing technology in quest for genetic susceptibility variants shaping the genomic landscape of TS. It is expected that at least part of the missing heritability of complex disorders, such as TS, will be attributable to low-frequency variants with intermediate penetrance effects (Manolio et al., 2009) and, if truly causative, they could account for a small proportion of TS cases.

In the present study, we identified and confirmed a rare novel *HDC* coding variant as well as two rare novel and two rare known *SLITRK1* coding variants, all confirmed by Sanger sequencing (**Table 2**). We did not extensively cover the regulatory regions of the genes; thus, regulatory variants may have been missed resulting in under-estimation of the contribution of these genes to TS risk.

The recent implication of the *L-histidine decarboxylase* (*HDC*) gene in TS etiology has raised the intriguing hypothesis of the involvement of histaminergic neural pathways in the onset of the disorder. Ercan-Sencicek et al. studied a family with a father and all eight of his children affected with TS, and found a rare premature termination codon mutation (p.W317X) in *HDC*, also absent in 3,000 control individuals. Due to the demonstrated dominant-negative mode of function of the mutant HDC enzyme, the authors concluded that histaminergic neurotransmission is most likely diminished in their patients (Ercan-Sencicek et al., 2010). However, *HDC* coding variants seem to be extremely rare since apart from the mutation identified in the original pedigree, *HDC* has not been found altered in other TS cases of Caucasian or Asian origin (Ercan-Sencicek et al., 2010; Lei et al., 2012). Interestingly, a preceding genome-wide study of 95 French Canadian trios with familial history of TS (Riviere et al., 2010) had also shown association to a microsatellite marker on chromosome 15 (D15S1016), lying within the same interval found to be linked with TS in the original study that implicated *HDC* in TS etiology. Finally, a recent genome-wide scan for *de novo* or transmitted rare copy number variants in TS found enrichment of genes within the histamine receptor signaling pathways (Fernandez et al., 2012). Even though in the present study we did not detect the rare variants previously reported in the literature, we did find a novel exonic nonsynonymous variant, chr15:g.50534882 (c.A1564C:p.I522L), in one TS case.

Histamine plays a central role in gastric acid secretion, innate, and acquired immunity and immunomodulation, bronchoconstriction, vasodilation and neurotransmission. The neuronal histaminergic system is involved in a number of basic physiological functions such as circadian rhythmicity, energy metabolism, neuro-endocrine homeostasis, stress, sensory, and motor functions, cognition, attention, learning,

TABLE 2 | Nonsynonymous variants confirmed by Sanger sequencing.

Location	Ref/Alt	Het	Gene	RefGene variant annotation	1000G	LRT	MutationTaster
chr13:84454582	C/G	1	*SLITRK1*	*SLITRK1*:NM_052910:exon1:c.G1061C:p.G354A	NA	D	D
chr13:84454485	C/A	1	*SLITRK1*	*SLITRK1*:NM_052910:exon1:c.G1158T:p.K386N	NA	D	D
chr13:84454751(rs146746846)	G/A	1	*SLITRK1*	*SLITRK1*:NM_052910:exon1:c.C892T:p.H298Y	NA	D	D
chr13:84454391(rs150504822)	T/A	2	*SLITRK1*	*SLITRK1*:NM_052910:exon1:c.A1252T:p.T418S	0.00019	D	D
chr15:50534882	T/G	1	*HDC*	*HDC*:NM_002112:exon12: c.A1564C:p.I522L	NA	N	D

Chr, chromosomal location; Ref, Reference allele; Alt, Alternative (rare) allele; Het, Number of heterozygous cases with the variant; 1000G, 1000 Genomes Project variant frequency (if available); LRT, Likelihood Ratio Test; LRT D, Deleterious; N, Neutral; MutationTaster D, Disease-causing; NA, Not available.

and memory. Histidine decarboxylase (HDC) is the key enzyme for histamine production from histidine and in the brain its mRNA is expressed exclusively in the posterior hypothalamus (Haas et al., 2008). So far, the histaminergic system has not received as much attention as other monoaminergic systems of the brain. Classically established as a "peripherally" important mediator of inflammation, the importance of histamine in neurotransmission, and its role in neuropsychiatric disorders is only recently starting to become appreciated (Tiligada et al., 2011) and deserves further investigation also in the context of TS. Interestingly, $Hdc^{-/-}$ deficient mice have several traits relevant to features of TS and have shown decreased brain histamine and increased sensitivity to stereotypic behaviors (i.e., hyperlocomotion) upon administration of dopamine agonists (Kubota et al., 2002) and repetitive grooming after induced fear (Xu et al., 2015). Such stimulant-induced movements, including rearing, sniffing, and biting have previously been proposed as a model of human tics (Saka and Graybiel, 2003; Castellan Baldan et al., 2014).

SLITRK1 has been extensively studied since its identification as a much promising TS candidate gene. However, with the exception of the variants reported by Abelson et al. (2005), additional novel non-synonymous mutations have not been identified in a large number of subsequent studies interrogating patient cohorts (Deng et al., 2006; Chou et al., 2007; Scharf et al., 2008; Zimprich et al., 2008) or single families (Robertson and Orth, 2006; Verkerk et al., 2006; Fabbrini et al., 2007; Pasquini et al., 2008). On the other hand, genetic association studies and haplotype analyses could not rule out the implication of *SLITRK1* in TS etiology either via the existence of risk factors in LD with *SLITRK1* (Miranda et al., 2009) or as of yet unidentified SLITRK1 regulatory variants (Karagiannidis et al., 2012). In our study, we did not detect the SLITRK1 variants that had been previously reported in association to TS but we report on the identification of two novel variants, chr13:g.84454582 and chr13:g.84454485, each found in one TS patient. We also identified two rare non-synonymous SLITRK1 variants (rs150504822 and rs146746846, identified in two TS cases and one TS case, respectively). Interestingly, rs150504822 was found in LD with rs6563353, a variant that has been previously associated with citalopram-induced general side-effect burden in patients with depression (Adkins et al., 2012). Citalopram, is a well-tolerated acute treatment drug conferring positive response in children and adolescents with OCD (Thomsen et al., 2001; Mukaddes et al., 2003).

Interestingly, *SLITRK1* encodes a transmembrane protein necessary for dendritic growth, axon guidance and branching of neuronal cells. It is expressed in both the embryonic and postnatal brain (cortex, thalamus, and basal ganglia), reflecting neuroanatomical regions most commonly affected in TS (Proenca et al., 2011), as well as in mature neurons with large axons (Aruga and Mikoshiba, 2003). $Slitrk1^{-/-}$ mice exhibited elevated anxiety and depression-like behaviour, consistent with TS symptoms, in which the anxiety-like behaviour was attenuated upon clonidine administration, a drug often used in TS treatment (Katayama et al., 2010).

Our previous and present studies suggest that *SLITRK1* and *HDC* may have an under-appreciated role in TS aetiology. Unarguably, the functional role of the identified variants warrants further investigation by a wide array of experiments. Next-generation sequencing technology is rapidly becoming a routine, albeit still costly approach to target patient genomes that is expected to significantly expedite the quest for rare variants with reduced penetrance, not only in TS susceptibility but also other complex neurodevelopmental and neuropsychiatric disorders.

AUTHOR CONTRIBUTIONS

JA, HP, JX, LD, and IK performed experimental procedures, data analysis and interpretation, and participated in manuscript writing. FT and PD participated in data analysis and interpretation, and in manuscript writing. ZT, RR, TW, LF, PN, US, CA, VT, AK, CB, PS, and CLB performed patient sample recruitment and ascertainment, and participated in data analysis and interpretation. JT, PP, GH, and MG designed the study, supervised experimental procedures, performed data analysis and interpretation, and wrote the manuscript. All authors read and approved the final version to be published and agreed to be accountable for all aspects of the work.

ACKNOWLEDGMENTS

We are indebted to the TS individuals and their families for accepting to participate in the studies of the genetic basis of TS. This study was made possible thanks to the collaborative efforts of Tourette Syndrome Genetics—Southern and Eastern Europe Initiative (TSGeneSEE) and COST Action BM905: European Network for the Study of GTS (EUNETGTS). This project was financed by FP7-PEOPLE-2012-ITN, project: TS-EUROTRAIN, grant number 316978, and grants from the National Institute of Mental Health [R01MH092293; U24MH068457] and the Human Genetics Institute of New Jersey. The collection of Canadian families for this study was supported by grants from The Tourette Syndrome Association of America, N.I.H. grant MS40024-01, the Ontario Mental Health Foundation, and The Tourette Syndrome Foundation of Canada. CB was supported by the Merit-prize scholarship of Semmelweis University and the János Bolyai Research Scholarship of the Hungarian Academy of Sciences BO/00987/16/5.

SUPPLEMENTARY MATERIAL

The Supplementary Material for this article can be found online at: http://journal.frontiersin.org/article/10.3389/fnins.2016.00428

REFERENCES

Abecasis, G. R., Auton, A., Brooks, L. D., DePristo, M. A., Durbin, R. M., Handsaker, R. E., et al. (2012). An integrated map of genetic variation from 1,092 human genomes. *Nature* 491, 56–65. doi: 10.1038/nature11632

Abelson, J. F., Kwan, K. Y., O'Roak, B. J., Baek, D. Y., Stillman, A. A., Morgan, T. M., et al. (2005). Sequence variants in SLITRK1 are associated with Tourette's syndrome. *Science* 310, 317–320. doi: 10.1126/science.1116502

Adkins, D. E., Clark, S. L., Åberg, K., Hettema, J. M., Bukszár, J., McClay, J. L., et al. (2012). Genome-wide pharmacogenomic study of citalopram-induced side effects in STAR*D. *Transl. Psychiatry* 2, e129. doi: 10.1038/tp.2012.57

Allen, R. P., Walters A. S., Montplaisir, J., Hening, W., Myers, A., Bell, T. J., et al. (2005). Restless legs syndrome prevalence and impact: REST general population study. *Arch. Intern. Med.* 165, 1286–1292. doi: 10.1001/archinte.165.11.1286

Aruga, J., and Mikoshiba, K. (2003). Identification and characterization of Slitrk, a novel neuronal transmembrane protein family controlling neurite outgrowth. *Mol. Cell. Neurosci.* 24, 117–129. doi: 10.1016/S1044-7431(03)00129-5

Castellan Baldan, L., Williams, K. A., Gallezot, J.-D., Pogorelov, V., Rapanelli, M., Crowley, M., et al. (2014). Histidine decarboxylase deficiency causes tourette syndrome: parallel findings in humans and mice. *Neuron* 81, 77–90. doi: 10.1016/j.neuron.2013.10.052

Cath, D. C., Hedderly, T., Ludolph, A. G., Stern, J. S., Murphy, T., Hartmann, A., et al. (2011). European clinical guidelines for Tourette syndrome and other tic disorders. *Eur. Child Adolesc. Psychiatry* 20, 155–171. doi: 10.1007/s00787-011-0164-6

Chou, I.-C., Wan, L. Liu, S.-C., Tsai, C.-H., and Tsai, F.-J. (2007). Association of the Slit and Trk-like 1 gene in Taiwanese patients with Tourette syndrome. *Pediatr. Neurol.* 37, 404–406. doi: 10.1016/j.pediatrneurol.2007.06.017

Deng, H., Le, W. D., Xie, W. J., and Jankovic, J. (2006). Examination of the SLITRK1 gene in Caucasian patients with Tourette syndrome. *Acta Neurol. Scand.* 114, 400–402. doi: 10.1111/j.1600-0404.2006.00706.x

Ercan-Sencicek, A. G., Stillman, A. A., Ghosh, A. K., Bilguvar, K., O'Roak, B. J., Mason, C. E., et al. (2010). L-histidine decarboxylase and Tourette's syndrome. *N. Engl. J. Med.* 362, 1901–1908. doi: 10.1056/NEJMoa0907006

Fabbrini, G., Pasquini, M., Aurilia, C., Berardelli, I., Breedveld, G., Oostra, B. A., et al. (2007). A large Italian family with Gilles de la Tourette syndrome: clinical study and analysis of the SLITRK1 gene. *Mov. Disord.* 22, 2229–2234. doi: 10.1002/mds.21697

Fernandez, T. V., Sanders, S. J., Yurkiewicz, I. R., Ercan-Sencicek, A. G., Kim, Y.-S., Fishman, D. O., et al. (2012). Rare copy number variants in tourette syndrome disrupt genes in histaminergic pathways and overlap with autism. *Biol. Psychiatry* 71, 392–402. doi: 10.1016/j.biopsych.2011.09.034

Guo, Y., Su, L., Zhang, J., Lei, J., Deng, X., Xu, H., et al. (2012). Analysis of the BTBD9 and HTR2C variants in Chinese Han patients with Tourette syndrome. *Psychiatr. Genet.* 22, 300–303. doi: 10.1097/YPG.0b013e32835862b1

Haas, H. L., Sergeeva, O. A., and Selbach, O. (2008). Histamine in the nervous system. *Physiol Rev.* 88, 1183–1241. doi: 10.1152/physrev.00043.2007

Hoekstra, P. J., Dietrich, A., Edwards, M. J., Elamin, I., and Martino, D. (2013). Environmental factors in Tourette syndrome. *Neurosci. Biobehav. Rev.* 37, 1040–1049. doi: 10.1016/j.neubiorev.2012.10.010

Hu, H., Huff, C. D., Moore, B., Flygare, S., Reese, M. G., and Yandell, M. (2013). VAAST 2.0: improved variant classification and disease-gene identification using a conservation-controlled amino acid substitution matrix. *Genet. Epidemiol.* 37, 622–634. doi: 10.1002/gepi.21743

Hu, X.-Z., Lipsky, R. H., Zhu, G., Akhtar, L. A., Taubman, J., Greenberg, B. D., et al. (2006). Serotonin transporter promoter gain-of-function genotypes are linked to obsessive-compulsive disorder. *Am. J. Hum. Genet.* 78, 815–826. doi: 10.1086/503850

Kalanithi, P. S., Zheng, W., Kataoka, Y., DiFiglia, M., Grantz, H., Saper, C. B., et al. (2005). Altered parvalbumin-positive neuron distribution in basal ganglia of individuals with Tourette syndrome. *Proc. Natl. Acad. Sci. U.S.A.* 102, 13307–13312. doi: 10.1073/pnas.0502624102

Karagiannidis, I., Dehning, S., Sandor, P., Tarnok, Z., Rizzo, R., Wolanczyk, T., et al. (2013). Support of the histaminergic hypothesis in Tourette syndrome: association of the histamine decarboxylase gene in a large sample of families. *J. Med. Genet.* 50, 760–764. doi: 10.1136/jmedgenet-2013-101637

Karagiannidis, I., Rizzo, R., Tarnok, Z., Wolanczyk, T., Hebebrand, J., Nöthen, M. M., et al. (2012). Replication of association between a SLITRK1 haplotype and Tourette Syndrome in a large sample of families. *Mol. Psychiatry* 17, 665–668. doi: 10.1038/mp.2011.151

Katayama, K., Yamada, K., Ornthanalai, V. G., Inoue, T., Ota, M., Murphy, N. P., et al. (2010). Slitrk1-deficient mice display elevated anxiety-like behavior and noradrenergic abnormalities. *Mol. Psychiatry* 15, 177–184. doi: 10.1038/mp.2008.97

Keen-Kim, D., Mathews, C. A., Reus, V. I., Lowe, T. L., Herrera, L. D., Budman, C. L., et al. (2006). Overrepresentation of rare variants in a specific ethnic group may confuse interpretation of association analyses. *Hum. Mol. Genet.* 15, 3324–3328. doi: 10.1093/hmg/ddl408

Kilic, F., Murphy, D. L., and Rudnick, G. (2003). A human serotonin transporter mutation causes constitutive activation of transport activity. *Mol. Pharmacol.* 64, 440–446. doi: 10.1124/mol.64.2.440

Kubota, Y., Ito, C., Sakurai, E., Sakurai, E., Watanabe, T., and Ohtsu, H. (2002). Increased methamphetamine-induced locomotor activity and behavioral sensitization in histamine-deficient mice. *J. Neurochem.* 83, 837–845. doi: 10.1046/j.1471-4159.2002.01189.x

Lei, J., Deng, X., Zhang, J., Su, L., Xu, H., Liang, H., et al. (2012). Mutation screening of the HDC gene in Chinese Han patients with Tourette syndrome. *Am. J. Med. Genet. B. Neuropsychiatr. Genet.* 159B, 72–76. doi: 10.1002/ajmg.b.32003

Li, H., and Durbin, R. (2009). Fast and accurate short read alignment with Burrows-Wheeler transform. *Bioinformatics* 25, 1754–1760. doi: 10.1093/bioinformatics/btp324

Li, H., Handsaker, B., Wysoker, A., Fennell, T., Ruan, J., Homer, N., et al. (2009). The Sequence Alignment/Map format and SAMtools. *Bioinformatics* 25, 2078–2079. doi: 10.1093/bioinformatics/btp352

Li, Y., Vinckenbosch, N., Tian, G., Huerta-Sanchez, E., Jiang, T., Jiang, H., et al. (2010). Resequencing of 200 human exomes identifies an excess of low-frequency non-synonymous coding variants. *Nat. Genet.* 42, 969–972. doi: 10.1038/ng.680

Lodato, M. A., Woodworth, M. B., Lee, S., Evrony, G. D., Mehta, B. K., Karger, A., et al. (2015). Somatic mutation in single human neurons tracks developmental and transcriptional history. *Science* 350, 94–98. doi: 10.1126/science.aab1785

Machiela, M. J., and Chanock, S. J. (2015). LDlink: a web-based application for exploring population-specific haplotype structure and linking correlated alleles of possible functional variants. *Bioinformatics* 31, 3555–3557. doi: 10.1093/bioinformatics/btv402

Manolio, T. A., Collins, F. S., Cox, N. J., Goldstein, D. B., Hindorff, L. A., Hunter, D. J., et al. (2009). Finding the missing heritability of complex diseases. *Nature* 461, 747–753. doi: 10.1038/nature08494

Mathews, C. A., and Grados, M. A. (2011). Familiality of Tourette syndrome, obsessive-compulsive disorder, and attention-deficit/hyperactivity disorder:

heritability analysis in a large sib-pair sample. *J. Am. Acad. Child Adolesc. Psychiatry* 50, 46–54. doi: 10.1016/j.jaac.2010.10.004

Mathews, C. A., Scharf, J. M., Miller, L. L., MacDonald-Wallis, C., Lawlor, D. A., and Ben-Shlomo, Y. (2014). Association between pre- and perinatal exposures and Tourette syndrome or chronic tic disorder in the ALSPAC cohort. *Br. J. Psychiatry* 204, 40–45. doi: 10.1192/bjp.bp.112.125468

McKenna, A., Hanna, M., Banks, E., Sivachenko, A., Cibulskis, K., Kernytsky, A., et al. (2010). The genome analysis toolkit: a MapReduce framework for analyzing next-generation DNA sequencing data. *Genome Res.* 20, 1297–1303. doi: 10.1101/gr.107524.110

Miranda, D. M., Wigg, K., Kabia, E. M., Feng, Y., Sandor, P., and Barr, C. L. (2009). Association of SLITRK1 to Gilles de la Tourette Syndrome. *Am. J. Med. Genet. B Neuropsychiatr. Genet.* 150B, 483–486. doi: 10.1002/ajmg.b.30840

Moya, P. R., Wendland, J. R., Rubenstein, L. M., Timpano, K. R., Heiman, G. A., Tischfield, J. A., et al. (2013). Common and rare alleles of the serotonin transporter gene, SLC6A4, associated with Tourette's disorder. *Mov. Disord.* 28, 1263–1270. doi: 10.1002/mds.25460

Mukaddes, N. M., Abali, O., and Kaynak, N. (2003). Citalopram treatment of children and adolescents with obsessive-compulsive disorder: a preliminary report. *Psychiatry Clin. Neurosci.* 57, 405–408. doi: 10.1046/j.1440-1819.2003.01139.x

Muller-Vahl, K. R., Meyer, G. J., Knapp, W. H., Emrich, H. M., Gielow, P., Brucke, T., et al. (2005). Serotonin transporter binding in Tourette Syndrome. *Neurosci. Lett.* 385, 120–125. doi: 10.1016/j.neulet.2005.05.031

O'Roak, B. J., Morgan, T. M., Fishman, D. O., Saus, E., Alonso, P., Gratacos, M., et al. (2010). Additional support for the association of SLITRK1 var321 and Tourette syndrome. *Mol. Psychiatry* 15, 447–450. doi: 10.1038/mp.2009.105

Pasquini, M., Fabbrini, G., Berardelli, I., Bonifati, V., Biondi, M., and Berardelli, A. (2008). Psychopathological features of obsessive-compulsive disorder in an Italian family with Gilles de la Tourette syndrome not linked to the SLITRK1 gene. *Psychiatry Res.* 161, 109–111. doi: 10.1016/j.psychres.2008.02.012

Pauls, D. L., Fernandez, T. V., Mathews, C. A., State, M. W., and Scharf, J. M. (2014). The Inheritance of Tourette Disorder: a review. *J. Obsessive Compuls. Relat. Disord.* 3, 380–385. doi: 10.1016/j.jocrd.2014.06.003

Pauls, D. L., Raymond, C. L., Stevenson, J. M., and Leckman, J. F. (1991). A family study of Gilles de la Tourette syndrome. *Am. J. Hum. Genet.* 48, 154–163.

Peterson, B. S., Thomas, P., Kane, M. J., Scahill, L., Zhang, H., Bronen, R., et al. (2003). Basal Ganglia volumes in patients with Gilles de la Tourette syndrome. *Arch. Gen. Psychiatry* 60, 415–424. doi: 10.1001/archpsyc.60.4.415

Price, R. A., Kidd, K. K., Cohen, D. J., Pauls, D. L., and Leckman, J. F. (1985). A twin study of Tourette syndrome. *Arch. Gen. Psychiatry* 42, 815–820. doi: 10.1001/archpsyc.1985.01790310077011

Proenca, C. C., Gao, K. P., Shmelkov, S. V., Rafii, S., and Lee, F. S. (2011). Slitrks as emerging candidate genes involved in neuropsychiatric disorders. *Trends Neurosci.* 34, 143–153. doi: 10.1016/j.tins.2011.01.001

Reese, M. G., Moore, B., Batchelor, C., Salas, F., Cunningham, F., Marth, G. T., et al. (2010). A standard variation file format for human genome sequences. *Genome Biol.* 11:R88. doi: 10.1186/gb-2010-11-8-r88

Riviere, J.-B., St-Onge, J., Gaspar, C., Diab, S., Dion, Y., Lesperance, P., et al. (2010). Genome-wide TDT analysis in French-Canadian families with Tourette syndrome. *Can. J. Neurol. Sci.* 37, 110–112. doi: 10.1017/S0317167100009744

Riviere, J.-B., Xiong, L., Levchenko, A., St-Onge, J., Gaspar, C., Dion, Y., et al. (2009). Association of intronic variants of the BTBD9 gene with Tourette syndrome. *Arch. Neurol.* 66, 1267–1272. doi: 10.1001/archneurol.2009.213

Robertson, M. M., and Orth, M. (2006). Behavioral and affective disorders in Tourette syndrome. *Adv. Neurol.* 99, 39–60.

Saka, E., and Graybiel, A. M. (2003). Pathophysiology of Tourette's syndrome: striatal pathways revisited. *Brain Dev.* 25(Suppl. 1), S15–S19. doi: 10.1016/S0387-7604(03)90002-7

Scharf, J. M., Moorjani, P., Fagerness, J., Platko, J. V., Illmann, C., Galloway, B., et al. (2008). Lack of association between SLITRK1var321 and Tourette syndrome in a large family-based sample. *Neurology* 70, 1495–1496. doi: 10.1212/01.wnl.0000296833.25484.bb

Schwarz, J. M., Rodelsperger, C., Schuelke, M., and Seelow, D. (2010). MutationTaster evaluates disease-causing potential of sequence alterations. *Nat. Methods* 7, 575–576. doi: 10.1038/nmeth0810-575

Thomsen, P. H., Ebbesen, C., and Persson, C. (2001). Long-term experience with citalopram in the treatment of adolescent OCD. *J. Am. Acad. Child Adolesc. Psychiatry* 40, 895–902. doi: 10.1097/00004583-200108000-00010

Tiligada, E., Kyriakidis, K., Chazot, P. L., and Passani, M. B. (2011). Histamine pharmacology and new CNS drug targets. *CNS Neurosci. Ther.* 17, 620–628. doi: 10.1111/j.1755-5949.2010.00212.x

TSAICG (2007). Genome scan for Tourette disorder in affected-sibling-pair and multigenerational families. *Am. J. Hum. Genet.* 80, 265–272. doi: 10.1086/511052

Turjanski, N., Lees, A. J., and Brooks, D. J. (1999). Striatal dopaminergic function in restless legs syndrome: 18F-dopa and 11C-raclopride PET studies. *Neurology* 52, 932–937. doi: 10.1212/WNL.52.5.932

Verkerk, A. J., Cath, D. C., van der Linde, H. C., Both, J., Heutink, P., Breedveld, G., et al. (2006). Genetic and clinical analysis of a large Dutch Gilles de la Tourette family. *Mol. Psychiatry* 11, 954–964. doi: 10.1038/sj.mp.4001877

Wang, K., Li, M., and Hakonarson, H. (2010). ANNOVAR: functional annotation of genetic variants from high-throughput sequencing data. *Nucleic Acids Res.* 38, e164. doi: 10.1093/nar/gkq603

Welter, D., MacArthur, J., Morales, J., Burdett, T., Hall, P., Junkins, H., et al. (2014). The NHGRI GWAS Catalog, a curated resource of SNP-trait associations. *Nucleic Acids Res.* 42, D1001–D1006. doi: 10.1093/nar/gkt1229

Wendland, J. R., DeGuzman, T. B., McMahon, F., Rudnick, G., Detera-Wadleigh, S. D., and Murphy, D. L. (2008). SERT Ileu425Val in autism, Asperger syndrome and obsessive-compulsive disorder. *Psychiatr. Genet.* 18, 31–39. doi: 10.1097/YPG.0b013e3282f08a06

Wendland, J. R., Kruse, M. R., and Murphy, D. L. (2006). Functional SLITRK1 var321, varCDfs and SLC6A4 G56A variants and susceptibility to obsessive-compulsive disorder. *Mol. Psychiatry* 11, 802–804. doi: 10.1038/sj.mp.4001848

Winkelmann, J., Schormair, B., Lichtner, P., Ripke, S., Xiong, L., Jalilzadeh, S., et al. (2007). Genome-wide association study of restless legs syndrome identifies common variants in three genomic regions. *Nat. Genet.* 39, 1000–1006. doi: 10.1038/ng2099

Xu, M., Li, L., Ohtsu, H., and Pittenger, C. (2015). Histidine decarboxylase knockout mice, a genetic model of Tourette syndrome, show repetitive grooming after induced fear. *Neurosci. Lett.* 595, 50–53. doi: 10.1016/j.neulet.2015.03.067

Yu, D., Mathews, C. A., Scharf, J. M., Neale, B. M., Davis, L. K., Gamazon, E. R., et al. (2015). Cross-disorder genome-wide analyses suggest a complex genetic relationship between Tourette's syndrome and OCD. *Am. J. Psychiatry* 172, 82–93. doi: 10.1176/appi.ajp.2014.13101306

Zimprich, A., Hatala, K., Riederer, F., Stogmann, E., Aschauer, H. N., and Stamenkovic, M. (2008). Sequence analysis of the complete SLITRK1 gene in Austrian patients with Tourette's disorder. *Psychiatr. Genet.* 18, 308–309. doi: 10.1097/YPG.0b013e3283060f6f

22

The Impact of a Cognitive–Behavioral Therapy on Event-Related Potentials in Patients with Tic Disorders or Body-Focused Repetitive Behaviors

Simon Morand-Beaulieu[1,2,3]*, Kieron P. O'Connor*[2,4]*, Maxime Richard*[1,2,3]*, Geneviève Sauvé*[1,2]*, Julie B. Leclerc*[2,5]*, Pierre J. Blanchet*[2,6] *and Marc E. Lavoie*[1,2,4]***

[1] Laboratoire de psychophysiologie cognitive et sociale, Montreal, QC, Canada, [2] Centre de recherche de l'Institut universitaire en sante mentale de Montréal, Montreal, QC, Canada, [3] Département de neurosciences, Faculté de médecine, Université de Montréal, Montreal, QC, Canada, [4] Département de psychiatrie, Faculté de médecine, Université de Montréal, Montreal, QC, Canada, [5] Département de psychologie, Faculté des sciences humaines, Université du Québec à Montréal, Montreal, QC, Canada, [6] Département de stomatologie, Faculté de médecine dentaire, Université de Montréal, Montreal, QC, Canada

Edited by:
Kirsten R. Müller-Vahl, Hannover Medical School, Hannover, Germany

Reviewed by:
Katja Biermann-Ruben, Institute of Clinical Neuroscience and Medical Psychology, Germany
Joseph Mcguire, UCLA, USA

Correspondence:
Marc E. Lavoie
marc.lavoie@umontreal.ca

Context: Tic disorders (TD) are characterized by the presence of non-voluntary contractions of functionally related groups of skeletal muscles in one or multiple body parts. Patients with body-focused repetitive behaviors (BFRB) present frequent and repetitive behaviors, such as nail biting or hair pulling. TD and BFRB can be treated with a cognitive–behavioral therapy (CBT) that regulates the excessive amount of sensorimotor activation and muscular tension. Our CBT, which is called the cognitive–psychophysiological (CoPs) model, targets motor execution and inhibition, and it was reported to modify brain activity in TD. However, psychophysiological effects of therapy are still poorly understood in TD and BFRB patients. Our goals were to compare the event-related potentials (ERP) of TD and BFRB patients to control participants and to investigate the effects of the CoPs therapy on the P200, N200, and P300 components during a motor and a non-motor oddball task.

Method: Event-related potential components were compared in 26 TD patients, 27 BFRB patients, and 27 control participants. ERP were obtained from 63 EEG electrodes during two oddball tasks. In the non-motor task, participants had to count rare stimuli. In the motor task, participants had to respond with a left and right button press for rare and frequent stimuli, respectively. ERP measures were recorded before and after therapy in both patient groups.

Results: CoPs therapy improved symptoms similarly in both clinical groups. Before therapy, TD and BFRB patients had reduced P300 oddball effect during the non-motor task, in comparison with controls participants. An increase in the P300 oddball effect was observed posttherapy. This increase was distributed over the whole cortex in BFRB patients, but localized in the parietal area in TD patients.

Discussion: These results suggest a modification of neural processes following CoPs therapy in TD and BFRB patients. CoPs therapy seems to impact patients' attentional processes and context updating capacities in working memory (i.e., P300 component). Our results are consistent with a possible role of the prefrontal cortex and corpus callosum in mediating interhemispheric interference in TD.

Keywords: Tourette syndrome, tic disorders, body-focused repetitive behaviors, habit disorder, cognitive–behavioral therapy, cognitive–psychophysiological therapy, event-related potentials, electrophysiology

INTRODUCTION

Tic disorders (TD) are characterized by repetitive non-voluntary contractions of functionally related groups of skeletal muscles in one or more parts of the body, including blinking, cheek twitches, and head or knee jerks among others. Tics can also be more complex and take the form of self-inflicted repetitive actions, such as teeth grinding, head slapping, or tense-release hand gripping cycles. They also appear as more purposive and stereotyped movements of longer duration, such as facial gestures and grooming-like movements. Furthermore, tics can be vocal, and they range from simple sounds, such as sniffing, coughing, or barking, to more complex vocalizations, such as echolalia or coprolalia. The tics may wax and wane over the course of weeks, months, and years. They can appear in bouts many times a day with onset longer than a year and arise prior to 18 years old with a peak in symptoms intensity around 12 years old. Tourette syndrome, which is the best known TD, involves multiple motor tics and at least one vocal tic. In comparison, persistent TD implies either motor or phonic tics, but not both. Tourette syndrome and persistent TD patients are often pooled together as a sole group, and the need for a distinction between both has been debated, since phonic tics have an inherent motor component (1).

Recent brain imaging investigations have revealed impairment in cortico-striato-thalamo-cortical (CSTC) pathways, which assure the communication between the basal ganglia and the motor cortex (2–4). At the cortical level, the overactivity of the supplementary motor area (SMA) was also observed in TD. The SMA is an important structure related, in large part, to the generation of tics and also to sensory urges (5, 6). Consistent with these findings, gray matter thinning was also found within the SMA, and this was also correlated to the severity of tics (7) and premonitory urges (8).

The large majority of patients with TD also face various comorbidities (9), which include obsessive–compulsive disorder (OCD) or at least some obsessive–compulsive symptoms (OCS), attention-deficit hyperactivity disorder (ADHD), depression, and anxiety disorders. Another pathology often associated with TD is body-focused repetitive behaviors (BFRB), also known as habit disorder. BFRB represent a clinical term that includes various diagnoses, such as trichotillomania, skin picking, and onychophagia. Despite the heterogeneity of symptoms comprised of the BFRB category, their main symptoms are directed toward the body, in reaction to feelings of discomfort, which is often present in TD. In the DSM-IV-TR, trichotillomania was categorized as an impulse control disorder, not elsewhere classified, and was associated with skin picking and onychophagia (10). In the DSM-V, trichotillomania and skin picking are now classified within the obsessive–compulsive and related disorders category, while onychophagia and dermatophagia are mentioned as "other specified obsessive–compulsive and related disorders." Despite the fact that these disorders have been relocated to the obsessive–compulsive category, impulse control and feeling of sensory discomfort remain an important communality of their profile. This incapacity to resist a specific impulse or urge is a characteristic shared with TD patients. Both groups also show heightened levels of sensorimotor activation (11–13). However, even though BFRB resemble to TD in certain ways and these two disorders sometimes co-occur with one another, it must be noted that are different diagnoses.

There is a clear benefit in distinguishing between TD and BFRB, for the reason that the relationship between these two entities is sometimes clinically unclear, because the presence of complex movements in BFRB can often be confounded with complex tics. We propose that a reasonable method of differentiating these two groups would be to compare directly their brain activity during the performance of contrasting tasks with different levels of motor demand. For instance, O'Connor et al. (14) reported that TD and BFRB patients both failed to adequately adjust their hand responses to automated or controlled movements. More precisely, TD patients had the most severe impairment in synchronizing motor-related brain activity with their actual response time, followed by the BFRB and the control groups. These findings give support to a dimensional model of classification with BFRB falling between TD and controls along a continuum of motor arousal.

Recent brain imaging investigations on trichotillomania suggest that BFRB could share common impaired neural networks with TD, affecting mainly motor processing. For instance, increased gray matter density in the left striatum, the left amygdalohippocampal formation, the cingulate gyrus, the SMA, and the frontal cortex was found in trichotillomania (15). Furthermore, BFRB patients with trichotillomania or skin picking as their main habit have less fractional anisotropy in the anterior cingulate and temporal areas, which indicate a lower fiber density, axonal diameter, and myelination in white matter tracts involved in motor habits generation and suppression (16, 17). Additional circuits seem affected in unmedicated TD, where engagement in habit formation behavior correlated with greater connectivity of motor structures in the right hemisphere and stronger structural connectivity between the SMA and the putamen, which predicted more severe tics (18). All in all, aberrant reinforcement signals to the sensorimotor cortex and the striatum might be crucial for habit formation and tic generation as well. These areas are all known to be involved in cognition and habit learning and could contribute to the development of pathological habits, but more research are needed to incorporate other types of impulse control disorders.

Another good reason to characterize TD and BFRB is mainly related to their response to treatment. Currently, cognitive–behavioral therapy (CBT) constitutes an effective line of treatment for adults with both TD (19, 20) and BFRB (21–24), but the cognitive–behavioral and physiological outcomes are not well understood. The therapy proposed by our group is based on the cognitive–psychophysiological (CoPs) model and aims at regulating the high level of sensorimotor activation present in these populations and preventing the build-up of tension that leads to tic bursts or to the compulsive habit related to BFRB (12, 25, 26). Its effectiveness in treating adults affected by either disorder has been demonstrated many times (26–28). The positive effects of the CoPs therapy in TD patients are also reflected at the cerebral level. This was first reported with a TD group, which showed reduced electrocortical activity related to the inhibition of automatic motor responses. It was shown that the motor-related brain response during automatic inhibition, normalized following successful CoPs therapy (29). These results are also consistent with fMRI recordings during a motor inhibition task, which found a significant decrease in putamen activation after cognitive–behavioral treatment in adult TD (30). More recently, the CoPs therapy induced a reduction of the lateralized readiness potentials, a brain electrical potential partly generated by the SMA and the basal ganglia (13). Thus, these results are strongly consistent with the cortical–striatal and basal ganglia impairment hypothesis in TD. More importantly, these results showed that psychological treatments have the potential to induce changes in behavior and cognitive processes that are followed by modification of brain activity. The next question to explore is the cerebral impact of therapy in the BFRB.

One effective way to follow various levels of cognitive and electrocortical activity within milliseconds accuracy is the use of event-related potentials (ERPs). Thus, we specifically aimed at the investigation of three ERP components, the P200, the N200, and the P300 recorded at pre- and posttherapy. The P200 is a component that indexes evaluation of stimulus salience and its task-related adequacy (31, 32). The N200 indexes target detection and conflict monitoring (33), whereas the P300 is related to stimulus evaluation and context updating in working memory (34). To the best of our knowledge, no study has, so far, investigated the ERPs in BFRB patients, although several have studied TD patients (35–42). Thus, our first goal is to compare specific ERP components in TD and BFRB patients before any treatment. Our second aim is to focus on cerebral changes that accompany behavioral and cognitive modification, after CoPs therapy. We expect an improvement in tics and habits symptoms in TD and BFRB patients, respectively. The main hypothesis predicts that TD and BFRB patients will show intact early evaluation of salience as reflected by the P200 (31, 32), while showing larger target detection and conflict monitoring as indexed by a larger N200 (33), which is consistent with earlier clinical findings with TD reporting an intact P200 amplitude (42), and larger N200 amplitude (39). Finally, we hypothesize a reduced P300 oddball effect in our clinical groups, which was also consistently found in TD patients with OCS (42), with OCD (43–46), and without comorbidity (39, 47). Such reduced P300 would indicate a decrease in memory updating processes (34) in both disorders. We propose to contrast ERPs across motor and non-motor oddball tasks, which will ascribe the contribution of motor responses. Earlier studies involving healthy participants with the counting and the motor oddball task showed activation of the SMA, the cerebellum, the thalamus, and the parietal cortex. However, activation of the middle frontal gyrus central opercular cortex and parietal operculum was specific to the motor oddball task, suggesting a specific contribution of these regions in action execution (48). Finally, we hypothesize an equivalent normalization of the P300 in both patient groups after treatment.

MATERIALS AND METHODS

Participants

Patients with either TD or BFRB were recruited from the *Centre d'études sur les troubles obsessionnels-compulsifs et les tics* from the *Centre de recherche de l'Institut universitaire en santé mentale de Montréal* to participate in this study. Patients with TD as their main concern were assigned to the TD group. Therefore, the TD group was composed of 26 patients who met the DSM-IV-TR criteria for either Tourette syndrome (307.23) or chronic TD (307.22) (10). Patients with BFRB as their main concern were assigned to the BFRB group. The latter group was composed of 27 patients with specific habit disorders, such as trichotillomania ($n = 12$), onychophagia ($n = 8$), skin picking ($n = 5$), and bruxism ($n = 2$). These two patients' groups were matched to a group of 27 healthy controls on the basis of age, intelligence (Raven), and laterality.[1] The project was approved by the ethics committee of the *Centre de recherche de l'Institut universitaire en santé mentale de Montréal*, and all participants granted their written informed consent, in accordance with the Declaration of Helsinki. Seven TD patients and four BFRB patients were under medication during the study. Those medication were α2-adrenergic agonists ($n = 1$), β_2-adrenergic agonists ($n = 1$), antidepressants ($n = 7$), benzodiazepine ($n = 3$), non-benzodiazepine ($n = 1$) hypnotics, neuroleptics ($n = 2$), and lithium ($n = 1$). However, to be included in our study, their medication had to remain stable throughout the entire process. Socio-demographic characteristics of our participants can be found in **Table 1**.

Exclusion criteria consisted of the presence of a psychiatric diagnosis, such as schizophrenia, mood disorders, somatoform disorders, dissociative disorders, and substance-related disorders. The presence of personality disorders was screened with the personality diagnostic questionnaire-fourth edition (49–51), and participants with personality disorders were excluded. Other medical conditions, such as neurological diseases, were screened by a neurologist (Pierre J. Blanchet) and were also a criterion for exclusion.

[1]Twenty of the 26 TS patients and 19 of the 27 controls included in this study were also included in one of our previous study, but with a different experimental task (13).

TABLE 1 | Socio-demographic and clinical characteristics.

	TD (n = 26)		BFRB (n = 27)		Controls (n = 27)				
	Mean	SD	Mean	SD	Mean	SD	F	p	Group difference
Age	38	11.9	40	14.4	36	13.0	0.48	ns	
Sex (% of males)	65%	N/A	26%	N/A	41%	N/A	**4.60***	**<0.05**	TD > BFRB
Intelligence (percentiles)	88	13.8	80	17.2	84	17.1	1.49	ns	
Laterality (R:L:A)	24:2:0	N/A	24:3:0	N/A	25:0:3	N/A	5.42[a]	ns	
OCS (Padua)	32	32.1	35	25.8	17	15.6	**4.14***	**<0.05**	BFRB > controls
Depression (BDI)	11	10.2	14	7.8	3	3.8	**15.70*****	**<0.001**	TD and BFRB > controls
Anxiety (BAI)	8	5.9	11	6.6	5	4.6	**7.19****	**<0.01**	BFRB > controls
Impulsivity (BIS-10)[b]	71	8.8	72	7.9	64	8.7	**5.82****	**<0.01**	TD and BFRB > controls

Laterality: R, right-handed; L, left-handed; A, ambidextrous. Intelligence: Raven's matrices percentiles; OCS, obsessive–compulsive symptoms; BDI, Beck depression inventory; BAI, Beck anxiety inventory; BIS-10, Barratt impulsiveness scale; ns, not statistically significant.

**p < 0.05.*

***p < 0.01.*

****p < 0.001.*

[a]Fisher's exact test was used to analyze categorical data with cells containing an expected count below 5.

[b]One TD patient and eight controls with missing data.

Every significant result is in bold.

Procedures

Clinical Assessment

Patients underwent a battery of psychological tests to assess symptoms. The Tourette Syndrome Global Scale [TSGS (52)] and the Yale Global Tic Severity Scale [YGTSS (53)] were used to assess tics symptoms in TD patients. We adapted the TSGS and the YGTSS to assess the presence of habit disorders in the BFRB group. In these adapted versions of both questionnaires, the word "tic" was replaced by the word "habit." These questionnaires were adapted to quantify both tics and habits on the same metric uniformly. This adaptation has been validated in a prior research from our group (54).

We also used the *Massachusetts General Hospital Hair Pulling Scale* [MGH-HPS (55)] to assess BFRB severity. The MGH-HPS is a seven-point inventory measuring the severity of trichotillomania symptoms. Again, an adaptation of this scale was proposed to assess onychophagia, skin picking, and skin scratching. Therefore, the current data reported in the MGH-scale column reflected the severity score of the principal habit of each BFRB patient. Good convergent validity was found between TSGS and MGH scales, as prior research found correlations between TSGS tic scores and the MGH-HPS (r = 0.49, p < 0.05), as well as the MGH scales adapted for nail biting and skin picking (r = 0.52, p < 0.05) (54).

Obsessive–compulsive symptoms were assessed with the Padua inventory (56). The 10th version of the Barratt Impulsiveness Scale (BIS-10) was administered to assess impulsivity in our participants (57). The Beck anxiety inventory [BAI (58)] and the Beck depression inventory [BDI (59)] were used to assess anxiety and depression symptomatology, respectively. The occurrence of anxiety disorders was assessed by a structured interview with the anxiety disorders interview schedule (60). Severe psychological stressors, time availability, and other psychological problems were also screened.

Cognitive–Behavioral Therapy Based on the Cognitive–Psychophysiological Model

The two clinical groups, which are composed of 26 patients with TD and 27 patients with BFRB, underwent the same CBT, based on the cognitive–psychophysiological (CoPs) model (12). This treatment, while including some classic principles of symptom awareness and habit reversal therapy, focuses on cognitive and behavioral restructuration in situations presenting a high risk for tic bouts. The therapy was delivered by two licensed psychologist (supervised by Kieron P. O'Connor) on a weekly one-to-one basis. The treatment program includes basic clinical steps, which are cumulative and administered over 14 60-min sessions: awareness training (psychoeducation, daily diary, video, situational profile), muscle discrimination (gradation of tension, normalize contractions), muscular relaxation, reducing sensorimotor activation, modifying background style of action, cognitive and behavioral restructuring (development of alternative goal driven responses using cognitive and behavioral strategies), generalization, and preventing relapse.[2] At the end of the 14th week, there is a home-based practice period lasting 4 weeks with weekly phone contact with the therapist to ensure compliance and deal with trouble shooting. Therefore, there was a time lapse of 18 weeks between the beginning of the program and the posttreatment evaluation. Conditions of treatment delivery, duration, homework, and treatment monitoring were equivalent and supervised for integrity.

Oddball Paradigms

Two types of oddball paradigms were used in this study. During both oddball tasks, 200 black letters (X and O on a white background) were randomly presented during 100 ms on a

[2]Contact the authors for more information about the CoPs program. Also, see Lavoie et al. (25) or O'Connor et al. (26) for further details.

computer screen (Viewsonic SVGA 17″ monitor), with a random 1700–2200 ms inter-trial interval. The frequent stimulus (the letter "O") was presented 80% of the time ($n = 160$), whereas the rare stimulus (the letter "X") was presented with a 20% probability ($n = 40$). The first task is a *counting oddball task*, which presented the same stimuli, but this time participants must only count the number of rare stimuli. At the end of the experiment, the participants had to report the exact amount of rare stimuli ($n = 40$). The second task is a *motor oddball task*, where participants pressed the keyboard left arrow key with their left index finger when frequent stimuli were presented and pressed the right arrow key with their right index finger, when the rare stimuli were presented. The order of presentation of the counting and the motor tasks was counterbalanced across participants.

Electrophysiological Recordings

The EEG was recorded during both oddball tasks, with a digital amplifier (Sensorium Inc., Charlotte, VT, USA). EEG signal was recorded from 63 Ag/AgCl electrodes mounted in a lycra cap (Electrode Arrays, El Paso, TX, USA)[3] and placed according to standard EEG guidelines (61). All electrodes were referenced to the nose. The signal was sampled continuously at 500 Hz and recorded with 0.01 Hz high-pass filter and a 100-Hz low-pass filter (60 Hz notch filter). Impedance was kept below 5 kΩ, using an electrolyte gel (JNetDirect Biosciences, Herndon, VA, USA). Bipolar electro-oculogram (EOG) was recorded to clear EEG from eye artifacts, such as blinks and eye movements. Electrodes were placed at the outer canthus of each eye (horizontal EOG) and below and above left eye (vertical EOG). The stimuli were monitored by Presentation (Neurobehavioral Systems, Albany, CA, USA),[4] and the signal was recorded with IWave (InstEP Systems, Montréal, QC, USA) running on two PCs.

ERP Extraction from Raw EEG Signal

Ocular artifacts were corrected offline with the Gratton algorithm (62). Raw signals were averaged offline and time-locked to the stimulus onset, in a time window of 100 ms prior to stimulus onset until 900 ms after stimulus onset. Stimuli were categorized across frequent and rare conditions. ERP data were filtered offline with a 0.30-Hz high-pass filter and a 30-Hz low-pass filter. During the averaging procedure, clippings due to amplifiers saturation and remaining epochs exceeding 100 μV were removed. Finally, participants had to have at least 20 valid trials in each condition to be included in the analyses.

The amplitude of the P200 was calculated as the maximum peak during the 150–300 ms interval, whereas the amplitude of the N200 was calculated as the lowest peak during the same interval. The amplitude of the P300 component was calculated as the mean amplitude in the 300–550 ms interval. Thirty electrodes were used to analyze each of these components: AF1, AF2, AF3, AF4, F1, F2, F3, F4, F5, F6 (frontal region), FC1, FC2, FC3, FC4, C1, C2, C3, C4, C5, C6 (central region), CP1, CP2, CP5, CP6, P1, P2, P3, P4, P5, and P6 (parietal region).

[3]http://www.sandsresearch.com/electrode-caps.html

[4]http://www.neurobs.com/

Statistical Analyses

Since the control group was only tested once, two separate sets of analyses were performed. The first set of analyses compared the TD, BFRB, and control groups at the baseline, whereas the second set of analyses compared the TD and BFRB groups at baseline and after CoPs therapy. Therefore, we performed each MANOVA twice, first with the between-group factor group (TD/BFRB/controls), and then the within-group factor therapy (pre/post) was added. The between-group factor Group only contained two levels in this second set of analyses (TD/BFRB). Independent samples t-tests were performed to compare the two groups on age, intelligence, depression, and anxiety scores. Paired samples t-tests were also performed to compare TSGS, YGTSS, BDI, and BAI scores before and after the therapy.

To compare TD and BFRB patients with controls on N200, P200, and P300 peak amplitude, repeated-measures MANOVAs were performed with the between-group factor Group (TD/BFRB/controls), and three within-group factors: condition (frequent/rare), region (frontal/central/parietal), and hemisphere (left/right). To assess the therapy effects, a within-group factor therapy was added (pre/post) in the second set of analyses. Significant interactions in all components were further analyzed with paired and independent samples t-tests. Further analyses were performed on each clinical group (TD and BFRB) to examine if the impact of CoPs therapy differed between groups. Huynh–Feldt corrections for repeated-measures analyses were performed when required. Tukey's test was used to assess differences between groups before therapy.

RESULTS

Impact of CoPs Therapy on Clinical Measures

The therapy induced a reduction in tics and habits symptoms in TD and BFRB patients, respectively. In both groups, there were reductions in TSGS [$F(1,51) = 67.09$, $p < 0.001$] and YGTSS total scores [$F(1,51) = 89.13$, $p < 0.001$]. Reductions in TSGS total score remained significant when covarying for depression [$F(1,51) = 26.39$, $p < 0.001$] and anxiety [$F(1,51) = 23.99$, $p < 0.001$]. With impulsivity as a covariant, there was a trend toward a significant reduction in TSGS score [$F(1,50) = 3.23$, $p = 0.078$]. Reductions in YGTSS total score remained significant when covarying for depression [$F(1,51) = 31.16$, $p < 0.001$], anxiety [$F(1,51) = 17.07$, $p < 0.001$], and impulsivity [$F(1,50) = 5.15$, $p < 0.05$].

There were also reductions in YTGSS tics/habits impairment [$F(1,51) = 60.42$, $p < 0.001$] and motor tics/habits subscales [$F(1,51) = 55.84$, $p < 0.001$]. Moreover, there was a therapy by group interaction on the YGTSS motor tics/habits subscale [$F(1,51) = 5.84$, $p < 0.05$], which showed that motor tics/habits severity decrease following CoPs therapy in both patient groups, but improvements were more pronounced in the BFRB group. Moreover, the therapy induced a significant improvement in YGTSS scores on the phonic tic subscale in TD patients [$F(1,25) = 19.30$, $p < 0.001$], as well as reduced MGH scales scores for BFRB patients [$F(1,23) = 25.90$, $p < 0.001$]. Following therapy, anxiety and depressive symptoms were also diminished

TABLE 2 | CBT impact on clinical scales.

	Pre				Post							
	TD (n = 26)		BFRB (n = 27)		TD (n = 26)		BFRB (n = 27)					
	Mean	SD	Mean	SD	Mean	SD	Mean	SD	F	p	d	Group difference
Depression (BDI)	11	10.2	14	*7.8*	6	6.5	7	*6.0*	**26.69***	**<0.001**	0.73	TD and BFRB: pre > post
Anxiety (BAI)	8	5.9	11	*6.6*	6	6.5	8	*4.7*	**6.29***	**<0.05**	0.41	TD and BFRB: pre > post
OCS (Padua)[a]	30	30.9	35	*25.8*	28	23.5	35	*24.4*	0.22	ns	0.04	
Tic severity TSGS total score	18	9.8	17	*9.7*	9	8.6	7	*7.0*	**67.09***	**<0.001**	1.06	TD and BFRB: pre > post
YGTSS Total	40	15.3	28	*10.8*	26	11.2	16	*9.3*	**89.13***	**<0.001**	1.04	TD and BFRB: pre > post
Tics/habits impairment	20	10.5	14	*5.9*	10	5.0	7	*5.2*	**60.42***	**<0.001**	1.11	TD and BFRB: pre > post
Motor tics/habits severity	13	4.3	13	*3.5*	11	4.6	8	*4.4*	**55.84***	**<0.001**	0.86	TD and BFRB: pre > post
Phonic tics severity[b]	7	5.6	N/A	N/A	5	4.7	N/A	N/A	**19.30***	**<0.001**	0.53	TD: pre > post
MGH scales[c]	N/A	N/A	17	*3.6*	N/A	N/A	10	*5.6*	**25.90***	**<0.001**	1.49	BFRB: pre > post
Impulsivity (BIS-10)[d]	71	8.8	72	*7.9*	69	9.0	71	*7.4*	2.76	ns	0.13	

BDI, Beck depression inventory; BAI, Beck anxiety inventory; OCS, obsessive–compulsive symptoms; TSGS, Tourette's syndrome global scale; YGTSS, Yale Global Tic Severity Scale; MGH scales, Massachusetts General Hospital Hairpulling Scale and its adapted versions for other BFRB; ns, not statistically significant; d, Cohen's d were calculated with both clinical groups pooled together, except for YGTSS phonic tics subscale (TD only) and MGH scales (BFRB only).
**p < 0.05.*
****p < 0.001.*
[a]11 TD patients and five BFRB patients with missing data.
[b]Only for TD patients.
[c]Only for BFRB patients. Three patients with missing data.
[d]One TD patient with missing data.
Every significant result is in bold.

in both patient groups, as shown by significant reductions in BAI [$F(1,51) = 6.29$, $p < 0.05$] and BDI scores [$F(1,51) = 26.69$, $p < 0.001$]. The CoPs therapy had no impact on impulsivity. Clinical results are shown in **Table 2**.

Counting Oddball Task

P200 Component

Before CoPs therapy, there were main effects of condition [$F(1,77) = 170.52$, $p < 0.001$], region [$F(2,76) = 7.30$, $p < 0.005$], and hemisphere [$F(1,77) = 15.80$, $p < 0.001$]. The rare–frequent oddball effect was larger over the central region in all groups, which lead to a condition by region interaction [$F(2,76) = 80.50$, $p < 0.001$]. There was no group main effect or interaction for that component. No therapy effect reached statistical significance. ERP waveforms for the counting oddball task are shown in **Figure 1**.

N200 Component

Before CoPs therapy, there was a region main effect [$F(2,76) = 12.71$, $p < 0.001$], as well as condition by region [$F(2,76) = 13.86$, $p < 0.001$] and region by hemisphere [$F(2,76) = 4.58$, $p < 0.05$] interactions. There was also a condition by region by hemisphere by group interaction [$F(3.89,149.63) = 23.65$, $p < 0.05$], which revealed that BFRB patients had a larger N200 amplitude than controls over the right-central region during frequent stimuli [$F(2,77) = 3.36$, $p < 0.05$, Tukey: $p < 0.05$], thus reducing the N200 oddball effect. No significant change due to therapy was noted.

P300 Component

Before CoPs therapy, there were main effects of condition [$F(1,77) = 97.94$, $p < 0.001$], region [$F(1.30,100.32) = 51.46$, $p < 0.001$], and hemisphere [$F(1,77) = 4.31$, $p < 0.05$], as well as condition by region [$F(1.34,103.02) = 45.58$, $p < 0.001$] and condition by hemisphere [$F(1,77) = 4.75$, $p < 0.05$] interactions.

Most importantly, there was a condition by group [$F(2,77) = 5.26$, $p < 0.01$] interaction, which revealed smaller P300 amplitude during rare trials for both clinical groups, in comparison with the control group (**Figure 2**). This interaction remained significant even when covarying for medication [$F(2,76) = 4.65$, $p < 0.05$]. There was also a condition by region by hemisphere by group four-way interaction [$F(3.34,128.65) = 3.20$, $p < 0.05$], which revealed that there were significant between-group differences during rare trials over the left frontal [$F(2,77) = 3.25$, $p < 0.05$], left [$F(2,77) = 3.56$, $p < 0.05$] and right-central [$F(2,77) = 3.34$, $p < 0.05$], and right parietal [$F(2,77) = 3.35$, $p < 0.05$] regions. There were no such group differences during frequent trials.

When clinical groups were pooled together, the TSGS global score was negatively correlated with the P300 oddball effect in the right-central ($r = -0.28$, $p < 0.05$) and the left ($r = -0.27$, $p < 0.05$) and right ($r = -0.28$, $p < 0.05$) parietal regions. In the TD group, the P300 oddball effect was positively correlated with the BIS-10 score in the left-central ($r = 0.43$, $p < 0.05$) and parietal regions ($r = 0.48$, $p < 0.05$). There was no such correlation in the BFRB or the control group.

There was a main effect of therapy [$F(1,51) = 5.20$, $p < 0.05$], and a therapy by condition interaction [$F(1,51) = 10.63$, $p < 0.005$], which revealed an increase in amplitude during rare trials following therapy (see **Figure 2**). When covarying with medication, the therapy main effect was no longer significant, but the therapy by condition interaction remained significant [$F(1,50) = 5.42$, $p < 0.05$]. Also, when we analyzed groups separately, there was

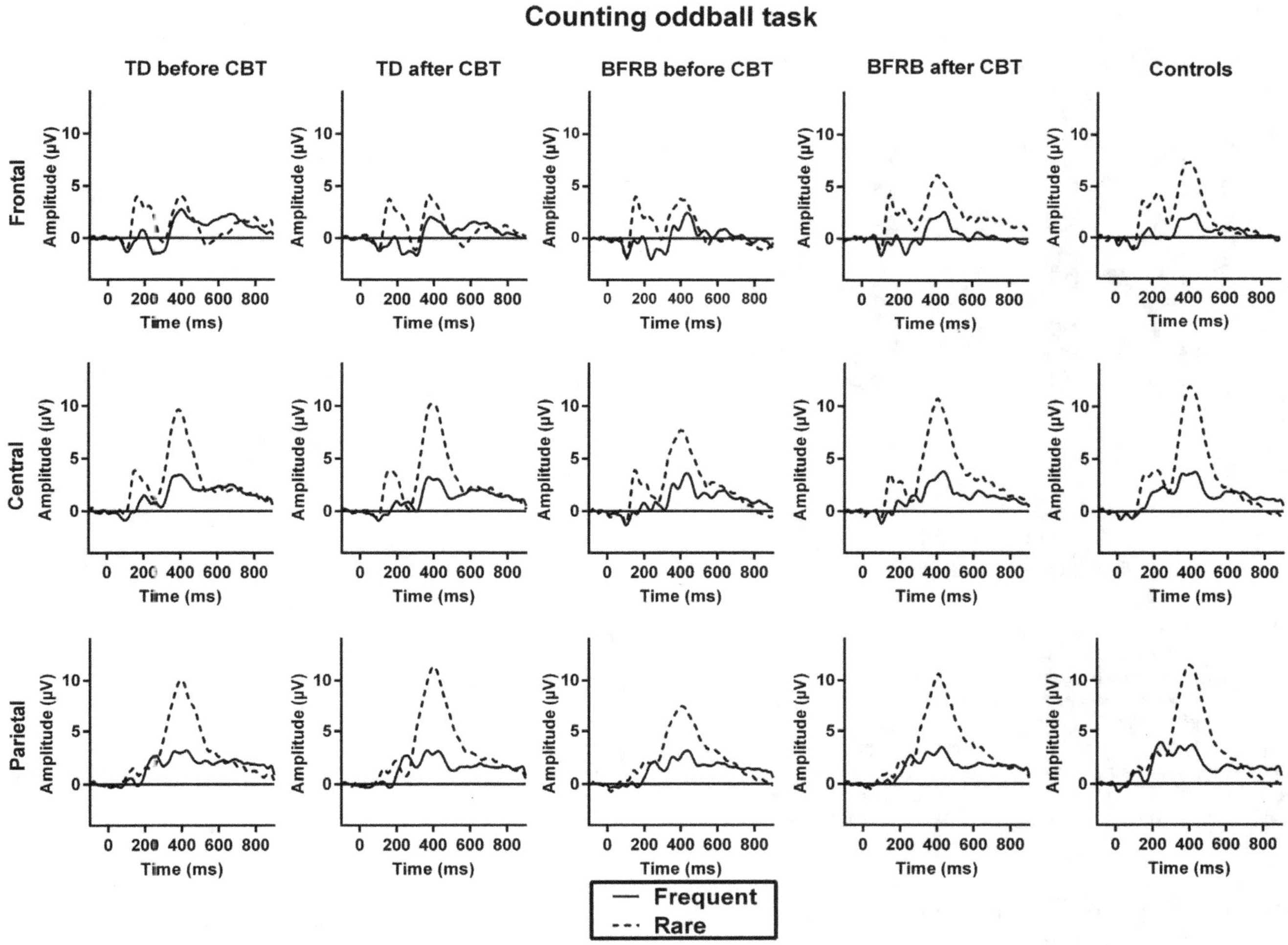

FIGURE 1 | ERP waveforms during the counting oddball task. The initial positive deflection that arises about 200 ms after stimulus presentation corresponds to the P200 component. The negative deflection that follows is the N200, which is then followed by the P300, a positive deflection that emerges 300 ms after stimulus presentation. The oddball effect is represented by the P300 amplitude to rare (dotted line) – frequent (solid line) stimuli. Before therapy, TD and BFRB patients had reduced P300 amplitude than controls during rare trials. A significant amplitude increase was induced by the CoPs therapy. This increase occurred in all three regions in BFRB patients but was more localized in the parietal region in TD patients.

a therapy main effect [$F(1,26) = 4.61$, $p < 0.05$] and a therapy by condition interaction [$F(1,26) = 8.17$, $p < 0.01$] in the BFRB group (which also revealed amplitude increase in rare trials). In comparison, there was only a trend toward a therapy by condition interaction in the TD group [$F(1,25) = 3,39$, $p = 0.078$], when analyzing the entire cortex. However, there was a localized therapy by condition interaction in the left parietal region [$F(1,25) = 3.88$, $p < 0.05$] in TD patients, revealing an amplitude increase during rare trials and thus, a larger oddball effect in this region after CoPs therapy (**Figure 3**).

Motor Oddball Task

Reaction Times

Before CoPs therapy, there was a main effect of condition [$F(1,77) = 169.37$, $p < 0.001$], which indicated that all participants responded faster to frequent than to rare stimuli. There was also a group main effect [$F(2,77) = 4.02$, $p < 0.05$] on median reaction times, which revealed that BFRB patients reaction times were delayed compared to the control group (Tukey: $p < 0.05$). There was no significant difference between TD patients and controls and no significant effect of therapy *per se* on reaction times.

P200

Event-related potentials waveforms for the motor oddball task are shown in **Figure 4**. Before CoPs therapy, there were condition by region [$F(2,76) = 98.10$, $p < 0.001$], condition by hemisphere [$F(1,77) = 16.45$, $p < 0.001$], and region by hemisphere [$F(2,76) = 10.87$, $p < 0.001$] interactions.

N200

Before CoPs therapy, there were condition by region [$F(2,76) = 10.44$, $p < 0.001$] and condition by hemisphere

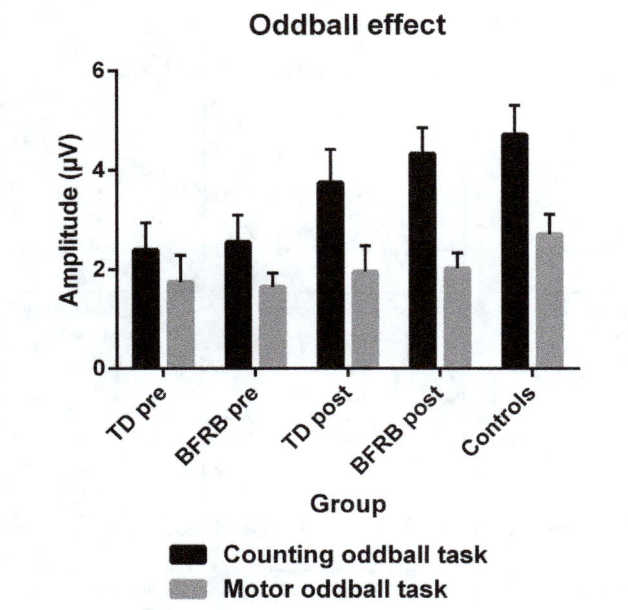

FIGURE 2 | The P300 oddball effect (therapy by condition). The P300 oddball effect represents the subtraction of frequent condition from the rare condition across all scalp regions. With the counting oddball task, the oddball effect was significantly reduced in both clinical groups at pretherapy (black). However, there were no significant differences across groups during the motor task (gray) and no effect of therapy reached significance. At posttherapy, a normalization of the oddball effect was induced during the counting oddball task (black), especially in BFRB patients, where it almost reaches the level of control participants. Note: error bars represent the SEM.

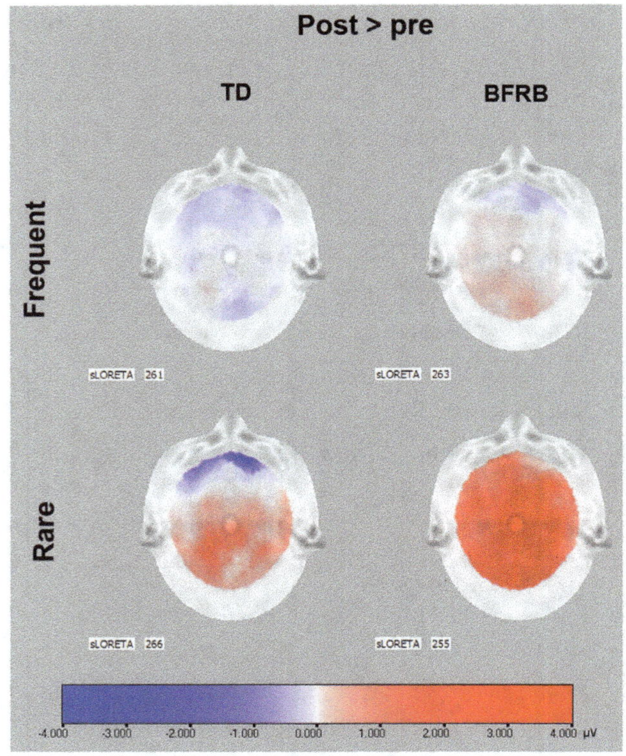

FIGURE 3 | P300 scalp topographies of activation changes induced by CoPs therapy. P300 data before therapy were subtracted from P300 data after CoPs therapy to illustrate the activation changes induced by CoPs therapy in frequent and rare conditions. Red color represents an activation increase following CoPs therapy, whereas blue color represents a decrease in activation in microvolts. The SLORETA number indicates the timeframe of each scalp. The timeframes were selected as the maximum peak during the 300–550 ms interval following stimulus presentation, for the frequent and rare condition. For both groups, scalp topographies show that most of the pre–posttherapy difference in P300 activation occurred during rare condition. In TD patients, the activation increase was localized in the parietal area, especially the central and left hemisphere. In BFRB patients, the increase was generalized to the whole cortex. Scalp topographies were obtained through LORETA (63).

[$F(1,77) = 12.62$, $p < 0.01$] interactions, which revealed a larger condition effect over the frontal left hemisphere.

P300

Before CoPs therapy, there were main effects of condition [$F(1,77) = 71.57$, $p < 0.001$] and region [$F(2,76) = 41.45$, $p < 0.001$] followed by condition by region [$F(2,76) = 13.65$, $p < 0.001$] and condition by hemisphere [$F(1,77) = 45.81$, $p < 0.001$] interactions. There was no significant group difference or effect of therapy in all three components during the motor oddball task (see **Figure 3**).

DISCUSSION

The main goal was to compare brain function in TD and BFRB patients during two oddball tasks and to record the effect of the CoPs therapy on clinical measures and brain functioning. To achieve this goal, we used ERP, a technique with high temporal resolution, which is well suited to follow complex stages of the processing stream. We expected that the CoPs therapy would induce a significant reduction in tic symptom severity in both clinical groups, whereas an increase in P300 amplitude was hypothesized to accompany that clinical improvement.

Our results showed that the P300 oddball effect was reduced in both clinical groups. Then, the CoPs therapy induced a normalization of the P300 oddball effect. The clinical change following therapy confirmed our hypothesis with a significant reduction in tics and habit disorders scale scores. Moreover, anxiety and depression symptoms also improved following therapy. These results were observed only in the counting oddball where no motor response was required.

Counting Oddball Task

Habit symptoms induced an increase in N200 amplitude over the right-central region, during the counting oddball task. Indeed, in BFRB patients, the N200 was larger for frequent stimuli, thus reducing the oddball effect. In an oddball paradigm, the N200 is traditionally representative of attention and detection processes (64). At a functional level, this central N200 is generated by the anterior cingulate cortex and is related to conflict monitoring and cognitive control (64, 65). The observed N200 asymmetry toward

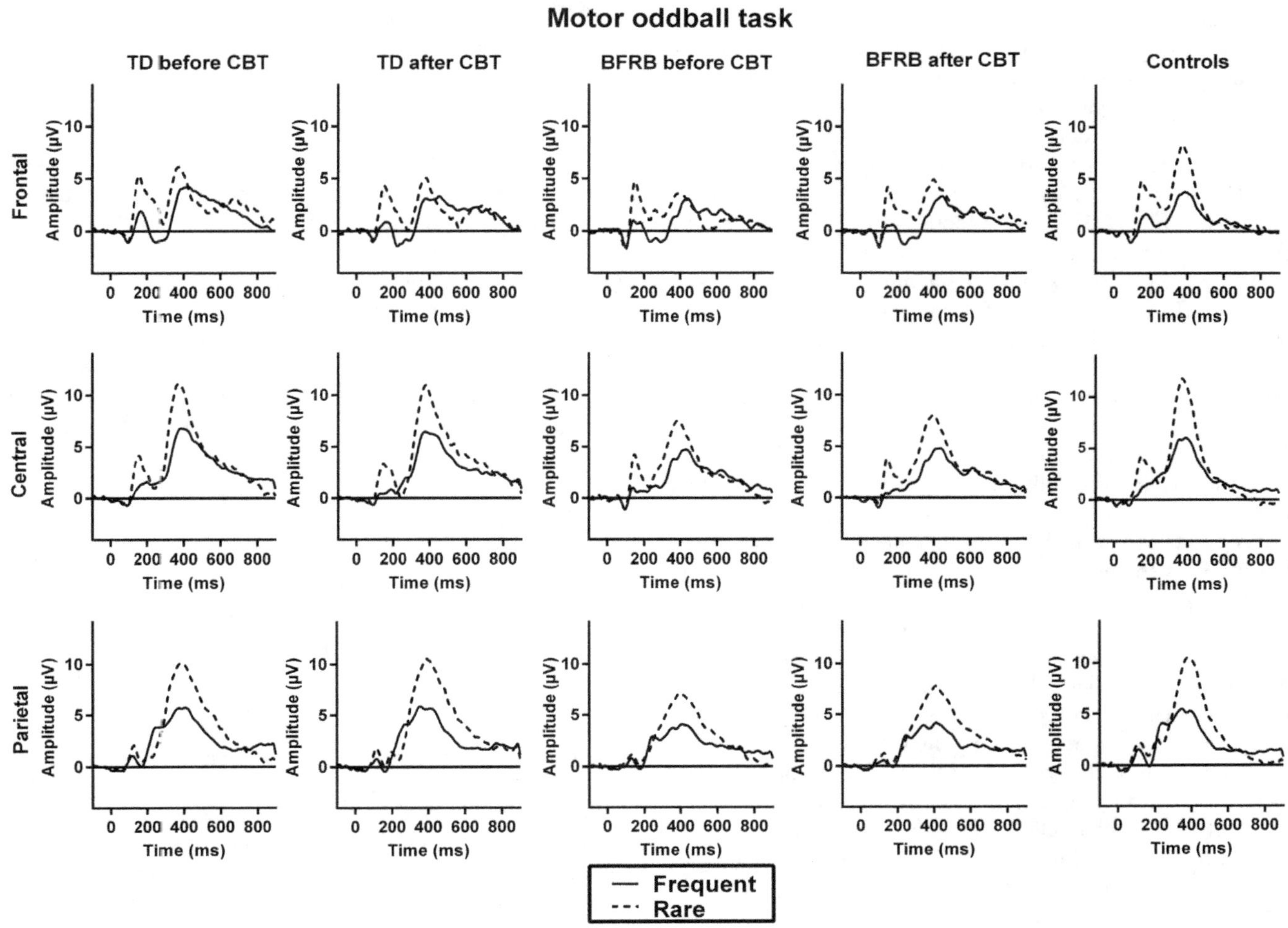

FIGURE 4 | ERP waveforms during the motor oddball task. No significant group differences were observed during the motor oddball task.

the right hemisphere could be caused by the impaired functioning of the corpus callosum (66). The corpus callosum and the prefrontal cortex have a role in mediating interhemispheric interference (67). Smaller corpus callosum could be due to accelerated pruning, whereas axonal pruning is reduced in the frontal cortex of TD patients (68). Therefore, such reports are consistent with our results of hemispheric discrepancy in the frontal and central regions, and the BFRB group seems to share that characteristic with the TD.

Since the N200 reflects monitoring and control, an increase in N200 amplitude could be considered as a function of the amount of effort that the individual put into regulating the urge to perform their habits and/or tics. However, the fact that the therapy failed to affect the N200 oddball effect could mean that despite better tics/habits awareness and modification of action style, this is not reflected by cerebral activity, at least in that ERP temporal window.

Later in the processing stream, for both patient group there was a significant reduction of the P300 oddball effect, particularly over the left anterior hemisphere (frontal and central) and the right posterior hemisphere (central and parietal). Moreover, the P300 oddball effect in the right-central region and bilaterally in the parietal region was negatively correlated with TSGS score, showing that the P300 oddball effect was reduced when tic/habits symptoms were more severe. Such correlation was not found with the YGTSS total score or one of its subscales. This could be explained by the fact that the TSGS has a more detailed behavioral subscale, including individual rating of learning problems, occupational problems, and motor restlessness (52). On the other side, the YGTSS has a 0–50 impairment subscale in which global impairment caused by TD is scored (53). Therefore, this difference between those two scales could explain why we found correlations between the P300 oddball effect with the TSGS, but not with the YGTSS.

The P300, which indexes processes of stimulus evaluation and categorization (69, 70), is generated by a network that includes the prefrontal cortex, the temporoparietal junction, the inferior parietal lobule, the supramarginal gyrus, and the cingulate gyrus (70, 71). In a study on a specific subtype of BFRB (i.e., trichotillomania) with MRI, it was reported that patients show higher levels of gray matter in the cingulate and parietal regions, in comparison with healthy controls (15). Trichotillomania patients also showed impairments in white matter tracts in the anterior cingulate gyrus, as shown by reduced fractional anisotropy in that region (16). In comparison, TD patients showed decrease gray matter in the anterior cingulate gyrus and the sensorimotor areas and reductions in white matter in the right cingulate gyrus (72). The P300 reduction has been related to impairments in gray matter of these regions (73), whereas another study reported positive correlations between P300 amplitude and white matter volumes in the prefrontal cortex and the temporoparietal junction, which were found in both healthy controls and patients at risk for psychosis (74). Therefore, P300 reduction could potentially reflect reduced white or gray matter of the prefrontal cortex and sensorimotor regions of the brain that in turn affect tics/habit symptoms.

Interestingly, the non-motor P300 oddball effect increased in both clinical groups following therapy. While this enhancement was found over the entire cortex in BFRB patients, it was localized to the parietal cortex in TD patients. One component of CoPs treatment model for tics and habits is awareness training, in which patients learn to better integrate information from the social, geographical, physical, and emotional context (12). Hence, the larger P300 oddball effect, found after therapy during a non-motor task, may depict enhance cognitive resources mobilized for working memory and contextual updating processes acquired through persistent training, during the CoPs therapy and practice sessions. Thus, the treatment may promote normalization of aberrant cortical pathways in adults with TD and BFRB. The change in P300 oddball effect could also represent an adaptive mechanism to update information in working memory despite reduced gray and white matter in sensorimotor and prefrontal areas (7, 8, 72, 75). Our findings are also consistent with recent findings in fMRI, which revealed that patients with greater tic severity reduction had higher activity in the inferior frontal gyrus (30). The authors argue that since the inferior frontal gyrus is involved in task-switching and set-shifting, greater activity of this region could be associated with less impairment in TD patients. However, these results were obtained from a motor inhibition priming task, which differ from our own non-motor oddball task that mobilize cerebral structures, such as the cerebellum, the thalamus, and the frontal and parietal cortex (48). Intriguingly, our posttherapy increase was found only with the counting oddball task, which could suggest that the non-motor P300 amplitude forms a good marker of tic/habits normalization that accompanies change in cortical activation.

Motor Oddball Task

Consistently, our ERP results during the motor oddball task confirmed that there were no significant group difference in all components during the motor oddball task and these ERP components, along with the reaction times, also were not affected by the CoPs therapy. While all participants showed delayed reaction times for rare than for frequent stimuli, which is expected with this type of motor oddball task, both clinical groups' reaction times were not significantly different from controls. This is consistent with prior findings with similar oddball paradigms in TD patients (39). Intact reaction times in adults with TD have also been found in Go/NoGo motor inhibition tasks (76, 77) and during a stimulus–response compatibility paradigm (13, 78).

As seen in **Figure 2**, the oddball effect is generally smaller in the motor than the counting task, in all groups. The amplitude of the P300 oddball effect during the motor task does not differ between groups. Motor-related potentials have been reported to overlap with the P300 and, thus, motor responses can have an attenuating effect on P300 component (79, 80). This could explain, in part, why that motor-related P300 was not significantly affected by tic/habit symptoms or by therapy in the motor oddball task. This suggests that TD and BFRB patients do not differ from healthy controls in the evaluation of stimuli salience and its task-related adequacy (N200/P200) in the context of a motor oddball task. Again, this is consistent with prior research on adults with TD that also showed intact P200 in counting oddball paradigm (42).

Limitations

The principal limitation of the current study is the fact that the control group was only tested once. Ideally, controls could have been tested a second time, with the same time interval between electrophysiological recordings than our patient groups. However, previous investigations showed good test–retest reliability of the P300 amplitude over time (81, 82), suggesting that control participants' electrocortical activity would not differ significantly in a second recording. Another limitation is that there were more males in the TD group and more females in the BFRB group, but this is consistent with the inherent gender ratio of both disorders (9, 83). Literature on this matter does not reveal significant gender difference on P300 amplitude in oddball paradigms (84–86).

Also, some patients were under medication, and others had sub-clinical comorbid disorders. Even though some of our results could be explained by these factors, we chose to include patients with comorbidities to have a better ecological validity, since comorbidities are the norm rather than the exception in TD (9, 87) and BFRB as well (88, 89). Finally, clinical scales were administered by unblinded clinicians, which could have affected the rating of symptom severity.

CONCLUSION

Our findings constitute one of many building blocks that seek integration of psychophysiological measures into evidence-based treatment of TD and BFRB. Consistent with that approach, the CoPs model considers the release of tension as a part of a general regulation system, which postulates that the evaluation of tics must focus further on situational triggers and on a particular style of action characterized by sensorimotor functioning that tends to increase muscular activation and tension. Our results allowed to improve the cerebral and cognitive outcome following the CoPs therapy, for these clinical groups. In conclusion, we demonstrated that TD and BFRB patients have smaller P300 oddball effect, reflecting impairments in attention and working memory. We also found a modification of this neural process after therapy, which was generalized throughout all brain regions in

BFRB patients and more localized in the parietal motor area in TD patients.

AUTHOR CONTRIBUTIONS

SMB has written this article in partial fulfillment for his doctoral thesis in neuroscience. KO is chief of the Tourette and OCD clinic, and he was responsible for English text revision for the current article. MR performed the analyses and wrote some sections of the manuscript. GS has co-written this article with SMB, particularly the pretherapy phase. JL was responsible, with KO, of the CoPs treatment. She also made editorial revisions. PB was responsible for the differential diagnosis. He also made editorial revisions. ML supervised all aspects of data acquisition and analysis with the first author. He also made editorial revisions.

ACKNOWLEDGMENTS

We wish to express our gratitude to Martine Germain for electrophysiological recordings, to Maite Hernandez for psychological testing, and to Karine Bergeron and Natalia Koszegi for clinical coordination. We also want to thank all the participants for their participation in our study.

FUNDING

This research was funded by an operating grant from the Canadian Institutes of Health Research (CIHR #93556) and a team grant from the Fonds de Recherche du Québec - Santé (FRQS #20573) awarded to ML, KO, and PB. SMB and GS both received doctoral scholarships from the FRQS for their work related to this article.

REFERENCES

1. Walkup JT, Ferrao Y, Leckman JF, Stein DJ, Singer H. Tic disorders: some key issues for DSM-V. *Depress Anxiety* (2010) **27**:600–10. doi:10.1002/da.20711
2. Miller AM, Bansal R, Hao X, Sanchez-Pena JP, Sobel LJ, Liu J, et al. Enlargement of thalamic nuclei in Tourette syndrome. *Arch Gen Psychiatry* (2010) **67**:955–64. doi:10.1001/archgenpsychiatry.2010.102
3. Felling RJ, Singer HS. Neurobiology of Tourette syndrome: current status and need for further investigation. *J Neurosci* (2011) **31**:12387–95. doi:10.1523/JNEUROSCI.0150-11.2011
4. Wang Z, Maia TV, Marsh R, Colibazzi T, Gerber A, Peterson BS. The neural circuits that generate tics in Tourette's syndrome. *Am J Psychiatry* (2011) **168**:1326–37. doi:10.1176/appi.ajp.2011.09111692
5. Bohlhalter S, Goldfine A, Matteson S, Garraux G, Hanakawa T, Kansaku K, et al. Neural correlates of tic generation in Tourette syndrome: an event-related functional MRI study. *Brain* (2006) **129**:2029–37. doi:10.1093/brain/awl050
6. Hampson M, Tokoglu F, King RA, Constable RT, Leckman JF. Brain areas coactivating with motor cortex during chronic motor tics and intentional movements. *Biol Psychiatry* (2009) **65**:594–9. doi:10.1016/j.biopsych.2008.11.012
7. Sowell ER, Kan E, Yoshii J, Thompson PM, Bansal R, Xu D, et al. Thinning of sensorimotor cortices in children with Tourette syndrome. *Nat Neurosci* (2008) **11**:637–9. doi:10.1038/nn.2121
8. Draper A, Jackson GM, Morgan PS, Jackson SR. Premonitory urges are associated with decreased grey matter thickness within the insula and sensorimotor cortex in young people with Tourette syndrome. *J Neuropsychol* (2016) **10**:143–53. doi:10.1111/jnp.12089
9. Freeman RD, Fast DK, Burd L, Kerbeshian J, Robertson MM, Sandor P. An international perspective on Tourette syndrome: selected findings from 3,500 individuals in 22 countries. *Dev Med Child Neurol* (2000) **42**:436–47. doi:10.1017/S0012162200000839
10. American Psychiatric Association. *Diagnostic and Statistic Manual of Mental Disorders*. Washington, DC: American Psychiatric Association (2000).
11. Biswal B, Ulmer JL, Krippendorf RL, Harsch HH, Daniels DL, Hyde JS, et al. Abnormal cerebral activation associated with a motor task in Tourette syndrome. *AJNR Am J Neuroradiol* (1998) **19**:1509–12.
12. O'Connor KP. A cognitive-behavioral/psychophysiological model of tic disorders. *Behav Res Ther* (2002) **40**:1113–42. doi:10.1016/S0005-7967(02)00048-7
13. Morand-Beaulieu S, O'Connor KP, Sauvé G, Blanchet PJ, Lavoie ME. Cognitive-behavioral therapy induces sensorimotor and specific electrocortical changes in chronic tic and Tourette's disorder. *Neuropsychologia* (2015) **79**(Pt B):310–21. doi:10.1016/j.neuropsychologia.2015.05.024
14. O'Connor KP, Lavoie ME, Robert M, Stip E, Borgeat F. Brain-behavior relations during motor processing in chronic tic and habit disorder. *Cogn Behav Neurol* (2005) **18**:79–88. doi:10.1097/01.wnq.0000151131.06699.af
15. Chamberlain SR, Menzies LA, Fineberg NA, Del Campo N, Suckling J, Craig K, et al. Grey matter abnormalities in trichotillomania: morphometric magnetic resonance imaging study. *Br J Psychiatry* (2008) **193**:216–21. doi:10.1192/bjp.bp.107.048314
16. Chamberlain SR, Hampshire A, Menzies LA, Garyfallidis E, Grant JE, Odlaug BL, et al. Reduced brain white matter integrity in trichotillomania: a diffusion tensor imaging study. *Arch Gen Psychiatry* (2010) **67**:965–71. doi:10.1001/archgenpsychiatry.2010.109
17. Grant JE, Odlaug BL, Hampshire A, Schreiber LR, Chamberlain SR. White matter abnormalities in skin picking disorder: a diffusion tensor imaging study. *Neuropsychopharmacology* (2013) **38**:763–9. doi:10.1038/npp.2012.241
18. Delorme C, Salvador A, Valabregue R, Roze E, Palminteri S, Vidailhet M, et al. Enhanced habit formation in Gilles de la Tourette syndrome. *Brain* (2015) **139**(Pt 2):605–15. doi:10.1093/brain/awv307
19. Wile DJ, Pringsheim TM. Behavior therapy for Tourette syndrome: a systematic review and meta-analysis. *Curr Treat Options Neurol* (2013) **15**:385–95. doi:10.1007/s11940-013-0238-5
20. McGuire JF, Piacentini J, Brennan EA, Lewin AB, Murphy TK, Small BJ, et al. A meta-analysis of behavior therapy for Tourette syndrome. *J Psychiatr Res* (2014) **50**:106–12. doi:10.1016/j.jpsychires.2013.12.009
21. Bloch MH, Landeros-Weisenberger A, Dombrowski P, Kelmendi B, Wegner R, Nudel J, et al. Systematic review: pharmacological and behavioral treatment for trichotillomania. *Biol Psychiatry* (2007) **62**:839–46. doi:10.1016/j.biopsych.2007.05.019
22. Gelinas BL, Gagnon MM. Pharmacological and psychological treatments of pathological skin-picking: a preliminary meta-analysis. *J Obsessive Compuls Relat Disord* (2013) **2**:167–75. doi:10.1016/j.jocrd.2013.02.003
23. McGuire JF, Ung D, Selles RR, Rahman O, Lewin AB, Murphy TK, et al. Treating trichotillomania: a meta-analysis of treatment effects and moderators for behavior therapy and serotonin reuptake inhibitors. *J Psychiatr Res* (2014) **58**:76–83. doi:10.1016/j.jpsychires.2014.07.015
24. Woods DW, Houghton DC. Evidence-based psychosocial treatments for pediatric body-focused repetitive behavior disorders. *J Clin Child Adolesc Psychol* (2015) **45**(3):227–40. doi:10.1080/15374416.2015.1055860
25. Lavoie ME, Leclerc J, O'Connor KP. Bridging neuroscience and clinical psychology: cognitive behavioral and psychophysiological models in the evaluation and treatment of Gilles de la Tourette syndrome. *Neuropsychiatry (London)* (2013) **3**:75–87. doi:10.2217/npy.12.70
26. O'Connor KP, Lavoie M, Blanchet P, St-Pierre-Delorme ME. Evaluation of a cognitive psychophysiological model for management of tic disorders: an open trial. *Br J Psychiatry* (2015). doi:10.1192/bjp.bp.114.154518
27. O'Connor KP, Brault M, Robillard S, Loiselle J, Borgeat F, Stip E. Evaluation of a cognitive-behavioural program for the management of chronic tic and habit disorders. *Behav Res Ther* (2001) **39**:667–81. doi:10.1016/S0005-7967(00)00048-6
28. O'Connor KP, Laverdure A, Taillon A, Stip E, Borgeat F, Lavoie M. Cognitive behavioral management of Tourette's syndrome and chronic tic disorder in medicated and unmedicated samples. *Behav Res Ther* (2009) **47**:1090–5. doi:10.1016/j.brat.2009.07.021

29. Lavoie ME, Imbriglio TV, Stip E, O'Connor KP. Neurocognitive changes following cognitive-behavioral treatment in Tourette syndrome and chronic tic disorder. *Int J Cogn Ther* (2011) **4**:34–50. doi:10.1521/ijct.2011.4.1.34
30. Deckersbach T, Chou T, Britton JC, Carlson LE, Reese HE, Siev J, et al. Neural correlates of behavior therapy for Tourette's disorder. *Psychiatry Res* (2014) **224**:269–74. doi:10.1016/j.pscychresns.2014.09.003
31. Potts GF, Tucker DM. Frontal evaluation and posterior representation in target detection. *Brain Res Cogn Brain Res* (2001) **11**:147–56. doi:10.1016/S0926-6410(00)00075-6
32. Potts GF, Patel SH, Azzam PN. Impact of instructed relevance on the visual ERP. *Int J Psychophysiol* (2004) **52**:197–209. doi:10.1016/j.ijpsycho.2003.10.005
33. Bocquillon P, Bourriez JL, Palmero-Soler E, Molaee-Ardekani B, Derambure P, Dujardin K. The spatiotemporal dynamics of early attention processes: a high-resolution electroencephalographic study of N2 subcomponent sources. *Neuroscience* (2014) **271**:9–22. doi:10.1016/j.neuroscience.2014.04.014
34. Donchin E, Coles MGH. Is the P300 component a manifestation of context updating? *Behav Brain Sci* (1988) **11**:357–74. doi:10.1017/S0140525X00058027
35. van de Wetering BJ, Martens CM, Fortgens C, Slaets JP, van Woerkom TC. Late components of the auditory evoked potentials in Gilles de la Tourette syndrome. *Clin Neurol Neurosurg* (1985) **87**:181–6. doi:10.1016/0303-8467(85)90004-6
36. van Woerkom TC, Fortgens C, Rompel-Martens CM, van de Wetering BJ. Auditory event-related potentials in adult patients with Gilles de la Tourette's syndrome in the oddball paradigm. *Electroencephalogr Clin Neurophysiol* (1988) **71**:443–9. doi:10.1016/0168-5597(88)90048-2
37. van Woerkom TC, Roos RA, van Dijk JG. Altered attentional processing of background stimuli in Gilles de la Tourette syndrome: a study in auditory event-related potentials evoked in an oddball paradigm. *Acta Neurol Scand* (1994) **90**:116–23. doi:10.1111/j.1600-0404.1994.tb02690.x
38. Oades RD, Dittmann-Balcar A, Schepker R, Eggers C, Zerbin D. Auditory event-related potentials (ERPs) and mismatch negativity (MMN) in healthy children and those with attention-deficit or Tourette/tic symptoms. *Biol Psychol* (1996) **43**:163–85. doi:10.1016/0301-0511(96)05189-7
39. Johannes S, Weber A, Muller-Vahl KR, Kolbe H, Dengler R, Munte TF. Event-related brain potentials show changed attentional mechanisms in Gilles de la Tourette syndrome. *Eur J Neurol* (1997) **4**:152–61. doi:10.1111/j.1468-1331.1997.tb00321.x
40. Johannes S, Wieringa BM, Mantey M, Nager W, Rada D, Muller-Vahl KR, et al. Altered inhibition of motor responses in Tourette syndrome and obsessive-compulsive disorder. *Acta Neurol Scand* (2001) **104**:36–43. doi:10.1034/j.1600-0404.2001.00308.x
41. Johannes S, Wieringa BM, Nager W, Muller-Vahl KR, Dengler R, Munte TF. Excessive action monitoring in Tourette syndrome. *J Neurol* (2002) **249**:961–6. doi:10.1007/s00415-002-0657-9
42. Thibault G, Felezeu M, O'Connor KP, Todorov C, Stip E, Lavoie ME. Influence of comorbid obsessive-compulsive symptoms on brain event-related potentials in Gilles de la Tourette syndrome. *Prog Neuropsychopharmacol Biol Psychiatry* (2008) **32**:803–15. doi:10.1016/j.pnpbp.2007.12.016
43. Towey JP, Tenke CE, Bruder GE, Leite P, Friedman D, Liebowitz M, et al. Brain event-related potential correlates of overfocused attention in obsessive-compulsive disorder. *Psychophysiology* (1994) **31**:535–43. doi:10.1111/j.1469-8986.1994.tb02346.x
44. Miyata A, Matsunaga H, Kiriike N, Iwasaki Y, Takei Y, Yamagami S. Event-related potentials in patients with obsessive-compulsive disorder. *Psychiatry Clin Neurosci* (1998) **52**:513–8. doi:10.1046/j.1440-1819.1998.00427.x
45. Sanz M, Molina V, Martin-Loeches M, Calcedo A, Rubia FJ. Auditory P300 event related potential and serotonin reuptake inhibitor treatment in obsessive-compulsive disorder patients. *Psychiatry Res* (2001) **101**:75–81. doi:10.1016/S0165-1781(00)00250-X
46. Kim MS, Kang SS, Youn T, Kang DH, Kim JJ, Kwon JS. Neuropsychological correlates of P300 abnormalities in patients with schizophrenia and obsessive-compulsive disorder. *Psychiatry Res* (2003) **123**:109–23. doi:10.1016/S0925-4927(03)00045-3
47. Johannes S, Wieringa BM, Nager W, Muller-Vahl KR, Dengler R, Munte TF. Electrophysiological measures and dual-task performance in Tourette syndrome indicate deficient divided attention mechanisms. *Eur J Neurol* (2001) **8**:253–60. doi:10.1046/j.1468-1331.2001.00199.x
48. Warbrick T, Reske M, Shah NJ. Do EEG paradigms work in fMRI? Varying task demands in the visual oddball paradigm: implications for task design and results interpretation. *Neuroimage* (2013) **77**:177–85. doi:10.1016/j.neuroimage.2013.03.026
49. Hyler SE. *Personality Questionnaire PDQ-41*. New York: New York State Psychiatric Institute (1994).
50. Wilberg T, Dammen T, Friis S. Comparing personality diagnostic questionnaire-4+ with longitudinal, expert, all data (LEAD) standard diagnoses in a sample with a high prevalence of axis I and axis II disorders. *Compr Psychiatry* (2000) **41**:295–302. doi:10.1053/comp.2000.0410295
51. Rodgers R, Callahan S, Chabrol H. [Revision of the translation of certain items in the French version of PDQ-4 (personality diagnostic questionnaire, Hyler, 1994)]. *Encephale* (2004) **30**:408–9.
52. Harcherik DF, Leckman JF, Detlor J, Cohen DJ. A new instrument for clinical studies of Tourette's syndrome. *J Am Acad Child Psychiatry* (1984) **23**:153–60. doi:10.1097/00004583-198403000-00006
53. Leckman JF, Riddle MA, Hardin MT, Ort SI, Swartz KL, Stevenson J, et al. The Yale Global Tic Severity Scale: initial testing of a clinician-rated scale of tic severity. *J Am Acad Child Adolesc Psychiatry* (1989) **28**:566–73. doi:10.1097/00004583-198907000-00015
54. O'Connor K, St-Pierre-Delorme ME, Leclerc J, Lavoie M, Blais MT. Meta-cognitions in Tourette syndrome, tic disorders, and body-focused repetitive disorder. *Can J Psychiatry* (2014) **59**:417–25. doi:10.1177/070674371405900804
55. Keuthen NJ, O'Sullivan RL, Ricciardi JN, Shera D, Savage CR, Borgmann AS, et al. The Massachusetts General Hospital (MGH) Hairpulling Scale: 1. Development and factor analyses. *Psychother Psychosom* (1995) **64**:141–5. doi:10.1159/000289003
56. Sanavio E. Obsessions and compulsions: the Padua inventory. *Behav Res Ther* (1988) **26**:169–77. doi:10.1016/0005-7967(88)90116-7
57. Bayle FJ, Bourdel MC, Caci H, Gorwood P, Chignon JM, Ades J, et al. [Factor analysis of French translation of the Barratt impulsivity scale (BIS-10)]. *Can J Psychiatry* (2000) **45**:156–65. doi:10.1177/070674370004500206
58. Beck AT, Epstein N, Brown G, Steer RA. An inventory for measuring clinical anxiety: psychometric properties. *J Consult Clin Psychol* (1988) **56**:893–7. doi:10.1037/0022-006X.56.6.893
59. Beck AT, Ward CH, Mendelson M, Mock J, Erbaugh J. An inventory for measuring depression. *Arch Gen Psychiatry* (1961) **4**:561–71. doi:10.1001/archpsyc.1961.01710120031004
60. Brown TA, DiNardo PA, Barlow DH. *Anxiety Disorders Interview Schedule for DSM-IV*. Boulder, CO: Graywind Publications (1994).
61. American EEG Society. Guideline thirteen: guidelines for standard electrode position nomenclature. *J Clin Neurophysiol* (1994) **11**:111–3. doi:10.1097/00004691-199401000-00014
62. Gratton G, Coles MG, Donchin E. A new method for off-line removal of ocular artifact. *Electroencephalogr Clin Neurophysiol* (1983) **55**:468–84. doi:10.1016/0013-4694(83)90135-9
63. Pascual-Marqui RD. Standardized low-resolution brain electromagnetic tomography (sLORETA): technical details. *Methods Find Exp Clin Pharmacol* (2002) **24**(Suppl D):5–12.
64. Folstein JR, Van Petten C. Influence of cognitive control and mismatch on the N2 component of the ERP: a review. *Psychophysiology* (2008) **45**:152–70. doi:10.1111/j.1469-8986.2007.00602.x
65. Warren CM, Tanaka JW, Holroyd CB. What can topology changes in the oddball N2 reveal about underlying processes? *Neuroreport* (2011) **22**:870–4. doi:10.1097/WNR.0b013e32834bbe1f
66. Plessen KJ, Lundervold A, Gruner R, Hammar A, Lundervold A, Peterson BS, et al. Functional brain asymmetry, attentional modulation, and interhemispheric transfer in boys with Tourette syndrome. *Neuropsychologia* (2007) **45**:767–74. doi:10.1016/j.neuropsychologia.2006.08.006
67. Margolis A, Donkervoort M, Kinsbourne M, Peterson BS. Interhemispheric connectivity and executive functioning in adults with Tourette syndrome. *Neuropsychology* (2006) **20**:66–76. doi:10.1037/0894-4105.20.1.66
68. Plessen KJ, Gruner R, Lundervold A, Hirsch JG, Xu D, Bansal R, et al. Reduced white matter connectivity in the corpus callosum of children with Tourette syndrome. *J Child Psychol Psychiatry* (2006) **47**:1013–22. doi:10.1111/j.1469-7610.2006.01639.x
69. Kok A. On the utility of P3 amplitude as a measure of processing capacity. *Psychophysiology* (2001) **38**:557–77. doi:10.1017/S0048577201990559
70. Bledowski C, Prvulovic D, Goebel R, Zanella FE, Linden DEJ. Attentional systems in target and distractor processing: a combined ERP and

fMRI study. *Neuroimage* (2004) **22**:530–40. doi:10.1016/j.neuroimage.2003.12.034

71. Linden DE. The P300: where in the brain is it produced and what does it tell us? *Neuroscientist* (2005) **11**:563–76. doi:10.1177/1073858405280524
72. Muller-Vahl KR, Kaufmann J, Grosskreutz J, Dengler R, Emrich HM, Peschel T. Prefrontal and anterior cingulate cortex abnormalities in Tourette syndrome: evidence from voxel-based morphometry and magnetization transfer imaging. *BMC Neurosci* (2009) **10**:47. doi:10.1186/1471-2202-10-47
73. Ford JM, Sullivan EV, Marsh L, White PM, Lim KO, Pfefferbaum A. The relationship between P300 amplitude and regional gray matter volumes depends upon the attentional system engaged. *Electroencephalogr Clin Neurophysiol* (1994) **90**:214–28. doi:10.1016/0013-4694(94)90093-0
74. Fusar-Poli P, Crossley N, Woolley J, Carletti F, Perez-Iglesias R, Broome M, et al. White matter alterations related to P300 abnormalities in individuals at high risk for psychosis: an MRI-EEG study. *J Psychiatry Neurosci* (2011) **36**:239–48. doi:10.1503/jpn.100083
75. Draganski B, Martino D, Cavanna AE, Hutton C, Orth M, Robertson MM, et al. Multispectral brain morphometry in Tourette syndrome persisting into adulthood. *Brain* (2010) **133**:3661–75. doi:10.1093/brain/awq300
76. Roessner V, Albrecht B, Dechent P, Baudewig J, Rothenberger A. Normal response inhibition in boys with Tourette syndrome. *Behav Brain Funct* (2008) **4**:29. doi:10.1186/1744-9081-4-29
77. Biermann-Ruben K, Miller A, Franzkowiak S, Finis J, Pollok B, Wach C, et al. Increased sensory feedback in Tourette syndrome. *Neuroimage* (2012) **63**:119–25. doi:10.1016/j.neuroimage.2012.06.059
78. Thibault G, O'Connor KP, Stip E, Lavoie ME. Electrophysiological manifestations of stimulus evaluation, response inhibition and motor processing in Tourette syndrome patients. *Psychiatry Res* (2009) **167**:202–20. doi:10.1016/j.psychres.2008.03.021
79. Kok A. Overlap between P300 and movement-related-potentials: a response to Verleger. *Biol Psychol* (1988) **27**:51–8. doi:10.1016/0301-0511(88)90005-1
80. Salisbury DF, Rutherford B, Shenton ME, McCarley RW. Button-pressing affects P300 amplitude and scalp topography. *Clin Neurophysiol* (2001) **112**:1676–84. doi:10.1016/S1388-2457(01)00607-1
81. Debener S, Kranczioch C, Herrmann CS, Engel AK. Auditory novelty oddball allows reliable distinction of top-down and bottom-up processes of attention. *Int J Psychophysiol* (2002) **46**:77–84. doi:10.1016/S0167-8760(02)00072-7
82. Williams LM, Simms E, Clark CR, Paul RH, Rowe D, Gordon E. The test-retest reliability of a standardized neurocognitive and neurophysiological test battery: "neuromarker". *Int J Neurosci* (2005) **115**:1605–30. doi:10.1080/00207450590958475
83. Siddiqui EU, Naeem SS, Naqvi H, Ahmed B. Prevalence of body-focused repetitive behaviors in three large medical colleges of Karachi: a cross-sectional study. *BMC Res Notes* (2012) **5**:614. doi:10.1186/1756-0500-5-614
84. Campanella S, Rossignol M, Mejias S, Joassin F, Maurage P, Debatisse D, et al. Human gender differences in an emotional visual oddball task: an event-related potentials study. *Neurosci Lett* (2004) **367**:14–8. doi:10.1016/j.neulet.2004.05.097
85. Rozenkrants B, Polich J. Affective ERP processing in a visual oddball task: arousal, valence, and gender. *Clin Neurophysiol* (2008) **119**:2260–5. doi:10.1016/j.clinph.2008.07.213
86. Wang R, Dong Z, Chen X, Zhang M, Yang F, Zhang X, et al. Gender differences of cognitive function in migraine patients: evidence from event-related potentials using the oddball paradigm. *J Headache Pain* (2014) **15**:6. doi:10.1186/1129-2377-15-6
87. Robertson MM. The Gilles de la Tourette syndrome: the current status. *Arch Dis Child Educ Pract Ed* (2012) **97**:166–75. doi:10.1136/archdischild-2011-300585
88. Stein DJ, Flessner CA, Franklin M, Keuthen NJ, Lochner C, Woods DW. Is trichotillomania a stereotypic movement disorder? An analysis of body-focused repetitive behaviors in people with hair-pulling. *Ann Clin Psychiatry* (2008) **20**:194–8. doi:10.1080/10401230802435625
89. Snorrason I, Ricketts EJ, Flessner CA, Franklin ME, Stein DJ, Woods DW. Skin picking disorder is associated with other body-focused repetitive behaviors: findings from an Internet study. *Ann Clin Psychiatry* (2012) **24**:292–9.

23

The First World Congress on Tourette Syndrome and Tic Disorders: Controversies and Hot Topics in Etiology and Treatment

Carol A. Mathews[1] *and Jeremy S. Stern*[2*]

[1] *Department of Psychiatry, College of Medicine, University of Florida, Gainesville, Florida, USA,* [2] *Department of Neurology, St George's University of London, London, UK*

Edited by:
Peristera Paschou,
Democritus University of Thrace, Greece

Reviewed by:
Natalie J. Forde,
University Medical Center Groningen, Netherlands
Luca Pagliaroli,
Semmelweis University, Hungary
Renata Rizzo,
Catania University, Italy

***Correspondence:**
Jeremy S. Stern
jestern@sgul.ac.uk

The first World Congress on Tourette Syndrome and Tic Disorders was held in London, June 2016 by the Tourette Association of America, Tourettes Action (UK), and the European Society for the Study of Tourette Syndrome. Presentations arising from large-scale collaborative projects were an important component of the scientific programme. This article focuses on areas raised in the hot topics session and two moderated debates, which covered emerging research in etiology and treatment. The hot topics ranged across genetics, arguably including the first confirmed Tourette Syndrome (TS) susceptibility gene *NRXN1,* neurocognition, and neurophysiology, including the possibility of a neurocognitive endophenotype for TS and the use of depth and cortical surface electrodes to investigate the neurophysiology of tics on the background of the evolving field of deep brain stimulation (DBS), to novel treatment approaches such as dental orthotics and an online behavioral intervention. The debates aired controversies in treatment; pharmacotherapy vs. behavioral treatment and the place of medical cannabinoids. These sessions demonstrate the vibrancy of a field that has considerably expanded in the last decade, the significant progress that has been made, and the direction that some of the most fruitful next phases of research will take.

Keywords: Tourette, tics, deep brain stimulation, dopamine, GWAS

INTRODUCTION

These sessions of the congress were devoted to late-breaking studies and hot topics, including controversies in the field of Tourette Syndrome (TS) research or treatment. The presentations fell into two main themes, the first, elucidating the etiology of TS, and the second, the identification of novel or controversial treatments for TS. These presentations highlight the importance of large-scale collaborative efforts in the study of TS and provide evidence that, after many years of incremental advances, with collaborative efforts more substantial discoveries may be just around the corner. This is best illustrated in the genetic studies, where nearly 100 clinicians and scientists contributed clinical samples and expertise, and in the studies of environmental risk factors, which took place using the Avon Longitudinal Study of Parents and Children (ALSPAC; Golding et al., 2001), a birth cohort in which data has been collected, curated, and studied for over 20 years by hundreds of researchers. Such large scale, collaborative efforts are also becoming the norm for studies examining the efficacy and safety of TS treatments, whether in the form of meta-analyses of multiple small investigator-initiated studies, or in the form of large, multi-institution investigations of a specific treatment.

TS has long been known to be a complex disorder etiologically, with both genetic and non-genetic contributors. However, clear specific risk factors for TS, either genetic or environmental, have been difficult to identify and/or replicate. The availability of large samples of individuals with extensive phenotype and/or genotype data, some population-based, and some clinically ascertained, have recently led to advances in our understanding of the causes of TS. Although, TS is one of the most heritable of the neurodevelopmental disorders (Pauls et al., 2014b), with heritability estimates of 60–80% (Davis et al., 2013), the last 30 years of genetic studies, including recent genome-wide association studies, have been inconclusive. These studies indicate that TS is highly polygenic; that is, hundreds (or perhaps thousands) of genes of small effect contribute to TS risk in an additive manner. For this reason, tens of thousands of samples will likely be needed to identify individual TS susceptibility variants using genome-wide approaches. However, the currently available sample sizes, while falling short of what is needed for comprehensive identification of the genes and gene variants responsible for TS, may be efficiently used for gene discovery using alternative approaches.

Genetic Studies

Two presentations in this session focused on such alternative approaches to dissecting the genetic etiology of TS, and demonstrate the value of complementary scientific approaches. In the first, Alden Huang (University of California, Los Angeles), working with the Tourette Syndrome Association International Consortium for Genetics (TSAICG), examined the relationship between TS and copy number variants (CNVs) in 2764 individuals with TS and 2853 ethnically matched controls. Analyses were limited to large (>400 kilobases), rare (<1% prevalence) CNVs, which are likely to be pathogenic. Huang identified multiple recurrent CNVs in genomic regions that have been previously implicated for TS, as well as substantial overlap with CNV regions that have been implicated in other neurodevelopmental disorders, including autism spectrum disorders (ASD) and intellectual disability(Grayton et al., 2012). Two of these regions showed an enrichment of CNVs in TS cases compared to controls. These were *NRXN1* (1-sided Fisher's exact, $p = 0.007$), which has been previously reported to be associated with TS and *CNTN4* ($p = 0.029$). All of the CNVs detected in *NRXN1* were deletions, consistent with the prior literature (Nag et al., 2013; McGrath et al., 2014), while both deletions and duplications were present in the *CNTN4* locus. At the time of the Congress *NRXN1* may be considered the first confirmed susceptibility gene for TS.

The second study used the same dataset to conduct gene pathway analyses. There are many forms of pathway analyses, but the basic idea is to identify enrichment of genetic variants within specific known gene pathways or gene sets. Like the CNV analyses discussed above, an advantage of pathway analyses is that they can be effective in relatively small sample sizes, typically requiring thousands rather than tens of thousands of samples. This work was conducted by Fotis Tsetsos (University of Thrace), in conjunction with the TSAICG. Tsetsos used two complementary statistical approaches to examine relationships between TS and gene pathways defined from multiple sources, including curated gene sets from the published literature, computational gene sets defined from cancer-oriented microarray data, genes annotated using the same GO search terms, genes that share a microRNA binding motif, etc. Variants associated with nervous system tissues, in particular, parietal cortex and basal ganglia, were enriched in these analyses. A gene set with promotor regions around TCF3 (transcription factor 3) was also implicated in TS etiology (corrected $p = 0.006$). TCF3 is a member of the HLH (helix-loop-helix) family of transcription factors, and is thought to regulate developmental patterning processes in the central nervous system. TCF3 also suppresses Wnt, a protein that is involved in neuronal differentiation and proliferation of neural development cells (Gribble et al., 2009).

Studies of Non-genetic Risk Factors

Genetic causation accounts for ~60% of TS risk, suggesting that other, non-genetic (environmental) factors are also very important in the development of this disorder. Previous work in both clinical and population-based samples have implicated a number of pre- and perinatal risk factors for TS, including prenatal maternal smoking, prenatal maternal alcohol use, and possibly maternal parity and weight gain during pregnancy (Mathews et al., 2006, 2014; Pringsheim et al., 2009; Motlagh et al., 2010). In the third study in this session to focus on the etiology of TS, Yoav Ben-Shlomo (University of Bristol), and his colleagues used the ALSPAC sample to examine another type of potential environmental risk factor for TS, maternal anxiety and depression during pregnancy. The ALSPAC cohort is a prospective pre-birth cohort that has followed children born in Avon, UK in 1992 and their parents for over 20 years, and has collected extensive phenotypic data (Golding et al., 2001). Ben-Shlomo compared self-reported anxiety and depressive symptoms for both mothers and fathers at four time points, two prenatal (18 and 32 weeks), and two postnatal (18 weeks and 8 months after delivery) for children with chronic tic disorders including TS (TS/CT) and a control sample of children without chronic tics (Ben-Shlomo et al., 2016). Socioeconomic measures and other relevant potential confounders were controlled for in the analysis. After correction for potential confounders, chronic maternal anxiety (present both pre- and post-birth) and pre-natal maternal depression (but not post-natal maternal depression) were significantly associated with TS/CT (odds ratio = 2.17, $p = 0.007$; odds ratio 1.86, $p = 0.04$, respectively). Paternal anxiety and depression were not significantly associated with TS/CT. These findings suggest that maternal psychopathology may be a risk factor for TS and other chronic tic disorders. Maternal chronic anxiety may in fact represent a shared genetic susceptibility for TS, as this variable was associated with TS/CT both pre-and post-natally. In contrast, maternal depression may represent a time-specific environmental risk factor for TS, perhaps representing medication use during pregnancy, or intra-uterine neuroendocrine effects of stress. It should be noted, however, that both associations require confirmation in independent datasets.

The final study pertaining to the etiology of TS in this session was a systematic review focused on neurocognitive performance in individuals with TS. This study contributes to a growing literature on potential endophenotypes for TS and other complex disorders. An endophenotype is a heritable, measurable trait or feature that is associated with a disorder of interest, but is state independent (e.g., manifests in individuals whether or not they are manifesting the disorder, including in unaffected family members). No endophenotypes have yet been identified for TS, but specific neurocognitive abnormalities have been suggested as potential endophenotypes for two related disorders that are highly comorbid with TS, obsessive compulsive disorder (OCD; Pauls et al., 2014a), and attention deficit hyperactivity disorder (ADHD; Pineda et al., 2011; Eddy and Cavanna, 2014; Peskin et al., 2015). The study by Beth Hobson (University of Birmingham), and her colleagues, takes the first step in identifying potential TS endophenotypes by investigating whether neurocognitive dysfunction is consistently associated with TS. A search of PubMed, Medline, and PsychINFO identified 12 relevant studies, four of which included children and/or adolescents. In general no consistent differences in neurocognitive function between TS cases and controls were found. The one possible exception was in the area of cognitive inhibitory control. Individuals with TS showed a trend toward verbal inhibitory deficits, although this finding did not reach the level of statistical significance. Inhibitory control in TS, typically motor inhibition, but also cognitive inhibition, may lie at the heart of the neurology of TS and is an active area of investigation requiring future study.

TREATMENT

Management of TS is challenging and has remained largely unsatisfactory through the last decade of intensifying clinical and scientific interest in the condition. In clinical terms, given the spectrum nature of the presentation, it is important to define the treatment target in each case, as comorbidities such as ADHD or OCD are commonly more impairing than are the tics themselves. Tics often improve over the course of adolescence and at present their treatment is overall less reliable and less evidence based than treatments for the commonly co-occurring disorders. However, tics can be extremely severe in up to 15% of cases, and their effect on functioning varies greatly between individuals. Where tics are severe or intrusive, pharmacotherapy can be considered. The index drug was haloperidol in the 1950s, and since then a variety of neuroleptics have been used, including newer or atypical agents (Hartmann and Worbe, 2013). The dopamine hypothesis as a substrate for TS essentially originated from this clinical association and has been variably substantiated in more recent functional imaging and other work (Singer et al., 1982; Segura and Strafella, 2013). An alpha-2 adrenergic agonist, clonidine, is well-established and other classes of drugs with some support for efficacy in TS treatment include the anticonvulsant Topiramate and the dopamine depleter tetrabenazine. Treatment efficacy for each option is variable. There is relatively little randomized controlled data, sparse head-to-head comparisons, and the available Class 1 evidence needs to be considered in the context of generally short-term trials conducted over the course of only weeks in a condition that is hard to objectively measure and naturally fluctuates, whereas in clinical practice an initial positive response with less benefit over time is commonly seen. There are several reviews and recommendations for drug treatment and the first truly systematic review and meta-analysis is in press (Roessner et al., 2011; Hollis et al., 2016).

The other conventional modality of treatment is behavioral. These have evolved from the early exploratory literature into evidence-based schedules based around strategies either designed to suppress tics by using competing responses to premonitory urges that precede tics (e.g., Habit Reversal Training; HRT) or to increase tolerance of the premonitory urges (e.g., Exposure with Response Prevention; ERP). HRT has been incorporated into a package called Comprehensive Behavioral Intervention for Tics (CBIT) which was effective in both children and adults in two influential randomized trials of 10 weeks therapy followed up for 6 months (Wilhelm et al., 2012).

In addition to the conventional treatments of pharmacotherapy and behavioral therapy, alternative approaches are also evolving, ranging from neurosurgical stereotactic deep brain stimulation (DBS), which has some evidence base, although not yet extensive, and other more controversial possibilities, such as oral orthotic devices and the use of medical cannabinoids. The treatment talks in this session focused on (1) the more controversial approaches to treating tics and (2) alternative approaches to delivering the more conventional treatments.

John Walkup (Cornell Weill Medical Center), presented the methodology and preliminary results from a TSA sponsored study of an oral orthotic device (an occlusal splint). This treatment evolved out of observations from the dental community that dental orthotics reduce tics anecdotally, with an underlying hypothesis that TS is caused by a brainstem response to dental factors rather than being a genetic neurodevelopmental syndrome (Sims and Stack, 2009). This hypothesis and corresponding treatment approach did not gain initial traction amongst neuropsychiatrists. However, patients and parents in a number of countries have been willing to try occlusal splints, sometimes at significant expense, leading to a real need for a high quality clinical trial. Walkup presented a double blind placebo controlled randomized study using the occlusal splint compared to sham orthotics over 2 weeks, with assessment of durability of effect over a further 4–6 weeks. Outcome measures include changes in tic severity, improvement in functioning, and assessments of acceptability and patient satisfaction. To date, open-label pilot studies of the intervention have found it to be feasible, acceptable and non-harmful. The first three participants had high satisfaction despite mild to moderate adverse effects (sore mouth, excess salivation etc.) and had reduced tic severity with two participants being very much improved on measures of functioning for the initial 2 weeks, although benefit was not sustained at this level for the remaining 4–6 weeks.

Michael Himle (University of Utah), presented the development of "TicHelper," a self-administered online tool for teaching or delivering CBIT from the team that have developed the treatment. If this mode of delivery is successful, there would be immediate potential impact on clinical practice, as specialist psychology resources are limited in most countries, particularly in non-urban areas, so that behavioral therapy often cannot be delivered. In a pilot study, the investigators selected 8 children to use the program for 2 weeks to target a single tic. 7/8 children showed a much increased awareness of tics and were able to demonstrate appropriate use of a competing response, all important components of successful CBIT. Longer term outcomes, including durable improvement of tics, are not yet available.

As noted previously, efforts are underway to understand the neurophysiology and etiology of TS, but much more work is yet to be done. Understanding the neurophysiology of the generation and control of tics and their neural correlates is relevant to identifying and refining appropriate treatments for this complex disorder. This is well-illustrated in the continuing questions over the most effective surgical target for DBS, the most radical of the existing treatments for TS, and the selection of patients likely to benefit. Non-invasive data mapping the neurological substrate for TS is available from functional radioisotope and magnetic resonance imaging and at an altogether different temporal and anatomical resolution by recording from DBS electrodes (Bour et al., 2015). On behalf of Shute et al., Aysegul Gunduz (University of Florida) presented a unique study examining two patients who were implanted with both subdural electrodes (primary motor, M1, and premotor, PM cortices) and depth electrodes (thalamic centromedian nucleus, Cm). Awake recordings were made of local field potentials (thalamus) and electrocorticograms (cortex) with the patient ticcing, suppressing tics, making voluntary movements, and imitating tics. Regionally specific activation patterns were suggested by phase amplitude coupling analysis (PAC). A dissociation was found between ticcing in which contralateral low frequency activity in all three areas was seen and for voluntary movements in which only the cortex was active. In one patient, tics could be detected electrophysiologically using this approach with 70% sensitivity and specificity. This complements the better established field of PAC changes in Parkinson's disease and its treatment with DBS and also opens further possibilities for capture and treatment of tics within closed loop adaptive DBS systems (Almeida et al., 2015).

Controversies in Treatment

In addition to the scientific presentations, the two congress debate sessions focused on treatment, and in particular, on controversies in treatment. The first explored CBIT vs. pharmacotherapy as first line treatment, and was chaired by Stanley Fahn (Columbia University), and presented by Douglas Woods (Texas A & M University; advocating CBIT) and Donald Gilbert (Cincinnati Children's Medical Center; advocating pharmacotherapy). Like all good conference debates, fair amounts of devil's advocacy and inventiveness were employed, reflecting the underlying truths that all clinicians are grappling with- drugs are not as reliably effective as we would like and commonly cause adverse effects (usually mild), CBIT and other behavioral interventions are not as accessible as they should be due to lack of funding and experienced practitioners within local reach. An important point that was raised during the debate was the fact that there are no comparative studies of the two modalities of treatment, and that such studies are necessary.

The other topic was the use of cannabinoids (including marijuana) in the treatment of TS, and was chaired by Joseph Jankovic (Baylor College of Medicine) and energetically debated by Kirsten Mueller-Vahl (Hannover School of Medicine; representing the pro-cannabinoid stance), and Paul Sandor (University of Toronto; representing the anti-cannabinoid stance). The underlying hypothesis was that neurotransmitters other than dopamine, including endocannabinoids, are likely to be important substrates of various aspects of TS. Endocannabinoids are thought to modulate many other classes of neurotransmitter, including monoamines with a high density of CB1 receptors in the basal ganglia. There are limited case reports and two controlled trials of Delta 9-tetrahydrocannabinol (THC; Muller-Vahl et al., 2002, 2003) which followed single dose studies. However, a comprehensive Cochrane review concluded there is insufficient evidence for clinical use (Curtis et al., 2009). As with the other controversial treatments, this area is worthy of further study. In clinical practice it is uncommon for adults in the UK to self-medicate with marijuana despite fairly frequent recreational use, which is in contrast to a German interview study (Muller-Vahl et al., 1997). Use of the medically isolated component of THC may offer different or more reliable effects, perhaps within the usual context of drug treatment of TS in which efficacy of all evidence-based options varies between individuals.

CONCLUSIONS AND FUTURE DIRECTIONS

As can be seen in the work presented in this session, research on the causes and treatment of TS is at a turning point. While much progress has been made in the last 10 years, there is still much to be done. In order to make substantial progress, collaboration is required, not only between investigators in similar fields, but also between scientists and clinicians across disciplines, and between scientists, clinicians, advocacy groups, and patients and families. Such collaborative efforts have been enormously successful in propelling forward breakthroughs in identifying genetic causes of ASD, new and novel treatments for cancer, to name two of many examples. Only with broad support and participation within and across constituencies, as well as a willingness to take risks, will we be able to make real strides forward toward a better understanding of this disorder, and toward effective identification and treatments.

AUTHOR CONTRIBUTIONS

JS part drafted and edited the manuscript. CM part drafted and edited the manuscript. JS and CM co-chaired the hot topics session at which some of the work was presented.

ACKNOWLEDGMENTS

This manuscript was motivated by the first World Congress for Tourette Syndrome and Tic Disorders (London, June 24–26, 2015) and was supported by the Tourette Association of America. We would like to acknowledge the contributions that the speakers and their research teams cited in this article made to the first World Congress on Tourette Syndrome and Tic Disorders.

REFERENCES

Almeida, L., Martinez-Ramirez, D., Rossi, P. J., Peng, Z., Gunduz, A., and Okun M. S. (2015). Chasing tics in the human brain: development of open, scheduled and closed loop responsive approaches to deep brain stimulation for tourette syndrome. *J. Clin. Neurol.* 11, 122–131. doi: 10.3988/jcn.2015.11.2.122

Ben-Shlomo, Y., Scharf, J. M., Miller, L. L., and Mathews, C. A. (2016). Parental mood during pregnancy and post-natally is associated with offspring risk of Tourette syndrome or chronic tics: prospective data from the Avon Longitudinal Study of Parents and Children (ALSPAC). *Eur. Child Adolesc. Psychiatry.* 25, 373–381. doi: 10.1007/s00787-015-0742-0

Bour, L. J., Ackermans, L., Foncke, E. M., Cath, D., van der Linden, C., and Tijssen V. (2015). Tic related local field potentials in the thalamus and the effect of deep brain stimulation in Tourette syndrome: report of three cases. *Clin. Neurophysiol.* 126, 1578–1588. doi: 10.1016/j.clinph.2014.10.217

Curtis, A., Clarke, C. E., and Rickards H. E. (2009). Cannabinoids for Tourette's syndrome. *Cochrane Database Syst. Rev.* 4:CD006565. doi: 10.1002/14651858.CD006565.pub2

Davis, L. K., Yu, D., Keenan, C. L., Gamazon, E. R., Konkashbaev, A. I., Derks, E. M., et al. (2013). Partitioning the heritability of Tourette syndrome and obsessive compulsive disorder reveals differences in genetic architecture. *PLoS Genet.* 9:e1003864. doi: 10.1371/journal.pgen.1003864

Eddy, C. M., and Cavanna, A. E. (2014). Set-shifting deficits: a possible neurocognitive endophenotype for Tourette syndrome without ADHD. *J. Atten. Disord.* doi: 10.1177/1087054714545536. [Epub ahead of print].

Golding, J., Pembrey, M., and Jones, R. (2001). ALSPAC–the Avon longitudinal study of parents and children. I. Study methodology. *Paediatr. Perinat. Epidemiol.* 15, 74–87. doi: 10.1046/j.1365-3016.2001.00325.x

Grayton, H. M., Fernandes, C., Rujescu, D., and Collier, D. A. (2012). Copy number variations in neurodevelopmental disorders. *Prog. Neurobiol.* 99, 81–91. doi: 10.1016/j.pneurobio.2012.07.005

Gribble, S. L., Kim, H. S., Bonner, J., Wang, X., and Dorsky, R. I. (2009). Tcf3 inhibits spinal cord neurogenesis by regulating sox4a expression. *Development* 136, 781–789. doi: 10.1242/dev.027995

Hartmann, A., and Worbe, Y. (2013). Pharmacological treatment of Gilles de la Tourette syndrome. *Neurosci. Biobehav. Rev.* 37, 1157–1161. doi: 10.1016/j.neubiorev.2012.10.014

Hollis, C., Pennant, M., Cuenca, J., Glazebrook, C., Kendall, T., Whittington, C., et al. (2016). Clinical effectiveness and patient perspectives of different treatment strategies for tics in children and adolescents with Tourette syndrome: a systematic review and qualitative analysis. *Health Technol. Assess.* 20, 1–450. doi: 10.3310/hta20040

Mathews, C. A., Bimson, B., Lowe, T. L., Herrera, L. D., Budman, C. L., Erenberg, G., et al. (2006). Association between maternal smoking and increased symptom severity in Tourette's syndrome. *Am. J. Psychiatry* 163, 1066–1073. doi: 10.1176/ajp.2006.163.6.1066

Mathews, C. A., Scharf, J. M., Miller, L. L., Macdonald-Wallis, C., Lawlor, D. A., and Ben-Shlomo, Y. (2014). Association between pre- and perinatal exposures and Tourette syndrome or chronic tic disorder in the ALSPAC cohort. *Br. J. Psychiatry* 204, 40–45. doi: 10.1192/bjp.bp.112.125468

McGrath, L. M., Yu, D., Marshall, C., Davis, L. K., Thiruvahindrapuram, B., Li, B., et al. (2014). Copy number variation in obsessive-compulsive disorder and Tourette syndrome: a cross-disorder study. *J. Am. Acad. Child Adolesc. Psychiatry* 53, 910–919. doi: 10.1016/j.jaac.2014.04.022

Motlagh, M. G., Katsovich, L., Thompson, N., Lin, H., Kim, Y. S., Scahill, L., et al. (2010). Severe psychosocial stress and heavy cigarette smoking during pregnancy: an examination of the pre- and perinatal risk factors associated with ADHD and Tourette syndrome. *Eur. Child Adolesc. Psychiatry* 19, 755–764. doi: 10.1007/s00787-010-0115-7

Muller-Vahl, K. R., Kolbe, H., and Dengler, R. (1997). [Gilles de la Tourette syndrome. Effect of nicotine, alcohol and marihuana on clinical symptoms]. *Nervenarzt* 68, 985–989.

Muller-Vahl, K. R., Schneider, U., Koblenz, A., Jobges, M., Kolbe, H., Daldrup, T., et al. (2002). Treatment of Tourette's syndrome with Delta 9-tetrahydrocannabinol (THC): a randomized crossover trial. *Pharmacopsychiatry* 35, 57–61. doi: 10.1055/s-2002-25028

Muller-Vahl, K. R., Schneider, U., Prevedel, H., Theloe, K., Kolbe, H., Daldrup, T., et al. (2003). Delta 9-tetrahydrocannabinol (THC) is effective in the treatment of tics in Tourette syndrome: a 6-week randomized trial. *J. Clin. Psychiatry* 64, 459–465. doi: 10.4088/JCP.v64n0417

Nag, A., Bochukova, E. G., Kremeyer, B., Campbell, D. D., Muller, H., Valencia-Duarte, A. V., et al. (2013). CNV analysis in Tourette syndrome implicates large genomic rearrangements in COL8A1 and NRXN1. *PLoS ONE* 8:e59061. doi: 10.1371/journal.pone.0059061

Pauls, D. L., Abramovitch, A., Rauch, S. L., and Geller, D. A. (2014a). Obsessive-compulsive disorder: an integrative genetic and neurobiological perspective. *Nat. Rev. Neurosci.* 15, 410–424. doi: 10.1038/nrn3746

Pauls, D. L., Fernandez, T. V., Mathews, C. A., State, M. W., and Scharf, J. M. (2014b). The inheritance of Tourette disorder: a review. *J. Obsessive Compuls. Relat. Disord.* 3, 380–385. doi: 10.1016/j.jocrd.2014.06.003

Peskin, V. A., Ordonez, A., Mackin, R. S., Delucchi, K., Monge, S., Mcgough, J. J., et al. (2015). Neuropsychological and dimensional behavioral trait profiles in Costa Rican ADHD sib pairs: potential intermediate phenotypes for genetic studies. *Am. J. Med. Genet. B Neuropsychiatr. Genet.* 168B, 247–257. doi: 10.1002/ajmg.b.32305

Pineda, D. A., Lopera, F., Puerta, I. C., Trujillo-Orrego, N., Aguirre-Acevedo, D. C., Hincapie-Henao, L., et al. (2011). Potential cognitive endophenotypes in multigenerational families: segregating ADHD from a genetic isolate. *Atten. Defic. Hyperact. Disord.* 3, 291–299. doi: 10.1007/s12402-011-0061-3

Pringsheim, T., Sandor, P., Lang, A., Shah, P., and O'connor, P. (2009). Prenatal and perinatal morbidity in children with Tourette syndrome and attention-deficit hyperactivity disorder. *J. Dev. Behav. Pediatr.* 30, 115–121. doi: 10.1097/DBP.0b013e31819e6a33

Roessner, V., Plessen, K. J., Rothenberger, A., Ludolph, A. G., Rizzo, R., Skov, L., et al. (2011). European clinical guidelines for Tourette syndrome and other tic disorders. Part II: pharmacological treatment. *Eur. Child Adolesc. Psychiatry* 20, 173–196. doi: 10.1007/s00787-011-0163-7

Segura, B., and Strafella, A. P. (2013). Functional imaging of dopaminergic neurotransmission in Tourette syndrome. *Int. Rev. Neurobiol.* 112, 73–93. doi: 10.1016/B978-0-12-411546-0.00003-2

Sims, A., and Stack, B. (2009). Tourette's syndrome: a pilot study for the discontinuance of a movement disorder. *Cranio* 27, 11–18. doi: 10.1179/crn.2009.003

Singer, H. S., Butler, I. J., Tune, L. E., Seifert, W. E. Jr., and Coyle, J. T. (1982). Dopaminergic dsyfunction in Tourette syndrome. *Ann. Neurol.* 12, 361–366. doi: 10.1002/ana.410120408

Wilhelm, S., Peterson, A. L., Piacentini, J., Woods, D. W., Deckersbach, T., Sukhodolsky, D. G., et al. (2012). Randomized trial of behavior therapy for adults with Tourette syndrome. *Arch. Gen. Psychiatry* 69, 795–803. doi: 10.1001/archgenpsychiatry.2011.1528

24

From Genetics to Epigenetics: New Perspectives in Tourette Syndrome Research

Luca Pagliaroli[1,2], Borbála Vető[2], Tamás Arányi[2,3] and Csaba Barta[1]**

[1] *Institute of Medical Chemistry, Molecular Biology and Pathobiochemistry, Semmelweis University, Budapest, Hungary,*
[2] *Research Centre for Natural Sciences, Institute of Enzymology, Hungarian Academy of Sciences, Budapest, Hungary,*
[3] *Centre National de la Recherche Scientifique UMR 6214, Institut National de la Santé et de la Recherche Médicale U1083, University of Angers, Angers, France*

Edited by:
Kirsten R. Müller-Vahl, Hannover Medical School, Germany

Reviewed by:
Munis Dundar, Erciyes University, Turkey
Thomas V. Fernandez, Yale University School of Medicine, USA

***Correspondence:**
Tamás Arányi
aranyi.tamas@ttk.mta.hu
Csaba Barta
barta.csaba@med.semmelweis-univ.hu

Gilles de la Tourette Syndrome (TS) is a neurodevelopmental disorder marked by the appearance of multiple involuntary motor and vocal tics. TS presents high comorbidity rates with other disorders such as attention deficit hyperactivity disorder (ADHD) and obsessive compulsive disorder (OCD). TS is highly heritable and has a complex polygenic background. However, environmental factors also play a role in the manifestation of symptoms. Different epigenetic mechanisms may represent the link between these two causalities. Epigenetic regulation has been shown to have an impact in the development of many neuropsychiatric disorders, however very little is known about its effects on Tourette Syndrome. This review provides a summary of the recent findings in genetic background of TS, followed by an overview on different epigenetic mechanisms, such as DNA methylation, histone modifications, and non-coding RNAs in the regulation of gene expression. Epigenetic studies in other neurological and psychiatric disorders are discussed along with the TS-related epigenetic findings available in the literature to date. Moreover, we are proposing that some general epigenetic mechanisms seen in other neuropsychiatric disorders may also play a role in the pathogenesis of TS.

Keywords: Tourette Syndrome, genetics, epigenetics, DNA methylation, non-coding RNA, neurological disorders, psychiatric disorders

INTRODUCTION

Gilles de la Tourette Syndrome (TS) is a neurodevelopmental disorder characterized by one vocal and multiple motor tics, lasting longer than a year (Robertson, 2000). The prevalence of TS is estimated to be ~1% and it occurs more in males than females, with a ratio of 4 to 1, without differences between social classes. Furthermore, in almost 90% of cases, TS arises along with comorbid neuropsychiatric disorders: in 45–60% with obsessive-compulsive disorder (OCD), while in 60% of cases with attention deficit hyperactivity disorder (ADHD). Anxiety, behavioral disorders, autism spectrum disorders, and learning disabilities are also quite common among individuals with TS (Baron-Cohen et al., 1999; Coffey et al., 2000; Kurlan et al., 2002; Burd et al., 2005; Robertson and Orth, 2006; Cavanna and Termine, 2012; Robertson, 2012).

Tics are defined as sudden movements or vocalizations that are recurrent, rapid, arrhythmic, and stereotyped. They decline in situations of distraction and relaxation, while they increase under stress and anxiety. It is generally preceded by premonitory urges or a sense of inner tension that is reduced or relieved by the performance of the tic (Kwak et al., 2003). Motor tics can be classified as (i) simple, involving single muscle or small group of muscles such as the case of blinking, eye rolling, nose twitching; or (ii) complex, requiring a coordinated pattern of movement or sound like touching, squatting, jumping. In the case of vocal tics, sniffing, throat clearing, snorting, gulping, and coughing are classified as simple; while barking, making of animal noises, and uttering strings of words are classified as complex (Robertson, 2012). The most common manifestation is the eye blinking, which is often the first to appear as well. The typical age of onset ranges from 2 to 21 years with a mean at 7 years. Tourette Syndrome is characterized by a waxing and waning course, peak symptom intensity is usually noted in late childhood. The decline of symptoms is usually in late adolescence or early adulthood (Fusco et al., 2006; Stillman et al., 2009).

THE GENETIC BACKGROUND OF TOURETTE SYNDROME

Like many other neuropsychiatric disorders, TS also has a complex etiology. Several environmental risk factors have been identified, such as perinatal hypoxia, maternal smoking during pregnancy, exposure to androgens, heat, and fatigue (Swain et al., 2007). These environmental factors may interact with many underlying genetic risk factors. To assess the overall genetic contribution in developing a disorder or trait, heritability estimates can be determined, which usually vary between different studies. Based on a recent meta-analysis of all human twin studies to date, the heritability of tics/tic disorders is 0.45 (Polderman et al., 2015). The two most recent studies on the heritability of TS and tic disorders estimated them to be 0.58 and 0.77, respectively (Davis et al., 2013; Mataix-Cols et al., 2015). The risk for first-degree relatives was significantly higher than for second-degree relatives (odds ratios 18.7 and 4.6, respectively). Despite this relatively large overall genetic contribution, most individual gene variants have only very small effects. Hence, most of the earlier studies attempting to unravel the genetic architecture of TS have been hampered by low statistical power due to small sample sizes and clinical heterogeneity. Linkage and candidate gene association studies have identified a number of chromosomal regions and gene polymorphisms possibly implicated in Tourette Syndrome. The candidates for these small scale studies have traditionally been variations in genes involved in the dopaminergic and serotonergic neurotransmitter systems, generally due to their suspected contribution to the etiology of other psychiatric disorders often comorbid with TS, such as ADHD, OCD, autism, etc.

The studied genetic variations are classified in different categories based on the extent of DNA alteration, including single nucleotide polymorphisms (SNPs), as well as shorter or longer repeat variants, such as variable number of tandem repeats (VNTRs) and copy number variations (CNVs). SNPs are the most common form of genetic variation in humans. A SNP represents the change of a single base-pair (bp) in the individual's DNA sequence. The frequency of a particular SNP can vary from private mutations (i.e., only one individual possesses the variation due to a *de novo* mutation) to very common polymorphisms found in almost half of the population. Millions of SNPs exist in an individual's genome, however, most of them are presumed to be neutral, but some may alter gene expression or cause structural changes in the encoded proteins (and other transcripts). Due to this, many SNPs are known to be associated with various human traits and diseases. VNTRs are polymorphisms in the genome where a short sequence of nucleotides (usually up to 100 bp) is organized in multiple copies, which are clustered together and oriented in the same direction. The copy number can vary between individuals and this may influence gene expression or protein structure. CNVs represent much larger genetic rearrangements (usually thousands to millions of base-pairs in length) and therefore change the copy number of genes within the region due to the deletion or duplication of a chromosomal segment. Gene variants implicated in TS are summarized in **Tables 1, 2**.

Most genetic findings implicated in the pathogenesis of Tourette Syndrome to date are inconsistent and studies yielding positive results lack replication in other independent cohorts. On the other hand, some nominally significant candidate gene associations might suffer from lack of proper statistical correction for multiple testing (e.g., Bonferroni correction). However, there are some examples for positive replications as well, these are summarized in **Table 1**. During the recent years meta-analyses confirmed the role of SLITRK1, NTN4, DRD2, DRD4 and AADAC gene polymorphisms in TS (Liu et al., 2014; Paschou et al., 2014; Yuan et al., 2015; Bertelsen et al., 2016). Here, we will review most of the genes that have been consistently replicated in TS. Single positive findings are summarized in **Table 2** and are not discussed in detail.

SLITRK1 is a member of the SLIT and TRK family, a type-I transmembrane protein with an extracellular leucine-rich repeat domain homologous to SLIT (Aruga and Mikoshiba, 2003). It is involved in the control of neurite outgrowth and it is expressed during both embryonic and postnatal development of the cortex, thalamus and the basal ganglia, the neuroanatomical structures believed to be affected in TS (Proenca et al., 2011). The gene coding for SLITRK1 is one of the most studied in relation with Tourette Syndrome. In 2005, a de novo inversion at chromosome 13q33.1 and two additional rare variants were identified in TS patients in the region including a single nucleotide deletion causing a frameshift and a truncated protein and a mutation in the 3′ untranslated region (3′UTR) at the putative binding site for microRNA hsa-miR-189 (Abelson et al., 2005). Since the original discovery several studies in various populations have attempted to replicate the association with controversial results. In a family study of Canadians, a common variation rs9593835 and two haplotypes were found to be associated with the disorder (Miranda et al., 2009). These results were also confirmed in a large sample of European trios with TS (Karagiannidis et al., 2012). A recent study on SLITRK1 found a significant difference in the distribution of haplotypes consisting of SNPs rs9546538, rs9531520, and rs9593835 between Japanese patients and controls (Inai et al., 2015).

Only one genome-wide association study (GWAS) has been published to date in TS by a large international consortium including a sample of 1285 cases and 4964 ancestry-matched

TABLE 1 | Multiple (positive) findings.

Gene	Full gene name	PUBMED ID	Type of analysis	Variation	Sample size	Ethnicity	References
AADAC	Arylacetamide deacetylase	13	CNV, meta-analysis	Deletion	243 TS patients, 1571 controls	European	Bertelsen et al., 2016
BTBD9	BTB domain containing 9	114781	SNP	rs9296249	110 TS patients, 440 controls	Han Chinese	Guo et al., 2012
			SNP	rs4714156, rs9296249, rs9357271	322 TS patients, 290 controls	French Canadian	Rivière et al., 2009
DRD2/ANKK1	Dopamine receptor D2/ankyrin repeat and kinase domain containing 1	1813/255239	SNP	Taq I A/ rs1800497	523 TS patients, 564 controls	European, Asian	Yuan et al., 2015
			SNP	rs6279, rs1079597, rs4648318	69 TS trios	Antioquian	Herzberg et al., 2010
			SNP	Taq I A/rs1800497	151 TS patients, 183 controls	Taiwanese	Lee et al., 2005
			SNP	Taq I A/rs1800497	274 TS patients, 714 controls	European	Comings et al., 1996b
			SNP	Taq I A/rs1800497	147 TS patients, 314 controls	European	Comings et al., 1991
DRD4	Dopamine receptor D4	1815	VNTR	48 bp exon 3 VNTR	291 TS patients (218 trios), 405 controls	Han Chinese	Liu et al., 2014
			VNTR	48 bp exon 3 VNTR	110 TS trios	French Canadian	Díaz-Anzaldúa et al., 2004
			VNTR	48 bp exon 3 VNTR	64 TS family trios	European	Grice et al., 1996
HDC	Histidine decarboxylase	3067	SNP	rs854150, rs1894236	520 TS families	European	Karagiannidis et al., 2013
			SNP	rare coding mutation (W317X)	720 TS patients, 360 controls	NA	Ercan-Sencicek et al., 2010
IMMP2L	IMP2 inner mitochondrial membrane peptidase-like (*S. cerevisiae*)	83943	CNV	Chromosomal deletion	188 TS patients, 316 controls	European (Danish)	Bertelsen et al., 2014
			CNV	Chromosomal translocation	1TS patient	European (British)	Patel et al., 2011
			SNP	rs112636940	258 TS trios	French Canadian	Díaz-Anzaldúa et al., 2004
			CNV	Chromosomal duplication	1 TS patient		Kroisel et al., 2001
			CNV	Chromosomal duplication	1 TS patient	NA	Petek et al., 2001
			CNV	Chromosomal translocation	1 TS patient	NA	Boghosian-Sell et al., 1996
MAOA	Monoamine oxidase A	4128	VNTR	Promoter	110 TS trios	French Canadian	Díaz-Anzaldúa et al., 2004
			VNTR	Exon	375 TS patients, 280 controls	European	Gade et al., 1998
NRXN1	Neurexin 1	9378	CNV	Chromosomal deletion	210 TS patients	Latin American	Nag et al., 2013
			CNV	Chromosomal deletion	111 TS patients, 73 controls		Sundaram et al., 2010
SLC6A3 (DAT1)	Solute carrier family 6 (neurotransmitter transporter), member 3	6531	VNTR	40 bp VNTR	103 TS trios	European (Hungarian)	Tarnok et al., 2007
			SNP	rs6347	266 TS patients, 236 controls	European	Yoon et al., 2007
			VNTR	40 bp VNTR	110 TS trios	French Canadian	Díaz-Anzaldúa et al., 2004
SLITRK1	SLIT and NTRK like family member 1	114798	SNP	rs9546538, rs9531520, rs9593835	NA	Japanese	Inai et al., 2015
			SNP	rs9593835, r9546538	375 TS families	European	Karagiannidis et al., 2012
			SNP, CNV	var321, chromosomal inversion,	174 TS patients, 2148 controls	European	O'Roak et al., 2010
			SNP	rs9593835	154 TS families	Canadian	Miranda et al., 2009
			SNP	var321	174 TS patients	European (Caucasian)	Abelson et al., 2005

TABLE 2 | Single (positive) findings.

Gene	Full gene name	PUBMED ID	Type of analysis	Variation	Sample size	Ethnicity	Reference
ADORA1	Adenosine A1 receptor	134	SNP	rs2228079	162 TS patients, 210 controls	European (Polish)	Janik et al., 2015
ADORA2A	Adenosine A2a receptor	135	SNP	rs5751876	162 TS patients, 210 controls	European (Polish)	Janik et al., 2015
BDNF	Brain-derived neurotrophic factor	627	SNP	rs6265	331 TS patients, 519 controls	Han Chinese	Liu et al., 2015a
CHRNA7	Cholinergic receptor, nicotinic, alpha 7 (neuronal)	1139	CNV	Chromosomal duplication	1 TS family	European (Danish)	Melchior et al., 2013
CNTNAP2	Contactin associated protein-like 2	26047	CNV	Chromosomal insertion/translocation	1 TS family	NA	Verkerk et al., 2003
COL8A1	Collagen, type VIII, alpha 1	1295	CNV	Chromosomal duplication	210 TS patients	Latin American	Nag et al., 2013
COMT	Catechol-O-methyltransferase	1312	CNV	Chromosomal duplication	1 TS patient	NA	Clarke et al., 2009
DLGAP3	Discs large homolog associated protein 3	28512	SNP	rs11264126	289 TS trios	NA	Crane et al., 2011
DPP6	Dipeptidyl-peptidase 6	1804	CNV	Chromosomal deletion	1 TS family	European (Italian)	Prontera et al., 2014
DRD3	Dopamine receptor D3	1814	SNP	Msc I polymorphism	139 TS patient, 91 controls	European	Comings et al., 1993
GDNF	Glial cell derived neurotrophic factor	2668	SNP	rs3096140	201 TS patients, 253 controls	American	Huertas-Fernández et al., 2015
GRIN2B	Glutamate receptor, ionotropic, N-methyl D-aspartate 2B	14812	SNP	rs1805476, rs1805502	261 TS nuclear families	Han Chinese	Che et al., 2015
GSTP1	Glutathione S-transferase pi 1	2950	SNP	rs6591256	121 TS patients, 105 controls	Taiwanese	Shen et al., 2014
HTR2C	5-hydroxytryptamine receptor 2C	3358	SNP	rs3813929, rs518147	87 TS patients, 311 controls	European	Dehning et al., 2010
IL1RN	Interleukin 1 receptor antagonist	3557	SNP	IL1B/IL1RN	159 TS patients, 175 controls	Taiwanese	Chou et al., 2010
LHX6	LIM homeobox 6	26468	SNP	rs3808901	222 TS trios	European	Paschou et al., 2012
NLGN4	Neuroligin 4, X-linked	57502	CNV	Chromosomal deletion	1 TS family	Irish-English	Lawson-Yuen et al., 2008
NTN4	Netrin 4	59277	SNP, meta-analysis	rs2060546	1008 TS patients, 1220 controls	European/French Canadian	Paschou et al., 2014
OLFM1	Olfactomedin 1	10439	CNV	Chromosomal translocation	176 TS patients	European (Danish)	Bertelsen et al., 2015
PARP1	Poly (ADP-ribose) polymerase 1	142	SNP	rs1805404	123 TS patients, 105 controls	Taiwanese	Wu et al., 2013a
RUNX1T1 (CBFA2T1)	Runt related transcription factor 1; translocated to, 1 (cyclin D related)	862	CNV	Chromosomal translocation	1 TS family	NA	Matsumoto et al., 2000
SLC6A4 (SERT)	Solute carrier family 6 member 4	6532	SNP	rs25531, rs25532	151 TS patients, 858 controls	European	Moya et al., 2013
TBCD	Tubulin folding cofactor D	6904	SNP	rs662669, rs3744161	4 TS families 105/357, 96 TS families	European	Paschou et al., 2004
TDO2	Tryptophan 2,3-dioxygenase	6999	SNP	Intron 6, G/T variant	NA	NA	Comings et al., 1996a
TDP1	Tyrosyl-DNA phosphodiesterase 1	55775	SNP	rs28365054	122 TS patients, 105 controls	Taiwanese	Wu et al., 2013b
TNF	Tumor necrosis factor	7124	SNP	rs1800629	117 TS patients, 405 controls	European	Keszler et al., 2014
TPH2	Tryptophan hydroxylase 2	121278	SNP	rs4565946	98 TS patients, 178 controls	European (German)	Mössner et al., 2007
XRCC1	X-ray repair complementing defective repair in Chinese hamster cells 1	7515	SNP	rs25487	73 TS patients, 158 controls	Han Chinese	Lin et al., 2012

controls (Scharf et al., 2013). After correction for multiple testing, none of the half a million studied SNPs reached genome wide significance ($p < 5*10^{-8}$), however top hits were enriched for gene variants expressed in the brain and some of them coincide with previous candidate genes. The top hit was rs7868992 ($p = 1.85*10^{-6}$), which is located in an intronic region of the *COL27A1* gene (collagen, type XXVII, alpha 1). COL27A1 is a fibrillar collagen primarily expressed in cartilage, but it is also expressed in the cerebellum during several stages of human development (Pace et al., 2003), however, its function in the developing nervous system is unknown (Fox, 2008). Another study in 260 Chinese trios assessed the preferential transmission of the rs7868992 and two other COL27A1 gene variants (rs4979357 and rs7868992) by transmission disequilibrium test (TDT) and found the latter two variants nominally significant, however these results did not survive correction for multiple testing (Liu et al., 2015b).

A replication study with the top 42 SNPs of the original GWAS was performed with a sample of over 600 cases and 600 controls and the meta-analysis yielded a top signal at rs2060546 with $p = 5.8*10^{-7}$ in proximity of the NTN4 gene on chromosome 12q22, which codes for netrin 4, an axon guidance protein expressed in the developing striatum. Many of the previous findings (26 out of 42) showed a similar trend underlining the reliability of the GWAS hits as true risk factors for TS (Paschou et al., 2014).

Dopamine receptors, especially DRD2 and DRD4 are two of the most widely studied candidate genes in the field of psychiatric genetics. The dopamine D2 receptor (DRD2) located on chromosome 11p23.2 was characterized previously with TaqIA, TaqIB and TaqID SNPs based on restriction digestion of these polymorphic sites with the TaqI restriction endonuclease enzyme (Vereczkei et al., 2013). Later it turned out that the TaqIA cleavage site is located ~10 kilobases downstream from the DRD2 gene, in exon 8 of the ANKK1 (ankyrin repeat and kinase domain containing 1) gene (Neville et al., 2004), which is a member of the serine/threonine kinase family. The TaqIA polymorphism (rs1800497) causes an amino acid change in ANKK1 (Glu713Lys), which seems to have a significant effect on the specificity of substrate binding. The protein product of the ANKK1 gene was considered as a negative regulator of the transcription factor NF-kB (Nuclear Factor-Kappa B) (Meylan and Tschopp, 2005). Moreover, the expression levels of NF-kB-regulated genes were shown to be altered by the TaqIA variant in an *in vitro* luciferase system (Huang et al., 2009). Since DRD2 is regulated by NF-kB (Fiorentini et al., 2002; Bontempi et al., 2007) it could be assumed that this ANKK1 variant can indirectly affect DRD2 receptor density. It is also possible, however, that the TaqIA SNP is only a marker of other functional DRD2 variants associated with a number of psychiatric disorders, such as the strongly linked TaqIB (Ponce et al., 2009).

A recent meta-analysis on the association of the TaqIA SNP rs1800497 and TS based on a number of previous case-control studies (**Table 1**) comprising a sample of over 500 cases and 500 controls, as well as TS trios concluded that this variant is indeed a risk factor for the development of the disorder (Yuan et al., 2015).

Another widely studied polymorphic dopamine receptor is thedopamine D4 receptor gene (DRD4) The DRD4 gene located on chromosome 11p15.5 is highly polymorphic, containing over 200 SNPs and several VNTRs. A 48 bp long VNTR ranging from 2 to 11 repeats in exon 3 of the gene changes the length of the third intracellular loop of the receptor (Vereczkei et al., 2013) with a possible effect on downstream signaling efficiency by inhibiting the adenylyl cyclase enzyme (Van Tol et al., 1992). The DRD4 7 repeat allele seems to show decreased sensitivity to dopamine compared to the 4 repeat allele (Asghari et al., 2002) and according to more recent neurobiological findings it does not form heteromers with D2 receptors in the striatum (Borroto-Escuela et al., 2011). The D4 receptor is mainly expressed in cortical and limbic regions in the CNS and carriers of the 7 repeat allele were shown to have higher susceptibility to various addictive behaviors, ADHD, as well as several other psychiatric traits.

A number of candidate gene studies have addressed the issue of possible relevance of the exon 3 VNTR in DRD4 in TS, and a couple of small family studies have found a positive association (**Table 1**). A combined family and case-control study in a Han Chinese TS population revealed significant transmission disequilibrium for the 2 repeat and the 7 repeat alleles. The results suggest that the 2 repeat allele might play a protective role, while the common 4 repeat may predispose to TS (Liu et al., 2014).

Arylacetamide deacetylase (AADAC) is an enzyme involved in neutral lipid lipolysis, detoxification, and drug metabolism and is mainly expressed in the liver (Quiroga and Lehner, 2011). However, its expression in different brain regions has also been confirmed with a so far unknown physiological relevance. A recent CNV-analysis in a smaller Danish TS cohort followed by a meta-analysis of a large European sample of over 1000 TS patients and 100,000 controls confirmed the role of AADAC deletions in TS pathogenesis (Bertelsen et al., 2016).

The IMMP2L gene located on chromosome 7q31 encodes a protein involved in processing the signal peptide sequences used to target mitochondrial proteins into the mitochondrium. Its association with TS was first discovered in a family with a balanced 7;18 translocation (Boghosian-Sell et al., 1996). A recent CNV study in a Danish cohort of 188 TS patients reported a 5′-end intragenic deletion of IMMP2L in seven of these patients (Bertelsen et al., 2014). Interestingly, in 4 of the 7 cases, the deletion was within intron 3. The frequency of this IMMP2L deletion was significantly higher than that of the control population. Notably, IMMP2L has been implicated in other neuropsychiatric disorders, such as autism and ADHD (International Molecular Genetic Study of Autism Consortium, 1998; Elia et al., 2010).

Histidine Decarboxylase (*HDC*), located on chromosome 15q21.2, encodes a member of the group II decarboxylase family that converts the amino acid L-histidine into histamine, a biogenic amine that can act as a local mediator released from mast cells during an immune reaction, as well as a monoaminergic neurotransmitter in the CNS. A premature termination codon (W317X) in the HDC gene was discovered in a large multigenerational family, where the father and all eight of his children were affected with TS had the non-sense variant (Ercan-Sencicek et al., 2010). On the other hand, a study of 100 Han Chinese TS patients failed to confirm the association of this non-sense mutation in HDC with the disorder (Lei et al., 2012). However, a subsequent large family study of 520 European trios with Tourette Syndrome transmission disequilibrium test (TDT) found SNPs rs854150 and rs1894236 to be over-transmitted in patients, confirming the role of HDC in the development of TS (Karagiannidis et al., 2013). Interestingly, HDC knockout mice have also been proposed as a genetic animal model of TS. The KO animals exhibited potentiated tic-like stereotypies, recapitulating a core phenomenology of the disorder (Castellan Baldan et al., 2014; Xu et al., 2015).

The NRXN1 gene located on chromosome 2p16.3 codes for an important mediator of cell-cell interactions in the central nervous system and it has been implicated in neuropsychiatric disorders, such as autism and schizophrenia (Vrijenhoek et al., 2008; Glessner et al., 2009). A rearrangement of ~400 Kb within exons 1-3 of NRXN1 was recently found in TS patients (Nag et al., 2013). Notably, this result is also consistent with a previous analysis reporting the presence of a CNV comprising NRXN1 in a Danish TS cohort (Sundaram et al., 2010).

For a more detailed review on the genetic background of TS and the description of candidate genes where no positive replications were published in the last few years, such as BTBD9, SLC6A3 (DAT1) and MAO-A, see recent review papers by (Paschou, 2013; Pauls et al., 2014).

FROM GENETICS TO EPIGENETICS

As described in the previous section, etiology of Tourette Syndrome has a considerable genetic component. However, it is evident that environment also plays an important role in TS, since discordance between monozygotic twins is not rare, while both prenatal (smoke, alcohol abuse, low birth weight, etc), and perinatal (complicated birth) risk factors were reported. Furthermore, it has also been hypothesized that TS might arise as a consequence of autoimmune mechanisms following Group A β-hemolytic streptococcal infection (GABHS) (Swedo et al., 1998; Snider and Swedo, 2003), a condition labeled as pediatric autoimmune neuropsychiatric disorder associated with streptococcal infection (PANDAS). Finally, the course of the disease is also influenced by environmental factors.

As seen earlier, based on family and twin studies the heritability of TS lies approximately between 50 and 80%, which is a figure often seen in case of other psychiatric disorders. However, gene polymorphisms reported by association studies of these disorders rarely account for more than just a fraction of the overall estimated genetic variance. This phenomenon of "missing heritability" may, in part, be explained by various epigenetic mechanisms arising from the dynamic interaction between the environment and an individual's genome.

Cells are reacting to acute and chronic environmental changes by altering their gene expression state, which can be considered as their adaptive reaction. The first step in this adaptive reaction is the modification of the chromatin structure. Chromatin is the macromolecular complex containing DNA and nuclear proteins/histones. The nucleosome is the building unit of chromatin. It consists of two of each of the four core histones (H3, H4, H2A, and H2B) forming an octamer wrapped around twice by DNA (**Figure 1**). The positively charged N-terminal histone tails are prone to undergo several modifications (acetylation, methylation, phosphorylation, etc.). Similarly, DNA can be methylated. These covalent modifications influence the chromatin structure and lead to changes of the transcriptional state of genes. Even though these changes are dynamic, they can be maintained through cell divisions and from one generation to the next. This mechanism, which does not involve the DNA sequence, but allows the transmission of acquired traits through mitosis and sometimes through a few generations, is called epigenetic inheritance. Another main but chromatin-independent epigenetic mechanism is via non-coding RNAs, which also play a crucial role in gene expression regulation often together with chromatin-related mechanisms.

EPIGENETIC MODIFICATIONS

DNA Methylation

The most common epigenetic modification of DNA is the covalent attachment of a methyl group to the C5 position of cytosines. In mammals methylation occurs almost exclusively in CpG dinucleotides (Ziller et al., 2011). Most of the CpG dinucleotides of the genome are present in regions with low GC abundance (Bird, 1993). These CG dinucleotides are generally methylated in all cell types. Methylation leads to high mutation rate, since the frequent oxidative deamination of 5-methyl-cytosine (5 mC) results in thymine (Antonarakis et al., 2000; Baba et al., 2011). This mutation is inefficiently repaired and thus its transmission rate is high. Therefore, low CpG frequency (10% of the expected) characterizes the non-coding part of the genome and CpG cytosines progressively disappear from these genomic regions. However, short CpG-rich sequences (CpG islands – CGI) are frequently found in gene regulatory regions (Bird et al., 1985; Deaton and Bird, 2011). CGIs often show tissue-specific methylation pattern and are frequently unmethylated (only) in germ cells (Smallwood et al., 2011; Zeng et al., 2014). Thus, the important gene regulatory sequences are preserved from a high mutation rate maintaining their biological function.

DNA methylation is tightly linked to gene expression. The more a regulatory region is methylated the less the gene is expressed. Several gene expression regulating DNA binding proteins (e.g., transcription factors) are sensitive to the methylation of their target sequence. Some of them cannot bind if the sequence is methylated (e.g., CTCF, E2F family, Myc, CREB; Hark et al., 2000; Blattler and Farnham, 2013), while others require methylated DNA for binding (e.g., MeCP2 methyl-CpG-binding protein 2 or Kaiso, a zinc finger protein; Lewis et al., 1992; Prokhortchouk et al., 2001; Arányi et al., 2005; Smith and Meissner, 2013). By the stabilization of different chromatin states, DNA methylation contributes to cell differentiation, cellular memory, X chromosome inactivation, and other nuclear processes. Although initially it was considered to be a static epigenetic mark, DNA methylation dynamically changes (Kangaspeska et al., 2008; Métivier et al., 2008; Yamagata

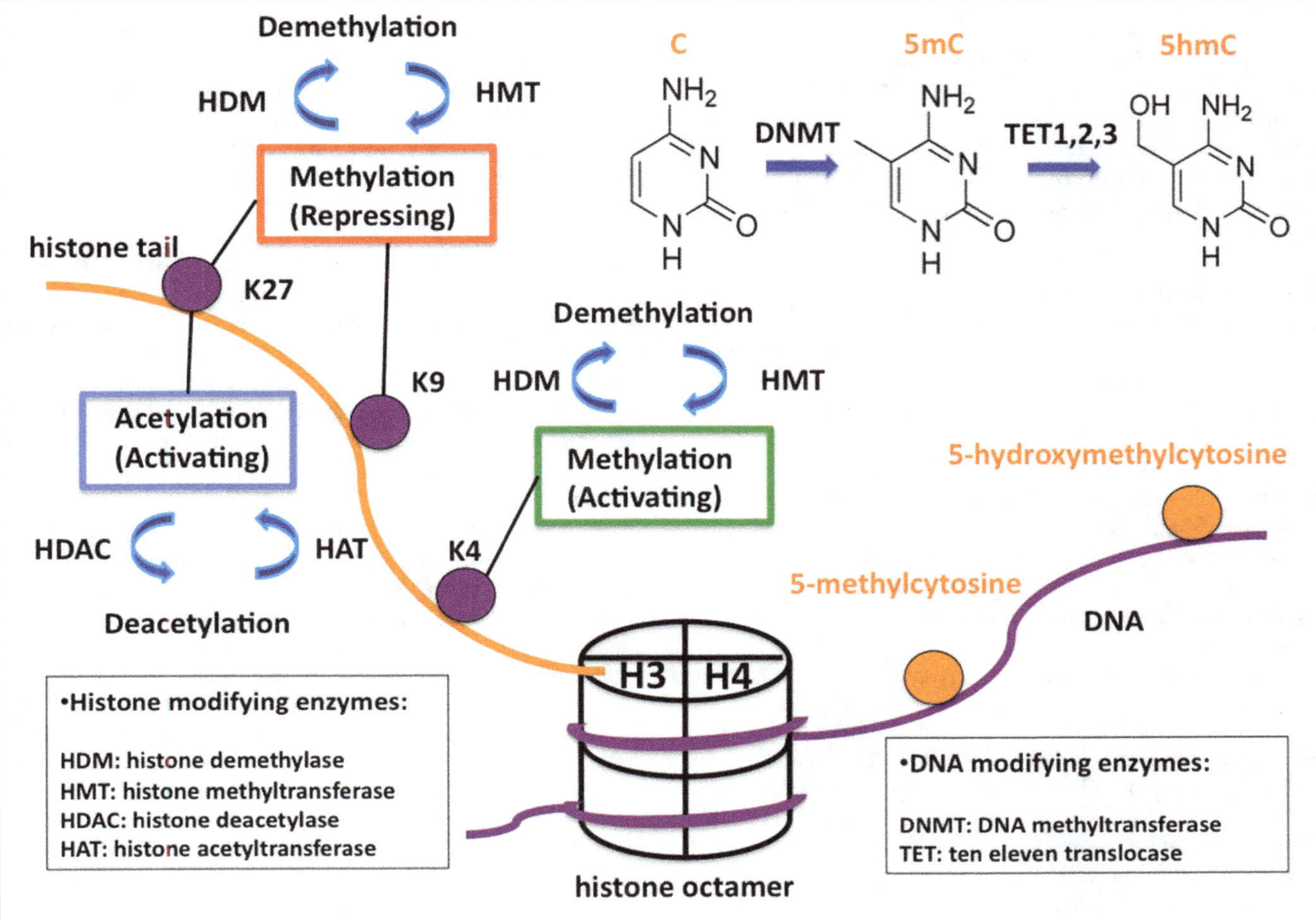

FIGURE 1 | Overview of common covalent epigenetic modifications. A schematic nucleosome and examples of potential epigenetic modifications are shown. The histone octamer is represented in a cylindrical form with one pair of histones H3/H4 indicated. The protruding H3 histone tail and DNA are indicated in orange and purple, respectively. Oppositely, histone and DNA modifications are shown in purple and orange. The functional roles of histone modifications are indicated in colored boxes. The enzyme families catalyzing the modifications are listed in boxes below. The enzymatic links between the different cytosine modifications are shown in the upper right corner of the figure.

et al., 2012b) and different enzymes ensure the equilibrium state.

DNA methylation is catalyzed by DNA methyl-transferase (DNMT) enzymes, which either establish or maintain the methylation pattern. DNMT1 is a maintenance methyl-transferase and it preferentially methylates DNA methylated only on one strand in order to preserve and reestablish the pattern of methylation after DNA replication (Pradhan et al., 1999; Mohan and Chaillet, 2013). By doing so, during DNA replication DNMT1 is enriched at the replication fork and reproduces the methylation pattern based on the original template strand (Schermelleh et al., 2007). DNMT3A and DNMT3B are *de novo* methyl-transferases capable of establishing new patterns of methylation. DNA demethylation is mainly performed by members of the ten-eleven-transferase (TET) enzyme family through the hydroxylation of the methyl group. This leads to the formation of 5-hydroxymethyl-cytosine (5 hmC), which is lost after further oxidation by the same enzyme (Hashimoto et al., 2015). While 5 mC nucleotides represent a few percent (typically between 3 and 7%) of all genomic cytosines in cells and cell lines, 5 hmC is much less abundant constituting only 0.01–1% of all cytosines (Globisch et al., 2010). Interestingly, 5 hmC is rather frequent in primary cells and particularly in the brain (Globisch et al., 2010). Different data also indicate that 5 hmC does not have a general transcriptional repression effect as 5 mC does (Wu et al., 2011; Kang et al., 2015; Li et al., 2016).

During development, genome-wide methylation changes occur before the differentiating cells acquire the adult-type methylation profiles. Similarly, induction of pluripotent stem cells or differentiation of stem cells in their physiological niches is accompanied by general DNA methylation changes. It is a dynamic and lifelong feature of DNA methylation. Local methylation changes happen in response to environmental factors, such as hormonal and metabolic effects or even early childhood stress (see later). The affected genes are silenced for long periods potentially through several generations. Toxic molecules, infections and hereditary or acquired diseases can have similar effects (Yamagata et al., 2012a). However, these alterations can undergo rapid reversion under appropriate environmental conditions. Due to the different environmental factors acting on each individual separately, DNA methylation changes throughout aging generate increasing methylation pattern differences between monozygotic twins, which leads to progressively appearing phenotypical variability (Fraga et al., 2005).

Histone Modifications

Histones are small, globular proteins, which are highly conserved in all eukaryotes. As mentioned earlier, the core histones building up the nucleosomes have N-terminal protruding tails, which are particularly prone to undergo posttranslational modifications (Allfrey et al., 1964). These epigenetic modifications include acetylation, methylation and phosphorylation. They play an important role in different nuclear processes, such as replication, DNA repair, transcription, and chromatin structure stabilization (Kouzarides, 2007; Bannister and Kouzarides, 2011). Although it was reported several decades ago that histones might undergo covalent modifications, their intensive investigation started only in the late 1990s.

The initial studies identified the lysine residues as targets of acetylation and revealed that they are essentially located on the H3 and H4 histone N-terminal tails. These modifications have rapid turnover (Zee et al., 2010). The reactions are catalysed by a high number of histone acetyl-transferases (HAT) and histone deacetylases (HDAC and Sirt) (Kuo and Allis, 1998; Legube and Trouche, 2003). Some complexes with HAT activity (e.g., p300 and CBP–CREB-binding protein) recruit also transcription factors and RNA PolII (Sakamoto et al., 2004). Thus, not surprisingly, lysine acetylation marks transcriptionally active euchromatic gene regulatory regions. For example, H3K27 (lysine 27 of histone H3) acetylation identifies active regulatory elements and separates active and inactive enhancers (ENCODE Project Consortium, 2012). H4 acetylation also indicates active chromatin territories; the acetylation of the two histones often occurs simultaneously. Acetylation profiles are inherited during DNA replication. The molecular mechanisms are still unclear and there might be several. According to one of them, histones with their epigenetic modifications are randomly distributed between the two new DNA molecules while the new chromatin is forming. Than newly synthesized histones are deposited and they rapidly acquire similar modifications to the old ones (Budhavarapu et al., 2013).

After understanding the role of histone acetylation, studies on histone methylation begun. Histone methylation has a much more complex pattern than acetylation since both arginines and lysines can be modified. Furthermore, arginines can be mono- or di-methylated, while lysines can be mono-, di-, or tri-methylated (Bannister and Kouzarides, 2011; Jahan and Davie, 2015; Greenblatt et al., 2016). Dozens of enzymes catalyse these post-translational modifications and their removal. The different enzymes are very selective and are capable to catalyse only one or two specific reactions (such as mono- and di-methylation of a specific lysine but not tri-methylation). Different histone methylations are specifically associated with various gene or chromatin regions. For example, H3K4me3 (trimethylation of lysine 4 of histone H3) marks transcription start sites (TSS) and it is characteristic of active promoters in the euchromatin (Santos-Rosa and Caldas, 2005). In addition, H3K36me3 is associated with actively transcribed gene bodies (Edmunds et al., 2008), while H3K27me3 typically occurs in transcriptionally repressed, heterochromatic regions (Bracken et al., 2006).

Networks of Epigenetic Modifications

In the different chromatin regions, complex patterns of histone and DNA modifications co-occur, which led to the formulation of the "histone code" hypothesis (Jenuwein and Allis, 2001). According to this hypothesis distinct patterns of chromatin modifications at any given genomic region would have the same meaning. These patterns are read by specific proteins, which then execute their local roles accordingly. However, it turned out that the histone code is most probably highly redundant.

Still, the epigenetic modifications are recognized by chromatin binding proteins. These proteins then often antagonize or promote the removal or catalysis of other covalent marks leading to the formation of complex patterns (Bannister and Kouzarides, 2011). Other proteins sensitive to the epigenetic pattern play important role in nuclear processes (e.g., γH2AX, a phosphorylated histone, participating in DNA repair). The proteins sensing and modifying the epigenetic marks are called readers, writers or erasers. Certainly, these proteins bind the chromatin with different affinity and therefore, they reside there for a shorter or longer time period depending on the local environmental context. The networks of modifications are therefore stochastically self-assembling and disassembling with various probability depending on the environmental conditions (Jeltsch and Jurkowska, 2014). This rapidly changing feature of the network makes the system particularly efficient in reacting to environmental stress (e.g., starvation, oxidative stress, or viral infection (Yamagata et al., 2012a) and modulating gene expression states in order to maintain the cellular homeostasis.

Therefore, it is not surprising that enzymes catalysing the addition or removal of covalent post-translational modifications of histones and DNA are closely linked to intermediary metabolism (**Figure 2**). To acetylate lysine residues, HAT enzymes use acetyl-CoA, a key molecule in carbohydrate and fat metabolism. Class III histone deacetylases (Sirt) need NAD+ for their activity (Vaquero et al., 2007). High level of energy intake leads to hyperacetylated histones, while low energy intake favors histone hypoacetylation. Methylation of histones and DNA needs S-adenosyl-methionin (SAM) as a cofactor, the methyl donor in biochemical reactions. The reaction also needs folate to regenerate SAM. The TeT (Ten-eleven Translocase) enzymes are oxygenases, which catalyse the demethylation reaction of DNA through the formation of 5-hydroxy-methyl cytosine. Jumonji family of histone demethylases have a similar reaction mechanism (Chen et al., 2006). Both TeT and Jumonji enzymes use α-ketoglutarate as a co-factor, which is a key metabolite of the citric-acid cycle. Enzymes catalysing the formation of α-ketoglutarate are different isoforms of isocitrate dehydrogenase (IDH). Some of the IDHs are mitochondrial, others are cytosolic,

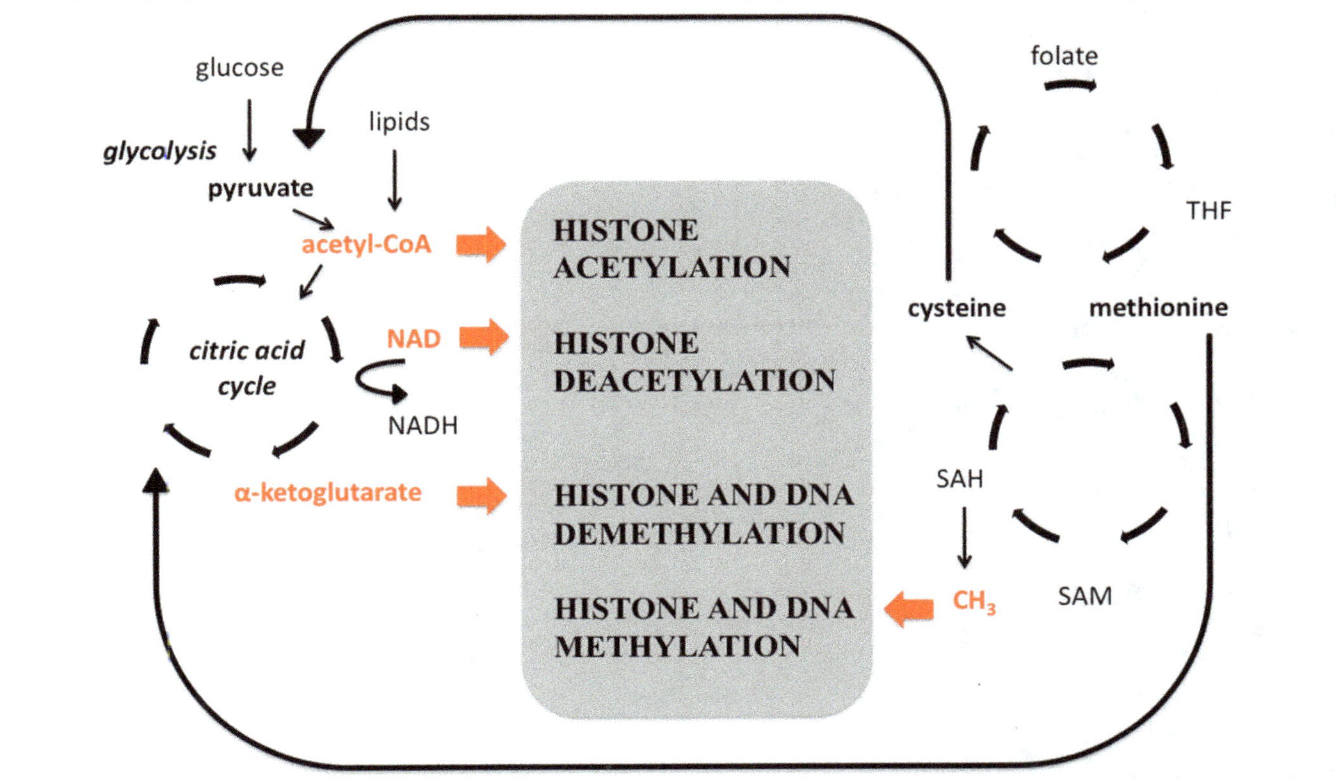

FIGURE 2 | The relationship between epigenetic modifications and intermediary metabolism. Glycolysis, lipid metabolism, citric acid cycle, amino acid metabolism, and folate/SAM cycles are tightly linked to epigenetic modifications (shown in the middle), since their products and cofactors (shown in red) are substrates of enzymes catalyzing the epigenetic modifications. Acetyl-coenzyme A and NAD contribute to histone acetylation and deacetylation, respectively. Methyl groups and alfa-ketoglutarate participate in the methylation and demethylation of both histones and DNA. NAD: nicotinamide adenine dinucleotide, THF: tetrahydrofolate, SAH: S-adenosylhomocysteine, SAM: S-adenosylmethionine.

and they depend on NADP and NAD, respectively. SNPs of these enzymes are associated with TS (see later), while their mutations show frequent occurrence in tumors (gliomas, AML) (Dang et al., 2010). The gain-of-function mutant enzymes catalyse the formation of 2-hydroxyglutarate (2-HG), a potent inhibitor of demethylases. Altogether these data suggest a tight link between environmental factors and epigenetic modifications.

Non-coding RNA(ncRNA)

Evidence from the Encyclopedia of DNA Elements (ENCODE) suggests that at least 80% of our genome is transcribed. The human genome encodes for less than 3% of protein-coding transcripts and consists primarily of the non-coding RNAs (ncRNAs), which was previously regarded as "junk" DNA (https://www.encodeproject.org/). Non-coding RNAs play a role in gene expression regulation (see below). For example they are implicated in the regulation of genes coding for enzymes catalyzing epigenetic modifications. Furthermore, non-coding RNAs are also involved in the regulation of chromosomal domains in tight interaction with epigenetic covalent modifications (e.g., X-chromosome inactivation).

An arbitrary threshold of 200 nucleotides of transcript length was drawn to classify two groups of ncRNAs into small or long ncRNAs. Small ncRNAs include microRNAs (miRNA), transfer RNAs (tRNA) and small nucleolar RNAs (snRNA). A microRNA (miRNA) is a small non-coding RNA molecule found in plants, animals and some viruses, which functions in transcriptional and post-transcriptional regulation of gene expression.

The biogenesis of microRNA involves two different cleavage steps by protein complexes taking place in the nucleus and in the cytoplasm leading to the development of an ~22 nucleotide long mature single-stranded miRNA (**Figure 3**; Filipowicz et al., 2008). First, the gene coding for miRNAs is transcribed by RNA Polimerase II resulting in a long precursor pri-miRNA characterized by a hairpin or fold-back structure with an imperfectly base-paired stem and a terminal loop (Miyoshi et al., 2010). Then, the hairpin structure of the pri-miRNA is cleaved and the ~70 nucleotide long precursor called pre-miRNA is released (Miyoshi et al., 2010). Subsequently, the pre-miRNA is exported into the cytoplasm (Kim et al., 2009). Once in the cytoplasm, the pre-miRNA is processed by RNase III Dicer generating a ~22 nucleotide miRNA-miRNA∗duplex. One strand of the duplex is loaded into a large multi-protein miRNA ribonucleoprotein complex (RISC complex), while the other strand, "passenger," is degraded. Once incorporated into RISC, the miRNA guides the complex to its messenger RNA targets

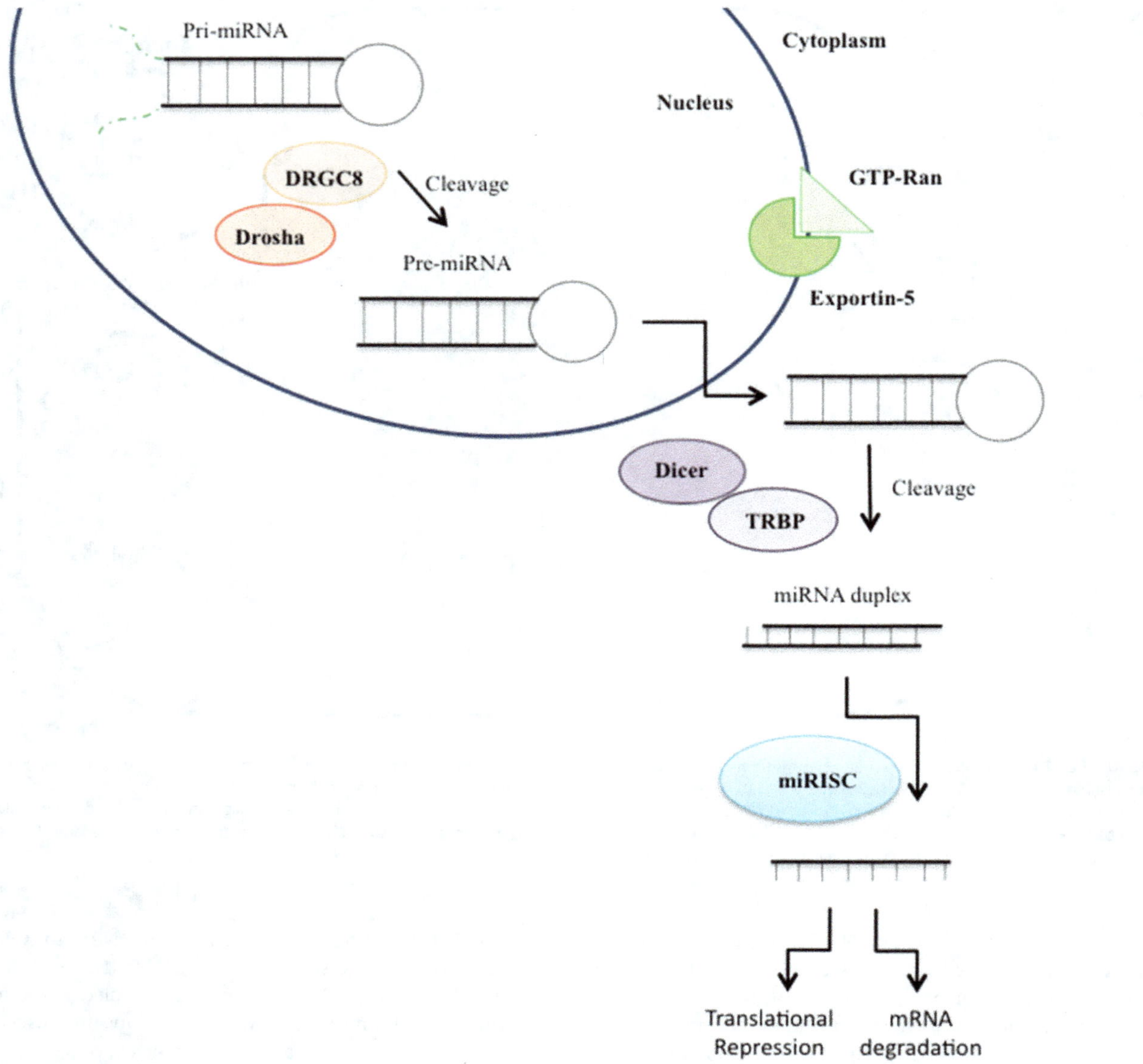

FIGURE 3 | miRNA biogenesis. MicroRNA (miRNA) genes are transcribed as primary miRNAs (pri-miRNAs) by RNA polymerase II (Pol II) in the nucleus. The long pri-miRNAs are cleaved by Microprocessor, which includes DROSHA and DiGeorge syndrome critical region 8 (DGCR8), to produce precursor miRNAs (pre-miRNAs), which are then exported to the cytoplasm by Exportin 5 and further processed by the DICER/TRPB complex to produce an miRNA duplex. One strand of the mature miRNA (the guide strand) is loaded into the miRNA-induced silencing complex (RISC) mediating gene suppression by targeted mRNA degradation or translational repression.

by base-pairing interactions. The binding to the miRNA target relies on the seed sequence, a 6–8 nucleotide domain located at the 5′ end of the miRNA. Based on the complementarity of the seed sequence and the target mRNA sequence located in the 3′UTRof the transcript, miRNAs down-regulate gene expression either through translational repression or mRNA degradation (Hutvágner and Zamore, 2002).

Longer RNAs include ribosomal RNAs (rRNA), natural antisense transcripts and other long non-coding RNAs (lncRNAs). Currently, about 2500 miRNAs and 50,000 lncRNAs have been annotated in the human genome, besides the ∼19,000 protein coding genes. As opposed to miRNAs, only a few lncRNAs show evolutionary conservation of the primary sequence, but most of them show tissue and cell type-specific expression, indicating that their expression must be tightly controlled. LncRNAs exhibit a diversity of molecular functions: they can act as transcriptional activators or repressors, as scaffolds for protein-protein interactions or as molecular decoys.

Genetic polymorphisms can involve both ncRNA sequences throughout the genome, as well as sequences in their target genes, which can affect ncRNA-mediated regulation. Polymorphisms in ncRNA genes can influence both their level of expression and the ncRNA function, thus resulting in differential regulation of their target genes.

Genetic variation may affect miRNA-mediated regulation in different ways. Altered miRNA transcription can be a result of polymorphisms in (a) miRNA promoters, (b) splice sites of the host gene where miRNAs reside, since many miRNAs are intronic, or (c) of polycistronic miRNA clusters (Calore et al., 2015). Mutations in the sequence of the transcribed miRNA may change its binding affinity to the biogenesis enzyme complexes, which changes their processing and may lead to misregulation of target genes. IsomiRs are variants within the processed miRNA sequence, which can affect specificity to their target, on the other hand target messenger RNA 3′UTR variants may either destroy existing miRNA seed regions or create new recognition sites. The presence of a SNP in the 3′UTR can theoretically result in three alterations in miRNA related regulation: (a) it can partially or completely disrupt the miRNA binding site, thus resulting in higher expression of the target gene, or (b) more rarely a SNP could either enhance the binding of a miRNA to the 3′UTR region through improvement of the original recognition site or (c) it may create a novel binding site for another miRNA. The latter will only affect the expression of the target gene if it coincides with the expression of the new miRNA spatially and temporally.

Although lncRNAs possess a much lower degree of conservation than miRNAs, their genetic polymorphisms may still be functional, i.e., SNPs within the lncRNA loci can change their expression or influence their downstream target genes. Altering lncRNA architecture may influence its ability to interact with proteins or other RNAs. In recent years, genetic variations in lncRNAs were implicated in several human diseases.

EPIGENETICS OF NEUROPSYCHIATRIC DISORDERS

Epimutations are epigenetic alterations, which have been linked to several diseases. These alterations can be classified as primary or secondary based on their origin (Oey and Whitelaw, 2014). Primary epimutations seem to be due to only environmental stress factors. It is often difficult to understand the pathomechanism of the resulting diseases or traits, which are generally less severe than in the case of secondary epimutations. Secondary epimutations are due to an initial genomic mutation. Most of these mutations target readers, writers and erasers of the epigenetic system and can lead to important changes of the global epigenetic profile (Lopez-Atalaya et al., 2014). In the following section we will describe some examples of epimutations leading to neuropsychiatric disorders (Plazas-Mayorca and Vrana, 2011).

Rubinstein-Taybi Syndrome

Rubinstein-Taybi syndrome has various clinical signs including moderate to severe learning difficulties (for a recent review see Lopez-Atalaya et al., 2014). The hereditary disease is autosomal dominant although very few documented cases of transmission exist. Most of the patients have *de novo* mutations. The development of the syndrome can be attributed to mutations in the CREB-binding protein (CBP) or more rarely in the highly homologous p300 protein encoding genes. Both proteins are transcriptional co-activators, have HAT activity and they bind the acetylated histones *via* their bromodomain. Thus, they provide platforms for other proteins (transcription factors and RNA PolII) necessary for transcription initiation.

Gliomas

Gliomas (Vigneswaran et al., 2015) are tumors arising from glial cells in the central nervous system (CNS). During tumor progression patients experience psychiatric, cognitive, and neurologic symptoms (Boele et al., 2015). Primary low-grade gliomas are typically diagnosed in the 40 s, and after treatment, these slow-growing tumors have a tendency to reappear and progress in grade to become grade III gliomas or glioblastomas (grade IV). In contrast to the secondary high-grade glioblastomas, the primary high-grade glioblastomas are diagnosed later and have very poor prognosis. Although histologically identical, the primary and secondary glioblastomas have different molecular characteristics.

Both primary low-grade and secondary high-grade gliomas are characterized by IDH1/2 mutation (see above). Approximately 90% of the mutations occur in the *IDH1* gene and almost all of them are the R132H variant (Vigneswaran et al., 2015). As mentioned earlier, this enzyme variant catalyzes the formation of an oncometabolite (2-HG), which inhibits DNA and histone demethylation leading to general (secondary) alteration of the epigenetic profile (Cohen et al., 2013). Nevertheless, gliomas with mutated *IDH1/2* gene have better prognosis than the others (Andronesi et al., 2013).

Rett Syndrome

Rett syndrome is a disease affecting only girls (1:10,000–15,000) (Chahrour and Zoghbi, 2007; Katz et al., 2012) and it is characterized by early onset (18 months) and variable neurological symptoms. Severe mental retardation and motor impairment such as ataxia, apraxia, and tremor (Chahrour and Zoghbi, 2007) accompanied by seizures and gastrointestinal symptoms are frequently present (Katz et al., 2012). Rett syndrome is an example of a severe disorder due to the mutation of the MeCP2 gene encoding an epigenetic "reader" i.e., a regulatory protein recognizing an epigenetic mark (Amir et al., 1999). Therefore, although Rett syndrome is considered to be a typical epigenetic disease, no major epigenetic alterations can be observed in the patients. Loss-of-function mutations of the gene coding for the transcriptional repressor *MeCP2* are responsible for the development of the disease (Amir et al., 1999). MeCP2 is a member of the methyl-CpG binding domain (MBD) protein family. Upon binding of methylated DNA, MeCP2 recruits transcriptional repressor complexes and HDACs. Interestingly, MeCP2 has recently been found to bind and repress long genes implicated in neuronal differentiation and modulation of neuronal functions (Gabel et al., 2015).

Autism Spectrum Disorder (ASD)

Rett syndrome is also considered to be a rare form of autism spectrum disorder (ASD) (Mbadiwe and Millis, 2013). ASD is clinically characterized by social communication deficits and repetitive behavior, which appears as early as 2 years of age and causes clinically significant impairment. ASD has high heritability rates suggesting a substantial genetic background. It has a polygenic origin with hundreds of susceptibility genes. Most of them are common variants with small effects, while some rare de novo variants with large effects also exist (Loke et al., 2015). Apart from *MeCP2*, *FMR1*, and *OXTR* also have profound effects and they were repeatedly reported in relation with ASD (Mbadiwe and Millis, 2013). Both of them are also linked to epigenetic alterations, which is clearly secondary in case of FMR1.

Fragile X syndrome

Approximately half of the patients with Fragile X syndrome meet the criteria of autism and it is a relatively frequent cause of ASD (5% of all monogenic cases). The *FMR1* gene encodes FMRP, a polyribosome associated protein playing an important role in protein translation (Penagarikano et al., 2007). The absence of the protein leads to perturbed neuronal development and intellectual disability (Contractor et al., 2015). Fragile X syndrome is caused by a CGG trinucleotide expansion in the regulatory region of the *FMR1* gene located on the chromosome X. This repeat expansion (>200) leads to the attraction of DNA methylation and the loss of expression of the gene (Oberlé et al., 1991; Penagarikano et al., 2007).

The oxytocin receptor (OXTR) gene is also a candidate gene for ASD (Loke et al., 2015). The neurotransmitter and hormone oxytocin was found to play a role in anxiety, aggressive behavior, and other neural functions. Several observations indicate that OXTR plays a role in the development of ASD. For instance, four SNPs in the gene were suggested to be associated with ASD. Furthermore, several studies reported higher DNA methylation level in patients than in controls in the promoter region of the gene (Gregory et al., 2009; Jack et al., 2012; Ziegler et al., 2015). Very important methylation increase (20–40%) was observed both in temporal cortex and peripheral blood. This temporal hypermethylation was also correlated with lower OXTR mRNA levels in autists (Gregory et al., 2009). Thus, it is not surprising that OXTR methylation has been associated with anxiety disorder and other traits characterizing ASD.

A recent genome-wide analysis of DNA methylation studied a sample of 50 monozygotic (MZ) twin pairs including twins discordant, as well as concordant for ASD. Within-twin and between-group analyses identified a number of differentially methylated regions associated with ASD. In addition, the authors reported significant correlations between DNA methylation and quantitatively measured autistic trait scores across the cohort implicating a role for altered DNA methylation in autism (Wong et al., 2014).

Finally, strong evidence shows that ASD has primary epigenetic origin, as well (Tordjman et al., 2014). Children with *in utero* exposure to the HDAC inhibitor valproic acid (an anticonvulsive and mood stabilizer drug) were found in several studies (Moore et al., 2000; Bromley et al., 2013; Christensen et al., 2013) to have a significantly increased risk to develop autism relative to those who were not treated. Other environmental factors during pregnancy can be considered as risk factors for ASD, such as viral infection (e.g., rubella) (Ornoy et al., 2015) and the dietary folic acid supplementation, which is regarded as controversial (Yang et al., 1989; Mbadiwe and Millis, 2013). Finally, several studies indicate that prenatal maternal stress is also a risk factor for developing ASD (Kinney et al., 2008 and references therein).

A considerable number of studies indicate that early life adversities (ELA) (e.g., childhood abuse or even prenatal and/or maternal stress) are severe risk factors for the development of psychiatric disorders such as major depression, suicidal behavior, etc. (Hoffmann and Spengler, 2014; Palma-Gudiel et al., 2015; Cattaneo and Riva, 2016). This seems to be due to a difficulty in coping with stress in these patients. During stress reactions the hypothalamus-pituitary-adrenal axis (HPA) is activated and glucocorticoids (cortisol in humans and corticosterone) are released, which in turn activate the pathways regulated by glucocorticoid and mineralocorticoid receptors. The axis is inhibited by the feedback activation of the glucocorticoid receptor (GR) in the hippocampus (Palma-Gudiel et al., 2015; Cattaneo and Riva, 2016).

The molecular mechanisms of the development of ELA-related alterations have been deciphered in a rat model system (Weaver et al., 2004). Weaver and colleagues have compared pups from "good" nursing and "bad" nursing females, two maternal behaviors generally occurring in rats (Liu et al., 1997; Caldji et al., 1998). Offsprings of "good moms" were less fearful and had a lower stress response in their adulthood than those of "bad moms." Weaver and colleagues observed higher DNA methylation levels in the hippocampus from early childhood (after postnatal day 1) until at least 3 months of age in the GR promoter in the offsprings of "bad moms" relative to those of "good moms." This difference concentrated at a certain region of the promoter and more precisely at a single CpG, located at the binding site of transcription factor NGFI-A regulating GR expression. They also observed the decreased binding of NGFI-A and hypoacetylation of histones in the methylated region of the promoter. These findings were accompanied by lower GR expression. Interestingly, but not surprisingly for an epigenetic mark, both the molecular and the behavioral phenotypes were reversible. Treatment with Trichostatin A, an HDAC inhibitor, reversed histone hypoacetylation, increased NGFI-A binding, GR expression, and decreased DNA methylation to some extent. Similarly, changing the environment had a similar effect as shown by cross-fostering, demonstrating that this phenotype is not determined by the genetic background and should be considered as having a primary epigenetic origin.

Based on these observations, several studies in animal models confirmed these findings (McGowan et al., 2011). In human cohorts a very small, but systematic methylation increase was reported from the same region of the GR promoter in individuals undergoing stressful events (Palma-Gudiel et al., 2015).

Non-coding RNAs are also associated with a wide range of neurodevelopmental, neurodegenerative, and psychiatric diseases both in humans and in animal models (Lin et al., 2011;

Johnson, 2012; Talkowski et al., 2012; Ziats and Rennert, 2012; Nishimoto et al., 2013; Petazzi et al., 2013; Barry et al., 2014). As a recent example, genetic variants of the long non-coding RNA MIAT were found to contribute to the risk of paranoid schizophrenia in a Han Chinese population (Rao et al., 2015). The authors performed a two-stage association analysis on 8 tagging SNPs covering the whole *MIAT* locus in two independent Han Chinese schizophrenia case–control cohorts. The discovery sample with over 1000 cases and 1000 controls yielded a significant increase of the minor T-allele of rs1894720 in patients and this association was confirmed in the replication cohort of a similar size.

MicroRNAs are also implicated in several neuropsychiatric disorders, such as schizophrenia and autism (Beveridge and Cairns, 2012; Mellios and Sur, 2012), neurodegenerative disorders like Alzheimer's and Parkinson's disease (Salta and De Strooper, 2012; Abe and Bonini, 2013; Tan et al., 2013), but also in other neurodevelopmental disorders such as Fragile X syndrome and Rett syndrome (Urdinguio et al., 2010; Wu et al., 2010; Im and Kenny, 2012; Sellier et al., 2013).

Epigenetics of Tourette Syndrome

As described earlier, the studies investigating TS mainly focused on the genetic background of the disease. Only few studies have been performed to date to investigate the role of epigenetic factors and non-coding RNA in the development of TS. One of these identified a nucleotide variant (var321) in the 3′ UTR of the *SLITRK1* gene leading to its stronger repression by miR-189. This variant has been investigated in several studies in Tourette patients and reported to be rare (Abelson et al., 2005). However, the role of this variant in TS pathogenesis is questionable due to its very low frequency (Keen-Kim et al., 2006). The unique study reported to date on the role of microRNAs in Tourette Syndrome profiled the expression of 754 miRNAs in the sera of six TS patients and three unaffected controls (Rizzo et al., 2015). The study found that miR-429, which is involved in midbrain and hindbrain differentiation and synaptic transmission was significantly underexpressed in TS patients. Measurement of circulating miR-429 may in the future be useful as a molecular biomarker to aid TS diagnosis.

Two association studies on DNA methylation related to TS have been conducted so far. The first showed no methylation alteration in TS patients relative to controls in a region on chromosome 8 in KCNK9 and TRAPPC9 genes (Sánchez Delgado et al., 2014). The regions were identified recently by genome-wide screens and by mapping mutations in single families. The other study was the first Epigenome-Wide Association Study (EWAS) investigating DNA methylation differences between hundreds of controls and patients from the Netherlands Twin Registry with tic phenotype (Zilhão et al., 2015). Very small methylation differences were observed, however, an enrichment of differentially methylated neural genes previously linked to neuropsychiatric disorders or with brain specific function was found among the top hits.

Finally, a recent promising study investigated GWAS results on gene sets. The association of TS and a gene set related to carbohydrate metabolism and more particularly a group of 33 genes involved in "astrocyte-neuron metabolic coupling," glycolysis and Krebs-cycle was demonstrated (de Leeuw et al., 2015). This is interesting because the genes identified include IDH2 (see above) and Malic enzyme 1, which is regulated by glucose level. Since these TS associated metabolic genes are known to play a role in epigenetic modifications, this suggeststhat the disorder is potentially characterized by altered neural epigenetic patterns.

Outlook

In the present review, we have shown that TS is a neuropsychiatric disorder with significant heritability. However, while very few rare genetic variants with large effects were described, it is plausible to assume that hundreds or even more frequent variants with small effects underlie the genetic susceptibility of the disorder. Furthermore, a considerable number of observations indicate that environmental factors also play a crucial role in the development of TS. As introduced above, environmental factors act *via* epigenetic modifications, including heritable covalent modifications of the chromatin and regulatory non-coding RNAs. In order to better understand the pathomechanism of TS, we propose here that more studies should be performed focusing on the role of epigenetics.

What questions should be asked? We think that since environmental (risk) factors are implicated in TS, these should be studied with particular interest. For instance, discordant monozygotic twins are very good candidates for finding epigenetic modifications implicated in the development of the disease, since they are genetically identical. Similarly, patients with known prenatal or perinatal antecedents probably also have important epigenetic grounding in the development of TS. We also consider that patients who developed TS due to streptococcus infection should also show epigenetic alteration relative to controls. Finally, since the disease is characterized by waxing and waning, kinetic analysis of epigenetic changes might also reflect important aspects of TS.

Animal models of TS or tic phenotype should also be studied for epigenetic alterations. While studies on human cohorts might be more descriptive, analyses of animal models could explain more directly the underlying molecular mechanisms.

How should these questions be addressed? Currently several techniques are available to study epigenetics. Genome-wide analyses are much more informative than investigations of single targets. These genome-wide approaches have recently become much less expensive and therefore affordable for most of the laboratories or consortia. Expression level and GWAS analyses can be performed on ncRNA, while chromatin immunoprecipitation (ChIP) followed by next generation sequencing (NGS) is useful for the investigation of histone modifications (Furey, 2012). Along with the ongoing technological advances in NGS, identifying genetic variation affecting ncRNA function associated with neuropsychiatric disease is likely to grow rapidly.

Finally, several genome-wide techniques exist for the study of DNA hydroxymethylation and DNA methylation. We propose to study DNA methylation rather than histone modifications, because it is more stable, than the latter one, although not as static as initially thought (Yamagata et al., 2012b). Furthermore, ChIP-like antibody-based techniques are much less quantitative than the chemical transformation (bisulfite conversion-based) techniques developed for DNA methylation. Therefore either array-based hybridization approaches after bisulfite conversion [Illumina 450 k (Bibikova et al., 2011) or the recent 850 k bead chips] or bisulfite conversion coupled to next generation sequencing could yield useful information (Kulis et al., 2012).

What cautions should be taken? First, we consider that the most important issues are sample size and tissue of origin. TS is a psychiatric disease mainly due to alterations in neuronal and potentially in glial cells. These cells in humans are rarely available for research, while blood cells and buccal or nasopharingeal epithelial cells have somewhat different epigenetic signatures. Although some of these cells can have similar epigenetic profiles in some genomic regions to the most important brain regions in TS (e.g., striatum), the results should always be interpreted cautiously (Hannon et al., 2015). In order to avoid such problems, brain samples should be investigated when possible, however that has obvious limitations in humans. Alternatively, as mentioned before discordant monozygotic twins can also be studied, finally, patients with TS presumably due to PANDAS origin are good candidates for blood sample analysis. It is hard to determine the ideal sample size. However, it is clear that already small sample sizes can be informative if repeated experiments give similar results and the samples are well-selected.

Second, new approaches available and proposed lead to the generation of "big data." Their correct analysis is necessary and requires the intensive collaboration of the biomedical and bioinformatitian scientists with profound knowledge of statistics.

Finally, when interpreting data, attention and caution should be exercised. Although biologically meaningful cutoffs for methylation differences between patients and controls is hard to determine, the value of very small but statistically significant changes is questionable. Furthermore, statistically significant hits showing association with the phenotype does not neccessarily mean causality. From a single descriptive experiment causality cannot be concluded, but further experiments should be performed.

In conclusion, we consider that introducing epigenetic studies in TS research has great potential. These investigations based on the previous results, the animal models and the twin and patients registries already existing will certainly identify new molecular mechanisms and hits playing an important role in the development of the disease. The discovery of the molecular details of ncRNA and epigenetic modification mediated regulation of gene expression, proteins and pathways is likely to provide novel insights into the pathogenesis of neuropsychiatric disease including Tourette Syndrome. This will also open new avenues for genetic diagnosis, as well as targeted and personalized therapeutic approaches. These studies will also strengthen the importance of some already known and suspected hits and altogether this will lead to the better understanding of TS and the opening of new avenues for the development of treatments.

AUTHOR CONTRIBUTIONS

LP, BV, TA, and CB were all involved in building up the concept of the paper, literature research, and writing of the manuscript.

ACKNOWLEDGMENTS

This project has been financed by FP7-People-2012-ITN, project: TS-Eurotrain, grant number 316978. CB was supported by the Merit-prize fellowship of Semmelweis University and the Bolyai János research fellowship of the Hungarian Academy of Sciences BO/00987/16/5.

REFERENCES

Abe, M., and Bonini, N. M. (2013). MicroRNAs and neurodegeneration: role and impact. *Trends Cell Biol.* 23, 30–36. doi: 10.1016/j.tcb.2012.08.013

Abelson, J. F., Kwan, K. Y., O'Roak, B. J., Baek, D. Y., Stillman, A. A., Morgan, T. M., et al. (2005). Sequence variants in SLITRK1 are associated with Tourette's syndrome. *Science* 310, 317–320. doi: 10.1126/science.1116502

Allfrey, V. G., Faulkner, R., and Mirsky, A. E. (1964). Acetylation and methylation of histones and their possible role in the regulation of RNA synthesis. *Proc. Natl. Acad. Sci. U.S.A.* 51, 786–794.

Amir, R. E., Van den Veyver, I. B., Wan, M., Tran, C. Q., Francke, U., and Zoghbi, H. Y. (1999). Rett syndrome is caused by mutations in X-linked MECP2, encoding methyl-CpG-binding protein 2. *Nat. Genet.* 23, 185–188. doi: 10.1038/13810

Andronesi, O. C., Rapalino, O., Gerstner, E., Chi, A., Batchelor, T. T., Cahill, D. P., et al. (2013). Detection of oncogenic IDH1 mutations using magnetic resonance spectroscopy of 2-hydroxyglutarate. *J. Clin. Invest.* 123, 3659–3663. doi: 10.1172/JCI67229

Antonarakis, S. E., Krawczak, M., and Cooper, D. N. (2000). Disease-causing mutations in the human genome. *Eur. J. Pediatr.* 159(Suppl. S173–S178). doi: 10.1007/PL00014395

Arányi, T., Faucheux, B. A., Khalfallah, O., Vodjdani, G., Biguet, N. F., Mallet, J., et al. (2005). The tissue-specific methylation of the human tyrosine hydroxylase gene reveals new regulatory elements in the first exon. *J. Neurochem.* 94, 129–139. doi: 10.1111/j.1471-4159.2005.03173.x

Aruga, J., and Mikoshiba, K. (2003). Identification and characterization of Slitrk, a novel neuronal transmembrane protein family controlling neurite outgrowth. *Mol. Cell. Neurosci.* 24, 117–129. doi: 10.1016/S1044-7431(03)00129-5

Asghari, V., Sanyal, S., Buchwaldt, S., Paterson, A., Jovanovic, V., and Van Tol, H. H. M. (2002). Modulation of intracellular cyclic AMP levels by different human dopamine D4 receptor variants. *J. Neurochem.* 65, 1157–1165. doi: 10.1046/j.1471-4159.1995.65031157.x

Baba, Y., Iida, A., and Watanabe, S. (2011). Sall3 plays essential roles in horizontal cell maturation through regulation of neurofilament expression levels. *Biochimie* 93, 1037–1046. doi: 10.1016/j.biochi.2011.02.016

Bannister, A. J., and Kouzarides, T. (2011). Regulation of chromatin by histone modifications. *Cell Res.* 21, 381–395. doi: 10.1038/cr.2011.22

Baron-Cohen, S., Mortimore, C., Moriarty, J., Izaguirre, J., and Robertson, M. (1999). The prevalence of Gilles de la Tourette's syndrome in children and adolescents with autism. *J. Child Psychol. Psychiatry* 40, 213–218.

Barry, G., Briggs, J. A., Vanichkina, D. P., Poth, E. M., Beveridge, N. J., Ratnu, V. S., et al. (2014). The long non-coding RNA Gomafu is acutely regulated in response to neuronal activation and involved in schizophrenia-associated alternative splicing. *Mol. Psychiatry* 19, 486–494. doi: 10.1038/mp.2013.45

Bertelsen, B., Melchior, L., Jensen, L. R., Groth, C., Glenthøj, B., Rizzo, R., et al. (2014). Intragenic deletions affecting two alternative transcripts of the IMMP2L gene in patients with Tourette syndrome. *Eur. J. Hum. Genet.* 22, 1283–1289. doi: 10.1038/ejhg.2014.24

Bertelsen, B., Melchior, L., Jensen, L. R., Groth, C., Nazaryan, L., Debes, N. M., et al. (2015). A t(3;9)(q25.1;q34.3) translocation leading to OLFM1 fusion transcripts in Gilles de la Tourette syndrome, OCD and ADHD. *Psychiatry Res.* 225, 268–275. doi: 10.1016/j.psychres.2014.12.028

Bertelsen, B., Stefánsson, H., Riff Jensen, L., Melchior, L., Mol Debes, N., Groth, C., et al. (2016). Association of AADAC Deletion and Gilles de la Tourette Syndrome in a Large European Cohort. *Biol. Psychiatry* 79, 383–391. doi: 10.1016/j.biopsych.2015.08.027

Beveridge, N. J., and Cairns, M. J. (2012). MicroRNA dysregulation in schizophrenia. *Neurobiol. Dis.* 46, 263–271. doi: 10.1016/j.nbd.2011.12.029

Bibikova, M., Barnes, B., Tsan, C., Ho, V., Klotzle, B., Le, J. M., et al. (2011). High density DNA methylation array with single CpG site resolution. *Genomics* 98, 288–295. doi: 10.1016/j.ygeno.2011.07.007

Bird, A. P. (1993). Functions for DNA methylation in vertebrates. *Cold Spring Harb. Symp. Quant. Biol.* 58, 281–285.

Bird, A., Taggart, M., Frommer, M., Miller, O. J., and Macleod, D. (1985). A fraction of the mouse genome that is derived from islands of nonmethylated, CpG-rich DNA. *Cell* 40, 91–99.

Blattler, A., and Farnham, P. J. (2013). Cross-talk between site-specific transcription factors and DNA methylation states. *J. Biol. Chem.* 288, 34287–34294. doi: 10.1074/jbc.R113.512517

Boele, F. W., Rooney, A. G., Grant, R., and Klein, M. (2015). Psychiatric symptoms in glioma patients from diagnosis to management. *Neuropsychiatr. Dis. Treat.* 11, 1413–1420. doi: 10.2147/NDT.S65874

Boghosian-Sell, L., Comings, D. E., and Overhauser, J. (1996). Tourette syndrome in a pedigree with a 7;18 translocation: identification of a YAC spanning the translocation breakpoint at 18q22.3. *Am. J. Hum. Genet.* 59, 999–1005.

Bontempi, S., Fiorentini, C., Busi, C., Guerra, N., Spano, P., and Missale, C. (2007). Identification and characterization of two nuclear factor-kappaB sites in the regulatory region of the dopamine D2 receptor. *Endocrinology* 148, 2563–2570. doi: 10.1210/en.2006-1618

Borroto-Escuela, D. O., Van Craenenbroeck, K., Romero-Fernandez, W., Guidolin, D., Woods, A. S., Rivera, A., et al. (2011). Dopamine D2 and D4 receptor heteromerization and its allosteric receptor-receptor interactions. *Biochem. Biophys. Res. Commun.* 404, 928–934. doi: 10.1016/j.bbrc.2010.12.083

Bracken, A. P., Dietrich, N., Pasini, D., Hansen, K. H., and Helin, K. (2006). Genome-wide mapping of Polycomb target genes unravels their roles in cell fate transitions. *Genes Dev.* 20, 1123–1136. doi: 10.1101/gad.381706

Bromley, R. L., Mawer, G. E., Briggs, M., Cheyne, C., Clayton-Smith, J., García-Fiñana, M., et al. (2013). The prevalence of neurodevelopmental disorders in children prenatally exposed to antiepileptic drugs. *J. Neurol. Neurosurg. Psychiatry* 84, 637–643. doi: 10.1136/jnnp-2012-304270

Budhavarapu, V. N., Chavez, M., and Tyler, J. K. (2013). How is epigenetic information maintained through DNA replication? *Epigenetics Chromatin* 6:32. doi: 10.1186/1756-8935-6-32

Burd, L., Freeman, R. D., Klug, M. G., and Kerbeshian, J. (2005). Tourette Syndrome and learning disabilities. *BMC Pediatr.* 5:34. doi: 10.1186/1471-2431-5-34

Caldji, C., Tannenbaum, B., Sharma, S., Francis, D., Plotsky, P. M., and Meaney, M. J. (1998). Maternal care during infancy regulates the development of neural systems mediating the expression of fearfulness in the rat. *Proc. Natl. Acad. Sci. U.S.A.* 95, 5335–5340.

Calore, M., De Windt, L. J., and Rampazzo, A. (2015). Genetics meets epigenetics: genetic variants that modulate noncoding RNA in cardiovascular diseases. *J. Mol. Cell. Cardiol* 89, 27–34. doi: 10.1016/j.yjmcc.2015.10.028

Castellan Baldan, L., Williams, K. A., Gallezot, J.-D., Pogorelov, V., Rapanelli, M., Crowley, M., et al. (2014). Histidine decarboxylase deficiency causes tourette syndrome: parallel findings in humans and mice. *Neuron* 81, 77–90. doi: 10.1016/j.neuron.2013.10.052

Cattaneo, A., and Riva, M. A. (2016). Stress-induced mechanisms in mental illness: a role for glucocorticoid signalling. *J. Steroid Biochem. Mol. Biol.* 160, 169–174. doi: 10.1016/j.jsbmb.2015.07.021

Cavanna, A. E., and Termine, C. (2012). Tourette syndrome. *Adv. Exp. Med. Biol.* 724, 375–383. doi: 10.1007/978-1-4614-0653-2_28

Chahrour, M., and Zoghbi, H. Y. (2007). The story of Rett syndrome: from clinic to neurobiology. *Neuron* 56, 422–437. doi: 10.1016/j.neuron.2007.10.001

Che, F., Zhang, Y., Wang, G., Heng, X., Liu, S., and Du, Y. (2015). The role of GRIN2B in Tourette syndrome: results from a transmission disequilibrium study. *J. Affect. Disord.* 187, 62–65. doi: 10.1016/j.jad.2015.07.036

Chen, Z., Zang, J., Whetstine, J., Hong, X., Davrazou, F., Kutateladze, T. G., et al. (2006). Structural insights into histone demethylation by JMJD2 family members. *Cell* 125, 691–702. doi: 10.1016/j.cell.2006.04.024

Chou, I.-C., Lin, H.-C., Wang, C.-H., Lin, W.-D., Lee, C.-C., Tsai, C.-H., et al. (2010). Polymorphisms of interleukin 1 gene IL1RN are associated with Tourette syndrome. *Pediatr. Neurol.* 42, 320–324. doi: 10.1016/j.pediatrneurol.2010.01.006

Christensen, J., Grønborg, T. K., Sørensen, M. J., Schendel, D., Parner, E. T., Pedersen, L. H., et al. (2013). Prenatal valproate exposure and risk of autism spectrum disorders and childhood autism. *JAMA* 309, 1696–1703. doi: 10.1001/jama.2013.2270

Clarke, R. A., Fang, Z. M., Diwan, A. D., and Gilbert, D. L. (2009). Tourette syndrome and klippel-feil anomaly in a child with chromosome 22q11 duplication. *Case Rep. Med.* 2009:361518. doi: 10.1155/2009/361518

Coffey, B. J., Biederman, J., Smoller, J. W., Geller, D. A., Sarin, P., Schwartz, S., et al. (2000). Anxiety disorders and tic severity in juveniles with Tourette's disorder. *J. Am. Acad. Child Adolesc. Psychiatry* 39, 562–568. doi: 10.1097/00004583-200005000-00009

Cohen, A. L., Holmen, S. L., and Colman, H. (2013). IDH1 and IDH2 mutations in gliomas. *Curr. Neurol. Neurosci. Rep.* 13:345. doi: 10.1007/s11910-013-0345-4

Comings, D. E., Comings, B. G., Muhleman, D., Dietz, G., Shahbahrami, B., Tast, D., et al. (1991). The dopamine D2 receptor locus as a modifying gene in neuropsychiatric disorders. *JAMA* 266, 1793–1800.

Comings, D. E., Gade, R., Muhleman, D., Chiu, C., Wu, S., To, M., et al. (1996a). Exon and intron variants in the human tryptophan 2,3-dioxygenase gene: potential association with Tourette syndrome, substance abuse and other disorders. *Pharmacogenetics* 6, 307–318.

Comings, D. E., Muhleman, D., Dietz, G., Dino, M., LeGro, R., and Gade, R. (1993). Association between Tourette's syndrome and homozygosity at the dopamine D3 receptor gene. *Lancet* 341, 906.

Comings, D. E., Wu, S., Chiu, C., Ring, R. H., Gade, R., Ahn, C., et al. (1996b). Polygenic inheritance of Tourette syndrome, stuttering, attention deficit hyperactivity, conduct, and oppositional defiant disorder: the additive and subtractive effect of the three dopaminergic genes–DRD2, D beta H, and DAT1. *Am. J. Med. Genet.* 67, 264–288. doi: 10.1002/(SICI)1096-8628(19960531)67:3<264::AID-AJMG4>3.0.CO;2-N

Contractor, A., Klyachko, V. A., and Portera-Cailliau, C. (2015). Altered neuronal and circuit excitability in Fragile X syndrome. *Neuron* 87, 699–715. doi: 10.1016/j.neuron.2015.06.017

Consortium, T. E. P. (2012). An integrated encyclopedia of DNA elements in the human genome. *Nature* 489, 57. doi: 10.1038/NATURE11247

Crane, J., Fagerness, J., Osiecki, L., Gunnell, B., Stewart, S. E., Pauls, D. L., et al. (2011). Family-based genetic association study of DLGAP3 in Tourette Syndrome. *Am. J. Med. Genet. B. Neuropsychiatr. Genet.* 156B, 108–114. doi: 10.1002/ajmg.b.31134

Dang, L., Jin, S., and Su, S. M. (2010). IDH mutations in glioma and acute myeloid leukemia. *Trends Mol. Med.* 16, 387–397. doi: 10.1016/j.molmed.2010.07.002

Davis, L. K., Yu, D., Keenan, C. L., Gamazon, E. R., Konkashbaev, A. I., Derks, E. M., et al. (2013). Partitioning the heritability of Tourette syndrome and obsessive compulsive disorder reveals differences in genetic architecture. *PLoS Genet.* 9:e1003864. doi: 10.1371/journal.pgen.1003864

de Leeuw, C., Goudriaan, A., Smit, A. B., Yu, D., Mathews, C. A., Scharf, J. M., et al. (2015). Involvement of astrocyte metabolic coupling in Tourette syndrome pathogenesis. *Eur. J. Hum. Genet.* 23, 1519–1522. doi: 10.1038/ejhg.2015.22

Deaton, A. M., and Bird, A. (2011). CpG islands and the regulation of transcription. *Genes Dev.* 25, 1010–1022. doi: 10.1101/gad.2037511

Dehning, S., Müller, N., Matz, J., Bender, A., Kerle, I., Benninghoff, J., et al. (2010). A genetic variant of HTR2C may play a role in the manifestation of Tourette syndrome. *Psychiatr. Genet.* 20, 35–38. doi: 10.1097/YPG.0b013e32833511ce

Díaz-Anzaldúa, A., Joober, R., Rivière, J.-B., Dion, Y., Lespérance, P., Chouinard, S., et al. (2004). Association between 7q31 markers and Tourette syndrome. *Am. J. Med. Genet. A* 127A, 17–20. doi: 10.1002/ajmg.a.20631

Edmunds, J. W., Mahadevan, L. C., and Clayton, A. L. (2008). Dynamic histone H3 methylation during gene induction: HYPB/Setd2 mediates all H3K36 trimethylation. *EMBO J.* 27, 406–420. doi: 10.1038/sj.emboj.7601967

Elia, J., Gai, X., Xie, H. M., Perin, J. C., Geiger, E., Glessner, J. T., et al. (2010). Rare structural variants found in attention-deficit hyperactivity disorder are preferentially associated with neurodevelopmental genes. *Mol. Psychiatry* 15, 637–646. doi: 10.1038/mp.2009.57

Ercan-Sencicek, A. G., Stillman, A. A., Ghosh, A. K., Bilguvar, K., O'Roak, B. J., Mason, C. E., et al. (2010). L-histidine decarboxylase and Tourette's syndrome. *N. Engl. J. Med.* 362, 1901–1908. doi: 10.1056/NEJMoa0907006

Filipowicz, W., Bhattacharyya, S. N., and Sonenberg, N. (2008). Mechanisms of post-transcriptional regulation by microRNAs: are the answers in sight? *Nat. Rev. Genet.* 9, 102–114. doi: 10.1038/nrg2290

Fiorentini, C., Guerra, N., Facchetti, M., Finardi, A., Tiberio, L., Schiaffonati, L., et al. (2002). Nerve growth factor regulates dopamine D(2) receptor expression in prolactinoma cell lines via p75(NGFR)-mediated activation of nuclear factor-kappaB. *Mol. Endocrinol.* 16, 353–366. doi: 10.1210/mend.16.2.0773

Fox, M. A. (2008). Novel roles for collagens in wiring the vertebrate nervous system. *Curr. Opin. Cell Biol.* 20, 508–513. doi: 10.1016/j.ceb.2008.05.003

Fraga, M. F., Ballestar, E., Paz, M. F., Ropero, S., Setien, F., Ballestar, M. L., et al. (2005). Epigenetic differences arise during the lifetime of monozygotic twins. *Proc. Natl. Acad. Sci. U.S.A.* 102, 10604–10609. doi: 10.1073/pnas.0500398102

Furey, T. S. (2012). ChIP-seq and beyond: new and improved methodologies to detect and characterize protein-DNA interactions. *Nat. Rev. Genet.* 13, 840–852. doi: 10.1038/nrg3306

Fusco, C., Bertani, G., Caricati, G., and Della Giustina, E. (2006). Stress fracture of the peroneal bone secondary to a complex tic. *Brain Dev.* 28, 52–54. doi: 10.1016/j.braindev.2005.03.009

Gabel, H. W., Kinde, B., Stroud, H., Gilbert, C. S., Harmin, D. A., Kastan, N. R., et al. (2015). Disruption of DNA-methylation-dependent long gene repression in Rett syndrome. *Nature* 522, 89–93. doi: 10.1038/nature14319

Gade, R., Muhleman, D., Blake, H., MacMurray, J., Johnson, P., Verde, R., et al. (1998). Correlation of length of VNTR alleles at the X-linked MAOA gene and phenotypic effect in Tourette syndrome and drug abuse. *Mol. Psychiatry* 3, 50–60.

Glessner, J. T., Wang, K., Cai, G., Korvatska, O., Kim, C. E., Wood, S., et al. (2009). Autism genome-wide copy number variation reveals ubiquitin and neuronal genes. *Nature* 459, 569–573. doi: 10.1038/nature07953

Globisch, D., Münzel, M., Müller, M., Michalakis, S., Wagner, M., Koch, S., et al. (2010). Tissue distribution of 5-hydroxymethylcytosine and search for active demethylation intermediates. *PLoS ONE* 5:e15367. doi: 10.1371/journal.pone.0015367

Greenblatt, S. M., Liu, F., and Nimer, S. D. (2016). Arginine methyltransferases in normal and malignant hematopoiesis. *Exp. Hematol.* 44, 435–441. doi: 10.1016/j.exphem.2016.03.009

Gregory, S. G., Connelly, J. J., Towers, A. J., Johnson, J., Biscocho, D., Markunas, C. A., et al. (2009). Genomic and epigenetic evidence for oxytocin receptor deficiency in autism. *BMC Med.* 7:62. doi: 10.1186/1741-7015-7-62

Grice, D. E., Leckman, J. F., Pauls, D. L., Kurlan, R., Kidd, K. K., Pakstis, A. J., et al. (1996). Linkage disequilibrium between an allele at the dopamine D4 receptor locus and Tourette syndrome, by the transmission-disequilibrium test. *Am. J. Hum. Genet.* 59, 644–652.

Guo, Y., Su, L., Zhang, J., Lei, J., Deng, X., Xu, H., et al. (2012). Analysis of the BTBD9 and HTR2C variants in Chinese Han patients with Tourette syndrome. *Psychiatr. Genet.* 22, 300–303. doi: 10.1097/YPG.0b013e32835862b1

Hannon, E., Lunnon, K., Schalkwyk, L., and Mill, J. (2015). Interindividual methylomic variation across blood, cortex, and cerebellum: implications for epigenetic studies of neurological and neuropsychiatric phenotypes. *Epigenetics* 10, 1024–1032. doi: 10.1080/15592294.2015.1100786

Hark, A. T., Schoenherr, C. J., Katz, D. J., Ingram, R. S., Levorse, J. M., and Tilghman, S. M. (2000). CTCF mediates methylation-sensitive enhancer-blocking activity at the H19/Igf2 locus. *Nature* 405, 486–489. doi: 10.1038/35013106

Hashimoto, H., Zhang, X., Vertino, P. M., and Cheng, X. (2015). The mechanisms of generation, recognition, and Erasure of DNA 5-Methylcytosine and Thymine oxidations. *J. Biol. Chem.* 290, 20723–20733. doi: 10.1074/jbc.R115.656884

Herzberg, I., Valencia-Duarte, A. V., Kay, V. A., White, D. J., Müller, H., Rivas, I. C., et al. (2010). Association of DRD2 variants and Gilles de la Tourette syndrome in a family-based sample from a South American population isolate. *Psychiatr. Genet.* 20, 179–183. doi: 10.1097/YPG.0b013e32833a215a

Hoffmann, A., and Spengler, D. (2014). DNA memories of early social life. *Neuroscience* 264, 64–75. doi: 10.1016/j.neuroscience.2012.04.003

Huang, W., Payne, T. J., Ma, J. Z., Beuten, J., Dupont, R. T., Inohara, N., et al. (2009). Significant association of ANKK1 and detection of a functional polymorphism with nicotine dependence in an African-American sample. *Neuropsychopharmacology* 34, 319–330. doi: 10.1038/npp.2008.37

Huertas-Fernández, I., Gómez-Garre, P., Madruga-Garrido, M., Bernal-Bernal, I., Bonilla-Toribio, M., Martín-Rodríguez, J. F., et al. (2015). GDNF gene is associated with tourette syndrome in a family study. *Mov. Disord.* 30, 1115–1120. doi: 10.1002/mds.26279

Hutvágner, G., and Zamore, P. D. (2002). A microRNA in a multiple-turnover RNAi enzyme complex. *Science* 297, 2056–2060. doi: 10.1126/science.1073827

Im, H.-I., and Kenny, P. J. (2012). MicroRNAs in neuronal function and dysfunction. *Trends Neurosci.* 35, 325–334. doi: 10.1016/j.tins.2012.01.004

Inai, A., Tochigi, M., Kuwabara, H., Nishimura, F., Kato, K., Eriguchi, Y., et al. (2015). Analysis of SLITRK1 in Japanese patients with Tourette syndrome using a next-generation sequencer. *Psychiatr. Genet.* 25, 256–258. doi: 10.1097/YPG.0000000000000104

International Molecular Genetic Study of Autism Consortium (1998). A full genome screen for autism with evidence for linkage to a region on chromosome 7q. *Hum. Mol. Genet.* 7, 571–578.

Jack, A., Connelly, J. J., and Morris, J. P. (2012). DNA methylation of the oxytocin receptor gene predicts neural response to ambiguous social stimuli. *Front. Hum. Neurosci.* 6:280. doi: 10.3389/fnhum.2012.00280

Jahan, S., and Davie, J. R. (2015). Protein arginine methyltransferases (PRMTs): role in chromatin organization. *Adv. Biol. Regul.* 57, 173–184. doi: 10.1016/j.jbior.2014.09.003

Janik, P., Berdyński, M., Safranow, K., and Żekanowski, C. (2015). Association of ADORA1 rs2228079 and ADORA2A rs5751876 Polymorphisms with Gilles de la Tourette Syndrome in the Polish Population. *PLoS ONE* 10:e0136754. doi: 10.1371/journal.pone.0136754

Jeltsch, A., and Jurkowska, R. Z. (2014). New concepts in DNA methylation. *Trends Biochem. Sci.* 39, 310–318. doi: 10.1016/j.tibs.2014.05.002

Jenuwein, T., and Allis, C. D. (2001). Translating the histone code. *Science* 293, 1074–1080. doi: 10.1126/science.1063127

Johnson, R. (2012). Long non-coding RNAs in Huntington's disease neurodegeneration. *Neurobiol. Dis.* 46, 245–254. doi: 10.1016/j.nbd.2011.12.006

Kang, J., Lienhard, M., Pastor, W. A., Chawla, A., Novotny, M., Tsagaratou, A., et al. (2015). Simultaneous deletion of the methylcytosine oxidases Tet1 and Tet3 increases transcriptome variability in early embryogenesis. *Proc. Natl. Acad. Sci. U.S.A.* 112, E4236–E4245. doi: 10.1073/pnas.1510510112

Kangaspeska, S., Stride, B., Métivier, R., Polycarpou-Schwarz, M., Ibberson, D., Carmouche, R. P., et al. (2008). Transient cyclical methylation of promoter DNA. *Nature* 452, 112–115. doi: 10.1038/nature06640

Karagiannidis, I., Dehning, S., Sandor, P., Tarnok, Z., Rizzo, R., Wolanczyk, T., et al. (2013). Support of the histaminergic hypothesis in Tourette syndrome: association of the histamine decarboxylase gene in a large sample of families. *J. Med. Genet.* 50, 760–764. doi: 10.1136/jmedgenet-2013-101637

Karagiannidis, I., Rizzo, R., Tarnok, Z., Wolanczyk, T., Hebebrand, J., Nöthen, M. M., et al. (2012). Replication of association between a SLITRK1 haplotype and Tourette Syndrome in a large sample of families. *Mol. Psychiatry* 17, 665–668. doi: 10.1038/mp.2011.151

Katz, D. M., Berger-Sweeney, J. E., Eubanks, J. H., Justice, M. J., Neul, J. L., Pozzo-Miller, L., et al. (2012). Preclinical research in Rett syndrome: setting the foundation for translational success. *Dis. Model. Mech.* 5, 733–745. doi: 10.1242/dmm.011007

Keen-Kim, D., Mathews, C. A., Reus, V. I., Lowe, T. L., Herrera, L. D., Budman, C. L., et al. (2006). Overrepresentation of rare variants in a specific ethnic group may confuse interpretation of association analyses. *Hum. Mol. Genet.* 15, 3324–3328. doi: 10.1093/hmg/ddl408

Keszler, G., Kruk, E., Kenezloi, E., Tarnok, Z., Sasvari-Szekely, M., and Nemoda, Z. (2014). Association of the tumor necrosis factor -308 A/G promoter polymorphism with Tourette syndrome. *Int. J. Immunogenet.* 41, 493–498. doi: 10.1111/iji.12147

Kim, V. N., Han, J., and Siomi, M. C. (2009). Biogenesis of small RNAs in animals. *Nat. Rev. Mol. Cell Biol.* 10, 126–139. doi: 10.1038/nrm2632

Kinney, D. K., Munir, K. M., Crowley, D. J., and Miller, A. M. (2008). Prenatal stress and risk for autism. *Neurosci. Biobehav. Rev.* 32, 1519–1532. doi: 10.1016/j.neubiorev.2008.06.004

Kouzarides, T. (2007). Chromatin modifications and their function. *Cell* 128, 693–705. doi: 10.1016/j.cell.2007.02.005

Kroisel, P. M., Petek, E., Emberger, W., Windpassinger, C., Wladika, W., and Wagner, K. (2001). Candidate region for Gilles de la Tourette syndrome at 7q31. *Am. J. Med. Genet.* 101, 259–261. doi: 10.1002/1096-8628(20010701)101:3<259::AID-AJMG1374>3.0.CO;2-#

Kulis, M., Heath, S., Bibikova, M., Queirós, A. C., Navarro, A., Clot, G., et al. (2012). Epigenomic analysis detects widespread gene-body DNA hypomethylation in chronic lymphocytic leukemia. *Nat. Genet.* 44, 1236–1242. doi: 10.1038/ng.2443

Kuo, M. H., and Allis, C. D. (1998). Roles of histone acetyltransferases and deacetylases in gene regulation. *Bioessays* 20, 615–626. doi: 10.1002/(SICI)1521-1878(199808)20:8<615::AID-BIES4>3.0.CO;2-H

Kurlan, R., Como, P. G., Miller, B., Palumbo, D., Deeley, C., Andresen, E. M., et al. (2002). The behavioral spectrum of tic disorders: a community-based study. *Neurology* 59, 414–420. doi: 10.1212/WNL.59.3.414

Kwak, C., Dat Vuong, K., and Jankovic, J. (2003). Premonitory sensory phenomenon in Tourette's syndrome. *Mov. Disord.* 18, 1530–1533. doi: 10.1002/mds.10618

Lawson-Yuen, A., Saldivar, J.-S., Sommer, S., and Picker, J. (2008). Familial deletion within NLGN4 associated with autism and Tourette syndrome. *Eur. J. Hum. Genet.* 16, 614–618. doi: 10.1038/sj.ejhg.5202006

Lee, C.-C., Chou, I.-C., Tsai, C.-H., Wang, T.-R., Li, T.-C., and Tsai, F.-J. (2005). Dopamine receptor D2 gene polymorphisms are associated in Taiwanese children with Tourette syndrome. *Pediatr. Neurol.* 33, 272–276. doi: 10.1016/j.pediatrneurol.2005.05.005

Legube, G., and Trouche, D. (2003). Regulating histone acetyltransferases and deacetylases. *EMBO Rep.* 4, 944–947. doi: 10.1038/sj.embor.embor941

Lei, J., Deng, X., Zhang, J., Su, L., Xu, H., Liang, H., et al. (2012). Mutation screening of the HDC gene in Chinese Han patients with Tourette syndrome. *Am. J. Med. Genet. B Neuropsychiatr. Genet.* 159B, 72–76. doi: 10.1002/ajmg.b.32003

Lewis, J. D., Meehan, R. R., Henzel, W. J., Maurer-Fogy, I., Jeppesen, P., Klein, F., et al. (1992). Purification, sequence, and cellular localization of a novel chromosomal protein that binds to methylated DNA. *Cell* 69, 905–914.

Li, S., Papale, L. A., Zhang, Q., Madrid, A., Chen, L., Chopra, P., et al. (2016). Genome-wide alterations in hippocampal 5-hydroxymethylcytosine links plasticity genes to acute stress. *Neurobiol. Dis.* 86, 99–108. doi: 10.1016/j.nbd.2015.11.010

Lin, M., Pedrosa, E., Shah, A., Hrabovsky, A., Maqbool, S., Zheng, D., et al. (2011). RNA-Seq of human neurons derived from iPS cells reveals candidate long non-coding RNAs involved in neurogenesis and neuropsychiatric disorders. *PLoS ONE* 6:e23356. doi: 10.1371/journal.pone.0023356

Lin, W.-Y., Lee, C.-C., Liu, H.-P., Chou, I.-C., Sheu, J. J.-C., Wan, L., et al. (2012). Association of genetic variations in X-ray repair cross-complementing group 1 and Tourette syndrome. *J. Clin. Lab. Anal.* 26, 321–324. doi: 10.1002/jcla.21525

Liu, D., Diorio, J., Tannenbaum, B., Caldji, C., Francis, D., Freedman, A., et al. (1997). Maternal care, hippocampal glucocorticoid receptors, and hypothalamic-pituitary-adrenal responses to stress. *Science* 277, 1659–1662.

Liu, S., Cui, J., Niu, Z., Yi, M., Zhang, X., Che, F., et al. (2015a). Do obsessive-compulsive disorder and Tourette syndrome share a common susceptibility gene? An association study of the BDNF Val66Met polymorphism in the Chinese Han population. *World J. Biol. Psychiatry* 16, 602–609. doi: 10.3109/15622975.2015.1012226

Liu, S., Cui, J., Zhang, X., Wu, W., Niu, H., Ma, X., et al. (2014). Variable number tandem repeats in dopamine receptor D4 in Tourette's syndrome. *Mov. Disord.* 29, 1687–1691. doi: 10.1002/mds.26027

Liu, S., Yu, X., Xu, Q., Cui, J., Yi, M., Zhang, X., et al. (2015b). Support of positive association in family-based genetic analysis between COL27A1 and Tourette syndrome. *Sci. Rep.* 5:12687. doi: 10.1038/srep12687

Loke, Y. J., Hannan, A. J., and Craig, J. M. (2015). The role of epigenetic change in Autism spectrum disorders. *Front. Neurol.* 6:107. doi: 10.3389/fneur.2015.00107

Lopez-Atalaya, J. P., Valor, L. M., and Barco, A. (2014). Epigenetic factors in intellectual disability: the Rubinstein-Taybi syndrome as a paradigm of neurodevelopmental disorder with epigenetic origin. *Prog. Mol. Biol. Transl. Sci.* 128, 139–176. doi: 10.1016/B978-0-12-800977-2.00006-1

Mataix-Cols, D., Isomura, K., Pérez-Vigil, A., Chang, Z., Rück, C., Larsson, K. J., et al. (2015). Familial risks of Tourette Syndrome and Chronic Tic disorders. A population-based cohort study. *JAMA Psychiatry* 72, 787–793. doi: 10.1001/jamapsychiatry.2015.0627

Matsumoto, N., David, D. E., Johnson, E. W., Konecki, D., Burmester, J. K., Ledbetter, D. H., et al. (2000). Breakpoint sequences of an 1;8 translocation in a family with Gilles de la Tourette syndrome. *Eur. J. Hum. Genet.* 8, 875–883. doi: 10.1038/sj.ejhg.5200549

Mbadiwe, T., and Millis, R. M. (2013). Epigenetics and Autism. *Autism Res. Treat.* 2013, 1–9. doi: 10.1155/2013/826156

McGowan, P. O., Suderman, M., Sasaki, A., Huang, T. C. T., Hallett, M., Meaney, M. J., et al. (2011). Broad epigenetic signature of maternal care in the brain of adult rats. *PLoS ONE* 6:e14739. doi: 10.1371/journal.pone.0014739

Melchior, L., Bertelsen, B., Debes, N. M., Groth, C., Skov, L., Mikkelsen, J. D., et al. (2013). Microduplication of 15q13.3 and Xq21.31 in a family with Tourette syndrome and comorbidities. *Am. J. Med. Genet. B Neuropsychiatr. Genet.* 162B, 825–831. doi: 10.1002/ajmg.b.32186

Mellios, N., and Sur, M. (2012). The Emerging Role of microRNAs in Schizophrenia and Autism Spectrum Disorders. *Front. Psychiatry* 3:39. doi: 10.3389/fpsyt.2012.00039

Métivier, R., Gallais, R., Tiffoche, C., Le Péron, C., Jurkowska, R. Z., Carmouche, R. P., et al. (2008). Cyclical DNA methylation of a transcriptionally active promoter. *Nature* 452, 45–50. doi: 10.1038/nature06544

Meylan, E., and Tschopp, J. (2005). The RIP kinases: crucial integrators of cellular stress. *Trends Biochem. Sci.* 30, 151–159. doi: 10.1016/j.tibs.2005.01.003

Miranda, D. M., Wigg, K., Kabia, E. M., Feng, Y., Sandor, P., and Barr, C. L. (2009). Association of SLITRK1 to Gilles de la Tourette Syndrome. *Am. J. Med. Genet. B Neuropsychiatr. Genet.* 150B, 483–486. doi: 10.1002/ajmg.b.30840

Miyoshi, K., Miyoshi, T., and Siomi, H. (2010). Many ways to generate microRNA-like small RNAs: non-canonical pathways for microRNA production. *Mol. Genet. Genomics* 284, 95–103. doi: 10.1007/s00438-010-0556-1

Mohan, K. N., and Chaillet, J. R. (2013). Cell and molecular biology of DNA methyltransferase 1. *Int. Rev. Cell Mol. Biol.* 306, 1–42. doi: 10.1016/B978-0-12-407694-5.00001-8

Moore, S. J., Turnpenny, P., Quinn, A., Glover, S., Lloyd, D. J., Montgomery, T., et al. (2000). A clinical study of 57 children with fetal anticonvulsant syndromes. *J. Med. Genet.* 37, 489–97. doi: 10.1136/jmg.37.7.489

Mössner, R., Müller-Vahl, K. R., Döring, N., and Stuhrmann, M. (2007). Role of the novel tryptophan hydroxylase-2 gene in Tourette syndrome. *Mol. Psychiatry* 12, 617–619. doi: 10.1038/sj.mp.4002004

Moya, P. R., Wendland, J. R., Rubenstein, L. M., Timpano, K. R., Heiman, G. A., Tischfield, J. A., et al. (2013). Common and rare alleles of the serotonin transporter gene, SLC6A4, associated with Tourette's disorder. *Mov. Disord.* 28, 1263–1270. doi: 10.1002/mds.25460

Nag, A., Bochukova, E. G., Kremeyer, B., Campbell, D. D., Muller, H., Valencia-Duarte, A. V., et al. (2013). CNV analysis in Tourette syndrome implicates large genomic rearrangements in COL8A1 and NRXN1. *PLoS ONE* 8:e59061. doi: 10.1371/journal.pone.0059061

Neville, M. J., Johnstone, E. C., and Walton, R. T. (2004). Identification and characterization of ANKK1: a novel kinase gene closely linked to DRD2 on chromosome band 11q23.1. *Hum. Mutat.* 23, 540–545. doi: 10.1002/humu.20039

Nishimoto, Y., Nakagawa, S., Hirose, T., Okano, H. J., Takao, M., Shibata, S., et al. (2013). The long non-coding RNA nuclear-enriched abundant transcript 1_2 induces paraspeckle formation in the motor neuron during the early phase of amyotrophic lateral sclerosis. *Mol. Brain* 6:31. doi: 10.1186/1756-6606-6-31

O'Roak, B. J., Morgan, T. M., Fishman, D. O., Saus, E., Alonso, P., Gratacòs, M., et al. (2010). Additional support for the association of SLITRK1 var321 and Tourette syndrome. *Mol. Psychiatry* 15, 447–450. doi: 10.1038/mp.2009.105

Oberlé, I., Rousseau, F., Heitz, D., Kretz, C., Devys, D., Hanauer, A., et al. (1991). Instability of a 550-base pair DNA segment and abnormal methylation in fragile X syndrome. *Science* 252, 1097–1102.

Oey, H., and Whitelaw, E. (2014). On the meaning of the word "epimutation". *Trends Genet.* 30, 519–520. doi: 10.1016/j.tig.2014.08.005

Ornoy, A., Weinstein-Fudim, L., and Ergaz, Z. (2015). Prenatal factors associated with autism spectrum disorder (ASD). *Reprod. Toxicol.* 56, 155–169. doi: 10.1016/j.reprotox.2015.05.007

Pace, J. M., Corrado, M., Missero, C., and Byers, P. H. (2003). Identification, characterization and expression analysis of a new fibrillar collagen gene, COL27A1. *Matrix Biol.* 22, 3–14. doi: 10.1016/S0945-053X(03)00007-6

Palma-Gudiel, H., Córdova-Palomera, A., Leza, J. C., and Fañanás, L. (2015). Glucocorticoid receptor gene (NR3C1) methylation processes as mediators of early adversity in stress-related disorders causality: a critical review. *Neurosci. Biobehav. Rev.* 55, 520–535. doi: 10.1016/j.neubiorev.2015.05.016

Paschou, P. (2013). The genetic basis of Gilles de la Tourette Syndrome. *Neurosci. Biobehav. Rev.* 37, 1026–1039. doi: 10.1016/j.neubiorev.2013.01.016

Paschou, P., Feng, Y., Pakstis, A. J., Speed, W. C., DeMille, M. M., Kidd, J. R., et al. (2004). Indications of linkage and association of Gilles de la Tourette syndrome in two independent family samples: 17q25 is a putative susceptibility region. *Am. J. Hum. Genet.* 75, 545–560. doi: 10.1086/424389

Paschou, P., Stylianopoulou, E., Karagiannidis, I., Rizzo, R., Tarnok, Z., Wolanczyk, T., et al. (2012). Evaluation of the LIM homeobox genes LHX6 and LHX8 as candidates for Tourette syndrome. *Genes. Brain. Behav.* 11, 444–451. doi: 10.1111/j.1601-183X.2012.00778.x

Paschou, P., Yu, D., Gerber, G., Evans, P., Tsetsos, F., Davis, L. K., et al. (2014). Genetic association signal near NTN4 in Tourette syndrome. *Ann. Neurol.* 76, 310–315. doi: 10.1002/ana.24215

Patel, C., Cooper-Charles, L., McMullan, D. J., Walker, J. M., Davison, V., and Morton, J. (2011). Translocation breakpoint at 7q31 associated with tics: further evidence for IMMP2L as a candidate gene for Tourette syndrome. *Eur. J. Hum. Genet.* 19, 634–639. doi: 10.1038/ejhg.2010.238

Pauls, D. L., Fernandez, T. V., Mathews, C. A., State, M. W., and Scharf, J. M. (2014). The inheritance of Tourette Disorder: a review. *J. Obsessive. Compuls. Relat. Disord.* 3, 380–385. doi: 10.1016/j.jocrd.2014.06.003

Penagarikano, O., Mulle, J. G., and Warren, S. T. (2007). The pathophysiology of fragile x syndrome. *Annu. Rev. Genomics Hum. Genet.* 8, 109–129. doi: 10.1146/annurev.genom.8.080706.092249

Petazzi, P., Sandoval, J., Szczesna, K., Jorge, O. C., Roa, L., Sayols, S., et al. (2013). Dysregulation of the long non-coding RNA transcriptome in a Rett syndrome mouse model. *RNA Biol.* 10, 1197–1203. doi: 10.4161/rna.24286

Petek, E., Windpassinger, C., Vincent, J. B., Cheung, J., Boright, A. P., Scherer, S. W., et al. (2001). Disruption of a novel gene (IMMP2L) by a breakpoint in 7q31 associated with Tourette syndrome. *Am. J. Hum. Genet.* 68, 848–858. doi: 10.1086/319523

Plazas-Mayorca, M. D., and Vrana, K. E. (2011). Proteomic investigation of epigenetics in neuropsychiatric disorders: a missing link between genetics and behavior? *J. Proteome Res.* 10, 58–65. doi: 10.1021/pr100463y

Polderman, T. J. C., Benyamin, B., de Leeuw, C. A., Sullivan, P. F., van Bochoven, A., Visscher, P. M., et al. (2015). Meta-analysis of the heritability of human traits based on fifty years of twin studies. *Nat. Genet.* 47, 702–709. doi: 10.1038/ng.3285

Ponce, G., Pérez-González, R., Aragüés, M., Palomo, T., Rodríguez-Jiménez, R., Jiménez-Arriero, M. A., et al. (2009). The ANKK1 kinase gene and psychiatric disorders. *Neurotox. Res.* 16, 50–59. doi: 10.1007/s12640-009-9046-9

Pradhan, S., Bacolla, A., Wells, R. D., and Roberts, R. J. (1999). Recombinant human DNA (cytosine-5) methyltransferase. I. Expression, purification, and comparison of de novo and maintenance methylation. *J. Biol. Chem.* 274, 33002–330010.

Proenca, C. C., Gao, K. P., Shmelkov, S. V., Rafii, S., and Lee, F. S. (2011). Slitrks as emerging candidate genes involved in neuropsychiatric disorders. *Trends Neurosci.* 34, 143–153. doi: 10.1016/j.tins.2011.01.001

Prokhortchouk, A., Hendrich, B., Jørgensen, H., Ruzov, A., Wilm, M., Georgiev, G., et al. (2001). The p120 catenin partner Kaiso is a DNA methylation-dependent transcriptional repressor. *Genes Dev.* 15, 1613–1618. doi: 10.1101/gad.198501

Prontera, P., Napolioni, V., Ottaviani, V., Rogaia, D., Fusco, C., Augello, B., et al. (2014). DPP6 gene disruption in a family with Gilles de la Tourette syndrome. *Neurogenetics* 15, 237–242. doi: 10.1007/s10048-014-0418-9

Quiroga, A. D., and Lehner, R. (2011). Role of endoplasmic reticulum neutral lipid hydrolases. *Trends Endocrinol. Metab.* 22, 218–225. doi: 10.1016/j.tem.2011.03.003

Rao, S.-Q., Hu, H.-L., Ye, N., Shen, Y., and Xu, Q. (2015). Genetic variants in long non-coding RNA MIAT contribute to risk of paranoid schizophrenia in a Chinese Han population. *Schizophr. Res.* 166, 125–130. doi: 10.1016/j.schres.2015.04.032

Rivière, J.-B., Xiong, L., Levchenko, A., St-Onge, J., Gaspar, C., Dion, Y., et al. (2009). Association of intronic variants of the BTBD9 gene with Tourette syndrome. *Arch. Neurol.* 66, 1267–1272. doi: 10.1001/archneurol.2009.213

Rizzo, R., Ragusa, M., Barbagallo, C., Sammito, M., Gulisano, M., Calì, P. V., et al. (2015). Circulating miRNAs profiles in tourette syndrome: molecular data and clinical implications. *Mol. Brain* 8, 44. doi: 10.1186/s13041-015-0133-y

Robertson, M. M. (2000). Tourette syndrome, associated conditions and the complexities of treatment. *Brain* 123, 425–462. doi: 10.1093/brain/123.3.425

Robertson, M. M. (2012). The Gilles de la Tourette syndrome: the current status. *Arch. Dis. Child. Educ. Pract. Ed.* 97, 166–175. doi: 10.1136/archdischild-2011-300585

Robertson, M. M., and Orth, M. (2006). Behavioral and affective disorders in Tourette syndrome. *Adv. Neurol.* 99, 39–60.

Sakamoto, S., Potla, R., and Larner, A. C. (2004). Histone deacetylase activity is required to recruit RNA polymerase II to the promoters of selected interferon-stimulated early response genes. *J. Biol. Chem.* 279, 40362–40367. doi: 10.1074/jbc.M406400200

Salta, E., and De Strooper, B. (2012). Non-coding RNAs with essential roles in neurodegenerative disorders. *Lancet. Neurol.* 11, 189–200. doi: 10.1016/S1474-4422(11)70286-1

Sánchez Delgado, M., Camprubí, C., Tümer, Z., Martínez, F., Milà, M., and Monk, D. (2014). Screening individuals with intellectual disability, autism and Tourette's syndrome for KCNK9 mutations and aberrant DNA methylation within the 8q24 imprinted cluster. *Am. J. Med. Genet. B Neuropsychiatr. Genet.* 165B, 472–478. doi: 10.1002/ajmg.b.32250

Santos-Rosa, H., and Caldas, C. (2005). Chromatin modifier enzymes, the histone code and cancer. *Eur. J. Cancer* 41, 2381–2402. doi: 10.1016/j.ejca.2005.08.010

Scharf, J. M., Yu, D., Mathews, C. A., Neale, B. M., Stewart, S. E., Fagerness, J. A., et al. (2013). Genome-wide association study of Tourette's syndrome. *Mol. Psychiatry* 18, 721–728. doi: 10.1038/mp.2012.69

Schermelleh, L., Haemmer, A., Spada, F., Rösing, N., Meilinger, D., Rothbauer, U., et al. (2007). Dynamics of Dnmt1 interaction with the replication machinery and its role in postreplicative maintenance of DNA methylation. *Nucleic Acids Res.* 35, 4301–4312. doi: 10.1093/nar/gkm432

Sellier, C., Freyermuth, F., Tabet, R., Tran, T., He, F., Ruffenach, F., et al. (2013). Sequestration of DROSHA and DGCR8 by expanded CGG RNA repeats alters microRNA processing in fragile X-associated tremor/ataxia syndrome. *Cell Rep.* 3, 869–880. doi: 10.1016/j.celrep.2013.02.004

Shen, C.-P., Chou, I.-C., Liu, H.-P., Lee, C.-C., Tsai, Y., Wu, B.-T., et al. (2014). Association of glutathione S-transferase P1 (GSTP1) polymorphism with Tourette syndrome in Taiwanese patients. *Genet. Test. Mol. Biomarkers* 18, 41–44. doi: 10.1089/gtmb.2013.0245

Smallwood, S. A., Tomizawa, S.-I., Krueger, F., Ruf, N., Carli, N., Segonds-Pichon, A., et al. (2011). Dynamic CpG island methylation landscape in oocytes and preimplantation embryos. *Nat. Genet.* 43, 811–814. doi: 10.1038/ng.864

Smith, Z. D., and Meissner, A. (2013). DNA methylation: roles in mammalian development. *Nat. Rev. Genet.* 14, 204–220. doi: 10.1038/nrg3354

Snider, L. A., and Swedo, S. E. (2003). Post-streptococcal autoimmune disorders of the central nervous system. *Curr. Opin. Neurol.* 16, 359–365. doi: 10.1097/01.wco.0000073938.19076.31

Stillman, A. A., Krsnik, Z., Sun, J., Rasin, M.-R., State, M. W., Sestan, N., et al. (2009). Developmentally regulated and evolutionarily conserved expression of SLITRK1 in brain circuits implicated in Tourette syndrome. *J. Comp. Neurol.* 513, 21–37. doi: 10.1002/cne.21919

Sundaram, S. K., Huq, A. M., Wilson, B. J., and Chugani, H. T. (2010). Tourette syndrome is associated with recurrent exonic copy number variants. *Neurology* 74, 1583–1590. doi: 10.1212/WNL.0b013e3181e0f147

Swain, J. E., Scahill, L., Lombroso, P. J., King, R. A., and Leckman, J. F. (2007). Tourette syndrome and tic disorders: a decade of progress. *J. Am. Acad. Child Adolesc. Psychiatry* 46, 947–968. doi: 10.1097/chi.0b013e318068fbcc

Swedo, S. E., Leonard, H. L., Garvey, M., Mittleman, B., Allen, A. J., Perlmutter, S., et al. (1998). Pediatric autoimmune neuropsychiatric disorders associated with streptococcal infections: clinical description of the first 50 cases. *Am. J. Psychiatry* 155, 264–271. doi: 10.1176/ajp.155.2.264

Talkowski, M. E., Maussion, G., Crapper, L., Rosenfeld, J. A., Blumenthal, I., Hanscom, C., et al. (2012). Disruption of a large intergenic noncoding RNA in subjects with neurodevelopmental disabilities. *Am. J. Hum. Genet.* 91, 1128–1134. doi: 10.1016/j.ajhg.2012.10.016

Tan, L., Yu, J.-T., Hu, N., and Tan, L. (2013). Non-coding RNAs in Alzheimer's disease. *Mol. Neurobiol.* 47, 382–393. doi: 10.1007/s12035-012-8359-5

Tarnok, Z., Ronai, Z., Gervai, J., Kereszturi, E., Gadoros, J., Sasvari-Szekely, M., et al. (2007). Dopaminergic candidate genes in Tourette syndrome: association between tic severity and 3′ UTR polymorphism of the dopamine transporter gene. *Am. J. Med. Genet. B Neuropsychiatr. Genet.* 144B, 900–905. doi: 10.1002/ajmg.b.30517

Tordjman, S., Somogyi, E., Coulon, N., Kermarrec, S., Cohen, D., Bronsard, G., et al. (2014). Gene × Environment interactions in autism spectrum disorders: role of epigenetic mechanisms. *Front. Psychiatry* 5:53. doi: 10.3389/fpsyt.2014.00053

Urdinguio, R. G., Fernandez, A. F., Lopez-Nieva, P., Rossi, S., Huertas, D., Kulis, M., et al. (2010). Disrupted microRNA expression caused by Mecp2 loss in a mouse model of Rett syndrome. *Epigenetics* 5, 656–663. doi: 10.4161/epi.5.7.13055

Van Tol, H. H., Wu, C. M., Guan, H. C., Ohara, K., Bunzow, J. R., Civelli, O., et al. (1992). Multiple dopamine D4 receptor variants in the human population. *Nature* 358, 149–152. doi: 10.1038/358149a0

Vaquero, A., Sternglanz, R., and Reinberg, D. (2007). NAD+-dependent deacetylation of H4 lysine 16 by class III HDACs. *Oncogene* 26, 5505–5520. doi: 10.1038/sj.onc.1210617

Vereczkei, A., Demetrovics, Z., Szekely, A., Sarkozy, P., Antal, P., Szilagyi, A., et al. (2013). Multivariate analysis of dopaminergic gene variants as risk factors of heroin dependence. *PLoS ONE* 8:e66592. doi: 10.1371/journal.pone.00 66592

Verkerk, A. J. M. H., Mathews, C. A., Joosse, M., Eussen, B. H. J., Heutink, P., and Oostra, B. A. (2003). CNTNAP2 is disrupted in a family with Gilles de la Tourette syndrome and obsessive compulsive disorder. *Genomics* 82, 1–9. doi: 10.1016/S0888-7543(03)00097-1

Vigneswaran, K., Neill, S., and Hadjipanayis, C. G. (2015). Beyond the World Health Organization grading of infiltrating gliomas: advances in the molecular genetics of glioma classification. *Ann. Transl. Med.* 3, 95. doi: 10.3978/j.issn.2305-5839.2015.03.57

Vrijenhoek, T., Buizer-Voskamp, J. E., van der Stelt, I., Strengman, E., Sabatti, C., Geurts van Kessel, A., et al. (2008). Recurrent CNVs disrupt three candidate genes in schizophrenia patients. *Am. J. Hum. Genet.* 83, 504–510. doi: 10.1016/j.ajhg.2008.09.011

Weaver, I. C. G., Cervoni, N., Champagne, F. A., D'Alessio, A. C., Sharma, S., Seckl, J. R., et al. (2004). Epigenetic programming by maternal behavior. *Nat. Neurosci.* 7, 847–854. doi: 10.1038/nn1276

Wong, C. C. Y., Meaburn, E. L., Ronald, A., Price, T. S., Jeffries, A. R., Schalkwyk, L. C., et al. (2014). Methylomic analysis of monozygotic twins discordant for autism spectrum disorder and related behavioural traits. *Mol. Psychiatry* 19, 495–503. doi: 10.1038/mp.2013.41

Wu, B.-T., Lin, W.-Y., Chou, I.-C., Liu, H.-P., Lee, C.-C., Tsai, Y., et al. (2013a). Association of poly(ADP-ribose) polymerase-1 polymorphism with Tourette syndrome. *Neurol. Sci.* 34, 1911–1916. doi: 10.1007/s10072-013-1405-x

Wu, B.-T., Lin, W.-Y., Chou, I.-C., Liu, H.-P., Lee, C.-C., Tsai, Y., et al. (2013b). Association of tyrosyl-DNA phosphodiesterase 1 polymorphism with Tourette syndrome in Taiwanese patients. *J. Clin. Lab. Anal.* 27, 323–327. doi: 10.1002/jcla.21606

Wu, H., D'Alessio, A. C., Ito, S., Wang, Z., Cui, K., Zhao, K., et al. (2011). Genome-wide analysis of 5-hydroxymethylcytosine distribution reveals its dual function in transcriptional regulation in mouse embryonic stem cells. *Genes Dev.* 25, 679–684. doi: 10.1101/gad.2036011

Wu, H., Tao, J., Chen, P. J., Shahab, A., Ge, W., Hart, R. P., et al. (2010). Genome-wide analysis reveals methyl-CpG-binding protein 2-dependent regulation of microRNAs in a mouse model of Rett syndrome. *Proc. Natl. Acad. Sci. U.S.A.* 107, 18161–18166. doi: 10.1073/pnas.1005595107

Xu, M., Li, L., Ohtsu, H., and Pittenger, C. (2015). Histidine decarboxylase knockout mice, a genetic model of Tourette syndrome, show repetitive grooming after induced fear. *Neurosci. Lett.* 595, 50–53. doi: 10.1016/j.neulet.2015.03.067

Yamagata, Y., Parietti, V., Stockholm, D., Corre, G., Poinsignon, C., Touleimat, N., et al. (2012a). Lentiviral transduction of CD34(+) cells induces genome-wide epigenetic modifications. *PLoS ONE* 7:e48943. doi: 10.1371/journal.pone.0048943

Yamagata, Y., Szabó, P., Szüts, D., Bacquet, C., Arànyi, T., and Páldi, A. (2012b). Rapid turnover of DNA methylation in human cells. *Epigenetics* 7, 141–145. doi: 10.4161/epi.7.2.18906

Yang, Y. C., Ricciardi, S., Ciarletta, A., Calvetti, J., Kelleher, K., and Clark, S. C. (1989). Expression cloning of cDNA encoding a novel human hematopoietic growth factor: human homologue of murine T-cell growth factor P40. *Blood* 74, 1880–1884.

Yoon, D. Y., Rippel, C. A., Kobets, A. J., Morris, C. M., Lee, J. E., Williams, P. N., et al. (2007). Dopaminergic polymorphisms in Tourette syndrome: association with the DAT gene (SLC6A3). *Am. J. Med. Genet. B Neuropsychiatr. Genet.* 144B, 605–610. doi: 10.1002/ajmg.b.30466

Yuan, A., Su, L., Yu, S., Li, C., Yu, T., and Sun, J. (2015). Association between DRD2/ANKK1 TaqIA Polymorphism and Susceptibility with Tourette Syndrome: a meta-analysis. *PLoS ONE* 10:e0131060. doi: 10.1371/journal.pone.0131060

Zee, B. M., Levin, R. S., Dimaggio, P. A., and Garcia, B. A. (2010). Global turnover of histone post-translational modifications and variants in human cells. *Epigenetics Chromatin* 3:22. doi: 10.1186/1756-8935-3-22

Zeng, J., Nagrajan, H. K., and Yi, S. V. (2014). Fundamental diversity of human CpG islands at multiple biological levels. *Epigenetics* 9, 483–491. doi: 10.4161/epi.27654

Ziats, M. N., and Rennert, O. M. (2012). Aberrant Expression of Long Noncoding RNAs in Autistic Brain. *J. Mol. Neurosci.* 49, 589–593. doi: 10.1007/s12031-012-9880-8

Ziegler, C., Dannlowski, U., Bräuer, D., Stevens, S., Laeger, I., Wittmann, H., et al. (2015). Oxytocin receptor gene methylation: converging multilevel evidence for a role in social anxiety. *Neuropsychopharmacology* 40, 1528–1538. doi: 10.1038/npp.2015.2

Zilhão, N. R., Padmanabhuni, S. S., Pagliaroli, L., Barta, C., Smit, D. J. A., Cath, D., et al. (2015). Epigenome-wide association study of Tic disorders. *Twin Res. Hum. Genet.* 18, 1–11. doi: 10.1017/thg.2015.72

Ziller, M. J., Müller, F., Liao, J., Zhang, Y., Gu, H., Bock, C., et al. (2011). Genomic distribution and inter-sample variation of non-CpG methylation across human cell types. *PLoS Genet.* 7:e1002389. doi: 10.1371/journal.pgen.1002389

Permissions

All chapters in this book were first published in TNGGTSNATLSCP, by Frontiers; hereby published with permission under the Creative Commons Attribution License or equivalent. Every chapter published in this book has been scrutinized by our experts. Their significance has been extensively debated. The topics covered herein carry significant findings which will fuel the growth of the discipline. They may even be implemented as practical applications or may be referred to as a beginning point for another development.

The contributors of this book come from diverse backgrounds, making this book a truly international effort. This book will bring forth new frontiers with its revolutionizing research information and detailed analysis of the nascent developments around the world.

We would like to thank all the contributing authors for lending their expertise to make the book truly unique. They have played a crucial role in the development of this book. Without their invaluable contributions this book wouldn't have been possible. They have made vital efforts to compile up to date information on the varied aspects of this subject to make this book a valuable addition to the collection of many professionals and students.

This book was conceptualized with the vision of imparting up-to-date information and advanced data in this field. To ensure the same, a matchless editorial board was set up. Every individual on the board went through rigorous rounds of assessment to prove their worth. After which they invested a large part of their time researching and compiling the most relevant data for our readers.

The editorial board has been involved in producing this book since its inception. They have spent rigorous hours researching and exploring the diverse topics which have resulted in the successful publishing of this book. They have passed on their knowledge of decades through this book. To expedite this challenging task, the publisher supported the team at every step. A small team of assistant editors was also appointed to further simplify the editing procedure and attain best results for the readers.

Apart from the editorial board, the designing team has also invested a significant amount of their time in understanding the subject and creating the most relevant covers. They scrutinized every image to scout for the most suitable representation of the subject and create an appropriate cover for the book.

The publishing team has been an ardent support to the editorial, designing and production team. Their endless efforts to recruit the best for this project, has resulted in the accomplishment of this book. They are a veteran in the field of academics and their pool of knowledge is as vast as their experience in printing. Their expertise and guidance has proved useful at every step. Their uncompromising quality standards have made this book an exceptional effort. Their encouragement from time to time has been an inspiration for everyone.

The publisher and the editorial board hope that this book will prove to be a valuable piece of knowledge for researchers, students, practitioners and scholars across the globe.

List of Contributors

Heike Eichele, Heidi van Wageningen and Lin Sørensen
Department of Biological and Medical Psychology, University of Bergen, Bergen, Norway

Tom Eichele
Department of Biological and Medical Psychology, University of Bergen, Bergen, Norway
K.G. Jebsen Centre for Research on Neuropsychiatric Disorders, University of Bergen, Bergen, Norway
Section for Neurophysiology, Department of Neurology, Haukeland University Hospital, Bergen, Norway

Ingvar Bjelland
Department of Psychiatry, Haukeland University Hospital, Bergen, Norway
Department of Clinical Medicine, Faculty of Medicine and Dentistry, University of Bergen, Bergen, Norway

Marie F. Høvik and Marius Kalsås Worren
Department of Clinical Medicine, Faculty of Medicine and Dentistry, University of Bergen, Bergen, Norway

Kenneth Hugdahl
Department of Biological and Medical Psychology, University of Bergen, Bergen, Norway
K.G. Jebsen Centre for Research on Neuropsychiatric Disorders, University of Bergen, Bergen, Norway
Department of Psychiatry, Haukeland University Hospital, Bergen, Norway

Kerstin J. Plessen
K.G. Jebsen Centre for Research on Neuropsychiatric Disorders, University of Bergen, Bergen, Norway
Child and Adolescent Mental Health Center, Mental Health Services Capital Region, Copenhagen, Denmark
Department of Clinical Medicine, Faculty of Health and Medical Sciences, University of Copenhagen, Copenhagen, Denmark

Tanvi Sambrani
Department of Education, Monash University, Melbourne, VIC, Australia
Clinic of Psychiatry, Social Psychiatry, and Psychotherapy, Hannover Medical School, Hannover, Germany

Ewgeni Jakubovski and Kirsten R. Müller-Vahl
Clinic of Psychiatry, Social Psychiatry, and Psychotherapy, Hannover Medical School, Hannover, Germany

Valsamma Eapen
School of Psychiatry, University of New South Wales, Sydney, NSW, Australia
Academic Unit of Child Psychiatry, Ingham Institute, Sydney South Western Local Health District, Sydney, NSW, Australia

Andrea E. Cavanna
Department of Neuropsychiatry, Birmingham and Solihull Mental Health NHS Foundation Trust, Birmingham, UK
Aston Brain Centre, School of Life and Health Sciences, Aston University, Birmingham, UK
Sobell Department of Motor Neuroscience and Movement Disorders, Institute of Neurology, University College London (UCL), London, UK

Mary M. Robertson
Neuropsychiatry, University College London (UCL), London, UK
St Georges Hospital and Medical School, London, UK
Department of Psychiatry, University of Cape Town, Cape Town, South Africa

Dorin Yael, Michal Israelashvili and Izhar Bar-Gad
The Leslie and Susan Goldschmied (Gonda) Multidisciplinary Brain Research Center, Bar-Ilan University, Ramat-Gan, Israel

Siyan Fan
Department of Anatomy and Neurosciences, VU University Medical Center, Amsterdam, Netherlands
Department of Psychiatry, VU University Medical Center, Amsterdam, Netherlands
Department of Social and Behavioural Science, Utrecht University, Utrecht, Netherlands

Odile A. van den Heuvel and Stella J. de Wit
Department of Anatomy and Neurosciences, VU University Medical Center, Amsterdam, Netherlands
Department of Psychiatry, VU University Medical Center, Amsterdam, Netherlands
Neuroscience Campus Amsterdam, VU/VU University Medical Center, Amsterdam, Netherlands
The OCD Team, Haukeland University Hospital, Bergen, Norway

Danielle C. Cath
Department of Social and Behavioural Science, Utrecht University, Utrecht, Netherlands
Academic Anxiety Center Altrecht, Utrecht, Netherlands

Ysbrand D. van der Werf
Department of Anatomy and Neurosciences, VU University Medical Center, Amsterdam, Netherlands
Neuroscience Campus Amsterdam, VU/VU University Medical Center, Amsterdam, Netherlands
Netherlands Institute for Neuroscience, Amsterdam, Netherlands

Froukje E. de Vries
Department of Anatomy and Neurosciences, VU University Medical Center, Amsterdam, Netherlands
Department of Psychiatry, VU University Medical Center, Amsterdam, Netherlands
Neuroscience Campus Amsterdam, VU/VU University Medical Center, Amsterdam, Netherlands

Dick J. Veltman
Department of Psychiatry, VU University Medical Center, Amsterdam, Netherlands
Neuroscience Campus Amsterdam, VU/VU University Medical Center, Amsterdam, Netherlands

Petra J. W. Pouwels
Neuroscience Campus Amsterdam, VU/VU University Medical Center, Amsterdam, Netherlands
Department of Physics and Medical Technology, VU University Medical Center, Amsterdam, Netherlands

Marianthi Georgitsi
Department of Molecular Biology and Genetics, Democritus University of Thrace, Alexandroupoli, Greece
Department of Medicine, Aristotle University of Thessaloniki, Thessaloniki, Greece

A. Jeremy Willsey and Matthew State
Department of Psychiatry, University of California, San Francisco, San Francisco, CA, USA

Carol A. Mathews
Department of Psychiatry, University of Florida School of Medicine, Gainesville, FL, USA

Jeremiah M. Scharf
Departments of Neurology and Psychiatry, Massachusetts General Hospital, Harvard Medical School, Boston, MA, USA

Peristera Paschou
Department of Molecular Biology and Genetics, Democritus University of Thrace, Alexandroupoli, Greece

Daphna Ruhrman, Ella Gev, Noa Benaroya-Milshtein, Silvana Fennig, Alan Apter and Tamar Steinberg
The Matta and Harry Freund Neuropsychiatric Tourette Clinic, Schneider Children's Medical Center of Israel, Petach Tikva, Israel
Sackler Faculty of Medicine, Tel Aviv University, Tel Aviv, Israel

Orit Krispin
The Matta and Harry Freund Neuropsychiatric Tourette Clinic, Schneider Children's Medical Center of Israel, Petach Tikva, Israel

Chiara Spinello, Giovanni Laviola and Simone Macrì
Section of Behavioural Neuroscience, Department of Cell Biology and Neuroscience, Istituto Superiore di Sanità, Roma, Italy

Wissam Deeb, Peter J. Rossi, Kyle Rizer and Michael S. Okun
Department of Neurology, University of Florida and Center for Movement Disorders and Neurorestoration, Gainesville, FL, USA

Mauro Porta
Tourette's Syndrome and Movement Disorders Center, Galeazzi Hospital, Milan, Italy

Veerle Visser-Vandewalle
Department of Stereotactic and Functional Neurosurgery, University of Cologne, Cologne, Germany

Domenico Servello
Neusurgical Department, IRCCS Galeazzi, Milan, Italy

Jean-Luc Houeto
Service de Neurologie, Institut National de la Santé et de la Recherche Médicale-Centres d'Investigation Clinique 1402, Centre Hospitalier Universitaire de Grenoble de Poitiers, Université de Poitiers, Poitiers, France

Joohi Shahed-Jimenez
Parkinson's Disease Center and Movement Disorders Clinic, Baylor College of Medicine, Houston, TX, USA

Fan-Gang Meng
Beijing Neurosurgical Institute, Capital Medical University, Beijing, China

Bryan T. Klassen
Department of Neurology, Mayo Clinic College of Medicine, Rochester, MN, USA

Jonathan W. Mink
Department of Neurology, University of Rochester Medical Center, Rochester, NY, USA

Douglas W. Woods
Department of Psychology, Marquette University, Milwaukee, WI, USA

Aysegul Gunduz
Department of Neurology, University of Florida and Center for Movement Disorders and Neurorestoration, Gainesville, FL, USA
J. Crayton Pruitt Family Department of Biomedical Engineering, University of Florida, Gainesville, FL, USA

Ester Nespoli
Competence in Neuro Spine Department, Boehringer Ingelheim Pharma GmbH & Co. KG, Biberach an der Riss, Germany
Department of Child and Adolescence Psychiatry/ Psychotherapy, University of Ulm, Ulm, Germany

Francesca Rizzo
Department of Child and Adolescence Psychiatry/ Psychotherapy, University of Ulm, Ulm, Germany
Institute of Anatomy and Cell Biology, University of Ulm, Ulm, Germany

Tobias M. Boeckers
Institute of Anatomy and Cell Biology, University of Ulm, Ulm, Germany

Bastian Hengerer
Competence in Neuro Spine Department, Boehringer Ingelheim Pharma GmbH & Co. KG, Biberach an der Riss, Germany

Andrea G. Ludolph
Department of Child and Adolescence Psychiatry/ Psychotherapy, University of Ulm, Ulm, Germany

Natalie J. Forde
Department of Psychiatry, University of Groningen, University Medical Center Groningen, Groningen, Netherlands
Department of Cognitive Neuroscience, Donders Institute for Brain, Cognition and Behaviour, Radboud University Medical Center, Nijmegen, Netherlands

Ahmad S. Kanaan
Clinic of Psychiatry, Social Psychiatry and Psychotherapy, Hannover Medical School, Hannover, Germany
Max Planck Institute for Human Cognitive and Brain Sciences, Leipzig, Germany

Joanna Widomska
Department of Cognitive Neuroscience, Donders Institute for Brain, Cognition and Behaviour, Radboud University Medical Center, Nijmegen, Netherlands

Michelle Dunlap
Tourette-Gesellschaft Deutschland e.V., Hannover, Germany

Sarah Gerasch
Clinic of Psychiatry, Social Psychiatry and Psychotherapy, Hannover Medical School, Hannover, Germany

Jeffrey Glennon
Department of Cognitive Neuroscience, Donders Institute for Brain, Cognition and Behaviour, Radboud University Medical Center, Nijmegen, Netherlands

Bastian Hengerer
Boehringer Ingelheim Pharma GmbH & Co. KG, CNS Research, Biberach an der Riss, Germany

Pieter J. Hoekstra
Department of Psychiatry, University of Groningen, University Medical Center Groningen, Groningen, Netherlands

Andrea Ludolph
Department of Child and Adolescent Psychiatry, University of Ulm, Ulm, Germany

Peristera Paschou
Department of Molecular Biology and Genetics, Democritus University of Thrace, Alexandropoulos, Greece

Shanmukha S. Padmanabhuni and Fotis Tsetsos
Department of Molecular Biology and Genetics, Democritus University of Thrace, Alexandroupoli, Greece

Rayan Houssari, Birgitte Bertelsen and Zeynep Tümer
Applied Human Molecular Genetics, Kennedy Center, Department of Clinical Genetics, Copenhagen University Hospital, Rigshospitalet, Glostrup, Denmark

Ann-Louise Esserlind and Jes Olesen
Danish Headache Center and Department of Neurology, Faculty of Health Sciences, University of Copenhagen, Glostrup Hospital, Glostrup, Denmark

Thomas M. Werge and Thomas F. Hansen
Institute of Biological Psychiatry, Mental Health Center Sct. Hans, Copenhagen University Hospital, Roskilde, Denmark

Peristera Paschou
Department of Molecular Biology and Genetics, Democritus University of Thrace, Alexandroupoli, Greece
Department of Biological Sciences, Purdue University, West Lafayette, IN, USA

Nawei Sun, Jay A. Tischfield and Gary A. Heiman
Department of Genetics, Rutgers University, Piscataway, NJ, USA
Human Genetics Institute of New Jersey, Piscataway, NJ, USA

Robert A. King
Child Study Center, Yale School of Medicine, New Haven, CT, USA

Nuno R. Zilhão
Department of Clinical and Health Psychology, Utrecht University, Utrecht, Netherlands
Department of Biological Psychology, Vrije Universiteit, Amsterdam, Netherlands

Dirk J. Smit
Department of Biological Psychology, Vrije Universiteit, Amsterdam, Netherlands
Neuroscience Campus Amsterdam, Vrije Universiteit, Amsterdam, Netherlands

Dorret I. Boomsma
Department of Biological Psychology, Vrije Universiteit, Amsterdam, Netherlands

Danielle C. Cath
Department of Clinical and Health Psychology, Utrecht University, Utrecht, Netherlands
Altrecht Academic Anxiety Center, Utrecht, Netherlands

Natalie J. Forde
Department of Psychiatry, University of Groningen, University Medical Center Groningen, Groningen, Netherlands
Department of Cognitive Neuroscience, Donders Institute for Brain, Cognition and Behaviour, Radboud University Medical Center, Nijmegen, Netherlands

Lisa Ronan
Brain Mapping Unit, Department of Psychiatry, University of Cambridge, Cambridge, UK

Marcel P. Zwiers
Department of Cognitive Neuroscience, Donders Institute for Brain, Cognition and Behaviour, Radboud University Medical Center, Nijmegen, Netherlands

Aaron F. Alexander-Bloch
Brain Mapping Unit, Department of Psychiatry, University of Cambridge, Cambridge, UK
Child Psychiatry Branch, National Institute of Mental Health, Bethesda, MD, USA

Stephen V. Faraone
Departments of Psychiatry and of Neuroscience and Physiology, SUNY Upstate Medical University, Syracuse, NY, USA
Department of Biomedicine, K.G. Jebsen Centre for Research on Neuropsychiatric Disorders, University of Bergen, Bergen, Norway

Jaap Oosterlaan
Clinical Neuropsychology Section, Department of Clinical, Neuro and Developmental Psychology, Vrije Universiteit Amsterdam, Amsterdam, Netherlands

Dirk J. Heslenfeld
Clinical Neuropsychology Section, Department of Clinical, Neuro and Developmental Psychology, Vrije Universiteit Amsterdam, Amsterdam, Netherlands
Department of Experimental and Applied Psychology, Vrije Universiteit Amsterdam, Amsterdam, Netherlands

Catharina A. Hartman and Pieter J. Hoekstra
Department of Psychiatry, University of Groningen, University Medical Center Groningen, Groningen, Netherlands

Jan K. Buitelaar
Department of Cognitive Neuroscience, Donders Institute for Brain, Cognition and Behaviour, Radboud University Medical Center, Nijmegen, Netherlands
Karakter Child and Adolescent Psychiatry University Centre, Nijmegen, Netherlands

Nicole Pedroarena-Leal and Diane Ruge
Department of Psychology and Neurosciences, Leibniz Research Centre for Working Environment and Human Factors, Technical University Dortmund, Dortmund, Germany

Joohi Jimenez-Shahed
Parkinson's Disease Center and Movement Disorders Clinic, Department of Neurology, Baylor College of Medicine, Houston, TX, USA

Ilknur Telkes and Nuri F. Ince
Department of Biomedical Engineering, University of Houston, Houston, TX, USA

Ashwin Viswanathan
Department of Neurosurgery, Baylor College of Medicine, Houston, TX, USA

Fotis Tsetsos, Shanmukha S. Padmanabhuni, John Alexander, Iordanis Karagiannidis, Margaritis Tsifintaris, Apostolia Topaloudi, Dimitrios Mantzaris and Peristera Paschou
Department of Molecular Biology and Genetics, Democritus University of Thrace, Alexandroupolis, Greece

Marianthi Georgitsi
Department of Molecular Biology and Genetics, Democritus University of Thrace, Alexandroupolis, Greece
Laboratory of General Biology, Department of Medicine, Aristotle University of Thessaloniki, Thessaloniki, Greece

Petros Drineas
Computer Science Department, Rensselaer Polytechnic Institute, Troy, NY, USA

Christina N. Lessov-Schlaggar
Department of Psychiatry, Washington University School of Medicine, St. Louis, MO, USA

Joshua B. Rubin
Department of Neurology, Washington University School of Medicine, St. Louis, MO, USA
Department of Pediatrics, Washington University School of Medicine, St. Louis, MO, USA

Bradley L. Schlaggar
Department of Psychiatry, Washington University School of Medicine, St. Louis, MO, USA
Department of Neurology, Washington University School of Medicine, St. Louis, MO, USA
Department of Pediatrics, Washington University School of Medicine, St. Louis, MO, USA
Department of Radiology, Washington University School of Medicine, St. Louis, MO, USA
Department of Neuroscience, Washington University School of Medicine, St. Louis, MO, USA

Valerie Cathérine Brandt, Valeria Sajin and Alexander Münchau
Department of Paediatric and Adult Movement Disorders and Neuropsychiatry, Center of Brain, Behavior and Metabolism, University of Lübeck, Lübeck, Germany
Department of Neurology, University of Lübeck, Lübeck, Germany

Christian Beck and Silke Anders
Department of Neurology, Institute of Social and Affective Neuroscience, University of Lübeck, Lübeck, Germany

John Alexander, Hera Potamianou, Iordanis Karagiannidis, Fotis Tsetsos and Peristera Paschou
Department of Molecular Biology and Genetics, Democritus University of Thrace, Alexandroupoli, Greece

Jinchuan Xing, Li Deng, Jay Tischfield and Gary A. Heiman
Department of Genetics, Rutgers, The State University of New Jersey, Piscataway, NJ, USA
Human Genetics Institute of New Jersey, Rutgers, The State University of New Jersey, Piscataway, NJ, USA

Petros Drineas
Computer Science Department, Purdue University, West Lafayette, USA

Zsanett Tarnok, Luca Farkas and Peter Nagy
Vadaskert Clinic for Child and Adolescent Psychiatry, Budapest, Hungary

Renata Rizzo
Department of Clinical and Experimental Medicine, University of Catania, Catania, Italy

Tomasz Wolanczyk and Urszula Szymanska
Department of Child Psychiatry, Medical University of Warsaw, Warsaw, Poland

Christos Androutsos, Vaia Tsironi and Anastasia Koumoula
Child and Adolescent Psychiatry Clinic, Sismanoglio General Hospital of Attica, Athens, Greece

Csaba Barta
Molecular Biology and Pathobiochemistry, Institute of Medical Chemistry, Semmelweis University, Budapest, Hungary

TSGeneSEE
Tourette Syndrome Genetics — Southern and Eastern Europe Initiative (TSGeneSEE Consortium)

Paul Sandor
Department of Psychiatry, University of Toronto, Toronto, ON, Canada

Cathy L. Barr
Genetics and Development Division, Krembil Research Institute, University Health Network, Toronto, ON, Canada
Program in Neurosciences and Mental Health, The Hospital for Sick Children, Toronto, ON, Canada

Marianthi Georgitsi
Department of Molecular Biology and Genetics, Democritus University of Thrace, Alexandroupoli, Greece
Laboratory of General Biology, Department of Medicine, Aristotle University of Thessaloniki, Thessaloniki, Greece

Simon Morand-Beaulieu and Maxime Richard
Laboratoire de psychophysiologie cognitive et sociale, Montreal, QC, Canada
Centre de recherche de l'Institut universitaire en santé mentale de Montréal, Montreal, QC, Canada
Département de neurosciences, Faculté de médecine, Université de Montréal, Montreal, QC, Canada

Kieron P. O'Connor
Centre de recherche de l'Institut universitaire en santé mentale de Montréal, Montreal, QC, Canada
Département de psychiatrie, Faculté de médecine, Université de Montréal, Montreal, QC, Canada

Geneviève Sauvé
Laboratoire de psychophysiologie cognitive et sociale, Montreal, QC, Canada
Centre de recherche de l'Institut universitaire en santé mentale de Montréal, Montreal, QC, Canada

Julie B. Leclerc
Centre de recherche de l'Institut universitaire en santé mentale de Montréal, Montreal, QC, Canada
Département de psychologie, Faculté des sciences humaines, Université du Québec à Montréal, Montreal, QC, Canada

Pierre J. Blanchet
Centre de recherche de l'Institut universitaire en santé mentale de Montréal, Montreal, QC, Canada
Département de stomatologie, Faculté de médecine dentaire, Université de Montréal, Montreal, QC, Canada

Marc E. Lavoie
Laboratoire de psychophysiologie cognitive et sociale, Montreal, QC, Canada
Centre de recherche de l'Institut universitaire en santé mentale de Montréal, Montreal, QC, Canada
Département de psychiatrie, Faculté de médecine, Université de Montréal, Montreal, QC, Canada

Carol A. Mathews
Department of Psychiatry, College of Medicine, University of Florida, Gainesville, Florida, USA

Jeremy S. Stern
Department of Neurology, St George's University of London, London, UK

Luca Pagliaroli
Institute of Medical Chemistry, Molecular Biology and Pathobiochemistry, Semmelweis University, Budapest, Hungary
Research Centre for Natural Sciences, Institute of Enzymology, Hungarian Academy of Sciences, Budapest, Hungary

Borbála Vető
Research Centre for Natural Sciences, Institute of Enzymology, Hungarian Academy of Sciences, Budapest, Hungary

Tamás Arányi
Research Centre for Natural Sciences, Institute of Enzymology, Hungarian Academy of Sciences, Budapest, Hungary
Centre National de la Recherche Scientifique UMR 6214, Institut National de la Santé et de la Recherche Médicale U1083, University of Angers, Angers, France

Csaba Barta
Institute of Medical Chemistry, Molecular Biology and Pathobiochemistry, Semmelweis University, Budapest, Hungary

Index

www.ingramcontent.com/pod-product-compliance
Lightning Source LLC
LaVergne TN
LVHW080931210926
848485LV00004B/773